Brain Disorders: Biological Mechanisms

Brain Disorders: Biological Mechanisms

Editor: Jake Williams

MURPHY & MOORE
www.murphy-moorepublishing.com

www.murphy-moorepublishing.com

MURPHY & MOORE

Cataloging-in-Publication Data

Brain disorders : biological mechanisms / edited by Jake Williams.
p. cm.
Includes bibliographical references and index.
ISBN 978-1-63987-081-3
1. Brain--Diseases. 2. Brain--Abnormalities. 3. Brain chemistry. 4. Biochemistry. I. Williams, Jake.
RC386 .B73 2022
616.8--dc23

Murphy & Moore Publishing,
1 Rockefeller Plaza,
New York City, NY 10020, USA

ISBN 978-1-63987-081-3 (Hardback)

Contents

Preface

I am honored to present to you this unique book which encompasses the most up-to-date data in the field. I was extremely pleased to get this opportunity of editing the work of experts from across the globe. I have also written papers in this field and researched the various aspects revolving around the progress of the discipline. I have tried to unify my knowledge along with that of stalwarts from every corner of the world, to produce a text which not only benefits the readers but also facilitates the growth of the field.

Brain disorders refer to the conditions which impair the normal functioning of the brain. These can range from trauma, tumors, infections and stroke. Trauma encompasses concussion and traumatic brain injury. A concussion causes a short term disruption in the brain while traumatic brain injury entails a permanent damage to the brain. Some of the different infections which can affect the brain are meningitis, brain abscess and encephalitis. Tumors in the brain can be either benign or malignant. Both of them can cause problems in the normal functioning of the brain by exerting pressure on it. They can also be classified as primary brain tumors and secondary tumors. While primary tumors can be either benign or malignant, secondary tumors are always malignant in nature. This book discusses the fundamentals as well as modern approaches of the study of brain disorders. It includes some of the vital pieces of work being conducted across the world, on various topics related to this field. This book will provide comprehensive knowledge to the readers.

Finally, I would like to thank all the contributing authors for their valuable time and contributions. This book would not have been possible without their efforts. I would also like to thank my friends and family for their constant support.

Editor

1

Six Years of Research on the National Institute of Mental Health's Research Domain Criteria (RDoC) Initiative

*Dean Carcone and Anthony C. Ruocco**

Departments of Psychology and Psychological Clinical Science, University of Toronto, Toronto, ON, Canada

Edited by:
Andrew Harkin,
Trinity College, Dublin, Ireland

Reviewed by:
Wen-Jun Gao,
Drexel University College of Medicine, USA
Vladeta Ajdacic-Gross,
University of Zurich, Switzerland

***Correspondence:**
Anthony C. Ruocco
anthony.ruocco@utoronto.ca

Six years have passed since the National Institute of Mental Health (NIMH) in the United States launched the Research Domain Criteria (RDoC) initiative. The RDoC introduces a framework for research on the biology of mental illness that integrates research findings across multiple levels of information. The framework outlines constructs that represent specific quantifiable dimensions of behavior (e.g., responses to acute threat, cognitive control) and corresponding units of analysis that can be used to study the constructs, beginning at the levels of genes, molecules, cells, circuits and physiology, and moving up to behaviors and self-reports. In this systematic review, a literature search was conducted to synthesize empirical research published since the proposal of the framework that incorporated the RDoC. Forty-eight peer-reviewed scholarly articles met eligibility criteria for the review. Studies differed according to whether they analyzed RDoC constructs and units of analysis within vs. between clinically-diagnosed and non-psychiatric samples. The most commonly studied constructs were subsumed within the domains of Negative Valence Systems, Positive Valence Systems and Cognitive Systems, providing initial results which primarily connected genetics, brain circuits and physiology research findings with behavior and self-reports. Prospects for future research adopting the RDoC matrix and utilizing a dimensional approach to studying the biology of mental illness are discussed.

Keywords: research domain criteria (RDoC), mental disorders, cells, circuits and systems, physiology, brain, neuroscience

INTRODUCTION

The Research Domain Criteria (RDoC) framework was unveiled by the National Institute of Mental Health (NIMH) in a commentary published in the American Journal of Psychiatry (Insel et al., 2010). In response to concerns over the validity of the diagnostic criteria espoused in the Diagnostic and Statistical Manual (DSM) and what some consider inadequate efforts to address these concerns in the process of revising the manual in the DSM-5, the RDoC was proposed as an alternate framework to conceptually organize and direct biological research on mental disorders (Cuthbert and Insel, 2013; Insel, 2013). This framework encourages research to be structured around five major domains: Negative Valence Systems, driving reactions to aversive stimuli; Positive Valence Systems, driving reactions to positive stimuli; Cognitive

Systems, including various mental processes; Social Processes, responsible for interpersonal behavior and cognition; and Arousal and Regulatory Systems, involved in context-based and homeostatic regulation or neural systems. Research on these systems and processes is organized around a dimensional approach incorporating and integrating the following levels or units of analysis: genes, molecules, cells, circuits, physiology, behavior and self-report. By re-orienting research away from DSM categories and toward a multimodal dimensional framework based on empirically validated constructs, the aim of the NIMH's RDoC initiative has been to progress further understanding of these domains such that a new diagnostic nosology can be developed.

The initial structure and five domains of the RDoC Matrix were the product of a series of workshops arranged by the NIMH (see Development of the RDoC Framework (2016) on the NIMH website). Each of the domains is subdivided into constructs representing specific functional dimensions of behavior. For example, the Cognitive Systems domain encompasses the constructs Attention, Perception, Declarative Memory, Language, Cognitive Control and Working Memory. Some of these constructs are further divided into subconstructs, such as the division of Perception into Visual Perception, Auditory Perception, and Olfactory/Somatosensory/Multimodal Perception. These constructs and subconstructs are crossed with the seven RDoC units of analysis to form the skeleton of the RDoC Matrix. Cells of this matrix are filled with relevant empirically supported *elements*, describing relevant research topics within a construct which can be investigated at a given unit of analysis. For example, dopamine and serotonin are molecular elements of the Reward Valuation subconstruct of Approach Motivation, under the Positive Valence Systems domain. For an illustration of all divisions within the matrix, please refer to The RDoC Matrix (2016) on the NIHM website. The organization of the RDoC Matrix remains flexible, having undergone additions, modifications, and a recent redesign since its launch (RDoC Launches User-Friendly Matrix Format, 2016).

Six years have passed since the proposal of the RDoC framework, conceivably allowing sufficient time for researchers to design, conduct, and publish initial studies that adopt this innovative new framework. The purpose of this brief systematic review is to summarize all peer-reviewed studies published since the proposal of the framework that explicitly purport to incorporate at least one domain, construct, or element of the RDoC. The aim of the review article is to provide an overview of research on the RDoC to identify patterns in the domains, constructs, and units of analysis most commonly studied and the research designs that have been employed.

METHOD

Database Search

The ProQuest search engine was used to access the PsycINFO and Medline databases to return all studies indexed using the term "Research Domain Criteria" and/or the acronym "RDoC". The results were restricted to peer-reviewed work published in a scholarly journal after April 2013, the date that the RDoC was officially proposed. This search was conducted on April 4, 2016, and returned 330 unique results. Abstracts for these 330 studies were initially screened to remove reviews, commentaries, and results erroneously returned by the search (e.g., those pertaining to Refractory Dissolved Organic Carbon). Following this screen, 61 potentially relevant articles were selected to pass through a second screen following review of the full text of each manuscript. Please refer to **Figure 1** for a visual representation of article screening and selection.

Article Inclusion and Exclusion

In order for an article to be selected for inclusion in this review, it must have met the following inclusion criteria: (1) empirically examined one or more identified RDoC domains, constructs, or elements; and (2) made direct reference to the RDoC framework as part of the study rationale, interpretation of results, or implications and future directions. In order to be retained, an article must also not have met any of the following exclusion criteria: (1) the article represented a proposal for RDoC-related research that had not yet been conducted; (2) the focus of an article was the empirical validation of a psychometric measure related to an RDoC construct, rather than the examination of the construct itself; and (3) the article centered around a case study. Of the 61 articles selected for full-text review, the majority (48 articles) were found to be relevant primary empirical studies which explored themes consistent with the RDoC framework. These articles have been included in this review. A summary of the constructs and units of analysis explored, as well as the key results of these studies, have been included in a Supplementary Table provided with this review article. It should be noted that additional research closely related to RDoC constructs, although not explicitly identifying use of the RDoC framework, has been conducted during the previous 6 years. These studies have not been included in this review article.

RESULTS

Common Experimental Designs

Many of the studies reviewed shared similar experimental designs and approaches to applying the RDoC framework.

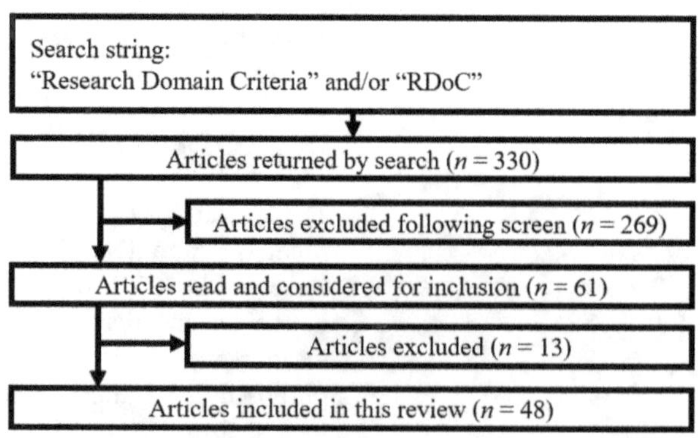

FIGURE 1 | Flowchart of articles screened and selected.

The most common approach was to explore an explicitly defined RDoC construct, subconstruct, or element using two or more units of analysis. This often resulted in describing relationships between higher level behaviors or traits and lower level biological underpinnings. Additionally, many of these studies overtly employed a transdiagnostic approach by examining a given construct across more than one group defined by clinical diagnosis. Another common approach was to explore associations between constructs or subconstructs within or across RDoC domains using one or more units of analysis. Alternatively, a number of studies employed a dimensional approach to study psychological or behavioral phenotypes related to established RDoC domains but focusing on constructs not explicitly defined within the RDoC matrix. Finally, two studies explored the application of the RDoC to the design of clinical interventions. Please refer to the Supplementary Table for additional information on the experimental designs and results of all studies reviewed.

Arousal and Regulatory Systems

Since the proposal of the RDoC framework, domains have not been equally represented in the literature. With the exception of six studies not specifying a particular domain of focus, almost all the research summarized in this review examined at least one construct in either the Cognitive Systems, Positive Valence Systems, or Negative Valence Systems domains. Only two studies (Tegeler et al., 2015; Olbrich et al., 2016) focused exclusively on the domain of Arousal and Regularity Systems, both targeting the Arousal construct. These studies also both used similar physiological measures to study clinical samples. Tegeler et al. (2015) demonstrated that hemispheric dominance in high-frequency brain activity was related to baroreflex sensitivity and higher resting heart rate. Olbrich et al. (2016) showed that pre-treatment physiological measures predict remission from major depressive disorder (MDD) and response to SSRI treatment. Both of these studies highlight the potential of the RDoC for studying arousal systems relevant to psychopathology.

Social Processes

Similar to the Arousal and Regulatory Systems, only two studies exclusively examined the Social Processes Domain (Fang et al., 2014; Lindberg et al., 2015). Both of these studies explored the Affiliation and Attachment construct, although the experimental paradigms employed by each were quite distinct. Fang et al. (2014) recorded behavior on a social exclusion task in males with social anxiety disorder following administration of oxytocin. For males with lower self-reported attachment avoidance, oxytocin promoted social affiliation and cooperation. In contrast, Lindberg et al. (2015) described how similar scales of the Attachment and Clinical Issues Questionnaire (Lindberg and Thomas, 2011) are associated with both current alcohol dependence in adults and risk of future alcohol dependence in high school students. Although research has now examined the Affiliation and Attachment construct within the context of the RDoC, the remaining constructs of Social Communication, Perception and Understanding of Self, and Perception and Understanding of Others have yet to be independently explored.

Positive Valence Systems

Twelve publications included in this review article, examined Positive Valence Systems, although none of these explored the constructs of Habit or Initial/Sustained Responsiveness to Reward Attainment. Rather, research has primarily focused on reward-related constructs such as approach motivation (Karalunas et al., 2014) and reward learning (Webb et al., 2016). For example, Sharp et al. (2014) used fMRI to compare brain activation patterns during a card-guessing reward task between three female groups: depressed adolescents with a maternal history of depression, never-depressed adolescents with a maternal history of depression, and never-depressed adolescents with no maternal history of depression. Lower right ventral striatal activity was observed for both currently depressed and at-risk adolescents. Additionally, activity in this region was inversely correlated with maternal Beck Depression Inventory (BDI) scores across all groups. These results highlight the potential for disruptions in Positive Valence Systems to be used as identifiable vulnerability factors for the development of MDD.

Arrondo et al. (2015) employed a similar transdiagnostic approach in the examination of circuitry related to the Expectancy construct. Patients with schizophrenia, MDD, and controls completed a task to induce anticipation of monetary reward while undergoing fMRI. Reduced activation associated with reward anticipation was observed in the bilateral ventral striatum for both patient groups compared to controls. This reduction in activation was related to self-reported anhedonia and overall depression symptoms for patients with schizophrenia but not MDD. Through their application of the RDoC, these two studies showcase the potential for transdiagnostic and dimensional examination of psychological constructs.

Cognitive Systems

Research on Cognitive Systems has been considerable and diverse, with eighteen studies published on four of the six constructs within the domain (e.g., Cognitive Control: Lopez-Garcia et al. (2016); Perception: Silverstein et al. (2015); Attention: Kleinman et al. (2015); and Working Memory: Francazio and Flessner (2015)). To elaborate on one example, Chan et al. (2015) demonstrated how a standard performance-monitoring event-related potential paradigm can be used within an RDoC framework to examine Cognitive Control and Performance Monitoring systems. Adults with a history of psychosis and a control group completed a flanker task while undergoing EEG. Reduced error-related negativity and error positivity amplitudes were observed for individuals with a history of psychosis compared to controls. Additionally, reduced error positivity amplitude was associated with schizotypal personality traits across both groups, suggesting that these disruptions in neural circuitry may represent a transdiagnostic phenotype.

As an additional example of a study employing multiple units of analysis to explore a Cognitive System, Newman et al. (2016)

focused on the Response Selection construct by examining the relationship between cortical thickness and performance on a go/no-go task. In a sample of 114 adults, 46% of which exhibited symptoms of Attention Deficit Hyperactivity Disorder (ADHD) persisting into adulthood, thickness of the caudal inferior frontal gyrus was associated with poorer response inhibition (i.e., more commission errors) regardless of ADHD symptoms or history of substance abuse. Of note, cortical thickness of this area was also inversely correlated with frequency of cannabis use and persistence of ADHD symptoms.

A transdiagnostic approach to the study of the Visual Perception Cognitive System was adopted by Silverstein et al. (2015). This work investigated disturbances in perceptual organization across patients with body dysmorphic disorder (BDD) and schizophrenia, which are two patient groups defined in part by perceptual distortions. Performance on tasks of perceptual organization was compared between these groups, non-patients, and an obsessive-compulsive disorder (OCD) group. Only patients with schizophrenia performed worse on these measures than comparison groups, while patients with BDD did not differ from non-patients or OCD patients. Consequently, it was suggested that the disturbances in visual perception found in BDD may be unrelated to problems in perceptual organization. Furthermore, these results are consistent with the conclusion that disturbances in perceptual organization may be more specific to schizophrenia and other neurodevelopmental disorders.

Rather than focusing on an RDoC *construct*, one study examined a single *element* of the Perception construct within the Cognitive Systems matrix. Chen et al. (2016) explored the relationship between the expression of the dysbindin protein, found in neural tissue, and disturbances in the regulation of lipid synthesis and synaptic plasticity. A reduction of sterol regulatory element binding protein-1 (SREBP1), a transcriptional regulator for lipid synthesis, was found in both deceased patients with schizophrenia and dysbindin-1 knockout mice. Additional results suggest that this disturbance in SREBP1 maturation may lead to a disruption in synaptic plasticity, and these disruptions may be corrected in knockout mice with the administration of the anti-psychotic drug clozapine. This multi-modal approach illustrates the goals of the RDoC framework, using multiple levels of analysis to provide a comprehensive empirical characterization of clinically relevant phenotypic variation.

Negative Valence Systems

The domain most commonly explored by the research collected in this systematic review was Negative Valence Systems, with 20 publications examining at least one construct within this domain. With the exception of Frustrative Non-Reward, four of the five constructs within this domain were investigated by at least one study (e.g., Acute Threat: Yancey et al. (2016); Potential Threat: Latzman et al. (2016); Sustained Threat: Weinberg et al. (2016); and Loss: Woody et al. (2014)), with Acute Threat the most commonly studied construct. As an example, Bauer et al. (2013) explored Acute Threat using both physiological and self-report measures. The Clinician Administered Posttraumatic Stress Disorder (PTSD) Scale (Blake et al., 1995) was administered to 36 adults reporting prior exposure to a traumatic event, a sample in which the Acute Threat system may be compromised. Additionally, these adults underwent physiological recordings, including heart rate, skin conductance, and eye-blinks, while performing a script-driven emotional imagery task. Measures of physiological reactivity, thought to be sensitive to disturbances in the Acute Threat system, correlated significantly with severity of PTSD symptoms at an initial visit and at a six-month follow-up assessment. This was taken to suggest that physiological reactivity is a stable and valid measure of disturbances in the Acute Threat construct associated with PTSD. Furthermore, Pineles et al. (2013) demonstrated that these physiological measures are a better predictor of PTSD diagnosis than self-report measures of emotional response.

An additional noteworthy study used a population of 76 captive chimpanzees to investigate the Potential Threat construct as it relates to genes, physiology and anxious behavior (Latzman et al., 2016). It was shown that scratching behavior, an indicator of negative arousal, exhibited a sex-specific association with both AVPR1A genotype, a gene related to mammalian social behavior, and brain morphometry in regions associated with this gene. Although only three studies (Chen et al., 2016; Kondo et al., 2016; Latzman et al., 2016) employed non-human mammals in their research, they highlight how animal research can contribute to the understanding of species-general elements within the RDoC matrix.

A number of studies explored topics related to established domains, but focused on constructs not explicitly defined as a construct in the RDoC matrix, such as neuroticism (i.e., the tendency to experience negative affect; Bedwell et al., 2014) and anhedonia (i.e., the inability to feel pleasure; Webb et al., 2016). One of these studies, Østergaard et al. (2014), overtly proposed that melancholia should be included as an additional construct within the Negative Valence Systems domain. Analysis of self-report measures of depression symptoms in a large treatment study of depression suggested a common and unidimensional construct reflecting melancholia is sensitive to pharmacological intervention. According to the authors, the results of this and prior work highlight how melancholia meets the criteria for inclusion as an RDoC construct, as stipulated in Cuthbert and Insel (2013). As the RDoC matrix is a work in progress, it will be interesting to see how proposals like this can influence its development.

Research Exploring More than One Domain

Ten of the studies reviewed examined more than one RDoC domain, commonly exploring associations between constructs or subconstructs across multiple domains. Verona and Bresin (2015), for example, examined the relationship between threat-related Negative Valence Systems and the Cognitive System subconstruct of Response Selection. Adults with a history of violent and criminal offences completed the Buss Perry Aggression Questionnaire (Buss and Perry, 1992), which was taken as an index of proneness to aggression associated with Sustained and Acute Threat responses. Participants then underwent EEG while completing an emotional-linguistic go/no-go task. During blocks presenting threatening words, self-reported anger and aggressive behavior each were associated with smaller P3 amplitude recorded during response inhibition, an electrophysiological marker that is taken to represent reduced inhibitory control processing. It is suggested that this relationship may indicate that sensitivity to acute or sustained threat may deteriorate cognitive control processes.

An additional example of research spanning across multiple domains is work which explored the application of the RDoC to the design of clinical interventions. "Engage", first described in Alexopoulos and Arean (2014), is a psychological intervention designed to specifically target disturbances in RDoC-defined Positive and Negative Valence Systems through *reward exposure*, the facilitation of meaningful and rewarding activities. A sample of older adults with MDD received 9 weeks of Engage (Alexopoulos et al., 2015). Symptom improvements within this group were compared to a patient group from a previous study (Alexopoulos et al., 2011), in which participants received problem-solving therapy (PST). The Engage intervention demonstrated comparable efficacy to PST in reducing symptoms and functional impairment associated with MDD. In order to explore the mechanism underlying this change, Alexopoulos et al. (2016) examined how MDD symptoms and a self-reported rating of behavioral activation influenced each other throughout Engage. In a sample of 48 older adults with MDD completing 9 weeks of Engage, greater increases in behavioral activation, taken as a broad index of Positive Valence Systems function, predicted change in depression severity during treatment and at a 36-week follow-up assessment. These investigations may mark the first of many treatment studies based on targeting dimensions included in the RDoC Matrix.

DISCUSSION

With 6 years having elapsed since the RDoC framework was introduced, it is timely to review findings from the first wave of research which adopted the framework. This systematic review identified 48 primary empirical articles published in the last 4 years (see Supplementary Table) which either directly examined an RDoC-defined construct, or interpreted their results in a manner consistent with the RDoC framework. As described above, the majority of these studies fall into common prototypes regarding their goals and their approach to applying the RDoC framework. At present, it seems that an "RDoC study" describes: (1) research on a single defined RDoC construct using multiple levels of analysis; (2) research which explores associations between separate RDoC constructs and/or elements; and/or (3) research which adopts a transdiagnostic perspective to investigate an RDoC construct by examining multiple categories of a disorder or symptom dimensions. Some additional studies purport to use approaches consistent with the RDoC framework but incorporate phenotypes which are not (or may not yet have been) specified within the RDoC matrix. We do not know if RDoC studies will continue to fall within these rough categories, but the approaches that they represent are informative for the design of subsequent research. The topics of focus for these future studies will likely be influenced by the growth and modification of the RDoC matrix and by significant advances in research made within this framework. Whether this pattern of research reflects the way future studies will be designed likely depends on subsequent modifications to the RDoC matrix and the progression of research during these formative years of the framework.

This systematic review highlights a notable scarcity of research explicitly intended to examine the RDoC domains of Social Processes and Arousal and Regulatory Systems. This is of course not to say that research in these and related areas has not been carried out but that the RDoC framework specifically has not been adopted in publications of this work. Conversely, a remarkable number of studies have been published which explore the domains of Cognitive Systems, Negative Valence Systems, and Positive Valence Systems. It is unlikely that this disparity is an artifact of the database search used in this review, as no domain-specific terms were included as search criteria. It may be speculated that constructs related to the more well-represented domains may currently be easier to cast within the RDoC framework, prompting a greater number of researchers to incorporate this new perspective. For example, research on attention may lend itself more easily to be examined from a multi-level biological and behavioral perspective, while work of this type may be less common when examining topics such as self-perception or non-verbal communication. Different fields of study may also have been quicker or slower to adopt the RDoC framework depending at least in part on the established theories in the field that emphasize or deemphasize biological contributions to the constructs of interest. This may be reflected in the relative number of unoccupied cells in the lower-level units of analysis present within the RDoC matrix at the time of this review (e.g., Cognitive Systems: 17% unoccupied vs. Social Processes: 34% unoccupied; see The RDoC Matrix (2016)). However, this does not explain the lack of research using the RDoC framework to investigate Arousal and Regulatory Systems, a domain that is well populated with respect to RDoC units of analysis. Rather, it can be argued that this domain is historically better understood than other domains (although perhaps not in relation to self-report constructs relevant to mental and neurological illness), and consequently has been the focus of fewer research studies since the introduction of the RDoC Framework only 6 years ago.

Although the transition to a dimensional and empirically-driven research framework on mental illness has been anticipated for many years (Krueger and Piasecki, 2002), the RDoC proposal has been met with a mixture of support, resistance and controversy. For a discussion of the challenges facing the RDoC framework, please refer to Patrick and Hajcak (2016). It has been suggested that all authoritative systems of nosology (including both the DSM and the RDoC) likely impeded the development of scientific theory by constraining competitive discourse (Markon, 2013). Additionally, having more than one active system of nosology may promote fractures in research continuity between funding bodies and geographic regions. Although researchers in the United States are in part incentivized to adopt an RDoC framework by receiving funding from the NIMH, researchers outside the region may not yet have as strong of an incentive to do so and therefore may be less likely to make the transition. Conversely, many researchers are optimistic about the promise of dimensional approaches to studying mental illness, components of which are inherent to many aspects of the RDoC framework. Indeed, there is potential for the framework to provide a useful alternative to structuring clinical research on mental illness (Casey et al., 2013), although the existing body of research incorporating this framework is relatively small and requires further advancement to refine the model and realize the potential of this transformative new approach.

AUTHOR CONTRIBUTIONS

DC and ACR conceptualized the topic, reviewed studies for eligibility in the review, and wrote the manuscript. DC conducted the literature search.

FUNDING

ACR is supported by a New Investigator Salary Award (MSH-130177) from the Canadian Institutes of Health Research and an Early Researcher Award (ER14-10-185) from the Ministry of Research and Innovation, Province of Ontario. DC is supported by an Ontario Graduate Scholarship.

REFERENCES

Alexopoulos, G. S., and Arean, P. (2014). A model for streamlining psychotherapy in the RDoC era: the example of 'Engage'. *Mol. Psychiatry* 19, 14–19. doi: 10.1038/mp.2013.150

Alexopoulos, G. S., Raue, P. J., Gunning, F., Kiosses, D. N., Kanellopoulos, D., Pollari, C., et al. (2016). "Engage" therapy: behavioral activation and improvement of late-life major depression. *Am. J. Geriatr. Psychiatry* 24, 320–326. doi: 10.1016/j.jagp.2015.11.006

Alexopoulos, G. S., Raue, P. J., Kiosses, D. N., Mackin, R. S., Kanellopoulos, D., McCulloch, C., et al. (2011). Problem-solving therapy and supportive therapy in older adults with major depression and executive dysfunction: effect on disability. *Arch. Gen. Psychiatry* 68, 33–41. doi: 10.1001/archgenpsychiatry.2010.177

Alexopoulos, G. S., Raue, P. J., Kiosses, D. N., Seirup, J. K., Banerjee, S., and Arean, P. A. (2015). Comparing engage with PST in late-life major depression: a preliminary report. *Am. J. Geriatr. Psychiatry* 23, 506–513. doi: 10.1016/j.jagp.2014.06.008

Arrondo, G., Segarra, N., Metastasio, A., Ziauddeen, H., Spencer, J., Reinders, N. R., et al. (2015). Reduction in ventral striatal activity when anticipating a reward in depression and schizophrenia: a replicated cross-diagnostic finding. *Front. Psychol.* 6:1280. doi: 10.3389/fpsyg.2015.01280

Bauer, M. R., Ruef, A. M., Pineles, S. L., Japuntich, S. J., Macklin, M. L., Lasko, N. B., et al. (2013). Psychophysiological assessment of PTSD: a potential research domain criteria construct. *Psychol. Assess.* 25, 1037–1043. doi: 10.1037/a0033432

Bebko, G., Bertocci, M., Chase, H., Dwojak, A., Bonar, L., Almeida, J., et al. (2015). Decreased amygdala-insula resting state connectivity in behaviorally and emotionally dysregulated youth. *Psychiatry Res.* 231, 77–86. doi: 10.1016/j.pscychresns.2014.10.015

Bedwell, J. S., Gooding, D. C., Chan, C. C., and Trachik, B. J. (2014). Anhedonia in the age of RDoC. *Schizophr. Res.* 160, 226–227. doi: 10.1016/j.schres.2014.10.028

Blake, D. D., Weathers, F. W., Nagy, L. M., Kaloupek, D. G., Gusman, F. D., Charney, D. S., et al. (1995). The development of a clinician-administered PTSD scale. *J. Trauma. Stress* 8, 75–90. doi: 10.1002/jts.2490080106

Buss, A. H., and Perry, M. (1992). The aggression questionnaire. *J. Pers. Soc. Psychol.* 63, 452–459.

Casey, B. J., Craddock, N., Cuthbert, B. N., Hyman, S. E., Lee, F. S., and Ressler, K. J. (2013). DSM-5 and RDoC: progress in psychiatry research? *Nat. Rev. Neurosci.* 14, 810–814. doi: 10.1038/nrn3621

Chan, C. C., Trachik, B. J., and Bedwell, J. S. (2015). An event-related potential investigation of error monitoring in adults with a history of psychosis. *Clin. Neurophysiol.* 126, 1717–1726. doi: 10.1016/j.clinph.2014.11.016

Chen, Y., Bang, S., McMullen, M. F., Kazi, H., Talbot, K., Ho, M.-X., et al. (2016). Neuronal activity-induced sterol regulatory element binding protein-1 (srebp1) is disrupted in dysbindin-null mice—potential link to cognitive impairment in schizophrenia. *Mol. Neurobiol.* doi: 10.1007/s12035-016-9773-x [Epub ahead of print].

Costa Dias, T. G., Iyer, S. P., Carpenter, S. D., Cary, R. P., Wilson, V. B., Mitchel, S. H., et al. (2015). Characterizing heterogeneity in children with and without ADHD based on reward system connectivity. *Dev. Cogn. Neurosci.* 11, 155–174. doi: 10.1016/j.dcn.2014.12.005

Cuthbert, B. N., and Insel, T. R. (2013). Toward the future of psychiatric diagnosis: the seven pillars of RDoC. *BMC Med.* 11:126. doi: 10.1186/1741-7015-11-126

Development of the RDoC Framework. (2016). National institute of mental health. Available online at: https://www.nimh.nih.gov/research-priorities/rdoc/development-of-the-rdoc-framework.shtml. [Accessed April 4, 2016].

Fang, A., Hoge, E. A., Heinrichs, M., and Hofmann, S. G. (2014). Attachment style moderates the effects of oxytocin on social behaviors and cognitions during social rejection: applying a research domain criteria framework to social anxiety. *Clin. Psychol. Sci.* 2, 740–747. doi: 10.1177/2167702614527948

Francazio, S. K., and Flessner, C. A. (2015). Cognitive flexibility differentiates young adults exhibiting obsessive-compulsive behaviors from controls. *Psychiatry Res.* 228, 185–190. doi: 10.1016/j.psychres.2015.04.038

Gruber, J., Mennin, D. S., Fields, A., Purcell, A., and Murray, G. (2015). Heart rate variability as a potential indicator of positive valence system disturbance: a proof of concept investigation. *Int. J. Psychophysiol.* 98, 240–248. doi: 10.1016/j.ijpsycho.2015.08.005

Hartmann, A. S., Thomas, J. J., Greenberg, J. L., Matheny, N. L., and Wilhelm, S. (2014). A comparison of self-esteem and perfectionism in anorexia nervosa and body dysmorphic disorder. *J. Nerv. Ment. Dis.* 202, 883–888. doi: 10.1097/NMD.0000000000000215

Insel, T. (2013). Transforming diagnosis [Online]. national institute of mental health. Available online at: http://www.nimh.nih.gov/about/director/2013/transforming-diagnosis.shtml. [Accessed April 4, 2016].

Insel, T., Cuthbert, B., Garvey, M., Heinssen, R., Pine, D. S., Quinn, K., et al. (2010). Research domain criteria (RDoC): toward a new classification framework for research on mental disorders. *Am. J. Psychiatry* 167, 748–751. doi: 10.1176/appi.ajp.2010.09091379

Jones, B. D. M., Chopra, K. K., Grummitt, J., Ravindran, A., Matthews, S. G., and Levitan, R. D. (2015). High reactivity of the cortisol awakening response predicts positive treatment outcome in heterogeneous depressed patients completing an alternate milieu inpatient program. *Gen. Hosp. Psychiatry* 37, 601–605. doi: 10.1016/j.genhosppsych.2015.06.006

Karalunas, S. L., Fair, D., Musser, E. D., Aykes, K., Iyer, S. P., and Nigg, J. T. (2014). Subtyping attention-deficit/hyperactivity disorder using temperament dimensions: toward biologically based nosologic. *JAMA Psychiatry* 71, 1015–1024. doi: 10.1001/jamapsychiatry.2014.763

Kleinman, A., Caetano, S. C., Brentani, H., Rocca, C. C., dos Santos, B., Andrade, E. R., et al. (2015). Attention-based classification pattern, a research domain criteria framework, in youths with bipolar disorder and attention-deficit/hyperactivity disorder. *Aust. N. Z. J. Psychiatry* 49, 255–265. doi: 10.1177/0004867414557957

Kondo, M. A., Fukudome, D., Smith, D. R., Gallagher, M., Kamiya, A., and Sawa, A. (2016). Dimensional assessment of behavioral changes in the cuprizone short-term exposure model for psychosis. *Neurosci. Res.* 107, 70–74. doi: 10.1016/j.neures.2016.01.006

Krueger, R. F., and Piasecki, T. M. (2002). Toward a dimensional and psychometrically-informed approach to conceptualizing psychopathology. *Behav. Res. Ther.* 40, 485–499. doi: 10.1016/s0005-7967(02)00016-5

Lang, P. J., McTeague, L. M., and Bradley, M. M. (2016). RDoC, DSM and the reflex physiology of fear: A biodimensional analysis of the anxiety disorders spectrum. *Psychophysiology* 53, 336–347. doi: 10.1111/psyp.12462

Latzman, R. D., Young, L. J., and Hopkins, W. D. (2016). Displacement behaviors in chimpanzees (*Pan troglodytes*): a neurogenomics investigation of the RDoC negative valence systems domain. *Psychophysiology* 53, 355–363. doi: 10.1111/psyp.12449

Leventhal, A. M., Strong, D. R., Sussman, S., Kirkpatrick, M. G., Unger, J. B., Barrington-Trimis, J. L., et al. (2016). Psychiatric comorbidity in adolescent electronic and conventional cigarette use. *J. Psychiatr. Res.* 73, 71–78. doi: 10.1016/j.jpsychires.2015.11.008

Lindberg, M. A., Fugett, A., and Carter, J. E. (2015). Tests of the attachment and clinical issues questionnaire as it applies to alcohol dependence. *J. Addict. Med.* 9, 286–295. doi: 10.1097/ADM.0000000000000131

Lindberg, M. A., and Thomas, S. W. (2011). The attachment and clinical issues questionnaire (ACIQ): scale development. *J. Genet. Psychol.* 172, 329–352. doi: 10.1080/00221325.2010.541382

Lopez-Garcia, P., Lesh, T. A., Salo, T., Barch, D. M., MacDonald, A. W. III, Gold, J. M., et al. (2016). The neural circuitry supporting goal maintenance during cognitive control: a comparison of expectancy AX-CPT and dot probe expectancy paradigms. *Cogn. Affect. Behav. Neurosci.* 16, 164–175. doi: 10.3758/s13415-015-0384-1

MacNamara, A., Kotov, R., and Hajcak, G. (2016). Diagnostic and symptom-based predictors of emotional processing in generalized anxiety disorder and major depressive disorder: an event-related potential study. *Cognit. Ther. Res.* 40, 275–289. doi: 10.1007/s10608-015-9717-1

Markon, K. E. (2013). Epistemological pluralism and scientific development: an argument against authoritative nosologies. *J. Pers. Disord.* 27, 554–579. doi: 10.1521/pedi.2013.27.5.554

Marquand, A. F., Rezek, I., Buitelaar, J., and Beckmann, C. F. (2016). Understanding heterogeneity in clinical cohorts using normative models: beyond case-control studies. *Biol. Psychiatry* 80, 552–561. doi: 10.1016/j.biopsych.2015.12.023

Moser, J. S., Durbin, C. E., Patrick, C. J., and Schmidt, N. B. (2015). Combining neural and behavioral indicators in the assessment of internalizing psychopathology in children and adolescents. *J. Clin. Child Adolesc. Psychol.* 44, 329–340. doi: 10.1080/15374416.2013.865191

Nelson, B. D., Hodges, A., Hajcak, G., and Shankman, S. A. (2015). Anxiety sensitivity and the anticipation of predictable and unpredictable threat: evidence from the startle response and event-related potentials. *J. Anxiety Disord.* 33, 62–71. doi: 10.1016/j.janxdis.2015.05.003

Nelson, L. D., Strickland, C., Krueger, R. F., Arbisi, P. A., and Patrick, C. J. (2016). Neurobehavioral traits as transdiagnostic predictors of clinical problems. *Assessment* 23, 75–85. doi: 10.1177/1073191115570110

Newman, E., Jernigan, T. L., Lisdahl, K. M., Tamm, L., Tapert, S. F., Potkin, S. G., et al. (2016). Go/no go task performance predicts cortical thickness in the caudal inferior frontal gyrus in young adults with and without ADHD. *Brain Imaging Behav.* 10, 880–892. doi: 10.1007/s11682-015-9453-x

Norrholm, S. D., Glover, E. M., Stevens, J. S., Fani, N., Galatzer-Levy, I. R., Bradley, B., et al. (2015). Fear load: the psychophysiological over-expression of fear as an intermediate phenotype associated with trauma reactions. *Int. J. Psychophysiol.* 98, 270–275. doi: 10.1016/j.ijpsycho.2014.11.005

Olbrich, S., Tränkner, A., Surova, G., Gevirtz, R., Gordon, E., Hegerl, U., et al. (2016). CNS- and ANS-arousal predict response to antidepressant medication: findings from the randomized iSPOT-D study. *J. Psychiatr. Res.* 73, 108–115. doi: 10.1016/j.jpsychires.2015.12.001

Østergaard, S. D., Bech, P., Trivedi, M. H., Wisniewski, S. R., Rush, A. J., and Fava, M. (2014). Brief, unidimensional melancholia rating scales are highly sensitive to the effect of citalopram and may have biological validity: implications for the research domain criteria (RDoC). *J. Affect. Disord.* 163, 18–24. doi: 10.1016/j.jad.2014.03.049

Patrick, C. J., and Hajcak, G. (2016). RDoC: translating promise into progress. *Psychophysiology* 53, 415–424. doi: 10.1111/psyp.12612

Patrick, C. J., Venables, N. C., Yancey, J. R., Hicks, B. M., Nelson, L. D., and Kramer, M. D. (2013). A construct-network approach to bridging diagnostic and physiological domains: application to assessment of externalizing psychopathology. *J. Abnorm. Psychol.* 122, 902–916. doi: 10.1037/a0032807

Pineles, S. L., Suvak, M. K., Liverant, G. I., Gregor, K., Wisco, B. E., Pitman, R. K., et al. (2013). Psychophysiologic reactivity, subjective distress and their associations with PTSD diagnosis. *J. Abnorm. Psychol.* 122, 635–644. doi: 10.1037/a0033942

Ryan, K. A., Dawson, E. L., Kassel, M. T., Weldon, A. L., Marshall, D. F., Meyers, K. K., et al. (2013). Shared dimensions of performance and activation dysfunction in cognitive control in females with mood disorders. *Brain* 138, 1424–1434. doi: 10.1093/brain/awv070

RDoC Launches User-Friendly Matrix Format. (2016). National Institute of Mental Health. Available online at: https://www.nimh.nih.gov/news/science-news/2016/rdoc-launches-user-friendly-matrix-format.shtml. [Accessed April 4, 2016].

Sharp, C., Kim, S., Herman, L., Pane, H., Reuter, T., and Strathearn, L. (2014). Major depression in mothers predicts reduced ventral striatum activation in adolescent female offspring with and without depression. *J. Abnorm. Psychol.* 123, 298–309. doi: 10.1037/a0036191

Siegle, G. J., D'Andrea, W., Jones, N., Hallquist, M. N., Stepp, S. D., Fortunato, A., et al. (2015). Prolonged physiological reactivity and loss: association of pupillary reactivity with negative thinking and feelings. *Int. J. Psychophysiol.* 98, 310–320. doi: 10.1016/j.ijpsycho.2015.05.009

Silverstein, S. M., Elliott, C. M., Feusner, J. D., Keane, B. P., Mikkilineni, D., Hansen, N., et al. (2015). Comparison of visual perceptual organization in schizophrenia and body dysmorphic disorder. *Psychiatry Res.* 229, 426–433. doi: 10.1016/j.psychres.2015.05.107

Stringaris, A., Vidal-Ribas Belil, P., Artiges, E., Lemaitre, H., Gollier-Briant, F., Wolke, S., et al. (2015). The brain's response to reward anticipation and depression in adolescence: dimensionality, specificity and longitudinal predictions in a community-based sample. *Am. J. Psychiatry* 172, 1215–1223. doi: 10.1176/appi.ajp.2015.14101298

Tegeler, C. H., Shaltout, H. A., Tegeler, C. L., Gerdes, L., and Lee, S. W. (2015). Rightward dominance in temporal high-frequency electrical asymmetry corresponds to higher resting heart rate and lower baroreflex sensitivity in a heterogeneous population. *Brain Behav.* 5:e00343. doi: 10.1002/brb3.343

The RDoC Matrix. (2016). National institute of mental health. Available online at: https://www.nimh.nih.gov/research-priorities/rdoc/constructs/rdoc-matrix.shtml. [Accessed October 23, 2016].

Van Meter, A. R., and Youngstrom, E. A. (2015). A tale of two diatheses: temperament, BIS, and BAS as risk factors for mood disorder. *J. Affect. Disord.* 180, 170–178. doi: 10.1016/j.jad.2015.03.053

Verona, E., and Bresin, K. (2015). Aggression proneness: transdiagnostic processes involving negative valence and cognitive systems. *Int. J. Psychophysiol.* 98, 321–329. doi: 10.1016/j.ijpsycho.2015.03.008

Webb, C. A., Dillon, D. G., Pechtel, P., Goer, F. K., Murray, L., Huys, Q. J. M., et al. (2016). Neural correlates of three promising endophenotypes of depression: evidence from the EMBARC study. *Neuropsychopharmacology* 41, 454–463. doi: 10.1038/npp.2015.165

Webb, C. A., Weber, M., Mundy, E. A., and Killgore, W. D. S. (2014). Reduced gray matter volume in the anterior cingulate, orbitofrontal cortex and thalamus as a function of mild depressive symptoms: a voxel-based morphometric analysis. *Psychol. Med.* 44, 2833–2843. doi: 10.1017/S0033291714000348

Weinberg, A., Meyer, A., Hale-Rude, E., Perlman, G., Kotov, R., Klein, D. N., et al. (2016). Error-related negativity (ERN) and sustained threat: conceptual framework and empirical evaluation in an adolescent sample. *Psychophysiology* 53, 372–385. doi: 10.1111/psyp.12538

Woody, M. L., McGeary, J. E., and Gibb, B. E. (2014). Brooding rumination and heart rate variability in women at high and low risk for depression: group differences and moderation by COMT genotype. *J. Abnorm. Psychol.* 123, 61–67. doi: 10.1037/a0035450

Wu, M.-J., Mwangi, B., Bauer, I. E., Passos, I. C., Sanches, M., Zunta-Soares, G. B., et al. (2017). Identification and individualized prediction of clinical phenotypes in bipolar disorders using neurocognitive data, neuroimaging scans and machine learning. *Neuroimage* 145, 254–264. doi: 10.1016/j.neuroimage.2016.02.016

Yancey, J. R., Vaidyanathan, U., and Patrick, C. J. (2015). Aversive startle potentiation and fear pathology: mediating role of threat sensitivity and moderating impact of depression. *Int. J. Psychophysiol.* 98, 262–269. doi: 10.1016/j.ijpsycho.2014.10.014

Yancey, J. R., Venables, N. C., and Patrick, C. J. (2016). Psychoneurometric operationalization of threat sensitivity: relations with clinical symptom and physiological response criteria. *Psychophysiology* 53, 393–405. doi: 10.1111/psyp.12512

2

Neonatal Hypoxia Ischaemia: Mechanisms, Models, and Therapeutic Challenges

Lancelot J. Millar[1], Lei Shi[1,2], Anna Hoerder-Suabedissen[1] and Zoltán Molnár[1]*

[1] *Molnár Group, Department of Physiology, Anatomy and Genetics, University of Oxford, Oxford, UK,* [2] *JNU-HKUST Joint Laboratory for Neuroscience and Innovative Drug Research, College of Pharmacy, Jinan University, Guangzhou, China*

Edited by:
Daniela Tropea,
Trinity College, Dublin, Ireland

Reviewed by:
Alla B. Salmina,
Krasnoyarsk State Medical University, Russia
Gunnar Naulaers,
KU Leuven, Belgium

***Correspondence:**
Lancelot J. Millar
lancelot.millar@univ.ox.ac.uk

Neonatal hypoxia-ischaemia (HI) is the most common cause of death and disability in human neonates, and is often associated with persistent motor, sensory, and cognitive impairment. Improved intensive care technology has increased survival without preventing neurological disorder, increasing morbidity throughout the adult population. Early preventative or neuroprotective interventions have the potential to rescue brain development in neonates, yet only one therapeutic intervention is currently licensed for use in developed countries. Recent investigations of the transient cortical layer known as subplate, especially regarding subplate's secretory role, opens up a novel set of potential molecular modulators of neonatal HI injury. This review examines the biological mechanisms of human neonatal HI, discusses evidence for the relevance of subplate-secreted molecules to this condition, and evaluates available animal models. Neuroserpin, a neuronally released neuroprotective factor, is discussed as a case study for developing new potential pharmacological interventions for use post-ischaemic injury.

Keywords: neonatal, hypoxia-ischemia, encephalopathy, subplate, neurodevelopment, neuroserpin, neuroprotection

INTRODUCTION: GLOBAL CLINICAL IMPACT OF NEONATAL HYPOXIA ISCHAEMIA

The clinical definition of neonatal HI injury is "asphyxia of the umbilical blood supply to the human fetus occurring at 36 gestational weeks or later" (Perlman, 1997, 2006; Volpe, 2001, 2012 Shah P.S. et al., 2006). Neonatal HI is synonymous with hypoxic-ischaemic encephalopathy (HIE) occurring in the term infant, where term is defined as 36 gestational weeks or later. This review addresses neonatal HI or HIE, any results concerning perinatal hypoxic-ischaemia injury will be clearly indicated in the text. This disorder encompasses a large range of physiological origins

---

Abbreviations: AMPA, alpha-amino-3-hydroxy-5-methyl-4-isoxazole propionic acid; BBB, blood brain barrier; CPR, cardiopulmonary resuscitation; CNS, central nervous system; CSF, cortico-spinal fluid; CSPG, chondroitin sulfate proteoglycan; CTGF, connective tissue growth factor; E(18), embryonic day (18); EM, electron microscopy; GABA, γ-aminobutyric acid; HI, hypoxia-ischaemia; HIF-1, hypoxia inducible factor 1; IL-1ß, interleukin-1ß; IL-6, interleukin-6; IL-9, interleukin-9; LPS, lipopolysaccharide; MRI, magnetic resonance imaging; MRS, magnetic resonance spectroscopy; NMDA, *N*-methyl-D-aspartate; OGD, oxygen glucose deprivation; P(8), postnatal day (8); poly(I:C), polyinosinic-polycytidylic acid; rER, rough endoplasmic reticulum; TNF-α, tumour-necrosis factor-α; tPA, tissue plasminogen activator; VEGF, vascular endothelial growth factor.

and clinical outcomes (Volpe, 1995). The diagnostic criteria for neonatal HI are based on a set of markers demonstrated to correlate with clinical outcome (Finer et al., 1981; Perlman, 1997; Richer et al., 2001). These include: 5-min Apgar score of less than 5 (Levene et al., 1986; Ruth and Raivio, 1988; Laptook et al., 2009); need for delivery room intubation or CPR (Richardson B.S. et al., 1996; Salhab et al., 2004a; Shalak and Perlman, 2004; Kattwinkel et al., 2010); umbilical cord arterial pH less than 7.00 (Ruth and Raivio, 1988; Perlman and Risser, 1993; Robertson N.J. et al., 2002; Salhab et al., 2004b); and abnormal neurological signs, such as hypotonic muscles or lack of sucking reflex (Levene et al., 1986; Robertson et al., 1989; Richer et al., 2001). Electroencephalography (EEG) has also proved helpful as a predictor of clinical outcome (reviewed in Walsh et al., 2011; van Laerhoven et al., 2013). Amplitude-integrated EEG (aEEG) in particular, a filtered time-compressed continuous one- or two-channel read-out, has been demonstrated a reliable predictor in meta-analyses up to 5 years after birth (al Naqeeb et al., 1999; Sinclair et al., 1999; Toet et al., 1999; Biagioni et al., 2001; Shah D.K. et al., 2006; Nash et al., 2011; Murray et al., 2016; Weeke et al., 2016), however, some report that aEEG remains less reliable than MRI, especially following hypothermia treatment (Doyle et al., 2010; Weeke et al., 2016). The Thompson score, an EEG measure of predictive neurodevelopment, is likely to remain useful to clinicians (Thompson et al., 1997; Horn et al., 2016). This is by no means an exhaustive list of risk factors and signs of clinical concern that can occur during the early postnatal period (Shalak and Perlman, 2004; Hagberg et al., 2015).

Neonatal HI is the most common cause of death and disability in human neonates (Grow and Barks, 2002; Ferriero, 2004; Shalak and Perlman, 2004), accounting for 23% of infant mortality worldwide, and affecting 0.7–1.2 million infants annually (Lawn et al., 2005; see **Figure 1**). In developed countries, incidence of HI injury has not decreased in the past two decades (Himmelmann et al., 2005; Vincer et al., 2006), remaining a significant cause of fatality and disability. The frequency of motor and cognitive disorders linked to perinatal and early postnatal brain injury actually increased during the 1990s, and currently remains stable (Vincer et al., 2006; Robertson and Iwata, 2007; Wilson-Costello et al., 2007). Progress in assisted respiratory and intensive care technology has led to greater than 90% survival of infants born after gestational week 23 (Larroque et al., 2004; Fellman et al., 2010), perhaps accounting for the increased burden of disability within the population as mortality rates have decreased substantially.

Amongst those who survive the initial injury, rates of disability remain high throughout life. Of patients surviving neonatal HI, 5–10% of infants demonstrate persistent motor deficits, and 20–50% display sensory or cognitive abnormalities that persist to adolescence (Hack et al., 1992; Vohr et al., 2000; Volpe, 2001, 2012; Lee et al., 2013). A meta-analysis of seven studies including 386 infant patients investigated the average incidence of mortality and morbidity: 5.9% of all patients across all studies died, 16.3% suffered neonatal seizures, and 17.2% experienced neurological deficits, with 14.2% qualifying for a diagnosis of cerebral palsy (Graham et al., 2008). Long-term outcomes in neonatal asphyxia infants have also been investigated. One meta-analysis found that 1–18% of patients were identified as having severe sensorimotor or learning disorders by the age of 2–5 years, with only 50–60% of patients reported as developmentally normal (Dilenge et al., 2001). This study covered a wide range of injury severities and follow-up ages. Disorders included seizures, hearing and vision loss (Robertson and Finer, 1985), language disorders, microcephaly, and muscle spasticity (Shankaran et al., 1991, 2012). Studies also report more severe neurological signs in patients suffering severe HI compared to those with milder HI injury (Robertson and Finer, 1985). Yet, many individuals who showed abnormal neurological signs at birth were normal at 2-year follow-up (De Souza and Richards, 1978). Clinical features and outcomes of neonatal HI are summarized in **Figure 1**.

Despite the high disability burden associated with surviving neonatal HI patients, there are very few preventative or protective treatments available for infants suspected to have suffered an HI event. The only licensed treatment currently available is hypothermia. This treatment involves subjecting either the infant's whole body or head-only to temperatures of around 33°C (Choi et al., 2012; Tagin et al., 2012). Hypothermia was first demonstrated to improve survival in cases of cardiac arrest (Bernard et al., 2002; Nikolov and Cunningham, 2003), and has since been applied as a neuroprotective treatment in acute neonatal HI injury patients (Gunn et al., 1997, 2005; Gunn and Gunn, 1998; Shankaran et al., 2002, 2005; Eicher et al., 2005; Gluckman et al., 2005; Jacobs et al., 2005, 2013; Shah et al., 2007; Azzopardi et al., 2009; Shah, 2010). A recent meta-analysis found that hypothermia carried out in over 1,200 infants reduced the rate of death and neurological handicaps at 18 months follow-up across all severity categories of neonatal HI injury (Tagin et al., 2012). However, hypothermia alone is not sufficient to prevent all brain injury or neurological symptoms, highlighting the need for additional therapies to use in conjunction. Xenon gas administration is currently being trialed as an additive therapy alongside hypothermia (Hobbs et al., 2008; Thoresen et al., 2009; Johnston et al., 2011). There are currently no other licensed treatments available for neonatal HI.

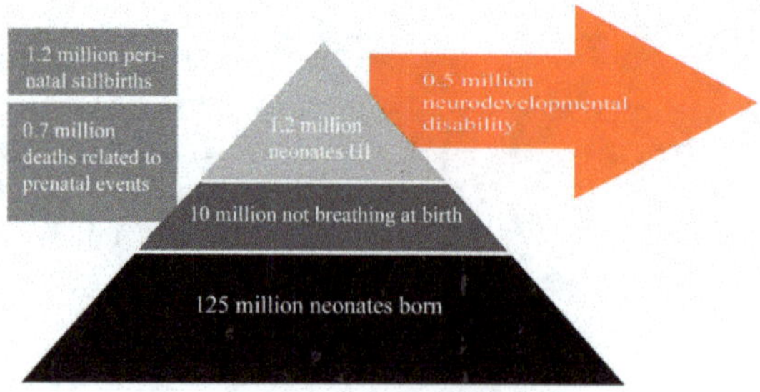

FIGURE 1 | Summary of Clinical Impact of Neonatal HI. This figures summarizes the number of neonates affected by neonatal HI annually across the globe relative to the number of live births per annum. Estimated figures for persistent disability associated with neonatal HI are also included. Estimates are based on data from studies references in this review (Hack et al., 1992; Vohr et al., 2000; Dilenge et al., 2001; Volpe, 2001, 2012; Graham et al., 2008; Lee et al., 2013).

Despite the efficiency of hypothermia (Tagin et al., 2012; Jacobs et al., 2013; Pauliah et al., 2013; Srinivasakumar et al., 2013; Kracer et al., 2014; Kali et al., 2015), death and disability remain a common feature of neonatal HI prognosis. Observations concerning global prevalence and poor long-term outcome reiterate the urgency of finding novel neuroprotective treatments for use during and directly following HI injury. This review examines the neuropathology resulting from neonatal HI injury in humans. The review then examines currently available animal models of neonatal HI and summarizes the strengths and weakness of such models for research into this complex human condition. Finally, the review will detail a potential approach toward identifying new pharmacological targets for neonatal HI therapies, focusing on the protein neuroserpin.

NEUROBIOLOGY OF NEONATAL HYPOXIA ISCHAEMIA IN HUMANS

There is ample evidence that brain damage occurs in human neonatal HI patients with poor clinical outcomes, documented in both imaging and histopathological studies (Mortola, 1999; Volpe, 2008, 2012; Northington et al., 2011). Neuropathology has been characterized in human post-mortem studies, concluding that most areas of the brain are vulnerable to some extent to neonatal HI injury (Miller et al., 2005; Triulzi et al., 2006; Billiards et al., 2008; Cohen and Scheimberg, 2008; de Vries and Groenendaal, 2010; Volpe, 2012). Gray and white matter lesions have been described at term after HI (Eken et al., 1994; Marin-Padilla, 1996, 1997, 1999). Localization and extent of neuropathology has been shown to be associated with neurodevelopmental symptoms, giving insights into the nature of disability the patients may present with.

Neuroanatomy: Structural Imaging

Infants who survive the initial HI insult display cerebral damage visible with structural imaging. Magnetic resonance imagining (MRI) studies of term infants with neurological signs and combinations of fetal distress, cord acidemia, and depressed Apgar scores have been carried out in over 1,000 infants (reviewed in Volpe, 2012). These studies report great variation in the anatomical areas involved between individual patients, yet most samples described either patients demonstrating predominant or substantial injury to cerebral cortex (Barkovich et al., 1995; Rutherford et al., 2004; Miller et al., 2005; Chau et al., 2008, 2012, 2013; Li et al., 2009), or basal ganglia and thalamus (Barkovich et al., 1995; Rutherford et al., 1998, 2004; Cowan et al., 2003; Kaufman et al., 2003; Miller et al., 2005; Chau et al., 2008) in partially overlapping subpopulations. These two patterns of injury are shown in **Figure 2**. Cerebral white matter has been described as selectively sensitive to term HI injury (Inder et al., 1999; Craig et al., 2003). Although less common, severe selective involvement of subcortical white matter has been documented (Neil et al., 2002; Vermeulen et al., 2003). One review described the literature concerning structural MRI scans in the acute phase (within 2 weeks after birth): approximately 15–30% of scans were normal, lesions in basal ganglia and thalamus are present in 40–80% of cases, with abnormalities of watershed white matter and cortex present in 40–60% of patients (Volpe, 2012). MRI anatomy has been shown to agree well with post-mortem studies (Cowan et al., 2003). Therefore, no single area of the brain is specifically damaged following neonatal HI. Any future treatments should take this diversity into account and provide neuroprotection to neurons throughout the brain.

The MRI scan is currently the method of choice for investigation of neonatal anatomy in both clinical and experimental circumstances (Perrin et al., 1997; Ment et al., 2002; Li et al., 2009). Diffusion-weighted MRI imaging has greatly improved identification of the time of onset of brain lesions (L'Abee et al., 2005; Chau et al., 2009). A reduced diffusion coefficient can be calculated, showing restricted diffusion during the first few days after the insult, with pseudonormalization by the end of the first week (McKinstry et al., 2002; Malik et al., 2006; Liauw et al., 2009). Sequential imaging has shown that lesions in the basal ganglia may increase in size during the first week after birth (Soul et al., 2001; Barkovich et al., 2006), and asymmetric diffusion within white matter has been correlated with clinical severity of hemiparesis (Glenn et al., 2007). Cranial ultrasound also remains a valuable clinical tool (Daneman et al., 2006). Another technique promising to add to understanding of neonatal HI is magnetic resonance spectroscopy (MRS), which allows brain metabolism to be imaged in real time (Kemp and Radda, 1994; Soares and Law, 2009). Full-term neonates with perinatal asphyxia have been studied, indicating that brain metabolism becomes abnormal after 6 to 12 h only to decrease even further after 24 h (Wyatt et al., 1989; Moorcraft et al., 1991; Roth et al., 1992). This coincided with clinical deterioration such as development of seizures. The concept of a delayed metabolic abnormality or 'secondary energy failure' has been elaborated in animal models (Lorek et al., 1994; Penrice et al., 1997; Groenendaal et al., 2006). Using MRS in these animal models, neuroprotective strategies could be tested. By using MRS data as real-time measurements of decreased brain metabolism in brain injury. ^{1}H-MRS and ^{31}P-MRS studied have demonstrated metabolic abnormalities following HI insult, which may persist for weeks (Groenendaal et al., 1994; Robertson et al., 1999). Unfortunately, with the magnetic field strength of current clinical systems, only large brain areas can be examined, limiting the use of this technique. Infants who have suffered neonatal HI often exhibit abnormal EEG activity (reviewed in Walsh et al., 2011; van Laerhoven et al., 2013). A range of abnormalities have been described, including: low voltage in isoelectric EEG (Finer et al., 1983; Legido et al., 1991), mild voltage depression (Watanabe et al., 1980; Toet et al., 2002; Murray et al., 2010), and asymmetry of trace (Aso et al., 1989; Zeinstra et al., 2001; Murray et al., 2009), although all of these criteria have been differently defined by different analysts (Rennie et al., 2004; Shellhaas et al., 2007). However, imaging techniques are constantly improving.

Lesions occur in many clinical patients, yet the effect on cognitive function is as diverse as the neuroanatomy. The area of cortex and basal ganglia damaged during the initial HI injury is directly predictive of language and motor outcome in childhood (Steinman et al., 2009; Martinez-Biarge et al., 2011). Examination

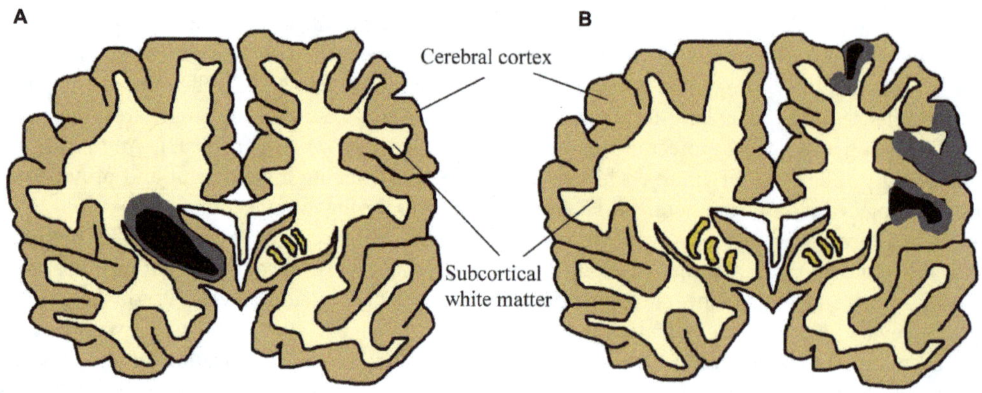

FIGURE 2 | Simplified Schematic of Brain Damage in Neonatal HI, approximately at the level of primary somatosensory and motor cortex. The two main patterns of injury, partially overlapping in patients, are shown separately for this schematic (adapted from Budday et al., 2014). Two colours have been used to show that many neonatal HI injuries consist of a centre of necrosis (black) and a penumbra of less acutely damaged tissue (gray). The exact location of these sites will vary depending on the nature of the injury. Black/gray areas represent the potential site of lesions, although those shown in this schematic are severe yet unilateral. **(A)** Primary basal-ganglia and thalamus injury pattern. **(B)** Primary watershed cortex and underlying white matter injury. Injury can primarily occur either to cortical gray matter or subcortical white matter depending on the nature of the injury. Severity also varies substantially between patients and within the brain of individuals. These have been documented in many human structural imaging studies (Barkovich et al., 1995; Cowan et al., 2003; Kaufman et al., 2003; Rutherford et al., 2004; Miller et al., 2005; Chau et al., 2008, 2012, 2013; Li et al., 2009).

of diffusion-tensor imaging of neonates was predictive of survival and motor outcome (Hunt et al., 2004; Ward et al., 2006). Children with basal-ganglia-thalamus pattern of injury tend to be severely disabled due to dyskinetic cerebral palsy and epilepsy (Himmelmann et al., 2007). Infants with predominant watershed white matter and cortex lesions have more prominent cognitive than motor deficits (Miller et al., 2005; Gonzalez and Miller, 2006; Steinman et al., 2009). Severe motor impairment is uncommon, and this group is often considered to have a normal outcome when seen at 12–18 months, although suboptimal head growth, behavioral problems, epilepsy, and a delay in language emerge during late childhood (Mercuri et al., 2000; Miller et al., 2002; Oguni et al., 2008; Sato et al., 2008; Steinman et al., 2009). Therefore, cortical damage appears to be relevant to functional outcome in surviving neonatal HI patients. This information could be used to predict future susceptibility to disability before it manifests, allowing social and educational supports to be put in place early.

Molecular Mechanisms of Cell Death

Anatomical studies describe loss of brain volume following moderate and severe neonatal HI. However, the underlying molecular mechanisms responsible for cell death are debated (McLean and Ferriero, 2004; Fatemi et al., 2009; Northington et al., 2011; Baburamani et al., 2012). Many pathways have been implicated in HI injury in the term brain, primarily: excitotoxicity, oxidative stress, and inflammation. Molecular studies have drawn attention to a fact essential for the development of successful new therapies that the neonatal brain and its injury is fundamentally different from that seen in adult HI stroke injury (McLean and Ferriero, 2004; Johnston et al., 2011; Baburamani et al., 2012; Semple et al., 2013).

There are many important differences between neonatal HI and adult ischaemic stroke. For example, severe HI events in the infant brain can lead to liquifactive disintegration, not seen after adult stroke (Larroche, 1977; Rorke, 1992). Newly formed blood vessels are fragile and prone to rupture (Trommer et al., 1987; Volpe, 1989; Ment et al., 1991; Jones et al., 2002), and surrounded by fewer astrocyte end-feet (El-Khoury et al., 2006). Another key site of difference is the BBB. Studies in rodents indicate that the BBB is compromised as a result of neonatal HI (Muramatsu et al., 1997; Svedin et al., 2007; Ferrari et al., 2010; Tu et al., 2011; Yang et al., 2012). Yet the common belief that the neonate BBB is less effective has recently come under revision (Saunders et al., 1999, 2012, 2014; McLean and Ferriero, 2004; Baburamani et al., 2012; Stolp et al., 2016). Tight junctions, the occlusive element of the BBB, are present as soon as embryonic vessels invade the brain (Schulze and Firth, 1992; Bauer et al., 1993; Stewart and Hayakawa, 1994; Kniesel et al., 1996), and are functional (Ek et al., 2003, 2006; Daneman et al., 2010). In a model of hypoxia in newborn piglet, BBB integrity was maintained (Stonestreet et al., 1992), yet other experiments have demonstrated damage to the BBB following neonatal HI (Alvarez-Diaz et al., 2007; Leonardo and Pennypacker, 2009).

Cerebrovascular autoregulation is another factor which must be considered in neonates. The concept that preterm infants have a 'pressure passive' cerebral circulation is widely accepted. However, sick term infants demonstrate impaired autoregulation (Pryds et al., 1990; Hardy et al., 1999; Boylan et al., 2000) and the range of blood pressure over which cerebrovascular autoregulation functions expands with maturity (Tuor and Grewal, 1994; Verma et al., 2000). Also, the concentrations and actions of various signaling molecules is different in the developing brain including; caspase-3 (Cheng et al., 1998), VEGF (Carmeliet and Storkebaum, 2002), and HIF-1 (Iyer et al., 1998), among others (reviewed in Baburamani et al., 2012).

One surprising difference is sexual dimorphism in response to neonatal HI. Male babies are at higher risk of cerebral palsy than females (Jarvis et al., 2005). Cognitive and motor outcomes are worse in male than in female low birth weight infants (Johnston and Hagberg, 2007). Quantitative imaging shows that male premature infants are more vulnerable to white matter injury, whereas females are more vulnerable to gray matter injury (Thompson et al., 2007). This sex difference has also been replicated in rodent *in vitro* models of hypoxic cell death (Zhu et al., 2006; Nijboer et al., 2007; Du et al., 2009). Although many molecular mechanisms are currently under investigation, this sexual dimorphism remains largely unexplained (Hill and Fitch, 2012; Chavez-Valdez et al., 2014; Demarest et al., 2016a,b; Waddell et al., 2016). Therefore, the unique state of the developmental brain should always be at the forefront of the researcher's minds.

Neonatal HI injury evolves over time (McLean and Ferriero, 2004). Injuries seen with MRI scans within the first few hours after asphyxia are subtle, restricted diffusion typically starting as small lesions in the putamen and thalami, progressing over the next 3 to 4 days to involve more extensive areas of the brain (Takeoka et al., 2002). Within the first few hours, regionally specific fluctuations in blood flow trigger excitotoxicity, free radical generation, and edema (Wigglesworth and Pape, 1978; Bennet et al., 1998; Jensen et al., 1999; Shalak and Perlman, 2004; Ferrari et al., 2010). A secondary phase of injury occurs during the following hours and days, resulting in neuroinflammation, mitochondrial permeabilization, and loss of cerebral autoregulation (Inder and Volpe, 2000; Hamrick and Ferriero, 2003; Scheepens et al., 2003; Hagberg et al., 2009; Leonardo and Pennypacker, 2009). A tertiary phase of brain injury has been proposed, which may exacerbate injury through persistent inflammation (Fleiss and Gressens, 2012).

The balance between molecular cell-death processes which cause this damage in neonatal HI remains debated. Early evidence indicates that the majority of cell death in neonatal HI is necrotic, however, all regions also undergo increased apoptotic death (Edwards and Mehmet, 1996; Edwards et al., 1997; Northington et al., 2001). Some studies suggest a more prominent role for apoptosis (Hill et al., 1995; Sidhu et al., 1997; Pulera et al., 1998; Hu et al., 2000; McLean and Ferriero, 2004). Immature neurons *in vitro* are more susceptible to apoptotic death than mature neurons (McDonald et al., 1997). Others report that necrosis is the major cellular pathology in humans and animals (Adamsons and Myers, 1973; Myers, 1975; Towfighi et al., 1995; Northington et al., 2001, 2005, 2011; Folkerth, 2005; Carloni et al., 2007; Stridh et al., 2013). Yet others recognize that both occur. Some report that necrosis predominates in severe cases, whereas apoptosis occurs in milder injury (Stroemer and Rothwell, 1998; Daval and Vert, 2004; Fatemi et al., 2009). Neurons often display morphologic features along an apoptosis-necrosis continuum (Portera-Cailliau et al., 1997a,b; Nakajima et al., 2000; Northington et al., 2007, 2011). In addition to apoptosis and necrosis, some neurons in the neonatal HI brain undergo autophagy (reviewed in Klionsky and Emr, 2000; Northington et al., 2011; Balduini et al., 2012). Neuronal autophagy occurs in rodent neonatal HI models (Lockshin and Zakeri, 1994; Carloni et al., 2008; Ginet et al., 2009). However, there is conflicting evidence as to whether the occurrence of autophagy augments brain damage (Koike et al., 2008; Puyal et al., 2009), or prevents the spread of necrotic cell death (Carloni et al., 2008). Artificially exclusive classification of cell death may hinder research and therapy development.

To add to this complexity, neonatal HI injury appears to activate several interacting molecular cascades. A simple schematic of the three major cascades is shown in **Figure 3**. The first is excitotoxicity, through which physiological glutamate neurotransmission leads to overactivation of postsynaptic receptors and cell death (reviewed in Hagberg et al., 1987; Choi, 1988, 1992; Hattori and Wasterlain, 1990; Danbolt, 2001). The *N*-methyl-D-aspartate (NMDA) receptor is relatively over-expressed in the developing brain (McDonald et al., 1989a; Represa et al., 1989; Fox et al., 1996). In P6 rats, the NMDA receptor is expressed at 150–200% of adult levels (Tremblay et al., 1988). The predominating combination of NMDA receptor subunits in the perinatal period seems to favor prolonged calcium influx for a given excitation (Danysz and Parsons, 1998). The same NMDA receptor that promotes plasticity can lead to massive Na^+ and water influx, cellular swelling, pathologically elevated intracellular calcium, and energy failure, leading to a 'spiral of death' (Choi, 1988). Oxygen glucose deprivation (OGD) in rat hippocampal neurons leads to a marked reduction in glutamate removal from the synapse (Jabaudon et al., 2000; Tao et al., 2001). Injection of NMDA into rat brain produces more extensive cell death in the neonate than in the adult (McDonald et al., 1988). Elevated glutamate has been documented in the cerebrospinal fluid (CSF) of infants who have suffered severe HI injury (Riikonen et al., 1992; Hagberg et al., 1993; Pu et al., 2008). The neonatal brain is much more prone to seizure activity than the mature brain (Holmes, 1991; Holmes and Ben-Ari, 2001), suggesting a prominent role for neuronal hyperexcitability and excitotoxicity although the molecular mechanisms behind this have not been fully elucidated (reviewed in Rakhade and Jensen, 2009). However, seizure activity could also be explained by paradoxical excitatory activity of the neurotransmitter gamma-amino butyric acid (GABA) in the developing brain (Staley et al., 1995). Drugs that block NMDA receptors are protective against HI injury in neonatal rodent models (McDonald et al., 1989a,b, 1990). Activation of AMPA receptors also contribute to injury (McDonald and Johnston, 1992; Deng et al., 2003; Talos et al., 2006), however, AMPA antagonists are not as protective (Ikonomidou et al., 1999; Noh et al., 2006). These findings are yet to be exploited in human clinical trials, as the integral role of glutamate receptors in healthy neuronal plasticity (Ikonomidou et al., 1999; Failor et al., 2010; Rocha-Ferreira and Hristova, 2015) could be damaged by the use of NMDA and AMPA antagonists at such a sensitive developmental stage.

An integrally linked cascade is that of oxidative stress. Excitotoxicity causes energy depletion, mitochondrial dysfunction, and cytosolic calcium accumulation, which in turn leads to generation of free radicals (Ferriero et al., 1996; Ferriero, 2001). Free radicals alter membrane pump function, allowing more glutamate release and NMDA receptor activation, leading to more excitotoxicity (Schanne et al., 1979; Robertson

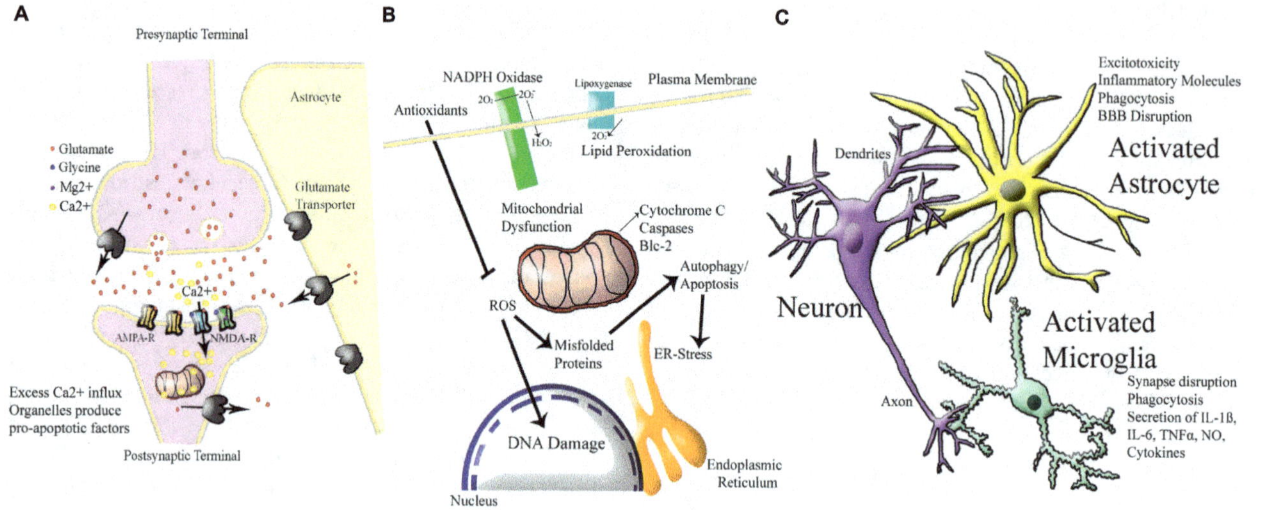

FIGURE 3 | Simplified Schematic of Major Molecular Injury Cascades involved in Neonatal HI. A vast number of molecules contribute to neonatal HI injury in the brain and all of these have been investigated in this disorder. These molecular targets can largely be split into the following three cascades. **(A)** Excitotoxicity (adapted from Vandenberg and Ryan, 2013) Ca^{2+} = calcium ion, Mg^{2+} = magnesium ion AMPA-R = α-amino-3-hydroxy-5-methyl-4-isoxazole propionic acid receptor, NMDA-R = *N*-methyl-D-aspartate receptor. **(B)** Oxidative Stress (adapted from http://www.enzolifesciences.com/platforms/cellular-analysis/oxidative-stress/). For simplicity, only free radicals are shown and physiological pathway substrates have been omitted. NADPH + Nicotinamide Adenine Dinucleotide Phosphate Hydrogen, O_2 = oxygen, O_2^- = negatively-charged oxygen free radiccal, H_2O_2 = hydrogen peroxide, ROS = ROS1 receptor tyrosine kinase encoded by the ROS1 gene, Blc = B cell leukaemia protein, ER = endoplasmic reticulum, DNA = deoxyribose nucleic acid. **(C)** Inflammation (adapted from Santiago et al., 2014). BBB = blood brain barrier, IL-6 = interleukin 6, IL-1B = interleukin 1 beta, TNFalpha = tumour necrosis factor alpha, NO = nitric oxide.

J.D. et al., 2002; Starkov et al., 2004). Oxidative stress is a general term for the increase in free radical production as a result of oxidative metabolism under pathologic conditions (Inder and Volpe, 2000; Ferriero, 2001). When oxygen floods the microenvironment of cells damaged by hypoxia, mitochondrial oxidative phosphorylation is overwhelmed and reactive oxygen species accumulate (Ferriero, 2001). Fetal life elapses in a low oxygen environment (East et al., 1998). In the first minutes of life, an abrupt increase in O_2 partial pressure occurs, which creates a pro-oxidant condition (Stiller et al., 2002). During birth asphyxia, excess calcium influx and other factors lead to severe oxidative stress (Forder and Tymianski, 2009). There is accumulation of hydrogen peroxide after HI in neonatal mice but not in adults (Lafemina et al., 2006). Because of its high lipid content, the brain is particularly susceptible to free radical attack (O'Brien and Sampson, 1965; Northington et al., 2001). The polyunsaturated fatty acid content of the brain increases during gestation (Crawford and Sinclair, 1971; Mishra and Delivoria-Papadopoulos, 1989). Lipid peroxidation may be a major factor in the white matter damage (Back et al., 1998; Baud et al., 2004). The developing brain's immature antioxidant defense also contributes to sensitivity to oxidative stress (Li et al., 1997; Mishra and Delivoria-Papadopoulos, 1999; Li and Jackson, 2002; Felderhoff-Mueser et al., 2002; Vannucci and Hagberg, 2004; Blomgren and Hagberg, 2006; Ikonomidou and Kaindl, 2011; Miller et al., 2012). Adequate stores of antioxidants are necessary to protect against oxidative injury. Specifically, depletion of neuronal reduced glutathione exacerbates oxidative injury (Chen and Liao, 2003; White and Cappai, 2003; Brongholi et al., 2006).

Finally, inflammation is a major component of neonatal HI injury. Low-dose treatment with intrauterine LPS dramatically increases severity of HI injury in neonatal mice, but protects against HI in adult rodents (Wang et al., 2007b). Intracerebral injection of NMDA receptor agonist produces a pattern of white matter injury, in which pretreatment with systemic IL-1ß, IL-6, IL-9, or TNF-α leads to a significant increase in lesion size (Marret et al., 1995; Dommergues et al., 2000). There is now substantial experimental evidence that intrauterine inflammation can exacerbate neonatal HI (Lehnardt et al., 2003; Eklind et al., 2005; Marini et al., 2007), which some have referred to as the "double-hit hypothesis" (reviewed in Agrawal and Hirsch, 2012; Hagberg et al., 2012; Dammann and Leviton, 2014). Microglia, the resident macrophages of the CNS, are among the first cells to become activated after HI (Fujimoto et al., 1989; Tahraoui et al., 2001; Kaur et al., 2007). Activated microglia migrate to damaged regions (Leonardo and Pennypacker, 2009) and produce inflammatory cytokines, glutamate, nitric oxide, and free radicals (Wood, 1995; Kaur and Ling, 2009). Drugs that block microglial activation protect the neonatal brain (Dommergues et al., 2003). Following hypoxia-ischemia, compromise of the BBB allows the entry of macrophages (Alvarez-Diaz et al., 2007; Leonardo and Pennypacker, 2009). Astrocytes also play a role in inflammation (Wang et al., 2003; Girard et al., 2008, 2009). CSF cytokines are elevated in term infants who later develop cerebral palsy (Savman et al., 1998; Dammann and O'Shea, 2008). The diverse network of interacting mechanisms demonstrate the molecular complexity of neonatal HI injury. Potential protective treatments should strive to tackle common mediators of these cascades relevant to all three pathways, otherwise full protection will not be achievable.

EVALUATION OF AVAILABLE ANIMAL MODELS OF NEONATAL HYPOXIA ISCHAEMIA

Neonatal hypoxia ischaemia has been modeled extensively in mice and rats (reviewed in Hagberg et al., 2002; van der Worp et al., 2007; Yager and Ashwal, 2009; Dean et al., 2015), with a minority of researchers also studying larger animals such as pigs, sheep (reviewed in Roohey et al., 1997; Dean et al., 2015) or primates (Fahn et al., 1979; Volpe, 2012). Models intending to replicate the clinical symptoms of neonatal human HI can be roughly divided into the four categories discussed below. All models have distinct advantages and disadvantages. A summary of available rodent models is shown in **Figure 4**.

Rice–Vannucci Model of Term Hypoxia Ischaemia

Most published studies modeling neonatal HI in animals have employed the Rice–Vannucci model (Rice et al., 1981). This model comprises unilateral carotid artery ligation, recovery with the dam for approximately 1 h, followed by exposure to 8% oxygen for 1–3 h at 37°C. Although, the model was initially described in rat (Rice et al., 1981), it has been successfully adapted for mouse with similar anatomical and behavioral effects (Ditelberg et al., 1996; Ferriero et al., 1996; Sheldon et al., 1998).

Rice' and Vannucci's model replicates anatomical damage seen in human neonates. Their initial study showed selective gray-matter sensitivity to neuronal necrosis, with gray matter injury observed in cortex, hippocampus, thalamus, and basal ganglia (Rice et al., 1981; Andine et al., 1990; Towfighi et al., 1995; Vannucci et al., 1999), encompassing the sites damaged in human neonatal HI. Histologically, there is a gradation of injury that correlates with the duration or severity of insult (Towfighi et al., 1991, 1995). White matter lesions have also been described in this model (de Torres et al., 1997; Ness et al., 2001; Liu et al., 2002; Drobyshevsky et al., 2005, 2007b), the extent of which correlate with the duration of exposure to hypoxia (Liu et al., 2002). However, bilateral common carotid artery ligation appears a stronger model of white matter damage (Jelinski et al., 1999; Uehara et al., 1999; Cai et al., 2001). Metabolic alterations in the Rice–Vannucci model include decreased cerebral blood flow (Sakurada et al., 1978; Vannucci et al., 1988), brain acidosis (Welsh et al., 1982; Yager et al., 1991), and decreased cerebral glucose uptake (Vannucci et al., 1989; Sokoloff et al., 1977). An inflammatory response has also been demonstrated (Bona et al., 1998).

Another convincing aspect of the Rice–Vannucci model is its ability to predict the therapeutic effect of hypothermia following the neonatal HI event. Mice treated with hypothermia showed smaller lesion volumes, in addition to better performance on the Morris water maze and circling tests (Yager et al., 1993; Lee et al., 2010; Kida et al., 2013; Lin et al., 2014). Many papers have investigated the behavioral outcomes of Rice–Vannucci injury in adult rodents. This model gives rise to well documented behavioral phenotypes including: impaired spatial learning and memory (Balduini et al., 2000, 2001; Ikeda et al., 2001; Wang et al., 2002; Arteni et al., 2003; Pereira et al., 2007; Cai et al., 2009; Greggio et al., 2011; Hill et al., 2012; Zheng and Weiss, 2013; Alexander et al., 2014; Gillani et al., 2015); impaired motor function as assessed by rotarod test, open field and motor reflexes (Barth and Stanfield, 1990; Jansen and Low, 1996a,b; Jansen et al., 1997; Balduini et al., 2000, 2001; Tomimatsu et al., 2002; Ådén et al., 2003; Lubics et al., 2005; Pazaiti et al., 2009; Im et al., 2010; Nijboer et al., 2010; Karalis et al., 2011; Chen et al., 2012; Ruiz et al., 2012; Sanches et al., 2012; Zheng et al., 2012; Xiong et al., 2013; Alexander et al., 2014; Gillani et al., 2014, 2015; Kim et al., 2014; Zhang Q. et al., 2014; Park D. et al., 2015; Park W.S. et al., 2015); sensory processing abnormalities (Alexander et al., 2014); and other cognitive phenotypes, such as reduced attention (Buwalda et al., 1995; Martin et al., 1997; Sanches et al., 2013; Perera et al., 2014; Miguel et al., 2015). Despite this broad range of documented effects, there are some contradictions between individual investigators (reviewed in Lubics et al., 2005), which suggest that different genetic backgrounds, severity, or experimenters can significantly affect the outcome of Rice–Vannucci model.

The Rice–Vannucci model of neonatal hypoxia ischaemia has several advantages. One is its prevalence, allowing direct comparisons with many other published papers (Vannucci et al., 1993, 2005; Yager and Ashwal, 2009; Dean et al., 2015). Another is that the contralateral hemisphere, exposed to hypoxia in the absence of ischemia, appears normal (Yager et al., 1991, 1992, 1996; Vannucci and Yager, 1992), providing a control hemisphere within the experimental brain. Thorough behavioral characterization (Arteni et al., 2003; Lubics et al., 2005) support the long term consequences of this model mimicking neonatal HI. One significant drawback of this model is the high variability in size and severity of infarct between animals, making comparisons between experimenters difficult (Vannucci and Hagberg, 2004; Vannucci and Vannucci, 2005). Additionally, the invasive nature of severing the common carotid artery does not replicate human injury; such severe vascular abnormalities occur rarely, if at all (Ment et al., 1984; Hill, 1991).

Hypoxia-Only Models

Some experimenters induce hypoxia in rodents exclusively using an oxygen deprivation chamber, without a preceding ischaemic procedure. These models are not as widely used as the Rice–Vannucci method, but have the potential to describe milder injuries and avoid the unphysiological occlusion of the common carotid artery. There are currently no published reviews or meta-analyses of hypoxia-only investigations, Supplementary Table 1 contains a brief summary of 122 published papers using hypoxia-only methodology compiled from Pubmed search results.

Historically, these methods have been used to investigate hypoxic brain biochemistry. Several studies have documented altered levels of neurotransmitters (Hedner et al., 1980; Kaneko et al., 1985; Yamamoto et al., 1985; Yamamoto and Kato,

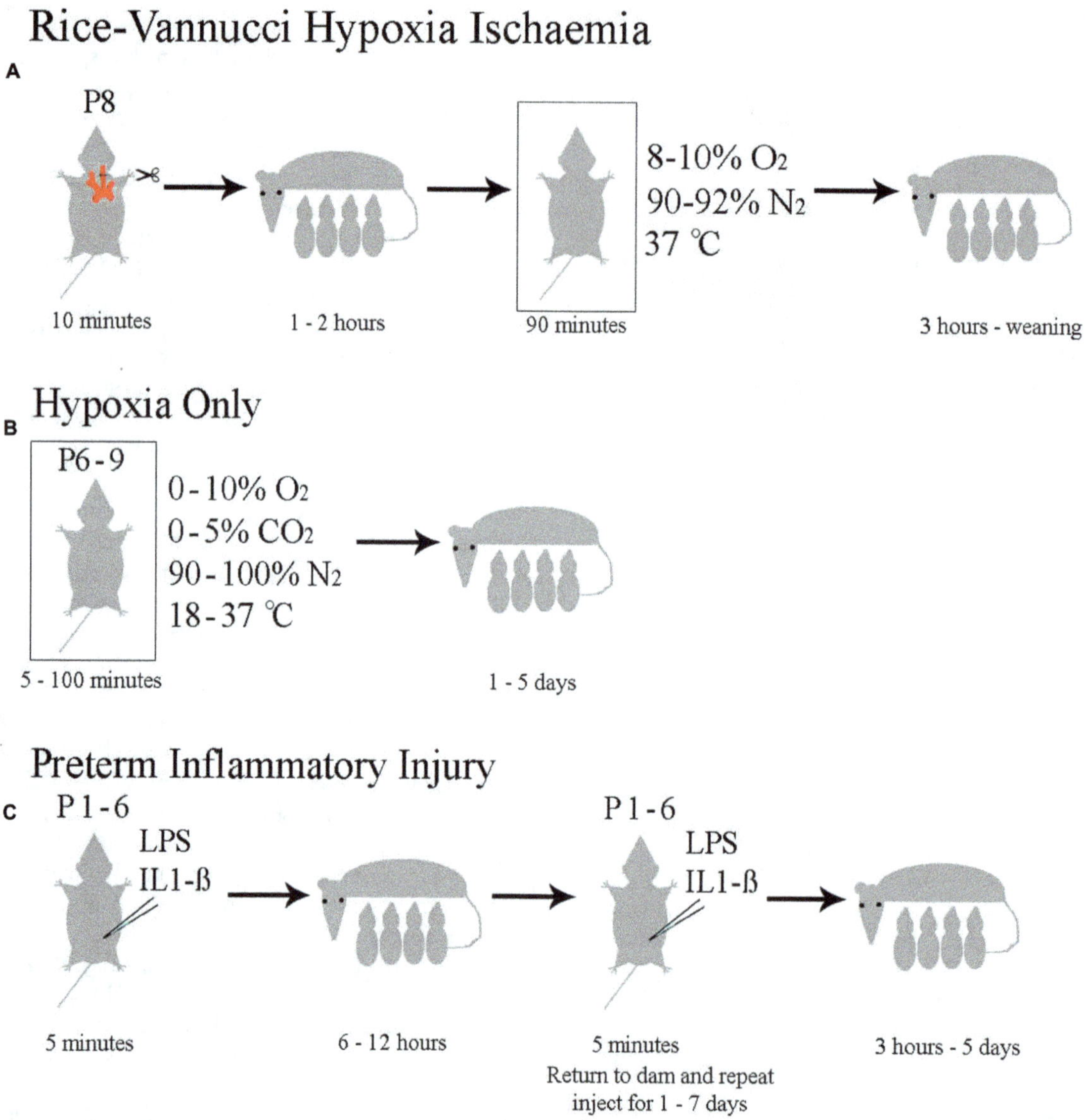

FIGURE 4 | Currently Used Rodent Models of Neonatal HI. (A) The Rice–Vannucci method as outlined in rats by Rice et al. (1981). **(B)** The general method with specifications taken from the pool of papers summarized in Supplementary Table 1. **(C)** The range of inflammatory models reviewed in Dean et al. (2015).

1986; Hadjiconstantinou et al., 1990; Seidler and Slotkin, 1990; Dell'Anna et al., 1993; Tanaka et al., 1995; Anju et al., 2010a,b; Anju and Paulose, 2011, 2013). However, there is little consensus over the direction or magnitude of changes (Decker M.J. et al., 2003; Decker et al., 2005). Hypoxia-only models have become an established model used to generate seizures in neonatal rats (Jensen et al., 1995; Applegate et al., 1996; Rodríguez-Alvárez et al., 2015; Sampath et al., 2015). In one such model, P6 rat pups were placed in chambers at 9% O_2 partial pressure and 20% CO_2 partial pressure for 60 min. Some pups were immediately restored to room air, whereas others underwent gradual reduction of CO_2 (Helmy et al., 2011; Tolner et al., 2011). Pups which underwent hypoxia with immediate restoration of CO_2 had a greater mortality rate and higher seizure frequency. However, subsequent anatomical analysis of these brains at P8 (Boss et al., 2005; Wang et al., unpublished), failed to show any differences in expression of cell death markers or layer-specific markers of healthy cortical neurons. Therefore, the hypoxia-only insult resulting in seizures appears to generate only subtle injury to the brain, far short of that seen in some human patients.

A range of behavioral phenotypes have been reported in hypoxia-only models, including hyperactivity (Shimomura and Ohta, 1988; Dell'Anna et al., 1991; Speiser et al., 1991; Decker et al., 2005); increased aggression (Mikati et al., 2005; Tang et al., 2006), altered ultrasonic vocalization (Venerosi et al., 2006), and disturbed sleep (Decker M.B. et al., 2003). Relatively few investigators have pursued standard tests of spatial memory and

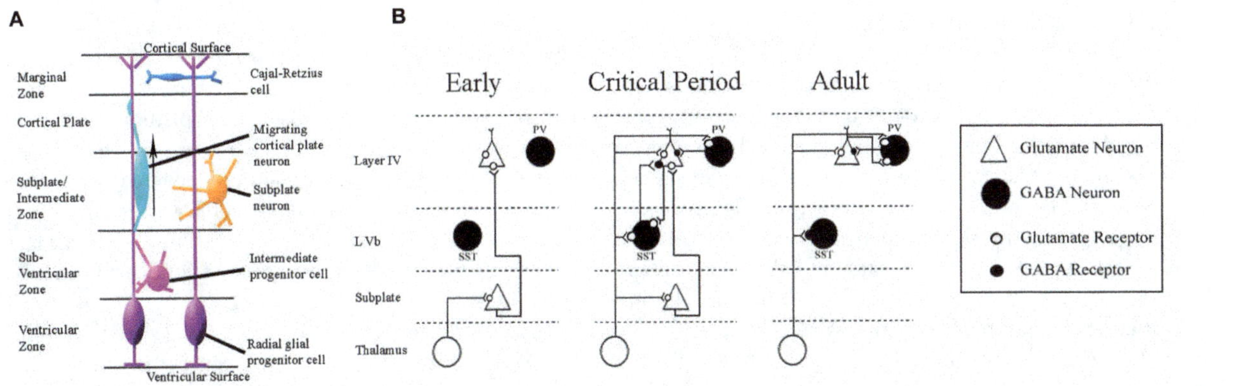

FIGURE 5 | Schematics of the anatomy and physiology of human subplate development. (A) Schematic coronal section showing the major cellular compartments within the developing human cortex at 26 post-conception weeks, reviewed in Hoerder-Suabedissen and Molnár (2015). The germinal zone (site of cell division) consists of the ventricular zone and subventricular zone. The subplate and intermediate zone lie between the germinal zone and the cortical plate (the site into which the permanent layers will migrate). The outermost layer is the early-born marginal zone. **(B)** Classical schematic of subplate architecture throughout development. In the earliest phase of thalamocortical circuit establishment subplate neurons (white) receive inputs from thalamus, and project axons to layer 4. At the onset of critical period, both subplate neurons and thalamus project to layer 4. In adult, subplate neurons have been eliminated by programmed cell death and layer 4 neurons receive inputs directly from thalamus. Adapted from Kanold (2009). This classical view has been augmented by the inclusion of GABA-ergic layer Vb interneurons which have been demonstrated to contribute to thalamocortical circuitry development in somatosensory mouse cortex (Marques-Smith et al., 2016).

locomotor behavior, and have obtained mixed results (Dell'Anna et al., 1991; Speiser et al., 1998; Rotstein et al., 2006; Coq et al., 2008; Raveendran and Skaria, 2013; Wang S. et al., 2015). The majority of hypoxia-only phenotypes are based on custom behavioral tests, making them difficult to compare to other established animal models. Additionally, some studies report no behavioral deficit following neonatal hypoxia alone (Buwalda et al., 1995; Iuvone et al., 1996; Casolini et al., 2005; Blaise et al., 2009; Mikhailenko et al., 2009; Anju et al., 2010c; Wang S. et al., 2015).

Although hypoxia-only models offer the potential to replicate the mechanism of hypoxia without major ischaemia seen in human neonatal HI patients, the models currently available are not ideal. One significant problem is the lack of methodological unity between different experimenters. There is little consensus on age of animal, background strain, oxygen partial pressure, time of exposure to hypoxia, or body temperature (see Supplementary Table 1). One example demonstrating the relevance of close control of these variables is temperature. P0 rat pups exposed to anoxia exhibit behavioral defects when anoxia was conducted at 39°C, yet not at 33 and 36°C (Rogalska et al., 2004, 2009; Caputa et al., 2005; reviewed in Rogalska et al., 2006). Therefore, far more care is needed to justify the design of hypoxia-only experiments before these models can be considered dependable models of human neonatal HI.

Inflammatory Models of Perinatal Brain Injury

Intrauterine infection is strongly associated with preterm birth and brain injury (Stoll et al., 2004; Mitha et al., 2013; Strunk et al., 2014; Dean et al., 2015). Many models have been described which introduce different inflammation-inducing molecules at different ages (Dean et al., 2015), many of which cause cerebral inflammation and white matter damage seen in human patients.

Administration of live *E. coli* into the uterus of pregnant rats can result in neutrophil infiltration in the fetal brain, increased fetal reabsorption and stillbirth, while surviving pups exhibit increased brain chemokines, cytokines, white matter injury, and behavioral phenotypes (Debillon et al., 2003; Rodts-Palenik et al., 2004; Pang et al., 2005; Yuan et al., 2005; Girard et al., 2009; Bergeron et al., 2013). The effects of bacterial mimetics such as the cell wall component lipopolysaccharide (LPS), have also been investigated. Intracervical injection in embryonic day 15 (E15) mice was associated with mild white matter injury but no behavioral deficits (Bell and Hallenbeck, 2002; Poggi et al., 2005; Wang et al., 2007a), whereas repeated intracervical LPS was associated with delayed neurosensory development (Toso et al., 2005; Rousset et al., 2006, 2013). Other inflammatory models include viral infection simulated by injection of poly(I:C), a synthetic double stranded viral RNA, injection of which is associated with long-term behavioral deficits (Shi et al., 2009; Richetto et al., 2013). Postnatal administration of inflammatory agents is widely used in rodents to model postnatal infection. Subcutaneous injection of live *E. coli* to P3 mouse pups was associated with microgliosis, loss of oligodendrocytes, and impaired motor coordination (Lieblein-Boff et al., 2013). However, most techniques which employ live bacterial injection have very high mortality rates (Rodewald et al., 1992; Tran and Weisman, 2004; Placencia et al., 2009; Loron et al., 2011). Postnatal intraperitoneal injection of LPS can also cause white matter damage and cerebral cytokine response (Brochu et al., 2011; Brehmer et al., 2012; Nobuta et al., 2012; Smith et al., 2014). Repeated daily injection of LPS in mice resulted in elevated serum IL-6, reduced gray matter volume, decreased oligodendrocyte numbers, and decreased myelin staining (Wang et al., 2009; Malaeb et al., 2014). Similarly, repeated IL-1β injection in

P1–P5 mice has been associated with impaired oligodendrocyte progenitor maturation, and severe memory deficits (Favrais et al., 2011).

One of the strengths of the inflammation model is that it reflects the exposure to infectious or inflammatory agents present outside of the highly sterile individually ventilated cages where many academic institutions keep experimental animals. Most of the inflammatory risk factors for increased severity of HI injury in human patients, such as maternal infection (Stoll et al., 2004; Girard et al., 2012; Dean et al., 2015), will result in systemic inflammation in addition to CNS-specific recruitment of microglia. However, there is currently debate concerning the relevance of maternal inflammation to fetal brain damage (Leviton et al., 1999; Redline and O'Riordan, 2000; Neufeld et al., 2005). The debate intensifies when fetal systemic inflammation is contrasted with neuroinflammation. Although the majority of publications cited above administer pro-inflammatory agents by intracerebral injection, some studies have administered LPS by intravenous injection (reviewed in Wang et al., 2006). In fetal sheep, intravenous LPS causes white-matter specific damage (Garnier et al., 2001, 2006; Duncan et al., 2002; Mallard et al., 2003; Peebles et al., 2003; Svedin et al., 2005), suggesting that systemic inflammation may be sufficient to trigger brain injury. However, the results of these experiments could be explained by a secondary neuroinflammatory response to systemic inflammation causing the white matter injury. Separating these parameters in future experiments will prove demanding.

Data suggest that gene expression in mouse models of inflammation closely corresponds to that seen in humans (Takao and Miyakawa, 2015), however, postnatal murine response to inflammation is likely different to that experienced by a human fetus. An important limitation of inflammatory studies is impact on cardiovascular function and the potential for secondary cerebral HI (Eklind et al., 2001; Favrais et al., 2011; Wang C.T. et al., 2015). Another is that varying results have been reported. This may be due to differences in LPS used between groups, purification method (Westphal, 1965; Lam et al., 2014), or dose (Fujihara et al., 2003). Alternatively, there is increasing evidence that the considerable individual variability in response to clinical sepsis between patients is related to host genetics (Christaki and Giamarellos-Bourboulis, 2014). Therefore, although inflammation is doubtless an important factor in neonatal brain injury, the variation between different models makes these methods difficult to evaluate.

Alternative Models

In many ways, non-rodent models are more representative of neonatal HI as it affects human patients. Here follows a brief flavor of techniques. Relatively few studies have investigated neonatal HI in primates. Classical studies asphyxiated term monkey fetuses by covering their heads with a rubber sac and clamping the umbilical cord (Fahn et al., 1979). Fetuses resuscitated after 20 min had extremely high mortality. However, 12 min of asphyxia were required to produce any neuropathologic injury. The fetuses displayed damage predominantly within the brainstem. In a model of partial ischemia (Fahn et al., 1979), pregnant females were rendered hypotensive during the third trimester. When blood oxygen saturation was reduced to 10% for 5 h, fetuses became profoundly acidemic. At birth, these displayed opisthotonus, decerebrate posturing, and convulsions. There is one model of white-matter injury based on baboons delivered prematurely by hysterotomy (Inder et al., 2004, 2005a,b). Premature baboons were treated in an intensive care setting. Approximately half displayed white-matter injury. Analysis of behavior has not been undertaken.

More work has been carried out in fetal sheep. Umbilical cord occlusion and term asphyxia has been carried out (Gunn et al., 1992; Williams et al., 1992; Mallard et al., 1993; Richardson B. et al., 1996; de Haan et al., 1997a,b,c; Richardson and Bocking, 1998; Dalitz et al., 2003), repeated asphyxia at 5-h intervals resulted in injury to the striatum almost exclusively, whereas episodes of asphyxia repeated every 5 min caused diffuse and extensive damage to cortex, thalamus, and cerebellum in 40% of animals, and selective neuronal necrosis in the remainder. White matter injury has also been investigated (Ting et al., 1983), only those fetuses in which the mean arterial blood pressure fell below 30 mmHg exhibit brain damage, irrespective of hypoxia. Neuropathologic injury after carotid artery occlusion for 30 min caused both gray and white matter involvement, with cortical damage and selective neuronal necrosis in thalamus and striatum (Reddy et al., 1998; Petersson et al., 2002). Several laboratories have developed models in sheep after systemic endotoxemia (Duncan et al., 2002; Mallard et al., 2003). Unfortunately, no behavioral outcomes are currently available in sheep.

Finally, other small laboratory animals have been investigated. Preterm rabbit fetuses exposed to sustained placental insufficiency via intrauterine occlusion of the descending aorta displayed significant alterations in motor responses to olfactory stimuli, coordination of suck and swallow, and marked hypertonia, reminiscent of spastic quadriplegia (Yoon et al., 1997; Derrick et al., 2004, 2007; Saadani-Makki et al., 2008). Diffusion-weighted imaging detected a threshold in white matter loss below which all rabbit kits developed hypertonia, (Drobyshevsky et al., 2005, 2007a). Another promising model is that of the spiny mouse, a rodent which shows a similar level of brain development to a human neonate at birth (Brunjes, 1985, 1989, 1990; Gozzo et al., 1985; D'Udine and Alleva, 1988; Brunjes et al., 1989), which also shows varied motor deficits (Ireland et al., 2008, 2009, 2010) and neuroanatomical pathology (Hutton et al., 2009; O'Connell et al., 2013) following neonatal HI.

In brief, large animals can better replicate the conditions of a single human fetus exposed to a non-sterile environment. However, none of these models have access to the same extent of transgenic manipulation or validated behavioral tests that are possible in rodent studies. These models are invaluable for aiding comparison of brain development at birth which occur between species (Clancy et al., 2007), whereas the relative immaturity of mouse and rat brains at birth introduce an unwelcome variable into these experiments. For the foreseeable future, insights from both rodent work and larger animals will be important for better understanding neonatal HI.

SUBPLATE: A REGION OF HYPER-SENSITIVITY TO NEONATAL HI?

One brain region exemplifying how much remains unknown about the developing brain's response to HI, and the uncertainties involved in interpreting results from animal studies, is subplate. The subplate is an early-born transitory neuronal layer of cerebral cortex which serves an important role in the establishment of thalamocortical connectivity during development (reviewed in Judas et al., 2010; Kanold and Luhmann, 2010; Kostovic and Judas, 2010; Hoerder-Suabedissen and Molnár, 2015) (see **Figure 4**). Thalamocortical axons associate with and grow alongside subplate neurons in the developing cortex (Herrmann et al., 1994; Molnár et al., 1998; Kostovic and Judas, 2006), and selective excitotoxic ablation of subplate disrupts thalamocortical connectivity in animal models (Ghosh et al., 1990; Ghosh and Shatz, 1992; Lein et al., 1999; Kanold et al., 2003; Kanold and Shatz, 2006; Magnani et al., 2013).

Subplate has been identified in a range of mammals by conserved molecular markers (Hoerder-Suabedissen et al., 2009; Hoerder-Suabedissen and Molnár, 2012; Oeschger et al., 2012; Pedraza et al., 2014). Neuronal death occurs in infant subplate during normal development (Chun et al., 1987; Al-Ghoul and Miller, 1989; Hamre et al., 1989; Kostovic and Rakic, 1990; Woo et al., 1991; Price et al., 1997). However, the molecular mechanisms behind this programmed cell-death remain unknown (McQuillen and Ferriero, 2005; Hoerder-Suabedissen and Molnár, 2015). Functional roles for subplate in thalamocortical (Allendoerfer and Shatz, 1994; Kanold and Luhmann, 2010) and corticothalamic (Grant et al., 2016) development have been described, demonstrating lasting significance of this transient population.

The susceptibility of subplate neurons to neonatal HI remains little understood. Early studies claimed subplate is selectively vulnerable. Cultured rat subplate neurons were more vulnerable to OGD compared to mixed cortical neurons (Nguyen and McQuillen, 2010). In rats exposed to systemic HI at E18, a significant decrease in Nurr1-expressing subplate neurons was documented by P2 (Jantzie et al., 2014, 2015a,b,c) and similarly in fetal sheep (Dean et al., 2011). However, Nurr1-expressing Layer VI neurons were also decreased. It is also possible that HI induced differential marker expression in subplate neurons, rather than cell death. *In vitro* electrophysiological recordings in neocortical slices from newborn rats have demonstrated a pronounced functional impairment of subplate neurons following OGD (Albrecht et al., 2005). Another influentiential study that claimed selective vulnerability of subplate to hypoxia used immunohistochemistry to detect cell-death in neurons labeled with BrdU at E10.5 following a modified Rice–Vannucci model in P1 rats (McQuillen et al., 2003; McQuillen and Ferriero, 2004, 2005). However, Layer VI neurons born at this date also expressed cell-death markers, suggesting subplate may not be selectively susceptible to HI injury. Conversely, a systematic quantification of cell death markers throughout subplate compared with other cortical layers was conducted using immunohistochemistry (Okusa et al., 2014). Three subplate-specific marker positive populations showed little co-staining with caspase-3 in brains with mild to moderate HI lesions. In severely damaged cases, caspase-3 staining was found throughout the cortex. Therefore, layer-specific sensitivity of cortical neurons to HI remains debated. A double birthdating study, targeting subplate and layer V or VI combined with HI could resolve this issue. However, such an experiment has not yet been performed.

Human literature supports the proposition that interstitial white matter, the equivalent of subplate in the postnatal human brain (Clancy et al., 2009; Suarez-Sola et al., 2009; Garcia-Marin et al., 2010; Hoerder-Suabedissen and Molnár, 2015), shows structural damage as a result of neonatal injury. Tissue from preterm human infants with periventricular leukomalacia showed a deficit in the number of MAP-2 expressing neurons throughout the interstitial white matter (Kinney et al., 2012). Scarring has been observed in interstitial white matter, alongside the expression of cell death markers, in brain tissue from human infants (Pogledic et al., 2014). The number of interstitial neurons present in white matter is known to peak at the developmental stage most sensitive to white matter injury (Kostovic et al., 2002; Kostovic and Judas, 2010). Immunohistochemical analysis on neonatal telencephalon samples obtained post-mortem from infants born at 25–32 weeks gestation showed a significant loss of GABA-ergic subplate neurons (Robinson et al., 2006). Many reviews have highlighted the interstitial white matter as a site which should be more thoroughly investigated in neonatal brain injury (Volpe et al., 1996; Leviton and Gressens, 2007; Volpe, 2009; Kostovic et al., 2011). Several of these reviews propose a role for subplate in resultant cognitive and behavioral deficits (Volpe, 2009, 1977; Kostovic et al., 2011), based on the established role of subplate in thalamocortical development. Unfortunately, post-mortem studies are unable to convey whether subplate pathology is responsible for any of the clinical outcomes in patients. The response of both human and rodent subplate to neonatal HI remains unclear, despite assertions of interest from the field. A systematic study of the subplate *in vitro* and *in vivo* following HI injury would provide valuable information. As subplate transiently integrates within the developing cortical circuitry (see **Figure 5**) interactions between subplate neurons and other cortical neurons, such as key interneuron populations, should also be further investigated (Marques-Smith et al., 2016).

There are several reasons for believing that subplate could be critical in neonatal HI. One is the proposed transient secretory function. Subplate is enriched in CSPGs, whereas the adjacent intermediate zone is not (Kostovic et al., 2014). Chondroitin sulfate proteoglycans (CSPGs) are generally secreted from cells, and the subplate transcriptome catalogs a plethora of genes involved in production of extracellular matrix and proteoglycans (Belgard et al., 2011; Hoerder-Suabedissen et al., 2013). Additional genes with subplate-restricted expression in the cortex encode secreted proteins, including neuroserpin (*Serpini1*), neuronal pentraxin 1 (*Nptx1*), and insulin-like growth factor binding protein 5 (*Igfbp5*) (Hoerder-Suabedissen et al., 2013), several of which have been validated by immunohistochemistry (Kondo et al., 2015). Connective tissue growth factor (CTGF), secreted extracellular matrix-associated protein involved in regulation of cellular adhesion, migration, mitogenesis, differentiation and survival (Brigstock, 1999; Stritt et al., 2009), is also detectable in the subplate at E18, increasing in intensity at P3 and P8 (Hoerder-Suabedissen et al., 2009, 2013). It is unknown whether subplate-secreted proteins serve a protective function in the developing brain or not. Related to this secretory function, subplate neurons express relatively mature rER (Kondo et al., 2015), an organelle essential for production of secreted proteins (reviewed in Novikoff, 1976; Pfeffer and Rothman, 1987; Lodish, 1988; Hurtley and Helenius, 1989; Pelham, 1989). As a result of the cellular pressures of high protein production, cells activate a series of mechanisms referred to as the ER stress response (Schroder and Kaufman, 2005; Wu and Kaufman, 2006; Kondo et al., 2011). Nissl staining demonstrates enriched protein production in subplate at P8 in mouse, although staining is much fainter in adult (Kondo et al., 2015). Morphology of subplate neurons is similar to that of rER-rich plasma cells under EM (Bloom, 1968; Kondo et al., 2015), and immunohistochemistry for ER stress marker binding immunoglobulin protein (BiP) confirmed that ER stress occurs in developing subplate (Okiyoneda et al., 2004; Kondo et al., 2005, 2012, 2015). BiP protein synthesis is up-regulated in whole brain under stress conditions, such as glucose deprivation, hypoxia, or the presence of toxins (Lee, 1987, 2001, 2005). It is not known exactly which proteins are secreted throughout development by the subplate, but this enhanced metabolic stress during hypoxia and the potential for neuroprotective secretion reinforce the value of further study of subplate in neonatal HI models and human patients.

NEUROSERPIN: A CASE FOR A NOVEL NEUROPROTECTIVE TREATMENT

The development of novel treatments to supplement the sole currently licensed therapy, hypothermia (Jacobs et al., 2005, 2013; Shah et al., 2007; Tagin et al., 2012), is imperative. Since the discovery of this groundbreaking treatment, little progress has been made in identifying additive pharmacological therapies. Few potential treatments have translated to human clinical trials. Resuscitation at room temperature (Vento et al., 2001a,b; Rabi et al., 2007) and xenon gas administration alongside hypothermia (Hobbs et al., 2008; Thoresen et al., 2009) are the only therapies shown to have any additive effect. However, more recent publications have questioned the efficacy of xenon as an additive therapy alongside hypothermia. For example, randomized clinical trials have demonstrated that although xenon gas is a safe treatment, there is little or no therapeutic effect of combined hypothermia and xenon gas in moderate and severe cases of neonatal HI at 18 months follow-up (Azzopardi et al., 2013, 2015; Dingley et al., 2014). A similar experiment in rats found that xenon treatment made no difference to lesion size or neuronal cell numbers in cases of severe HI (Sabir et al., 2016). Barbiturate anticonvulsants have no effect on long-term neurological development when given following neonatal HI (reviewed in Goldberg et al., 1986; Hall et al., 1998; Singh et al., 2004; Vargas-Origel et al., 2004; Evans et al., 2007). Recent clinical studies suggest that high dose erythropoietin (EPo) treatment in term HI neonates reduces disability (Strunk et al., 2008; Zhu et al., 2009; McPherson and Juul, 2010). However, even proponents of this potential treatment advise caution in interpreting these early results, and the therapeutic effect by no means completely prevents disability. Combination therapy of *N*-acetylcysteine, a free radical scavenger, and systemic hypothermia reduces infarct volume after focal HI injury (Jatana et al., 2006). Another free radical scavenger, allopurinol, reduces cerebral edema and neuropathological damage (Palmer et al., 1990). However, these treatments have only been trialed in animals, and the field is still awaiting a candidate neuroprotectice molecule which is both safe and effective in neonatal humans (Lai and Yang, 2011; Pazos et al., 2012).

Another therapeutic approach under development for neonatal HI is stem cell therapy (reviewed in Parolini et al., 2010; Zhang X. et al., 2014; Douglas-Escobar and Weiss, 2015; González-Portillo et al., 2015; Ruiz et al., 2017). These therapies make use of evidence that transplantation of human bone-marrow derived stem cells into the lesion can assist brain plasticity (Bonifacio et al., 2011; Tajiri et al., 2013). Results of this therapy have been promising in animal models (Jendelová et al., 2004; Daadi et al., 2009a,b), however, the technique awaits validation in a clinical setting. Additionally, the use of stem cell therapy for cerebral palsy in human patients has produced mixed results (Li et al., 2012; Liao et al., 2013; Sharma, 2014).

Therefore, new approaches are required to identify potential neuroprotective molecules as treatments for neonatal HI (Tuor et al., 1995; Ferriero, 2004; Fan et al., 2010). Drawing on our detailed yet incomplete knowledge of the physiology of neonatal HI, several factors must be satisfied in a new potential therapy. All potential treatments should be safe for vulnerable neonates and not interfere with essential developmental milestones. This challenges the NMDA-inhibition strategies (Meldrum, 1990; Johnston, 2001, 2005), as the glutamate system is essential for setting up normal synaptic plasticity within the developing brain (Hattori and Wasterlain, 1990; Ikonomidou et al., 1999; Johnston, 2009). Treatments should also be specific, to avoid extreme adverse effects in these vulnerable infants. The ideal treatment would target molecules common to the excitotoxicity, oxidative stress and inflammation pathways (Chaudhari et al., 2014; Fischer and Maier, 2015; Chamorro et al., 2016; Burd et al., 2016). Targeting these common mediators would allow a single therapy to be efficacious against multiple mediators of brain damage, instead of merely eliciting a reshuffle of pathways to favor a different method of cell death. Here follows an outline of one potential therapy under development which may satisfy these theoretical restraints as a model to incite debate concerning how future therapies are identified. Enter: neuroserpin.

Neuroserpin's Molecular Pedigree

Neuroserpin is a neuronally secreted serine-protease inhibitor enzyme with roles in cell death, neural plasticity, and microglial activation. Neuroserpin was first identified in the secreted product of cultured neuronal axons (Osterwalder et al., 1996). Protein expression is primarily localized to neurons (Osterwalder et al., 1996; Hastings et al., 1997; Lee et al., 2015b). The protein neuroserpin is encoded in mouse and human by the gene *Serpini1*. *Serpini1* mRNA expression is specific to the CNS, both in mouse (Krueger et al., 1997) and human (Teesalu et al., 2004). *In situ* hybridization studies have demonstrated expression of *Serpini1* throughout cortex, hippocampus, and olfactory bulbs, with scattered expression in cerebellum, pons, and thalamus from birth until adulthood (Krueger et al., 1997). High *Serpini1* expression has been identified in subplate relative to Layer VI of cortex in P8 mouse brain by microarray (Hoerder-Suabedissen et al., 2009), confirmed by immunohistochemistry (Kondo et al., 2015). Although *Serpini1* expression has been demonstrated in human brain tissue (Teesalu et al., 2004), detailed maps of expression are currently missing. This highly specific localisation suggests that *Serpini1*/neuroserpin modulatory treatments may not create dangerous side effects in other vulnerable organs such as the cardiovascular and pulmonary systems.

Neuroserpin is an inhibitory enzyme. Its primary target is the adult human stroke treatment, tissue plasminogen activator (tPA) (Osterwalder et al., 1996, 1998; Barker-Carlson et al., 2002; Yepes and Lawrence, 2004a; Miranda and Lomas, 2006; Ricagno et al., 2009, 2010). Neuroserpin has also been shown to exhibit weak inhibition of plasmin and urokinase plasminogen activator (Osterwalder et al., 1998). This function is conserved across species (Schrimpf et al., 1997; Hill et al., 2001; Ellisdon et al., 2014). Through inhibition of tPA, neuroserpin has the potential to influence many distinct molecular cascades (Yepes and Lawrence, 2004b,c; Benarroch, 2007; Yepes, 2015). tPA, also secreted by neurons (Krystosek and Seeds, 1981a,b; Lochner et al., 2006), has been shown to interact with a large number of pathways; activating NMDA receptors (Qian et al., 1993; Nicole et al., 2001), activating microglia (Benchenane et al., 2004), and recruitment of cell death related cascades (Yepes and Lawrence, 2004a; Zhao et al., 2007), in addition to its function of cleaving vascular thrombosis (Rijken et al., 1979, 1980). The known components of the neuroserpin/tPA molecular cascade are summarized in **Figure 6**.

Other, tPA-independent enzymatic pathways for neuroserpin have also been described (Ma et al., 2012a). Cell lines over-expressing neuroserpin demonstrate an increase in *N*-cadherin protein expression and related cell adhesion, maintained when the tPA binding site of neuroserpin is mutated (Lee et al., 2008). *In vitro*, neuroserpin has been shown to prevent excitotoxic neuronal death induced by plasmin and kainic acid (Wu et al., 2010), and the 20 methionine residues present within neuroserpin have been claimed to convey protection against oxidative stress (Mohsenifar et al., 2007), and exogenous neuroserpin has been shown to possess anti-inflammatory properties (Munuswamy-Ramanujam et al., 2010). The molecular cascades behind these tPA independent functions are not well understood (Ma et al., 2012a). Therefore, neuroserpin has the pedigree to target multiple cell death pathways occurring in the brain during neonatal HI.

Cell Death, Inflammation, and Plasticity

Neuroserpin's physiological actions can be broadly categorized into three major pathways: cell death, neuronal plasticity, and immune cell activation. These closely follow the major classes of molecular change proposed by pathological theories of neonatal HI, suggesting that neuroserpin offers the potential to target multiple brain-damage pathways.

Neuroserpin has been implicated in protection against neuronal death (Galliciotti and Sonderegger, 2006). Exogenous neuroserpin administration *in vitro* decreases apoptosis caused by tPA, NMDA, kainic acid, and OGD (Lebeurrier et al., 2005a,b; Mohsenifar et al., 2007; Lee et al., 2008; Wu et al., 2010; Rodríguez-González et al., 2011a; Ma et al., 2012b). In addition, aberrant initiation of neuroserpin expression in cancer cells preserves the tumor and has been linked with increased treatment-resistance in prostate cancer (Chang et al., 2000; Hasumi et al., 2005; Valiente et al., 2014). Exogenous neuroserpin reduces spread of kainate-induced seizures in mouse, and decreases the expression of cell death markers (Yepes et al., 2002).

Of the three classes of neuroserpin function, its role in inflammation is the least well understood. When applied to vascular plaques *in vitro*, recombinant neuroserpin reduced T-Cell lymphocyte invasion (Munuswamy-Ramanujam et al., 2010). Administration of intracerebral neuroserpin directly following adult HI stroke in mouse, showed a qualitative decrease in the volume of infarct infiltrated by activated microglia (Yepes et al., 2000), and lower microglial inflammatory marker expression (Gelderblom et al., 2013). In human adult stroke patients, higher levels of neuroserpin in blood samples correlate with lower levels of immune marker proteins (Rodríguez-González et al., 2011c). There is considerable debate whether microglial activation is beneficial or detrimental in neonatal HI (McRae et al., 1995; Mallard et al., 2013; Kaur et al., 2013), so understanding the role of neuroserpin in balancing this cascade could provide important data. The lack of a complete molecular network explaining these anti-inflammatory effects highlights the complexity of the pathways involved in cell death and inflammation. Understanding the underlying explanation for these changes will be an important preliminary to administration in human infants who do not live in the highly sterile environments maintained for experimental animals.

In addition, neuroserpin is involved in neuronal plasticity. This could be problematic in the development of neuroserpin as a neonatal HI treatment for human patients, as the neonatal human brain circuitry is undergoing a great deal of developmental plasticity modifications (reviewed in Aoki and Siekevitz, 1988; Partanen et al., 2013; Simpson et al., 2014). The first evidence that neuroserpin may have a role in neuronal plasticity originated from studies of endocrine cell lines, which grow neurite-like processes when neuroserpin is administered to their media (Hill et al., 2001; Jacovina et al., 2001; Borges et al., 2010). At the molecular level, neuroserpin secretion from dense core vesicles is enhanced by depolarisation in cultured neurons (Berger et al., 1999; Ishigami et al., 2007). Monocular

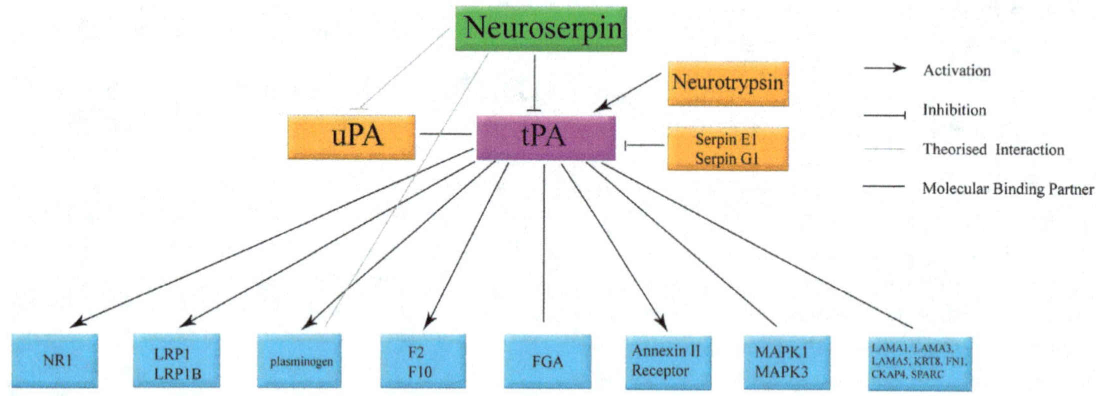

FIGURE 6 | Classical binding cascade for neuroserpin protein. The main molecular target of neuroserpin is inhibition of tPA. Confirmed molecular binding partners are shown with a black line. Arrows denote confirmed activation. Orthogonal lines denote confirmed inactivation. Lines without caps denote confirmed binding with no documented physiological data. tPA, tissue plasminogen activator; uPA, urokinase plasminogen activator. All other abbreviations denote standard gene names.

enucleation at P11 in mouse led to decreased *Serpini1* mRNA expression in contralateral primary visual cortex compared to the control hemisphere (Wannier-Morino et al., 2003). The relative importance of this molecular cascade for human plasticity is as yet unclear.

Neuroserpin in *In Vitro* and Adult Hypoxia Ischaemia

Neuroserpin has been studied extensively in cell culture models of HI stroke. Administration of neuroserpin protects mouse cortical neurons *in vitro* against NMDA-induced excitotoxicity, but not AMPA-induced excitotoxicity (Lebeurrier et al., 2005a,b; Ma et al., 2012b). Further, neuroserpin is protective in an *in vitro* model of HI, OGD (Wu et al., 2010; Rodríguez-González et al., 2011a; Ma et al., 2012b). Both neurons and astrocytes cultured in OGD undergo less apoptosis and do not exhibit damaged neural processes when exogenous neuroserpin is administered following OGD (Rodríguez-González et al., 2011a; Ma et al., 2012b). Hippocampal neurons from both wild-type and tPA knockout mice were protected from OGD, plasmin-mediated cell death and kainic acid by neuroserpin administration (Wu et al., 2010), demonstrating that neuroserpin's neuroprotective role is not exclusively dependent on tPA inhibition.

Neuroserpin is also neuroprotective *in vivo*. The major model used to simulate hypoxic-ischaemic stroke in adult rodents is analogous to the Rice–Vannucci model described above for neonates (Eklöf and Siesjö, 1973; Rice et al., 1981; Bederson et al., 1986). Adult rats injected with neuroserpin before left common carotid artery ligation followed by acute hypoxia showed a decrease in infarct volume compared to controls, in addition to a decrease in expression of apoptosis markers (Yepes et al., 2000). Neuroserpin knockout mice show increased lesion volumes following adult HI (Cinelli et al., 2001; Gelderblom et al., 2013), whereas transgenic mice expressing six-times normal neuroserpin expression demonstrate smaller infarct volumes (Cinelli et al., 2001). Exogenous neuroserpin injection is also protective against NMDA injection in live adult rat (Lebeurrier et al., 2005a). Currently, the only evidence for this has come from adults models of HI stroke, far from conclusive evidence of neonatal protection due to the differences in neuroanatomy and neurochemistry between the developing and adult brain. However, this work remains of utility, as at the very least investigating the neuroserpin-tPA system in neonatal models will add to understanding of the differences between neonatal and adult response to HI.

Neuroserpin administration in rats increases the window for effective tPA treatment in a model of adult stroke (Zhang et al., 2002). Increased tPA expression is found in neuroserpin knockout mice undergoing adult HI injury compared to controls (Cinelli et al., 2001; Gelderblom et al., 2013). However, exogenous neuroserpin is neuroprotective in tPA knockout mice (Wu et al., 2010). Ischaemic-reperfusion-induced injury in the retina of tPA knockout mice demonstrated rescued retinal apoptotic marker expression when injected with neuroserpin (Gu et al., 2015). Therefore, the neuroprotective properties of neuroserpin in adult HI appear to involve both neuroserpin's tPA-dependent and tPA-independent molecular cascades.

A role for neuroserpin in human adult HI stroke has also been described. Correlative studies have shown that high concentrations of neuroserpin in blood samples from human patients are associated with better functional outcome (Rodríguez-González et al., 2011b) and reduced inflammation (Rodríguez-González et al., 2011c). However, attempts to find a relationship between neuroserpin polymorphisms in humans and likelihood of stroke have produced little evidence of protective neuroserpin variants (Cole et al., 2007; Tjärnlund-Wolf et al., 2011). Mutations in the neuroserpin gene have been associated with two rare hereditary disorders (Galliciotti and Sonderegger, 2006); individuals present either with epilepsy (Yepes et al., 2002; Coutelier et al., 2008) or dementia with neuroserpin inclusion bodies (Davis et al., 1999a,b, 2002; Yazaki et al., 2001; Ricagno et al., 2010). It is not currently known whether these disorders are caused by novel functions of the mutated protein or by loss of physiological functions (Lee et al., 2015a).

Neuroserpin in Neonatal Hypoxia-Ischaemia

The evidence above from adult models of HI stroke is far from conclusive evidence of neonatal protection due to differences between the developing and adult brain. However, this work remains of utility, as at the very least investigating neuroserpin in neonatal models will add to understanding of the differences between neonatal and adult response to HI.

Evidence for a role of neuroserpin in neonatal HI is not entirely absent. A patent application published online claims that neuroserpin injection 4 h after neonatal HI in rat pups reduced infarct volume, but had no effect on LPS-sensitized HI (Kuan et al., 2010). However, the small number of published rodent microarrays following neonatal HI have failed to detect significant changes in *Serpini1* expression (Carmel et al., 2004; Hedtjarn et al., 2004a,b; Juul et al., 2009; Nagel et al., 2012; Rognlien et al., 2014). This could be explained by the delay between HI injury and sample collection, 6 h to 7 days post injury in this sample, which may be too early or too late to expect to see genomic changes in *Serpini1* expression. Also, microarray studies cannot reveal whether neonatal HI causes differences in neuroserpin translation or secretion, neither of which have yet been studied in neonatal HI.

Despite the lack of evidence for neuroserpin's direct role in neonatal HI, substantially more has been published documenting effects of its primary molecular target, tPA, in neonatal HI. tPA is broadly considered to be deleterious to cerebral recovery from neonatal HI (Adhami et al., 2008; Omouendze et al., 2013). In P7 rats which underwent unilateral common carotid artery ligation, tPA treatment was found to impair blood flow throughout the brain, an effect which was rescued by injection of the tPA inhibitor α2-antiplasmin (Adhami et al., 2008). Release of tPA by the cerebral microvasculature, as seen following neonatal HI, has also been shown to compromise the glucose content of the extracellular medium in neonatal mouse cortical culture (Henry et al., 2013). Administration of tPA inhibitor Plasminogen-activator-inhibitor 1 (PAI1) reduces locomotor disorder and white matter damage in LPS-sensitized neonatal HI rats (Yang et al., 2013a,b; Yang and Kuan, 2015). This pathway is relatively understudied in neonatal HI research, despite the potential to target a multitude of injury-relevant molecules. Drawing attention to molecules like neuroserpin and tPA, potential common moderators of injury pathways, will be essential to the development of new efficacious pharmacological treatments.

CONCLUSION

Neonatal HI remains the most common cause of infant death and disability globally. Reducing the burden of morbidity should be a high priority for biomedical research. A dearth of treatments are currently available postnatally for these vulnerable infants, restricted to only hypothermia, a breakthrough treatment which is not fully effective in all cases, with no currently licensed additive pharmacological treatments. A complex network of interacting molecular cascades, including excitotoxicity, oxidative stress, and inflammation contribute to the gradually developing pattern of neuronal cell death seen in asphyxiated neonates. Targeting common mediators of these pathways with specific targets linked to far-reaching effects offers a potential approach to generating new pharmacological treatments to exact neuroprotection in these neonatal patients.

AUTHOR CONTRIBUTIONS

All authors listed have made substantial, direct, and intellectual contribution to this work, and approved its final version for publication. LM, LS, AH-S, and ZM: conceived the review focus, conducted literature review, evaluated the literature. LM: reviewed literature, wrote first draft, critically revised the first draft, and finalized the manuscript. LS, AH-S, and ZM: gave feedback, and finalized the manuscript. All authors approved final version of manuscript.

FUNDING

This work was supported by the Department of Physiology, Anatomy and Genetics, University of Oxford, Oxford UK. LM is funded by the Clarendon Fund, Oxford, UK; University College, University of Oxford, UK; and the Department of Physiology, Anatomy and Genetics, University of Oxford, Oxford, UK. ZM is funded by the Department of Physiology, Anatomy and Genetics, University of Oxford, Oxford, UK. LS, AH-S and ZM are funded by the Medical Research Council Grant numbers: G00700311 and G00900901. LS and ZM are funded by The Academy of Medical Sciences Newton Advanced Fellowship in partnership with The Royal Society and The National Natural Science Foundation of China for collaborative projects (UK/China grant numbers: NA160314/8161101585).

ACKNOWLEDGMENTS

We thank Prof. David Edwards, Prof. Pierre Gressens, Dr. Bobbi Fleiss, Dr. Claire Thornton, and Dr. Ana Baburamani for informative discussions on neonatal hypoxia ischaemia and its models.

REFERENCES

Adamsons, K., and Myers, R. E. (1973). Perinatal asphyxia, causes, detection and neurologic sequelae. *Pediatr. Clin. North Am.* 20, 465–480. doi: 10.1016/S0031-3955(16)32855-3

Ådén, U., Halldner, L., Lagercrantz, H., Dalmau, I., Ledent, C., and Fredholm, B. B. (2003). Aggravated brain damage after hypoxic ischemia in immature adenosine A2A knockout mice. *Stroke* 34, 739–744. doi: 10.1161/01.STR.0000060204.67672.8B

Adhami, F., Yu, D., Yin, W., Schloemer, A., Burns, K. A., Liao, G., et al. (2008). Deleterious effects of plasminogen activators in neonatal cerebral hypoxia-ischemia. *Am. J. Pathol.* 172, 1704–1716. doi: 10.2353/ajpath.2008.070979

Agrawal, V., and Hirsch, E. (2012). Intrauterine infection and preterm labor. *Semin. Fetal Neonatal Med.* 17, 12–19. doi: 10.1016/j.siny.2011.09.001

al Naqeeb, N., Edwards, A. D., Cowan, F. M., and Azzopardi, D. (1999). Assessment of neonatal encephalopathy by amplitude-integrated electroencephalography. *Pediatrics* 103, 1263–1271. doi: 10.1542/peds.103.6.1263

Albrecht, J., Hanganu, I. L., Heck, N., and Luhmann, H. J. (2005). Oxygen and glucose deprivation induces major dysfunction in the somatosensory cortex of the newborn rat. *Eur. J. Neurosci.* 22, 2295–2305. doi: 10.1111/j.1460-9568.2005.04398.x

Alexander, M., Garbus, H., Smith, A., Rosenkrantz, T., and Fitch, R. (2014). Behavioral and histological outcomes following neonatal HI injury in a preterm (P3) and term (P7) rodent model. *Behav. Brain Res.* 259, 85–96. doi: 10.1016/j.bbr.2013.10.038

Al-Ghoul, W. M., and Miller, M. W. (1989). Transient expression of Alz-50 immunoreactivity in developing rat neocortex: a marker for naturally occurring neuronal death? *Brain Res.* 481, 361–367. doi: 10.1016/0006-8993(89)90815-9

Allendoerfer, K. L., and Shatz, C. J. (1994). The subplate, a transient neocortical structure: its role in the development of connections between thalamus and cortex. *Annu. Rev. Neurosci.* 17, 185–218. doi: 10.1146/annurev.ne.17.030194.001153

Alsharnoubi, J. M., Odland, H. H., and Saugstad, O. D. (2012). Nicotine does not influence NF-kappaB activity in neonatal mice reoxygenated with room-air or 100% oxygen. *J. Mater. Fetal Neonatal Med.* 25, 2102–2105. doi: 10.3109/14767058.2012.678434

Alvarez-Diaz, A., Hilario, E., de Cerio, F. G., Valls-i-Soler, A., and Alvarez-Diaz, F. J. (2007). Hypoxic-ischemic injury in the immature brain–key vascular and cellular players. *Neonatology* 92, 227–235. doi: 10.1159/000103741

Andine, P., Thordstein, M., Kjellmer, I., Nordborg, C., Thiringer, K., Wennberg, E., et al. (1990). Evaluation of brain damage in a rat model of neonatal hypoxic-ischemia. *J. Neurosci. Methods* 35, 253–260. doi: 10.1016/0165-0270(90)90131-X

Anju, T. R., Abraham, P. M., Antony, S., and Paulose, C. S. (2010a). Alterations in cortical GABAB receptors in neonatal rats exposed to hypoxic stress: role of glucose, oxygen, and epinephrine resuscitation. *Mol. Cell. Biochem.* 343, 1–11. doi: 10.1007/s11010-010-0491-9

Anju, T. R., Ajayan, M. S., and Paulose, C. S. (2013a). Disruption of cerebellar cholinergic system in hypoxic neonatal rats and its regulation with glucose, oxygen and epinephrine resuscitations. *Neuroscience* 236, 253–261. doi: 10.1016/j.neuroscience.2012.12.056

Anju, T. R., Binoy, J., Anitha, M., and Paulose, C. S. (2012a). Striatal GABA receptor alterations in hypoxic neonatal rats: role of glucose, oxygen and epinephrine treatment. *Neurochem. Res.* 37, 629–638. doi: 10.1007/s11064-011-0654-4

Anju, T. R., Jayanarayanan, S., and Paulose, C. S. (2011a). Decreased GABAB receptor function in the cerebellum and brain stem of hypoxic neonatal rats: role of glucose, oxygen and epinephrine resuscitation. *J. Biomed. Sci.* 18:31. doi: 10.1186/1423-0127-18-31

Anju, T. R., Korah, P. K., Jayanarayanan, S., and Paulose, C. S. (2011b). Enhanced brain stem 5HT(2)A receptor function under neonatal hypoxic insult: role of glucose, oxygen, and epinephrine resuscitation. *Mol. Cell. Biochem.* 354, 151–160. doi: 10.1007/s11010-011-0814-5

Anju, T. R., Mathew, J., Jayanarayanan, S., and Paulose, C. S. (2010b). Cerebellar 5HT2A receptor function under hypoxia in neonatal rats: role of glucose, oxygen, and epinephrine resuscitation. *Respir. Physiol. Neurobiol.* 172, 147–153. doi: 10.1016/j.resp.2010.05.009

Anju, T. R., Naijil, G., Shilpa, J., Roshni, T., and Paulose, C. S. (2013b). Neonatal hypoxic insult-mediated cholinergic disturbances in the brain stem: effect of glucose, oxygen and epinephrine resuscitation. *Neurol. Sci.* 34, 287–296. doi: 10.1007/s10072-012-0989-x

Anju, T. R., Nandhu, M. S., Jes, P., and Paulose, C. S. (2011c). Endocrine regulation of neonatal hypoxia: role of glucose, oxygen, and epinephrine supplementation. *Fetal Pediatr. Pathol.* 30, 338–349. doi: 10.3109/15513815.2011.587498

Anju, T. R., Peeyush Kumar, T., and Paulose, C. S. (2010c). Decreased GABAA receptors functional regulation in the cerebral cortex and brainstem of hypoxic neonatal rats: effect of glucose and oxygen supplementation. *Cell Mol. Neurobiol.* 30, 599–606. doi: 10.1007/s10571-009-9485-0

Anju, T. R., Smijin, S., Chinthu, R., and Paulose, C. S. (2012b). Decreased cholinergic function in the cerebral cortex of hypoxic neonatal rats: role of glucose, oxygen and epinephrine resuscitation. *Respir. Physiol. Neurobiol.* 180, 8–13. doi: 10.1016/j.resp.2011.08.013

Anju, T. R., Smijin, S., Korah, P. K., and Paulose, C. S. (2011d). Cortical 5HT 2A receptor function under hypoxia in neonatal rats: role of glucose, oxygen, and epinephrine resuscitation. *J. Mol. Neurosci.* 43, 350–357. doi: 10.1007/s12031-010-9449-3

Anju, T. R., and Paulose, C. S. (2011). Amelioration of hypoxia-induced striatal 5-HT(2A) receptor, 5-HT transporter and HIF1 alterations by glucose, oxygen and epinephrine in neonatal rats. *Neurosci. Lett.* 502, 129–132. doi: 10.1016/j.neulet.2011.05.236

Anju, T. R., and Paulose, C. S. (2013). Striatal cholinergic functional alterations in hypoxic neonatal rats: role of glucose, oxygen, and epinephrine resuscitation. *Biochem. Cell Biol.* 91, 350–356. doi: 10.1139/bcb-2012-0102

Aoki, C., and Siekevitz, P. (1988). Plasticity in brain development. *Sci. Am.* 259, 56–64. doi: 10.1038/scientificamerican1288-56

Applegate, C. D., Jensen, F., Burchfiel, J. L., and Lombroso, C. (1996). The effects of neonatal hypoxia on kindled seizure development and electroconvulsive shock profiles. *Epilepsia* 37, 723–727. doi: 10.1111/j.1528-1157.1996.tb00642.x

Arteni, N. S., Salgueiro, J., Torres, I., Achaval, M., and Netto, C. A. (2003). Neonatal cerebral hypoxia–ischemia causes lateralized memory impairments in the adult rat. *Brain Res.* 973, 171–178. doi: 10.1016/S0006-8993(03)02436-3

Aso, K., Scher, M. S., and Barmada, M. A. (1989). Neonatal electroencephalography and neuropathology. *J. Clin. Neurophysiol.* 6, 103–123. doi: 10.1097/00004691-198904000-00001

Aujla, P. K., Fetell, M. R., and Jensen, F. E. (2009). Talampanel suppresses the acute and chronic effects of seizures in a rodent neonatal seizure model. *Epilepsia* 50, 694–701. doi: 10.1111/j.1528-1167.2008.01947.x

Autheman, D., Sheldon, R. A., Chaudhuri, N., von Arx, S., Siegenthaler, C., Ferriero, D. M., et al. (2012). Glutathione peroxidase overexpression causes aberrant ERK activation in neonatal mouse cortex after hypoxic preconditioning. *Pediatr. Res.* 72, 568–575. doi: 10.1038/pr.2012.124

Azzopardi, D., Robertson, N. J., Bainbridge, A., Cady, E., Charles-Edwards, G., Deierl, A., et al. (2015). Moderate hypothermia within 6 h of birth plus inhaled xenon versus moderate hypothermia alone after birth asphyxia (TOBY-Xe): a proof-of-concept, open-label, randomised controlled trial. *Lancet Neurol.* doi: 10.1016/S1474-4422(15)00347-6 [Epub ahead of print].

Azzopardi, D., Robertson, N. J., Kapetanakis, A., Griffiths, J., Rennie, J. M., Mathieson, S. R., et al. (2013). Anticonvulsant effect of xenon on neonatal asphyxial seizures. *Arch. Dis. Child. Fetal Neonatal Ed.* 98, F437–F439. doi: 10.1136/archdischild-2013-303786

Azzopardi, D. V., Strohm, B., Edwards, A. D., Dyet, L., Halliday, H. L., Juszczak, E., et al. (2009). Moderate hypothermia to treat perinatal asphyxial encephalopathy. *N. Engl. J. Med.* 361, 1349–1358. doi: 10.1056/NEJMoa0900854

Baburamani, A. A., Ek, C. J., Walker, D. W., and Castillo-Melendez, M. (2012). Vulnerability of the developing brain to hypoxic-ischemic damage: contribution of the cerebral vasculature to injury and repair? *Front. Physiol.* 3:424. doi: 10.3389/fphys.2012.00424

Back, S. A., Gan, X., Li, Y., Rosenberg, P. A., and Volpe, J. J. (1998). Maturation-dependent vulnerability of oligodendrocytes to oxidative stress-induced death caused by glutathione depletion. *J. Neurosci.* 18, 6241–6253.

Balduini, W., Carloni, S., and Buonocore, G. (2012). Autophagy in hypoxia-ischemia induced brain injury. *J. Matern. Fetal Neonatal Med.* 25(Suppl. 1), 30–34. doi: 10.3109/14767058.2012.663176

Balduini, W., De Angelis, V., Mazzoni, E., and Cimino, M. (2000). Long-lasting behavioral alterations following a hypoxic/ischemic brain injury in neonatal rats. *Brain Res.* 859, 318–325. doi: 10.1016/S0006-8993(00)01997-1

Balduini, W., De Angelis, V., Mazzoni, E., and Cimino, M. (2001). Simvastatin protects against long-lasting behavioral and morphological consequences of neonatal hypoxic/ischemic brain injury. *Stroke* 32, 2185–2191. doi: 10.1161/hs0901.094287

Barker-Carlson, K., Lawrence, D. A., and Schwartz, B. S. (2002). Acyl-enzyme complexes between tissue-type plasminogen activator and neuroserpin are short-lived in vitro. *J. Biol. Chem.* 277, 46852–46857. doi: 10.1074/jbc.M207740200

Barkovich, A. J., Miller, S. P., Bartha, A., Newton, N., Hamrick, S. E., Mukherjee, P., et al. (2006). MR imaging, MR spectroscopy, and diffusion tensor imaging of sequential studies in neonates with encephalopathy. *AJNR Am. J. Neuroradiolo.* 27, 533–547.

Barkovich, A. J., Westmark, K., Partridge, C., Sola, A., and Ferriero, D. M. (1995). Perinatal asphyxia: MR findings in the first 10 days. *AJNR Am. J. Neuroradiol.* 16, 427–438.

Barth, T. M., and Stanfield, B. B. (1990). The recovery of forelimb-placing behavior in rats with neonatal unilateral cortical damage involves the remaining hemisphere. *J. Neurosci.* 10, 3449–3459.

Baud, O., Daire, J. L., Dalmaz, Y., Fontaine, R. H., Krueger, R. C., Sebag, G., et al. (2004). Gestational hypoxia induces white matter damage in neonatal rats: a new model of periventricular leukomalacia. *Brain Pathol.* 14, 1–10. doi: 10.1111/j.1750-3639.2004.tb00492.x

Bauer, H. C., Bauer, H., Lametschwandtner, A., Amberger, A., Ruiz, P., and Steiner, M. (1993). Neovascularization and the appearance of morphological characteristics of the blood-brain barrier in the embryonic mouse central nervous system. *Brain Res. Dev. Brain Res.* 75, 269–278. doi: 10.1016/0165-3806(93)90031-5

Bederson, J. B., Pitts, L. H., Tsuji, M., Nishimura, M. C., Davis, R. L., and Bartkowski, H. (1986). Rat middle cerebral artery occlusion: evaluation of the model and development of a neurologic examination. *Stroke* 17, 472–476. doi: 10.1161/01.STR.17.3.472

Belgard, T. G., Marques, A. C., Oliver, P. L., Abaan, H. O., Sirey, T. M., Hoerder-Suabedissen, A., et al. (2011). A transcriptomic atlas of mouse neocortical layers. *Neuron* 71, 605–616. doi: 10.1016/j.neuron.2011.06.039

Bell, M. J., and Hallenbeck, J. M. (2002). Effects of intrauterine inflammation on developing rat brain. *J. Neurosci. Res.* 70, 570–579. doi: 10.1002/jnr.10423

Benarroch, E. E. (2007). Tissue plasminogen activator: beyond thrombolysis. *Neurology* 69, 799–802. doi: 10.1212/01.wnl.0000269668.08747.78

Benchenane, K., López-Atalaya, J. P., Fernández-Monreal, M., Touzani, O., and Vivien, D. (2004). Equivocal roles of tissue-type plasminogen activator in stroke-induced injury. *Trends Neurosci.* 27, 155–160. doi: 10.1016/j.tins.2003.12.011

Bennet, L., Peebles, D. M., Edwards, A. D., Rios, A., and Hanson, M. A. (1998). The cerebral hemodynamic response to asphyxia and hypoxia in the near-term fetal sheep as measured by near infrared spectroscopy. *Pediatr. Res.* 44, 951–957. doi: 10.1203/00006450-199812000-00022

Berger, P., Kozlov, S. V., Cinelli, P., Krüger, S. R., Vogt, L., and Sonderegger, P. (1999). Neuronal depolarization enhances the transcription of the neuronal serine protease inhibitor neuroserpin. *Mol. Cell. Neurosci.* 14, 455–467. doi: 10.1006/mcne.1999.0804

Bergeron, J. D., Deslauriers, J., Grignon, S., Fortier, L. C., Lepage, M., Stroh, T., et al. (2013). White matter injury and autistic-like behavior predominantly affecting male rat offspring exposed to group B streptococcal maternal inflammation. *Dev. Neurosci.* 35, 504–515. doi: 10.1159/000355656

Bernard, S. A., Gray, T. W., Buist, M. D., Jones, B. M., Silvester, W., Gutteridge, G., et al. (2002). Treatment of comatose survivors of out-of-hospital cardiac arrest with induced hypothermia. *N. Engl. J. Med.* 346, 557–563. doi: 10.1056/NEJMoa003289

Biagioni, E., Mercuri, E., Rutherford, M., Cowan, F., Azzopardi, D., Frisone, M. F., et al. (2001). Combined use of electroencephalogram and magnetic resonance imaging in full-term neonates with acute encephalopathy. *Pediatrics* 107, 461–468. doi: 10.1542/peds.107.3.461

Billiards, S. S., Haynes, R. L., Folkerth, R. D., Borenstein, N. S., Trachtenberg, F. L., Rowitch, D. H., et al. (2008). Myelin abnormalities without oligodendrocyte loss in periventricular leukomalacia. *Brain Pathol.* 18, 153–163. doi: 10.1111/j.1750-3639.2007.00107.x

Blaise, S. A., Nedelec, E., Alberto, J. M., Schroeder, H., Audonnet, S., Bossenmeyer-Pourie, C., et al. (2009). Short hypoxia could attenuate the adverse effects of hyperhomocysteinemia on the developing rat brain by inducing neurogenesis. *Exp. Neurol.* 216, 231–238. doi: 10.1016/j.expneurol.2008.11.020

Blomgren, K., and Hagberg, H. (2006). Free radicals, mitochondria, and hypoxia-ischemia in the developing brain. *Free Radic. Biol. Med.* 40, 388–397. doi: 10.1016/j.freeradbiomed.2005.08.040

Bloom, W. (1968). *DW Fawcett A Textbook of Histology*. Amsterdam: Saunders, 582.

Boksa, P., Zhang, Y., and Nouel, D. (2015). Maternal oxytocin administration before birth influences the effects of birth anoxia on the neonatal rat brain. *Neurochem. Res.* 40, 1631–1643. doi: 10.1007/s11064-015-1645-7

Bona, E., Hagberg, H., Løberg, E. M., Bågenholm, R., and Thoresen, M. (1998). Protective effects of moderate hypothermia after neonatal hypoxia-ischemia: short-and long-term outcome. *Pediatr. Res.* 43, 738–745. doi: 10.1203/00006450-199806000-00005

Bonifacio, S. L., Glass, H. C., Peloquin, S., and Ferriero, D. M. (2011). A new neurological focus in neonatal intensive care. *Nat. Rev. Neurol.* 7, 485–494. doi: 10.1038/nrneurol.2011.119

Borges, V. M., Lee, T. W., Christie, D. L., and Birch, N. P. (2010). Neuroserpin regulates the density of dendritic protrusions and dendritic spine shape in cultured hippocampal neurons. *J. Neurosci. Res.* 88, 2610–2617. doi: 10.1002/jnr.22428

Boss, V., Sola, A., Wen, T. C., and Decker, M. J. (2005). Mild intermittent hypoxia does not induce stress responses in the neonatal rat brain. *Biol. Neonate* 88, 313–320. doi: 10.1159/000087629

Boylan, G. B., Young, K., Panerai, R. B., Rennie, J. M., and Evans, D. H. (2000). Dynamic cerebral autoregulation in sick newborn infants. *Pediatr. Res.* 48, 12–17. doi: 10.1203/00006450-200007000-00005

Brackmann, F. A., Link, A. S., Jung, S., Richter, M., Zoglauer, D., Walkinshaw, G., et al. (2013). Activin A regulation under global hypoxia in developing mouse brain. *Brain Res.* 1531, 65–74. doi: 10.1016/j.brainres.2013.07.039

Brehmer, F., Bendix, I., Prager, S., van de Looij, Y., Reinboth, B. S., Zimmermanns, J., et al. (2012). Interaction of inflammation and hyperoxia in a rat model of neonatal white matter damage. *PLoS ONE* 7:e49023. doi: 10.1371/journal.pone.0049023

Brigstock, D. R. (1999). The Connective Tissue Growth Factor/Cysteine-Rich 61/Nephroblastoma Overexpressed (CCN) Family 1. *Endocr. Rev.* 20, 189–206. doi: 10.1210/er.20.2.189

Brochu, M. E., Girard, S., Lavoie, K., and Sebire, G. (2011). Developmental regulation of the neuroinflammatory responses to LPS and/or hypoxia-ischemia between preterm and term neonates: an experimental study. *J. Neuroinflamm.* 20, 55. doi: 10.1186/1742-2094-8-55

Brongholi, K., Souza, D. G., Bainy, A. C., Dafre, A. L., and Tasca, C. I. (2006). Oxygen-glucose deprivation decreases glutathione levels and glutamate uptake in rat hippocampal slices. *Brain Res.* 1083, 211–218. doi: 10.1016/j.brainres.2006.02.003

Brooks, K. J., Clark, J. B., and Bates, T. E. (1996). Assessment of energy metabolism in the developing brain following aglycemic hypoxia by1H and31P NMR. *Neurochem. Res.* 21, 1089–1095. doi: 10.1007/BF02532419

Brunjes, P. C. (1985). A stereological study of neocortical maturation in the precocial mouse, *Acomys cahirinus*. *Brain Res.* 351, 279–287. doi: 10.1016/0165-3806(85)90199-3

Brunjes, P. C. (1989). A comparative study of prenatal development in the olfactory bulb, neocortex and hippocampal region of the precocial mouse *Acomys cahirinus* and rat. *Brain Res. Dev. Brain Res.* 49, 7–25. doi: 10.1016/0165-3806(89)90055-2

Brunjes, P. C. (1990). The precocial mouse, *Acomys cahirinus*. *Psychobiology* 18, 339–350.

Brunjes, P. C., Korol, D. L., and Stern, K. G. (1989). Prenatal neurogenesis in the telencephalon of the precocial mouse *Acomys cahirinus*. *Neurosci. Lett.* 107, 114–119. doi: 10.1016/0304-3940(89)90801-x

Budday, S., Raybaud, C., and Kuhl, E. (2014). A mechanical model predicts morphological abnormalities in the developing human brain. *Sci. Rep.* 4:5644. doi: 10.1038/srep05644

Burd, I., Welling, J., Kannan, G., and Johnston, M. V. (2016). Chapter five-excitotoxicity as a common mechanism for fetal neuronal injury with hypoxia and intrauterine inflammation. *Adv. Pharmacol.* 76, 85–101. doi: 10.1016/bs.apha.2016.02.003

Bustamante, D., Morales, P., Pereyra, J. T., Goiny, M., and Herrera-Marschitz, M. (2007). Nicotinamide prevents the effect of perinatal asphyxia on dopamine release evaluated with in vivo microdialysis 3 months after birth. *Exp. Brain Res.* 177, 358–369. doi: 10.1007/s00221-006-0679-0

Buwalda, B., Nyakas, C., Vosselman, H. J., and Luiten, P. G. (1995). Effects of early postnatal anoxia on adult learning and emotion in rats. *Behav. Brain Res.* 67, 85–90. doi: 10.1016/0166-4328(94)00108-R

Cai, J., Kang, Z., Liu, K., Liu, W., Li, R., Zhang, J. H., et al. (2009). Neuroprotective effects of hydrogen saline in neonatal hypoxia–ischemia rat model. *Brain Res.* 1256, 129–137. doi: 10.1016/j.brainres.2008.11.048

Cai, Z., Pang, Y., Xiao, F., and Rhodes, P. G. (2001). Chronic ischemia preferentially causes white matter injury in the neonatal rat brain. *Brain Res.* 898, 126–135. doi: 10.1016/S0006-8993(01)02180-1

Caputa, M., Rogalska, J., Wentowska, K., and Nowakowska, A. (2005). Perinatal asphyxia, hyperthermia and hyperferremia as factors inducing behavioural disturbances in adulthood: a rat model. *Behav. Brain Res.* 163, 246–256. doi: 10.1016/j.bbr.2005.05.015

Carloni, S., Buonocore, G., and Balduini, W. (2008). Protective role of autophagy in neonatal hypoxia-ischemia induced brain injury. *Neurobiol. Dis.* 32, 329–339. doi: 10.1016/j.nbd.2008.07.022

Carloni, S., Carnevali, A., Cimino, M., and Balduini, W. (2007). Extended role of necrotic cell death after hypoxia-ischemia-induced neurodegeneration in the neonatal rat. *Neurobiol. Dis.* 27, 354–361. doi: 10.1016/j.nbd.2007.06.009

Carlos, R., Seidler, F. J., Lappi, S., and Slotkin, T. A. (1991a). Fetal dexamethasone exposure affects basal ornithine decarboxylase activity in developing rat brain regions and alters acute responses to hypoxia and maternal separation. *Neonatology* 59, 69–77.

Carlos, R., Seidler, F. J., and Slotkin, T. A. (1991b). Fetal dexamethasone exposure sensitizes neonatal rat brain to hypoxia: effects on protein and DNA synthesis. *Dev. Brain Res.* 64, 161–166.

Carmel, J. B., Kakinohana, O., Mestril, R., Young, W., Marsala, M., and Hart, R. P. (2004). Mediators of ischemic preconditioning identified by microarray analysis of rat spinal cord. *Exp. Neurol.* 185, 81–96. doi: 10.1016/j.expneurol.2003.09.007

Carmeliet, P., and Storkebaum, E. (2002). Vascular and neuronal effects of VEGF in the nervous system: implications for neurological disorders. *Semin. Cell Dev. Biol.* 13, 39–53. doi: 10.1006/scdb.2001.0290

Casolini, P., Zuena, A. R., Cinque, C., Matteucci, P., Alema, G. S., Adriani, W., et al. (2005). Sub-neurotoxic neonatal anoxia induces subtle behavioural changes and specific abnormalities in brain group-I metabotropic glutamate receptors in rats. *J. Neurochem.* 95, 137–145. doi: 10.1111/j.1471-4159.2005.03349.x

Chamorro, A., Dirnagl, U., Urra, X., and Planas, A. M. (2016). Neuroprotection in acute stroke: targeting excitotoxicity, oxidative and nitrosative stress, and inflammation. *Lancet Neurol.* 15, 869–881. doi: 10.1016/S1474-4422(16)00114-9

Chang, W. W., Chang, N., Lin, S., Wu, C., and Wu, F. Y. (2000). Tissue-specific cancer-related serpin gene cluster at human chromosome band 3q26. *Genes Chromosomes Cancer* 29, 240–255. doi: 10.1002/1098-2264(2000)9999:9999<::AID-GCC1029>3.0.CO;2-A

Chau, V., Clément, J., Robitaille, Y., D'Anjou, G., and Vanasse, M. (2008). Congenital axonal neuropathy and encephalopathy. *Pediatr. Neurol.* 38, 261–266. doi: 10.1016/j.pediatrneurol.2007.11.005

Chau, V., Poskitt, K. J., and Miller, S. P. (2012). Magnetic resonance imaging in hypoxic-ischemic encephalopathy: still a cool test. *Arch. Pediatr. Adolesc. Med.* 166, 669–671. doi: 10.1001/archpediatrics.2012.579

Chau, V., Poskitt, K. J., Sargent, M. A., Lupton, B. A., Hill, A., Roland, E., et al. (2009). Comparison of computer tomography and magnetic resonance imaging scans on the third day of life in term newborns with neonatal encephalopathy. *Pediatrics* 123, 319–326. doi: 10.1542/peds.2008-0283

Chau, V., Synnes, A., Grunau, R. E., Poskitt, K. J., Brant, R., and Miller, S. P. (2013). Abnormal brain maturation in preterm neonates associated with adverse developmental outcomes. *Neurology* 81, 2082–2089. doi: 10.1212/01.wnl.0000437298.43688.b9

Chaudhari, P., Ye, Z., and Jang, Y. Y. (2014). Roles of reactive oxygen species in the fate of stem cells. *Antioxid. Redox Signal.* 20, 1881–1890. doi: 10.1089/ars.2012.4963

Chavez-Valdez, R., Martin, L. J., Razdan, S., Gauda, E. B., and Northington, F. J. (2014). Sexual dimorphism in BDNF signaling after neonatal hypoxia-ischemia and treatment with necrostatin-1. *Neuroscience* 260, 106–119. doi: 10.1016/j.neuroscience.2013.12.023

Chen, C. J., and Liao, S. L. (2003). Zinc toxicity on neonatal cortical neurons: involvement of glutathione chelation. *J. Neurochem.* 85, 443–453. doi: 10.1046/j.1471-4159.2003.01691.x

Chen, H., Spagnoli, F., Burris, M., Rolland, W. B., Fajilan, A., Dou, H., et al. (2012). Nanoerythropoietin is 10-times more effective than regular erythropoietin in neuroprotection in a neonatal rat model of hypoxia and ischemia. *Stroke* 43, 884–887. doi: 10.1161/STROKEAHA.111.637090

Cheng, Y., Deshmukh, M., D'Costa, A., Demaro, J. A., Gidday, J. M., Shah, A., et al. (1998). Caspase inhibitor affords neuroprotection with delayed administration in a rat model of neonatal hypoxic-ischemic brain injury. *J. Clin. Invest.* 101, 1992–1999. doi: 10.1172/JCI2169

Chiappe-Gutierrez, M., Kitzmueller, E., Labudova, O., Fuerst, G., Hoeger, H., Hardmeier, R., et al. (1998). mRNA levels of the hypoxia inducible factor (HIF-1) and DNA repair genes in perinatal asphyxia of the rat. *Life Sci.* 63, 1157–1167. doi: 10.1016/S0024-3205(98)00377-4

Choi, D. W. (1988). Calcium-mediated neurotoxicity: relationship to specific channel types and role in ischemic damage. *Trends Neurosci.* 11, 465–469. doi: 10.1016/0166-2236(88)90200-7

Choi, D. W. (1992). Excitotoxic cell death. *J. Neurobiol.* 23, 1261–1276. doi: 10.1002/neu.480230915

Choi, H. A., Badjatia, N., and Mayer, S. A. (2012). Hypothermia for acute brain injury—mechanisms and practical aspects. *Nat. Rev. Neurol.* 8, 214–222. doi: 10.1038/nrneurol.2012.21

Christaki, E., and Giamarellos-Bourboulis, E. J. (2014). The beginning of personalized medicine in sepsis: small steps to a bright future. *Clin. Genet.* 86, 56–61. doi: 10.1111/cge.12368

Chun, J. J., Nakamura, M. J., and Shatz, C. J. (1987). Transient cells of the developing mammalian telencephalon are peptide-immunoreactive neurons. *Nature* 325, 617–620. doi: 10.1038/325617a0

Cinelli, P., Madani, R., Tsuzuki, N., Vallet, P., Arras, M., Zhao, C. N., et al. (2001). Neuroserpin, a neuroprotective factor in focal ischemic stroke. *Mol. Cell. Neurosci.* 18, 443–457. doi: 10.1006/mcne.2001.1028

Clancy, B., Finlay, B. L., Darlington, R. B., and Anand, K. J. (2007). Extrapolating brain development from experimental species to humans. *Neurotoxicology* 28, 931–937. doi: 10.1016/j.neuro.2007.01.014

Clancy, B., Teague-Ross, T. J., and Nagarajan, R. (2009). Cross-species analyses of the cortical GABAergic and subplate neural populations. *Front. Neuroanat.* 3:20. doi: 10.3389/neuro.05.020.2009

Cleary, R. T., Sun, H., Huynh, T., Manning, S. M., Li, Y., Rotenberg, A., et al. (2013). Bumetanide enhances phenobarbital efficacy in a rat model of hypoxic neonatal seizures. *PLoS ONE* 8:e57148. doi: 10.1371/journal.pone.0057148

Cohen, M. C., and Scheimberg, I. (2008). Evidence of occurrence of intradural and subdural hemorrhage in the perinatal and neonatal period in the context of hypoxic ischemic encephalopathy: an observational study from two referral institutions in the United Kingdom. *Pediatr. Dev. Pathol.* 12, 169–176. doi: 10.2350/08-08-0509.1

Cole, J. W., Naj, A. C., O'Connell, J. R., Stine, O. C., Sorkin, J. D., Wozniak, M. A., et al. (2007). Neuroserpin polymorphisms and stroke risk in a biracial population: the stroke prevention in young women study. *BMC Neurol.* 7:1. doi: 10.1186/1471-2377-7-37

Coq, J. O., Strata, F., Russier, M., Safadi, F. F., Merzenich, M. M., Byl, N. N., et al. (2008). Impact of neonatal asphyxia and hind limb immobilization on musculoskeletal tissues and S1 map organization: implications for cerebral palsy. *Exp. Neurol.* 210, 95–108. doi: 10.1016/j.expneurol.2007.10.006

Coutelier, M., Andries, S., Ghariani, S., Dan, B., Duyckaerts, C., van Rijckevorsel, K., et al. (2008). Neuroserpin mutation causes electrical status epilepticus of slow-wave sleep. *Neurology* 71, 64–66. doi: 10.1212/01.wnl.0000316306.08751.28

Cowan, F., Rutherford, M., Groenendaal, F., Eken, P., Mercuri, E., Bydder, G. M., et al. (2003). Origin and timing of brain lesions in term infants with neonatal encephalopathy. *Lancet* 361, 736–742. doi: 10.1016/S0140-6736(03)12658-X

Craig, A., Ling Luo, N., Beardsley, D. J., Wingate-Pearse, N., Walker, D. W., Hohimer, A. R., et al. (2003). Quantitative analysis of perinatal rodent oligodendrocyte lineage progression and its correlation with human. *Exp. Neurol.* 181, 231-240. doi: 10.1016/S0014-4886(03)00032-3

Crawford, M. A., and Sinclair, A. J. (1971). "Nutritional influences in the evolution of mammalian brain," in *Proceedings of the Lipids, Malnutrition & the Developing Brain. Ciba Foundation Symposium*, Amsterdam, 267–292.

Daadi, M. M., Lee, S. H., Arac, A., Grueter, B. A., Bhatnagar, R., Maag, A. L., et al. (2009a). Functional engraftment of the medial ganglionic eminence cells in experimental stroke model. *Cell Transplant.* 18, 815–826. doi: 10.3727/096368909X470829

Daadi, M. M., Li, Z., Arac, A., Grueter, B. A., Sofilos, M., Malenka, R. C., et al. (2009b). Molecular and magnetic resonance imaging of human embryonic stem cell-derived neural stem cell grafts in ischemic rat brain. *Mol. Ther.* 17, 1282–1291. doi: 10.1038/mt.2009.104

Dalitz, P., Harding, R., Rees, S. M., and Cock, M. L. (2003). Prolonged reductions in placental blood flow and cerebral oxygen delivery in preterm fetal sheep exposed to endotoxin: possible factors in white matter injury after acute infection. *J. Soc. Gynecol. Investig.* 10, 283–290. doi: 10.1016/S1071-5576(03)00090-X

Dammann, O., and Leviton, A. (2014). Intermittent or sustained systemic inflammation and the preterm brain. *Pediatr. Res.* 75, 376–380. doi: 10.1038/pr.2013.238

Dammann, O., and O'Shea, T. M. (2008). Cytokines and perinatal brain damage. *Clin. Perinatol.* 35, 643–663. doi: 10.1016/j.clp.2008.07.011

Danbolt, N. C. (2001). Glutamate uptake. *Prog. Neurobiol.* 65, 1–105. doi: 10.1016/S0301-0082(00)00067-8

Daneman, A., Epelman, M., Blaser, S., and Jarrin, J. R. (2006). Imaging of the brain in full-term neonates: does sonography still play a role? *Pediatr. Radiol.* 36, 636–646. doi: 10.1007/s00247-006-0201-7

Daneman, A., Navarro, O. M., Somers, G. R., Mohanta, A., Jarrín, J. R., and Traubici, J. (2010). Renal pyramids: focused sonography of normal and pathologic processes 1. *Radiographics* 30, 1287–1307. doi: 10.1148/rg.305095222

Danysz, W., and Parsons, C. G. (1998). Glycine and N-methyl-D-aspartate receptors: physiological significance and possible therapeutic applications. *Pharmacol. Rev.* 50, 597–664.

Daval, J. L., Pourie, G., Grojean, S., Lievre, V., Strazielle, C., Blaise, S., et al. (2004). Neonatal hypoxia triggers transient apoptosis followed by neurogenesis in the rat CA1 hippocampus. *Pediatr. Res.* 55, 561–567. doi: 10.1203/01.PDR.0000113771.51317.37

Daval, J. L., and Vert, P. (2004). Apoptosis and neurogenesis after transient hypoxia in the developing rat brain. *Semin. Perinatol.* 28, 257–263. doi: 10.1053/j.semperi.2004.08.002

Davis, R. L., Holohan, P. D., Shrimpton, A. E., Tatum, A. H., Daucher, J., Collins, G. H., et al. (1999a). Familial encephalopathy with neuroserpin inclusion bodies. *Am. J. Pathol.* 155, 1901–1913. doi: 10.1016/S0002-9440(10)65510-1

Davis, R. L., Shrimpton, A. E., Holohan, P. D., Bradshaw, C., Feiglin, D., Collins, G. H., et al. (1999b). Familial dementia caused by polymerization of mutant neuroserpin. *Nature* 401, 376–379.

Davis, R. L., Shrimpton, A. E., Carrell, R. W., Lomas, D. A., Gerhard, L., Baumann, B., et al. (2002). Association between conformational mutations in neuroserpin and onset and severity of dementia. *Lancet* 359, 2242–2247. doi: 10.1016/S0140-6736(02)09293-0

de Haan, H. H., Gunn, A. J., and Gluckman, P. D. (1997a). Fetal heart rate changes do not reflect cardiovascular deterioration during brief repeated umbilical cord occlusions in near-term fetal lambs. *Am. J. Obstet. Gynecol.* 176(1 Pt 1), 8–17. doi: 10.1016/S0002-9378(97)80004-X

de Haan, H. H., Gunn, A. J., Williams, C. E., and Gluckman, P. D. (1997b). Brief repeated umbilical cord occlusions cause sustained cytotoxic cerebral edema and focal infarcts in near-term fetal lambs. *Pediatr. Res.* 41, 96–104.

de Haan, H. H., Gunn, A. J., Williams, C. E., Heymann, M. A., and Gluckman, P. D. (1997c). Magnesium sulfate therapy during asphyxia in near-term fetal lambs does not compromise the fetus but does not reduce cerebral injury. *Am. J. Obstet. Gynecol.* 176(1 Pt 1), 18–27.

De Souza, S. W., and Richards, B. (1978). Neurological sequelae in newborn babies after perinatal asphyxia. *Arch. Dis. Child.* 53, 564–569. doi: 10.1136/adc.53.7.564

de Torres, C., Munell, F., Ferrer, I., Reventós, J., and Macaya, A. (1997). Identification of necrotic cell death by the TUNEL assay in the hypoxic-ischemic neonatal rat brain. *Neurosci. Lett.* 230, 1–4. doi: 10.1016/S0304-3940(97)00445-X

de Vries, L. S., and Groenendaal, F. (2010). Patterns of neonatal hypoxic-ischaemic brain injury. *Neuroradiology* 52, 555–566. doi: 10.1007/s00234-010-0674-9

Dean, J. M., Shi, Z., Fleiss, B., Gunn, K. C., Groenendaal, F., van Bel, F., et al. (2015). A critical review of models of perinatal infection. *Dev. Neurosci.* 37, 289–304. doi: 10.1159/000370309

Dean, J. M., van de Looij, Y., Sizonenko, S. V., Lodygensky, G. A., Lazeyras, F., Bolouri, H., et al. (2011). Delayed cortical impairment following lipopolysaccharide exposure in preterm fetal sheep. *Ann. Neurol.* 70, 846–856. doi: 10.1002/ana.22480

Debillon, T., Gras-Leguen, C., Leroy, S., Caillon, J., Roze, J. C., and Gressens, P. (2003). Patterns of cerebral inflammatory response in a rabbit model of intrauterine infection-mediated brain lesion. *Brain Res. Dev. Brain Res.* 145, 39–48. doi: 10.1016/S0165-3806(03)00193-7

Decker, M. B., Breitburg, D. L., and Marcus, N. H. (2003). Geographical differences in behavioral responses to hypoxia: local adaptation to an anthropogenic stressor? *Ecol. Appl.* 13, 1104–1109. doi: 10.1890/1051-0761(2003)13[1104:gdibrt]2.0.co;2

Decker, M. J., Hue, G., Caudle, W., Miller, G., Keating, G., and Rye, D. (2003). Episodic neonatal hypoxia evokes executive dysfunction and regionally specific alterations in markers of dopamine signaling. *Neuroscience* 117, 417–425. doi: 10.1016/S0306-4522(02)00805-9

Decker, M. J., Jones, K. A., Solomon, I. G., Keating, G. L., and Rye, D. B. (2005). Reduced extracellular dopamine and increased responsiveness to novelty: neurochemical and behavioral sequelae of intermittent hypoxia. *Sleep* 28, 169–176.

Dell'Anna, E., Geloso, M. C., Magarelli, M., and Molinari, M. (1996). Development of GABA and calcium binding proteins immunoreactivity in the rat hippocampus following neonatal anoxia. *Neurosci. Lett.* 211, 93–96. doi: 10.1016/0304-3940(96)12733-6

Dell'Anna, M., Calzolari, S., Molinari, M., Iuvone, L., and Calimici, R. (1991). Neonatal anoxia induces transitory hyperactivity, permanent spatial memory deficits and CA1 cell density reduction in developing rats. *Behav. Brain Res.* 45, 125–134. doi: 10.1016/S0166-4328(05)80078-6

Dell'Anna, M. E., Geloso, M. C., Draisci, G., and Luthman, J. (1995). Transient changes in Fos and GFAP immunoreactivity precede neuronal loss in the rat hippocampus following neonatal anoxia. *Exp. Neurol.* 131, 144–156. doi: 10.1016/0014-4886(95)90016-0

Dell'Anna, M. E., Luthman, J., Lindqvist, E., and Olson, L. (1993). Development of monoamine systems after neonatal anoxia in rats. *Brain Res. Bull.* 32, 159–170. doi: 10.1016/0361-9230(93)90070-R

Demarest, T. G., Schuh, R. A., Waite, E. L., Waddell, J., McKenna, M. C., and Fiskum, G. (2016a). Sex dependent alterations in mitochondrial eectron transport chain proteins following neonatal rat cerebral hypoxic-ischemia. *J. Bioenerg. Biomembr.* 48, 591–598. doi: 10.1007/s10863-016-9678-4

Demarest, T. G., Waite, E. L., Kristian, T., Puche, A. C., Waddell, J., McKenna, M. C., et al. (2016b). Sex-dependent mitophagy and neuronal death following rat neonatal hypoxia-ischemia. *Neuroscience* 335, 103–113. doi: 10.1016/j.neuroscience.2016.08.026

Deng, W., Rosenberg, P. A., Volpe, J. J., and Jensen, F. E. (2003). Calcium-permeable AMPA/kainate receptors mediate toxicity and preconditioning by oxygen-glucose deprivation in oligodendrocyte precursors. *Proc. Natl. Acad. Sci. U.S.A.* 100, 6801–6806. doi: 10.1073/pnas.1136624100

Deng, Y. Y., Lu, J., Ling, E. A., and Kaur, C. (2009). Monocyte chemoattractant protein-1 (MCP-1) produced via NF-kappaB signaling pathway mediates migration of amoeboid microglia in the periventricular white matter in hypoxic neonatal rats. *Glia* 57, 604–621. doi: 10.1002/glia.20790

Derrick, M., Drobyshevsky, A., Ji, X., and Tan, S. (2007). A model of cerebral palsy from fetal hypoxia-ischemia. *Stroke* 38(Suppl.), 731–735. doi: 10.1161/01.STR.0000251445.94697.64

Derrick, M., Luo, N. L., Bregman, J. C., Jilling, T., Ji, X., Fisher, K., et al. (2004). Preterm fetal hypoxia-ischemia causes hypertonia and motor deficits in the neonatal rabbit: a model for human cerebral palsy? *J. Neurosci.* 24, 24–34. doi: 10.1523/JNEUROSCI.2816-03.2004

Dilenge, M. E., Majnemer, A., and Shevell, M. I. (2001). Long-term developmental outcome of asphyxiated term neonates. *J. Child Neurol.* 16, 781–792. doi: 10.1177/088307380101600110201

Dingley, J., Tooley, J., Liu, X., Scull-Brown, E., Elstad, M., Chakkarapani, E., et al. (2014). Xenon ventilation during therapeutic hypothermia in neonatal encephalopathy: a feasibility study. *Pediatrics* 133, 809–818. doi: 10.1542/peds.2013-0787

Ditelberg, J. S., Sheldon, R. A., Epstein, C. J., and Ferriero, D. M. (1996). Brain injury after perinatal hypoxia-ischemia is exacerbated in copper/zinc superoxide dismutase transgenic mice. *Pediatr. Res.* 39, 204–208. doi: 10.1203/00006450-199602000-00003

Dommergues, M., Plaisant, F., Verney, C., and Gressens, P. (2003). Early microglial activation following neonatal excitotoxic brain damage in mice: a potential target for neuroprotection. *Neuroscience* 121, 619–628. doi: 10.1016/S0306-4522(03)00558-X

Dommergues, M. A., Patkai, J., Renauld, J. C., Evrard, P., and Gressens, P. (2000). Proinflammatory cytokines and interleukin-9 exacerbate excitotoxic lesions of the newborn murine neopallium. *Ann. Neurol.* 47, 54–63. doi: 10.1002/1531-8249(200001)47:1<54::AID-ANA10>3.0.CO;2-Y

Douglas-Escobar, M., and Weiss, M. D. (2015). Hypoxic-ischemic encephalopathy: a review for the clinician. *JAMA Pediatr.* 169, 397–403. doi: 10.1001/jamapediatrics.2014.3269

Doyle, O., Temko, A., Murray, D., Lightbody, G., Marnane, W., and Boylan, G. (2010). "Predicting the neurodevelopmental outcome in newborns with hypoxic-ischaemic injury," in *Proceedings of the Engineering in Medicine and Biology Society (EMBC), 2010 Annual International Conference of the IEEE*, Buenos Aires, 1370–1373. doi: 10.1109/IEMBS.2010.5626736

Drobyshevsky, A., Derrick, M., Prasad, P. V., Ji, X., Englof, I., and Tan, S. (2007a). Fetal brain magnetic resonance imaging response acutely to hypoxia-ischemia predicts postnatal outcome. *Ann. Neurol.* 61, 307–314.

Drobyshevsky, A., Derrick, M., Wyrwicz, A. M., Ji, X., Englof, I., Ullman, L. M., et al. (2007b). White matter injury correlates with hypertonia in an animal model of cerebral palsy. *J. Cereb. Blood Flow Metab.* 27, 270–281.

Drobyshevsky, A., Song, S. K., Gamkrelidze, G., Wyrwicz, A. M., Derrick, M., Meng, F., et al. (2005). Developmental changes in diffusion anisotropy coincide with immature oligodendrocyte progression and maturation of compound action potential. *J. Neurosci.* 25, 5988–5997. doi: 10.1523/JNEUROSCI.4983-04.2005

Du, L., Hickey, R. W., Bayir, H., Watkins, S. C., Tyurin, V. A., Guo, F., et al. (2009). Starving neurons show sex difference in autophagy. *J. Biol. Chem.* 284, 2383–2396. doi: 10.1074/jbc.M804396200

D'Udine, B., and Alleva, E. (1988). The *Acomys cahirinus* (spiny mouse) as a new model for biological and neurobehavioural studies. *Pol. J. Pharmacol. Pharm.* 40, 525–534.

Duncan, J. R., Cock, M. L., Scheerlinck, J. P., Westcott, K. T., McLean, C., Harding, R., et al. (2002). White matter injury after repeated endotoxin exposure in the preterm ovine fetus. *Pediatr. Res.* 52, 941–949. doi: 10.1203/00006450-200212000-00021

East, C. E., Dunster, K. R., and Colditz, P. B. (1998). Fetal oxygen saturation and uterine contractions during labor. *Am. J. Perinatol.* 15, 345–349. doi: 10.1055/s-2007-993955

Edwards, A., and Mehmet, H. (1996). Apoptosis in perinatal hypoxic-ischaemic cerebral damage. *Neuropathol. Appl. Neurobiol.* 22, 494–498. doi: 10.1111/j.1365-2990.1996.tb01122.x

Edwards, A., Yue, X., Cox, P., Hope, P., Azzopardi, D., Squier, M., et al. (1997). Apoptosis in the brains of infants suffering intrauterine cerebral injury. *Pediatr. Res.* 42, 684–689. doi: 10.1203/00006450-199711000-00022

Eicher, D. J., Wagner, C. L., Katikaneni, L. P., Hulsey, T. C., Bass, W. T., Kaufman, D. A., et al. (2005). Moderate hypothermia in neonatal encephalopathy: efficacy outcomes. *Pediatr. Neurol.* 32, 11–17. doi: 10.1016/j.pediatrneurol.2004.06.014

Ek, C. J., Dziegielewska, K. M., Stolp, H., and Saunders, N. R. (2006). Functional effectiveness of the blood-brain barrier to small water-soluble molecules in developing and adult opossum (*Monodelphis domestica*). *J. Comp. Neurol.* 496, 13–26. doi: 10.1002/cne.20885

Ek, C. J., Habgood, M. D., Dziegielewska, K. M., and Saunders, N. R. (2003). Structural characteristics and barrier properties of the choroid plexuses in developing brain of the opossum (*Monodelphis domestica*). *J. Comp. Neurol.* 460, 451–464. doi: 10.1002/cne.10661

Eken, P., Jansen, G. H., Groenendaal, F., Rademaker, K. J., and de Vries, L. S. (1994). Intracranial lesions in the fullterm infant with hypoxic ischaemic encephalopathy: ultrasound and autopsy correlation. *Neuropediatrics* 25, 301–307. doi: 10.1055/s-2008-1073044

Eklind, S., Mallard, C., Arvidsson, P., and Hagberg, H. (2005). Lipopolysaccharide induces both a primary and a secondary phase of sensitization in the developing rat brain. *Pediatr. Res.* 58, 112–116. doi: 10.1203/01.PDR.0000163513.03619.8D

Eklind, S., Mallard, C., Leverin, A. L., Gilland, E., Blomgren, K., Mattsby-Baltzer, I., et al. (2001). Bacterial endotoxin sensitizes the immature brain to hypoxic–ischaemic injury. *Eur. J. Neurosci.* 13, 1101–1106. doi: 10.1046/j.0953-816x.2001.01474.x

Eklöf, B., and Siesjö, B. K. (1973). Cerebral blood flow in ischemia caused by carotid artery ligation in the rat. *Acta Physiol. Scand.* 87, 69–77. doi: 10.1111/j.1748-1716.1973.tb05367.x

El-Khoury, N., Braun, A., Hu, F., Pandey, M., Nedergaard, M., Lagamma, E. F., et al. (2006). Astrocyte end-feet in germinal matrix, cerebral cortex, and white matter in developing infants. *Pediatr. Res.* 59, 673–679. doi: 10.1203/01.pdr.0000214975.85311.9c

Ellisdon, A. M., Zhang, Q., Henstridge, M. A., Johnson, T. K., Warr, C. G., Law, R. H., et al. (2014). High resolution structure of cleaved Serpin 42 Da from *Drosophila melanogaster*. *BMC Struct. Biol.* 14:1. doi: 10.1186/1472-6807-14-14

Eskiocak, S., Tutunculer, F., Basaran, U. N., Taskiran, A., and Cakir, E. (2007). The effect of melatonin on protein oxidation and nitric oxide in the brain tissue of hypoxic neonatal rats. *Brain Dev.* 29, 19–24. doi: 10.1016/j.braindev.2006.05.007

Evans, D. J., Levene, M. I., and Tsakmakis, M. (2007). Anticonvulsants for preventing mortality and morbidity in full term newborns with perinatal asphyxia. *Cochrane Database Syst. Rev.* 3:CD001240. doi: 10.1002/14651858.CD001240.pub2

Ezquer, M. E., Valdez, S. R., and Seltzer, A. M. (2006). Inflammatory responses of the substantia nigra after acute hypoxia in neonatal rats. *Exp. Neurol.* 197, 391–398. doi: 10.1016/j.expneurol.2005.10.015

Ezquer, M. E., Valdez, S. R., Seltzer, A. M., and Jahn, G. A. (2008). Advancement of reproductive senescence and changes in the early expression of estrogen, progesterone and micro-opioid receptors induced by neonatal hypoxia in the female rat. *Brain Res.* 1214, 73–83. doi: 10.1016/j.brainres.2008.03.029

Fahn, S., Davis, J. N., and Rowland, L. P. (1979). *Cerebral Hypoxia and Its Consequences*. New York, NY: Raven Press.

Failor, S., Nguyen, V., Darcy, D. P., Cang, J., Wendland, M. F., Stryker, M. P., et al. (2010). Neonatal cerebral hypoxia-ischemia impairs plasticity in rat visual cortex. *J. Neurosci.* 30, 81–92. doi: 10.1523/JNEUROSCI.5656-08.2010

Fan, X., Kavelaars, A., Heijnen, C. J., Groenendaal, F., and van Bel, F. (2010). Pharmacological neuroprotection after perinatal hypoxic-ischemic brain injury. *Curr. Neuropharmacol.* 8, 324–334. doi: 10.2174/157015910793358150

Fatemi, A., Wilson, M. A., and Johnston, M. V. (2009). Hypoxic-ischemic encephalopathy in the term infant. *Clin. Perinatol.* 36, 835–vii. doi: 10.1016/j.clp.2009.07.011

Favrais, G., van de Looij, Y., Fleiss, B., Ramanantsoa, N., Bonnin, P., Stoltenburg-Didinger, G., et al. (2011). Systemic inflammation disrupts the developmental program of white matter. *Ann. Neurol.* 70, 550–565. doi: 10.1002/ana.22489

Felderhoff-Mueser, U., Sifringer, M., Pesditschek, S., Kuckuck, H., Moysich, A., Bittigau, P., et al. (2002). Pathways leading to apoptotic neurodegeneration following trauma to the developing rat brain. *Neurobiol. Dis.* 11, 231–245. doi: 10.1006/nbdi.2002.0521

Fellman, V., Hellström-Westas, L., Norman, M., Westgren, M., Källén, K., Lagercrantz, H., et al. (2010). One-year survival of extremely preterm infants after active perinatal care in Sweden. *Obstet. Anesth. Dig.* 30, 22–23. doi: 10.1097/01.aoa.0000367003.25266.35

Ferrari, D. C., Nesic, O., and Perez-Polo, J. R. (2010). Perspectives on neonatal hypoxia/ischemia-induced edema formation. *Neurochem. Res.* 35, 1957–1965. doi: 10.1007/s11064-010-0308-y

Ferriero, D. M. (2001). Oxidant mechanisms in neonatal hypoxia-ischemia. *Dev. Neurosci.* 23, 198–202. doi: 10.1159/000046143

Ferriero, D. M. (2004). Neonatal brain injury. *N. Engl. J. Med.* 351, 1985–1995. doi: 10.1056/NEJMra041996

Ferriero, D. M., Holtzman, D. M., Black, S. M., and Sheldon, R. A. (1996). Neonatal mice lacking neuronal nitric oxide synthase are less vulnerable to hypoxic–ischemic injury. *Neurobiol. Dis.* 3, 64–71. doi: 10.1006/nbdi.1996.0006

Finer, N., Robertson, C., Richards, R., Pinnell, L., and Peters, K. (1981). Hypoxic-ischemic encephalopathy in term neonates: perinatal factors and outcome. *J. Pediatr.* 98, 112–117. doi: 10.1016/S0022-3476(81)80555-0

Finer, N. N., Robertson, C. M., Peters, K. L., and Coward, J. H. (1983). Factors affecting outcome in hypoxic-ischemic encephalopathy in term infants. *Am. J. Dis. Child.* 137, 21–25. doi: 10.1001/archpedi.1983.02140270017006

Fischer, R., and Maier, O. (2015). Interrelation of oxidative stress and inflammation in neurodegenerative disease: role of TNF. *Oxid. Med. Cell. Longev.* 2015:610813. doi: 10.1155/2015/610813

Fleiss, B., and Gressens, P. (2012). Tertiary mechanisms of brain damage: a new hope for treatment of cerebral palsy? *Lancet Neurol.* 11, 556–566. doi: 10.1016/S1474-4422(12)70058-3

Folkerth, R. D. (2005). Neuropathologic substrate of cerebral palsy. *J. Child Neurol.* 20, 940–949. doi: 10.1177/08830738050200120301

Forder, J. P., and Tymianski, M. (2009). Postsynaptic mechanisms of excitotoxicity: involvement of postsynaptic density proteins, radicals, and oxidant molecules. *Neuroscience* 158, 293–300. doi: 10.1016/j.neuroscience.2008.10.021

Fox, K., Schlaggar, B. L., Glazewski, S., and O'Leary, D. D. (1996). Glutamate receptor blockade at cortical synapses disrupts development of thalamocortical and columnar organization in somatosensory cortex. *Proc. Natl. Acad. Sci. U.S.A.* 93, 5584–5589. doi: 10.1073/pnas.93.11.5584

Fujihara, M., Muroi, M., Tanamoto, K., Suzuki, T., Azuma, H., and Ikeda, H. (2003). Molecular mechanisms of macrophage activation and deactivation by lipopolysaccharide: roles of the receptor complex. *Pharmacol. Ther.* 100, 171–194. doi: 10.1016/j.pharmthera.2003.08.003

Fujimoto, E., Miki, A., and Mizoguti, H. (1989). Histochemical study of the differentiation of microglial cells in the developing human cerebral hemispheres. *J. Anat.* 166, 253–264.

Galliciotti, G., and Sonderegger, P. (2006). Neuroserpin. *Front. Biosci.* 11:33–45. doi: 10.2741/1778

Garcia-Marin, V., Blazquez-Llorca, L., Rodriguez, J. R., Gonzalez-Soriano, J., and DeFelipe, J. (2010). Differential distribution of neurons in the gyral white matter of the human cerebral cortex. *J. Comp. Neurol.* 518, 4740–4759. doi: 10.1002/cne.22485

Garnier, Y., Berger, R., Alm, S., von Duering, M. U., Coumans, A. B., Michetti, F., et al. (2006). Systemic endotoxin administration results in increased S100B protein blood levels and periventricular brain white matter injury in the preterm fetal sheep. *Eur. J. Obstet. Gynecol. Reprod. Biol.* 124, 15–22. doi: 10.1016/j.ejogrb.2005.05.014

Garnier, Y., Coumans, A., Berger, R., Jensen, A., and Hasaart, T. H. (2001). Endotoxemia severely affects circulation during normoxia and asphyxia in immature fetal sheep. *J. Soc. Gynecol. Investig.* 8, 134–142. doi: 10.1016/S1071-5576(01)00101-0

Gelderblom, M., Neumann, M., Ludewig, P., Bernreuther, C., Krasemann, S., Arunachalam, P., et al. (2013). Deficiency in serine protease inhibitor neuroserpin exacerbates ischemic brain injury by increased postischemic inflammation. *PLoS ONE* 8:e63118. doi: 10.1371/journal.pone.0063118

Ghosh, A., Antonini, A., McConnell, S. K., and Shatz, C. J. (1990). Requirement for subplate neurons in the formation of thalamocortical connections. *Nature* 347, 179–181. doi: 10.1038/347179a0

Ghosh, A., and Shatz, C. J. (1992). Involvement of subplate neurons in the formation of ocular dominance columns. *Science* 255, 1441–1443. doi: 10.1126/science.1542795

Gillani, Q. A., Akbar, A., Ali, M., and Iqbal, F. (2015). Gender-specific effects of CGP 55845, GABAB receptor antagonist, on neuromuscular coordination, learning and memory formation in albino mouse following neonatal hypoxia–ischemia insult. *Neurol. Sci.* 36, 961–969. doi: 10.1007/s10072-015-2205-2

Gillani, Q. A., Iqbal, S., Arfa, F., Khakwani, S., Akbar, A., Ullah, A., et al. (2014). Effect of GABA B receptor antagonist (CGP35348) on learning and memory in albino mice. *Sci. World J.* 2014:983651. doi: 10.1155/2014/983651

Ginet, V., Puyal, J., Clarke, P. G., and Truttmann, A. C. (2009). Enhancement of autophagic flux after neonatal cerebral hypoxia-ischemia and its region-specific relationship to apoptotic mechanisms. *Am. J. Pathol.* 175, 1962–1974. doi: 10.2353/ajpath.2009.090463

Girard, S., Kadhim, H., Beaudet, N., Sarret, P., and Sebire, G. (2009). Developmental motor deficits induced by combined fetal exposure to lipopolysaccharide and early neonatal hypoxia/ischemia: a novel animal model for cerebral palsy in very premature infants. *Neuroscience* 158, 673–682. doi: 10.1016/j.neuroscience.2008.10.032

Girard, S., Kadhim, H., Larouche, A., Roy, M., Gobeil, F., and Sebire, G. (2008). Pro-inflammatory disequilibrium of the IL-1 beta/IL-1ra ratio in an experimental model of perinatal brain damages induced by lipopolysaccharide and hypoxia-ischemia. *Cytokine* 43, 54–62. doi: 10.1016/j.cyto.2008.04.007

Girard, S., Sebire, H., Brochu, M. E., Briota, S., Sarret, P., and Sebire, G. (2012). Postnatal administration of IL-1Ra exerts neuroprotective effects following perinatal inflammation and/or hypoxic-ischemic injuries. *Brain Behav. Immun.* 26, 1331–1339. doi: 10.1016/j.bbi.2012.09.001

Glenn, O. A., Ludeman, N. A., Berman, J. I., Wu, Y. W., Lu, Y., Bartha, A. I., et al. (2007). Diffusion tensor MR imaging tractography of the pyramidal tracts correlates with clinical motor function in children with congenital hemiparesis. *AJNR. Am. J. Neuroradiol.* 28, 1796–1802. doi: 10.3174/ajnr.A0676

Gluckman, P. D., Wyatt, J. S., Azzopardi, D., Ballard, R., Edwards, A. D., Ferriero, D. M., et al. (2005). Selective head cooling with mild systemic hypothermia after neonatal encephalopathy: multicentre randomised trial. *Lancet* 365, 663–670. doi: 10.1016/S0140-6736(05)17946-X

Goldberg, R. N., Moscoso, P., Bauer, C. R., Bloom, F. L., Curless, R. G., Burke, B., et al. (1986). Use of barbiturate therapy in severe perinatal asphyxia: a randomized controlled trial. *J. Pediatr.* 109, 851–856. doi: 10.1016/S0022-3476(86)80713-2

Gonzalez, F. F., and Miller, S. P. (2006). Does perinatal asphyxia impair cognitive function without cerebral palsy? *Arch. Dis. Child. Fetal Neonatal Ed.* 91, F454–F459.

González-Portillo, A., Domínguez-Antolínez, I., and Muniategui-Azkona, E. (2015). Crisis of the welfare state: an analysis of the responses from social work. *Rev. Cercetare Interventie Soc.* 49, 173–186.

Gozzo, S., Dimitrieva, N., Iacopino, C., and D'Udine, B. (1985). A comparative study of mossy fiber distribution in the brain of the precocial *Acomys cahirinus* and of the altricial *Rattus norvegicus*: neuroanatomical bases and behavioral correlates. *Int. J. Neurosci.* 28, 163–172. doi: 10.3109/00207458508985387

Graham, E. M., Ruis, K. A., Hartman, A. L., Northington, F. J., and Fox, H. E. (2008). A systematic review of the role of intrapartum hypoxia-ischemia in the causation of neonatal encephalopathy. *Am. J. Obstet. Gynecol.* 199, 587–595. doi: 10.1016/j.ajog.2008.06.094

Grant, E., Hoerder-Suabedissen, A., and Molnár, Z. (2016). The regulation of corticofugal fiber targeting by retinal inputs. *Cereb. Cortex* 26, 1336–1348. doi: 10.1093/cercor/bhv315

Greggio, S., de Paula, S., de Oliveira, I. M., Trindade, C., Rosa, R. M., Henriques, J. A., et al. (2011). NAP prevents acute cerebral oxidative stress and protects against long-term brain injury and cognitive impairment in a model of neonatal hypoxia–ischemia. *Neurobiol. Dis.* 44, 152–159. doi: 10.1016/j.nbd.2011.06.018

Greggio, S., Rosa, R. M., Dolganov, A., de Oliveira, I. M., Menegat, F. D., Henriques, J. A., et al. (2009). NAP prevents hippocampal oxidative damage in neonatal rats subjected to hypoxia-induced seizures. *Neurobiol. Dis.* 36, 435–444. doi: 10.1016/j.nbd.2009.08.008

Groenendaal, F., de Vries, L. S., and van Bel, F. (2006). Favourable results with surgical treatment in 43 children with hypoplastic left-heart syndrome or similar disorders, 1999-2005. *Ned. Tijdschr. Geneeskd.* 150, 2731–2732.

Groenendaal, F., Meiners, L. C., Gooskens, R., and de Vries, L. S. (1994). Cerebral proton magnetic resonance spectroscopic imaging in a neonate with tuberous sclerosis. *Neuropediatrics* 25, 154–157. doi: 10.1055/s-2008-1073014

Grow, J., and Barks, J. D. (2002). Pathogenesis of hypoxic-ischemic cerebral injury in the term infant: current concepts. *Clin. Perinatol.* 29, 585–602. doi: 10.1016/S0095-5108(02)00059-3

Gu, R., Fu, L., Jiang, C., Xu, Y., Wang, X., and Yu, J. (2015). Retina is protected by neuroserpin from ischemic/reperfusion-induced injury independent of tissue-type plasminogen activator. *PLoS ONE* 10:e0130440. doi: 10.1371/journal.pone.0130440

Gunn, A. J., Battin, M., Gluckman, P. D., Gunn, T. R., and Bennet, L. (2005). Therapeutic hypothermia: from lab to NICU. *J. Perinat. Med.* 33, 340–346. doi: 10.1515/JPM.2005.061

Gunn, A. J., and Gunn, T. R. (1998). Thepharmacology'of neuronal rescue with cerebral hypothermia. *Early Hum. Dev.* 53, 19–35. doi: 10.1016/S0378-3782(98)00033-4

Gunn, A. J., Gunn, T. R., de Haan, H. H., Williams, C. E., and Gluckman, P. D. (1997). Dramatic neuronal rescue with prolonged selective head cooling after ischemia in fetal lambs. *J. Clin. Invest.* 99, 248–256. doi: 10.1172/JCI119153

Gunn, A. J., Parer, J. T., Mallard, E. C., Williams, C. E., and Gluckman, P. D. (1992). Cerebral histologic and electrocorticographic changes after asphyxia in fetal sheep. *Pediatr. Res.* 31, 486–491. doi: 10.1203/00006450-199205000-00016

Hack, M., Breslau, N., Aram, D., Weissman, B., Klein, N., and Borawski-Clark, E. (1992). The effect of very low birth weight and social risk on neurocognitive abilities at school age. *J. Dev. Behav. Pediatr.* 13, 412–420. doi: 10.1097/00004703-199212000-00005

Hadjiconstantinou, M., Yates, A. J., and Neff, N. H. (1990). Hypoxia-induced neurotransmitter deficits in neonatal rats are partially corrected by exogenous GM1 ganglioside. *J. Neurochem.* 55, 864–869. doi: 10.1111/j.1471-4159.1990.tb04571.x

Hagberg, H., Andersson, P., Kjellmer, I., Thiringer, K., and Thordstein, M. (1987). Extracellular overflow of glutamate, aspartate, GABA and taurine in the cortex and basal ganglia of fetal lambs during hypoxia-ischemia. *Neurosci. Lett.* 78, 311–317. doi: 10.1016/0304-3940(87)90379-X

Hagberg, H., Gressens, P., and Mallard, C. (2012). Inflammation during fetal and neonatal life: implications for neurologic and neuropsychiatric disease in children and adults. *Ann. Neurol.* 71, 444–457. doi: 10.1002/ana.22620

Hagberg, H., Mallard, C., Ferriero, D. M., Vannucci, S. J., Levison, S. W., Vexler, Z. S., et al. (2015). The role of inflammation in perinatal brain injury. *Nat. Rev. Neurol.* 11, 192–208. doi: 10.1038/nrneurol.2015.13

Hagberg, H., Mallard, C., Rousset, C. I., and Xiaoyang, W. (2009). Apoptotic mechanisms in the immature brain: involvement of mitochondria. *J. Child Neurol.* 24, 1141–1146. doi: 10.1177/0883073809338212

Hagberg, H., Peebles, D., and Mallard, C. (2002). Models of white matter injury: comparison of infectious, hypoxic-ischemic, and excitotoxic insults. *Ment. Retard. Dev. Disabil. Res. Rev.* 8, 30–38. doi: 10.1002/mrdd.10007

Hagberg, H., Thornberg, E., Blennow, M., Kjellmer, I., Lagercrantz, H., Thiringer, K., et al. (1993). Excitatory amino acids in the cerebrospinal fluid of asphyxiated infants: relationship to hypoxic-ischemic encephalopathy. *Acta Paediatr.* 82, 925–929. doi: 10.1111/j.1651-2227.1993.tb12601.x

Hall, R. T., Hall, F. K., and Daily, D. K. (1998). High-dose phenobarbital therapy in term newborn infants with severe perinatal asphyxia: a randomized, prospective study with three-year follow-up. *J. Pediatr.* 132, 345–348. doi: 10.1016/S0022-3476(98)70458-5

Hamre, K. M., Hyman, B. T., Goodlett, C. R., West, J. R., and Van Hoesen, G. W. (1989). Alz-50 immunoreactivity in the neonatal rat: changes in development and co-distribution with MAP-2 immunoreactivity. *Neurosci. Lett.* 98, 264–271. doi: 10.1016/0304-3940(89)90411-4

Hamrick, S. E., and Ferriero, D. M. (2003). The injury response in the term newborn brain: can we neuroprotect? *Curr. Opin. Neurol.* 16, 147–154. doi: 10.1097/00019052-200304000-00005

Hardy, P., Nuyt, A. M., Dumont, I., Peri, K. G., Hou, X., Varma, D. R., et al. (1999). Developmentally increased cerebrovascular NO in newborn pigs curtails cerebral blood flow autoregulation. *Pediatr. Res.* 46, 375–382. doi: 10.1203/00006450-199910000-00004

Hasegawa, K., Yoshioka, H., Sawada, T., and Nishikawa, H. (1991). Lipid peroxidation in neonatal mouse brain subjected to two different types of hypoxia. *Brain Dev.* 13, 101–103. doi: 10.1016/S0387-7604(12)80115-X

Hasegawa, K., Yoshioka, H., Sawada, T., and Nishikawa, H. (1993). Direct measurement of free radicals in the neonatal mouse brain subjected to hypoxia: an electron spin resonance spectroscopic study. *Brain Res.* 607, 161–166. doi: 10.1016/0006-8993(93)91502-J

Hastings, G. A., Coleman, T. A., Haudenschild, C. C., Stefansson, S., Smith, E. P., Barthlow, R., et al. (1997). Neuroserpin, a brain-associated inhibitor of tissue plasminogen activator is localized primarily in neurons. Implications for the regulation of motor learning and neuronal survival. *J. Biol. Chem.* 272, 33062–33067. doi: 10.1074/jbc.272.52.33062

Hasumi, H., Ishiguro, H., Nakamura, M., Sugiura, S., Osada, Y., Miyoshi, Y., et al. (2005). Neuroserpin (PI-12) is upregulated in high-grade prostate cancer and is associated with survival. *Int. J. Cancer* 115, 911–916. doi: 10.1002/ijc.20967

Hattori, H., and Wasterlain, C. G. (1990). Excitatory amino acids in the developing brain: ontogeny, plasticity, and excitotoxicity. *Pediatr. Neurol.* 6, 219–228. doi: 10.1016/0887-8994(90)90111-D

Hedner, T., Bergman, B., and Holmgren, M. (1980). Adrenal catecholamines during and following hypoxia in neonatal rats. *Med. Biol.* 58, 228–231.

Hedner, T., and Lundborg, P. (1980a). 5-HIAA levels in brain and cerebrospinal fluid of the neonatal rat during oxygen deprivation. *Neurosci. Lett.* 19, 315–318.

Hedner, T., and Lundborg, P. (1980b). Catecholamine metabolism in neonatal rat brain during asphyxia and recovery. *Acta Physiol. Scand.* 109, 169–175. doi: 10.1111/j.1748-1716.1980.tb06583.x

Hedner, T., and Lundborg, P. (1980c). Serotonin metabolism in neonatal rat brain during asphyxia and recovery. *Acta Physiol. Scand.* 109, 163–168.

Hedtjarn, M., Mallard, C., Eklind, S., Gustafson-Brywe, K., and Hagberg, H. (2004a). Global gene expression in the immature brain after hypoxia-ischemia. *J. Cereb. Blood Flow Metab.* 24, 1317–1332. doi: 10.1097/01.WCB.0000141558.40491.75

Hedtjarn, M., Mallard, C., and Hagberg, H. (2004b). Inflammatory gene profiling in the developing mouse brain after hypoxia-ischemia. *J. Cereb. Blood Flow Metab.* 24, 1333–1351.

Helmy, M. M., Tolner, E. A., Vanhatalo, S., Voipio, J., and Kaila, K. (2011). Brain alkalosis causes birth asphyxia seizures, suggesting therapeutic strategy. *Ann. Neurol.* 69, 493–500. doi: 10.1002/ana.22223

Henry, V. J., Lecointre, M., Laudenbach, V., Ali, C., Macrez, R., Jullienne, A., et al. (2013). High tPA release by neonate brain microvascular endothelial cells under glutamate exposure affects neuronal fate. *Neurobiol. Dis.* 50, 201–208. doi: 10.1016/j.nbd.2012.10.020

Herrmann, K., Antonini, A., and Shatz, C. J. (1994). Ultrastructural evidence for synaptic interactions between thalamocortical axons and subplate neurons. *Eur. J. Neurosci.* 6, 1729–1742. doi: 10.1111/j.1460-9568.1994.tb00565.x

Hida, K., Suzuki, N., Kwee, I. L., and Nakada, T. (1991). pH-lactate dissociation in neonatal anoxia: proton and 31P NMR spectroscopic studies in rat pups. *Magn. Reson. Med.* 22, 128–132. doi: 10.1002/mrm.1910220113

Hill, A. (1991). Current concepts of hypoxic-ischemic cerebral injury in the term newborn. *Pediatr. Neurol.* 7, 317–325. doi: 10.1016/0887-8994(91)90060-X

Hill, C. A., Alexander, M. L., McCullough, L. D., and Fitch, R. H. (2012). Inhibition of X-linked inhibitor of apoptosis with embelin differentially affects male versus female behavioral outcome following neonatal hypoxia-ischemia in rats. *Dev. Neurosci.* 33, 494–504. doi: 10.1159/000331651

Hill, C. A., and Fitch, R. H. (2012). Sex differences in mechanisms and outcome of neonatal hypoxia-ischemia in rodent models: implications for sex-specific neuroprotection in clinical neonatal practice. *Neurol. Res. Int.* 2012:867531. doi: 10.1155/2012/867531

Hill, I. E., MacManus, J. P., Rasquinha, I., and Tuor, U. I. (1995). DNA fragmentation indicative of apoptosis following unilateral cerebral hypoxia-ischemia in the neonatal rat. *Brain Res.* 676, 398–403. doi: 10.1016/0006-8993(95)00145-G

Hill, R. M., Brennan, S. O., and Birch, N. P. (2001). Expression, purification, and functional characterization of the serine protease inhibitor neuroserpin expressed in Drosophila S2 cells. *Protein Expr. Purif.* 22, 406–413. doi: 10.1006/prep.2001.1463

Himmelmann, K., Hagberg, G., Beckung, E., Hagberg, B., and Uvebrant, P. (2005). The changing panorama of cerebral palsy in Sweden. IX. Prevalence and origin in the birth-year period 1995–1998. *Acta Paediatr.* 94, 287–294. doi: 10.1111/j.1651-2227.2005.tb03071.x

Himmelmann, K., Hagberg, G., Wiklund, L. M., Eek, M. N., and Uvebrant, P. (2007). Dyskinetic cerebral palsy: a population-based study of children born between 1991 and 1998. *Dev. Med. Child Neurol.* 49, 246–251. doi: 10.1111/j.1469-8749.2007.00246.x

Hisanaga, K., Onodera, H., and Kogure, K. (1986). Changes in levels of purine and pyrimidine nucleotides during acute hypoxia and recovery in neonatal rat brain. *J. Neurochem.* 47, 1344–1350. doi: 10.1111/j.1471-4159.1986.tb00763.x

Hobbs, C., Thoresen, M., Tucker, A., Aquilina, K., Chakkarapani, E., and Dingley, J. (2008). Xenon and hypothermia combine additively, offering long-term functional and histopathologic neuroprotection after neonatal hypoxia/ischemia. *Stroke* 39, 1307–1313. doi: 10.1161/STROKEAHA.107.499822

Hoerder-Suabedissen, A., and Molnár, Z. (2012). Morphology of mouse subplate cells with identified projection targets changes with age. *J. Comp. Neurol.* 520, 174–185. doi: 10.1002/cne.22725

Hoerder-Suabedissen, A., and Molnár, Z. (2015). Development, evolution and pathology of neocortical subplate neurons. *Nat. Rev. Neurosci.* 16, 133–146. doi: 10.1038/nrn3915

Hoerder-Suabedissen, A., Oeschger, F. M., Krishnan, M. L., Belgard, T. G., Wang, W. Z., Lee, S., et al. (2013). Expression profiling of mouse subplate reveals a dynamic gene network and disease association with autism and schizophrenia. *Proc. Natl. Acad. Sci. U.S.A.* 110, 3555–3560. doi: 10.1073/pnas.1218510110

Hoerder-Suabedissen, A., Wang, W. Z., Lee, S., Davies, K. E., Goffinet, A. M., Rakic, S., et al. (2009). Novel markers reveal subpopulations of subplate neurons in the murine cerebral cortex. *Cereb. Cortex* 19, 1738–1750. doi: 10.1093/cercor/bhn195

Holmes, G. L. (1991). The long-term effects of seizures on the developing brain: clinical and laboratory issues. *Brain Dev.* 13, 393–409. doi: 10.1016/S0387-7604(12)80037-4

Holmes, G. L., and Ben-Ari, Y. (2001). The neurobiology and consequences of epilepsy in the developing brain. *Pediatr. Res.* 49, 320–325. doi: 10.1203/00006450-200103000-00004

Horn, E. P., Bein, B., Broch, O., Iden, T., Bohm, R., Latz, S. K., et al. (2016). Warming before and after epidural block before general anaesthesia for major abdominal surgery prevents perioperative hypothermia: a randomised controlled trial. *Eur. J. Anaesthesiol.* 33, 334–340. doi: 10.1097/EJA.0000000000000369

Hou, S. T., Jiang, S. X., Huang, D., and Desbois, A. (2007). A novel adenoviral vector-mediated neuronal selective gene expression in neonatal mouse brain in response to hypoxia. *Neurosci. Lett.* 419, 23–27. doi: 10.1016/j.neulet.2007.03.059

Hou, X., Ding, H., Teng, Y., Zhou, C., Tang, X., Li, S., et al. (2007). Research on the relationship between brain anoxia at different regional oxygen saturations and brain damage using near-infrared spectroscopy. *Physiol. Meas.* 28, 1251–1265. doi: 10.1088/0967-3334/28/10/010

Hou, X. L., Ding, H. Y., Zhou, C. L., Tang, X. Y., Ding, H. S., Teng, Y. C., et al. (2007). Correlation of brain hypoxia at different degrees with brain function and brain damage investigated using near infrared spectroscopy. *Zhonghua Er Ke Za Zhi* 45, 523–528.

Hu, B. R., Liu, C. L., Ouyang, Y., Blomgren, K., and Siesjo, B. K. (2000). Involvement of caspase-3 in cell death after hypoxia-ischemia declines during brain maturation. *J. Cerebral Blood Flow Metab.* 20, 1294–1300. doi: 10.1097/00004647-200009000-00003

Hu, C. J., Wang, L. Y., Chodosh, L. A., Keith, B., and Simon, M. C. (2003). Differential roles of hypoxia-inducible factor 1alpha (HIF-1alpha) and HIF-2alpha in hypoxic gene regulation. *Mol. Cell. Biol.* 23, 9361–9374. doi: 10.1128/MCB.23.24.9361-9374.2003

Hu, X., Qiu, J., Grafe, M. R., Rea, H. C., Rassin, D. K., and Perez-Polo, J. R. (2003). Bcl-2 family members make different contributions to cell death in hypoxia and/or hyperoxia in rat cerebral cortex. *Int. J. Dev. Neurosci.* 21, 371–377. doi: 10.1016/S0736-5748(03)00089-3

Hunt, R. W., Neil, J. J., Coleman, L. T., Kean, M. J., and Inder, T. E. (2004). Apparent diffusion coefficient in the posterior limb of the internal capsule predicts outcome after perinatal asphyxia. *Pediatrics* 114, 999–1003. doi: 10.1542/peds.2003-0935-L

Hurtley, S. M., and Helenius, A. (1989). Protein oligomerization in the endoplasmic reticulum. *Annu. Rev. Cell Biol.* 5, 277–307. doi: 10.1146/annurev.cb.05.110189.001425

Hutton, L. C., Abbass, M., Dickinson, H., Ireland, Z., and Walker, D. W. (2009). Neuroprotective properties of melatonin in a model of birth asphyxia in the spiny mouse (*Acomys cahirinus*). *Dev. Neurosci.* 31, 437–451. doi: 10.1159/000232562

Ikeda, K., Tanihara, H., Honda, Y., Tatsuno, T., Noguchi, H., and Nakayama, C. (1999). BDNF attenuates retinal cell death caused by chemically induced hypoxia in rats. *Invest. Ophthalmol. Vis. Sci.* 40, 2130–2140.

Ikeda, T., Mishima, K., Yoshikawa, T., Iwasaki, K., Fujiwara, M., Xia, Y. X., et al. (2001). Selective and long-term learning impairment following neonatal hypoxic-ischemic brain insult in rats. *Behav. Brain Res.* 118, 17–25. doi: 10.1016/S0166-4328(00)00287-4

Ikonomidou, C., Bosch, F., Miksa, M., Bittigau, P., Vockler, J., Dikranian, K., et al. (1999). Blockade of NMDA receptors and apoptotic neurodegeneration in the developing brain. *Science* 283, 70–74. doi: 10.1126/science.283.5398.70

Ikonomidou, C., and Kaindl, A. M. (2011). Neuronal death and oxidative stress in the developing brain. *Antioxid. Redox Signal.* 14, 1535–1550. doi: 10.1089/ars.2010.3581

Im, S., Yu, J., Park, E., Lee, J., Kim, H., Park, K., et al. (2010). Induction of striatal neurogenesis enhances functional recovery in an adult animal model of neonatal hypoxic-ischemic brain injury. *Neuroscience* 169, 259–268. doi: 10.1016/j.neuroscience.2010.04.038

Inder, T., Neil, J., Kroenke, C., Dieni, S., Yoder, B., and Rees, S. (2005a). Investigation of cerebral development and injury in the prematurely born primate by magnetic resonance imaging and histopathology. *Dev. Neurosci.* 27, 100–111.

Inder, T., Neil, J., Yoder, B., and Rees, S. (2005b). Patterns of cerebral injury in a primate model of preterm birth and neonatal intensive care. *J. Child Neurol.* 20, 965–967.

Inder, T. E., Hunt, R. W., Morley, C. J., Coleman, L., Stewart, M., Doyle, L. W., et al. (2004). Randomized trial of systemic hypothermia selectively protects the cortex on MRI in term hypoxic-ischemic encephalopathy. *J. Pediatr.* 145, 835–837. doi: 10.1016/j.jpeds.2004.07.034

Inder, T. E., Huppi, P. S., Warfield, S., Kikinis, R., Zientara, G. P., Barnes, P. D., et al. (1999). Periventricular white matter injury in the premature infant is followed by reduced cerebral cortical gray matter volume at term. *Ann. Neurol.* 46, 755–760. doi: 10.1002/1531-8249(199911)46:5<755::AID-ANA11>3.0.CO;2-0

Inder, T. E., and Volpe, J. J. (2000). Mechanisms of perinatal brain injury. *Semin. Neonatol.* 5, 3–16. doi: 10.1053/siny.1999.0112

Ireland, Z., Dickinson, H., Fleiss, B., Hutton, L. C., and Walker, D. W. (2010). Behavioural effects of near-term acute fetal hypoxia in a small precocial animal, the spiny mouse (*Acomys cahirinus*). *Neonatology* 97, 45–51. doi: 10.1159/000227293

Ireland, Z., Dickinson, H., Snow, R., and Walker, D. W. (2008). Maternal creatine: does it reach the fetus and improve survival after an acute hypoxic episode in the spiny mouse (*Acomys cahirinus*)? *Am. J. Obstet. Gynecol.* 198, 431.e1–6. doi: 10.1016/j.ajog.2007.10.790

Ireland, Z., Russell, A. P., Wallimann, T., Walker, D. W., and Snow, R. (2009). Developmental changes in the expression of creatine synthesizing enzymes and creatine transporter in a precocial rodent, the spiny mouse. *BMC Dev. Biol.* 9:39. doi: 10.1186/1471-213X-9-39

Ishigami, S., Sandkvist, M., Tsui, F., Moore, E., Coleman, T. A., and Lawrence, D. A. (2007). Identification of a novel targeting sequence for regulated secretion in the serine protease inhibitor neuroserpin. *Biochem. J.* 402, 25–34. doi: 10.1042/BJ20061170

Iuvone, L., Geloso, M. C., and Dell'Anna, E. (1996). Changes in open field behavior, spatial memory, and hippocampal parvalbumin immunoreactivity following enrichment in rats exposed to neonatal anoxia. *Exp. Neurol.* 139, 25–33. doi: 10.1006/exnr.1996.0077

Iyer, N. V., Leung, S. W., and Semenza, G. L. (1998). The human hypoxia-inducible factor 1alpha gene: HIF1A structure and evolutionary conservation. *Genomics* 52, 159–165. doi: 10.1006/geno.1998.5416

Jabaudon, D., Scanziani, M., Gahwiler, B. H., and Gerber, U. (2000). Acute decrease in net glutamate uptake during energy deprivation. *Proc. Natl. Acad. Sci. U.S.A.* 97, 5610–5615. doi: 10.1073/pnas.97.10.5610

Jacobs, S., Hunt, R., Tarnow-Mordi, W., Inder, T., and Davis, P. (2005). 181 cooling for newborns with hypoxic ischaemic encephalopathy. *Pediatr. Res.* 58, 385–385. doi: 10.1016/j.arcped.2012.11.007

Jacobs, S. E., Berg, M., Hunt, R., Tarnow-Mordi, W. O., Inder, T. E., and Davis, P. G. (2013). Cooling for newborns with hypoxic ischaemic encephalopathy. *Cochrane Database Syst. Rev.* 4, CD003311. doi: 10.1002/14651858.CD003311.pub3

Jacovina, A. T., Zhong, F., Khazanova, E., Lev, E., Deora, A. B., and Hajjar, K. A. (2001). Neuritogenesis and the nerve growth factor-induced differentiation of PC-12 cells requires annexin II-mediated plasmin generation. *J. Biol. Chem.* 276, 49350–49358. doi: 10.1074/jbc.M106289200

Jansen, E. M., and Low, W. C. (1996a). Long-term effects of neonatal ischemic-hypoxic brain injury on sensorimotor and locomotor tasks in rats. *Behav. Brain Res.* 78, 189–194.

Jansen, E. M., and Low, W. C. (1996b). Quantitative analysis of contralateral hemisphere hypertrophy and sensorimotor performance in adult rats following unilateral neonatal ischemic-hypoxic brain injury. *Brain Res.* 708, 93–99.

Jansen, E. M., Solberg, L., Underhill, S., Wilson, S., Cozzari, C., Hartman, B. K., et al. (1997). Transplantation of fetal neocortex ameliorates sensorimotor and locomotor deficits following neonatal ischemic–hypoxic brain injury in rats. *Exp. Neurol.* 147, 487–497. doi: 10.1006/exnr.1997.6596

Jantzie, L. L., Corbett, C. J., Berglass, J., Firl, D. J., Flores, J., Mannix, R., et al. (2014). Complex pattern of interaction between in utero hypoxia-ischemia and intra-amniotic inflammation disrupts brain development and motor function. *J. Neuroinflammation* 11:131. doi: 10.1186/1742-2094-11-131

Jantzie, L. L., Corbett, C. J., Firl, D. J., and Robinson, S. (2015a). Postnatal erythropoietin mitigates impaired cerebral cortical development following subplate loss from prenatal hypoxia-ischemia. *Cereb.Cortex* 25, 2683–2695. doi: 10.1093/cercor/bhu066

Jantzie, L. L., Hu, M. Y., Park, H. K., Jackson, M. C., Yu, J., Maxwell, J. R., et al. (2015b). Chloride cotransporter NKCC1 inhibitor bumetanide protects against white matter injury in a rodent model of periventricular leukomalacia. *Pediatr. Res.* 77, 554–562. doi: 10.1038/pr.2015.9

Jantzie, L. L., Winer, J. L., Maxwell, J. R., Chan, L. A., and Robinson, S. (2015c). Modeling encephalopathy of prematurity using prenatal Hypoxia-ischemia with Intra-amniotic lipopolysaccharide in rats. *J. Vis. Exp.* 105:e53196. doi: 10.3791/53196

Jarvis, S., Glinianaia, S. V., Arnaud, C., Fauconnier, J., Johnson, A., McManus, V., et al. (2005). Case gender and severity in cerebral palsy varies with intrauterine growth. *Arch. Dis. Child.* 90, 474–479. doi: 10.1136/adc.2004.052670

Jatana, M., Singh, I., Singh, A. K., and Jenkins, D. (2006). Combination of systemic hypothermia and N-acetylcysteine attenuates hypoxic-ischemic brain injury in neonatal rats. *Pediatr. Res.* 59, 684–689. doi: 10.1203/01.pdr.0000215045.91122.44

Jelinski, S. E., Yager, J. Y., and Juurlink, B. H. (1999). Preferential injury of oligodendroblasts by a short hypoxic–ischemic insult. *Brain Res.* 815, 150–153. doi: 10.1016/S0006-8993(98)01053-1

Jendelová, P., Herynek, V., Urdzikova, L., Glogarová, K., Kroupová, J., Andersson, B., et al. (2004). Magnetic resonance tracking of transplanted bone marrow and embryonic stem cells labeled by iron oxide nanoparticles in rat brain and spinal cord. *J. Neurosci. Res.* 76, 232–243. doi: 10.1002/jnr.20041

Jensen, A., Garnier, Y., and Berger, R. (1999). Dynamics of fetal circulatory responses to hypoxia and asphyxia. *Eur. J. Obstet. Gynecol. Reprod. Biol.* 84, 155–172. doi: 10.1016/S0301-2115(98)00325-X

Jensen, F. (1995). An animal model of hypoxia-induced perinatal seizures. *Ital. J. Neurol. Sci.* 16, 59–68. doi: 10.1007/BF02229075

Jensen, F., Blume, H., Alvarado, S., Firkusny, I., and Geary, C. (1995). NBQX blocks acute and late epileptogenic effects of perinatal hypoxia. *Epilepsia* 36, 966–972. doi: 10.1111/j.1528-1157.1995.tb00954.x

Johnston, M. V. (2001). Excitotoxicity in neonatal hypoxia. *Ment. Retard. Dev. Disabil. Res. Rev.* 7, 229–234. doi: 10.1002/mrdd.1032

Johnston, M. V. (2005). Excitotoxicity in perinatal brain injury. *Brain Pathol.* 15, 234–240. doi: 10.1111/j.1750-3639.2005.tb00526.x

Johnston, M. V. (2009). Plasticity in the developing brain: implications for rehabilitation. *Dev. Disab. Res. Rev.* 15, 94–101. doi: 10.1002/ddrr.64

Johnston, M. V., Fatemi, A., Wilson, M. A., and Northington, F. (2011). Treatment advances in neonatal neuroprotection and neurointensive care. *Lancet Neurol.* 10, 372–382. doi: 10.1016/S1474-4422(11)70016-3

Johnston, M. V., and Hagberg, H. (2007). Sex and the pathogenesis of cerebral palsy. *Dev. Med. Child Neurol.* 49, 74–78. doi: 10.1017/S001216220700 0199.x

Jones, M. K., Szabo, I. L., Kawanaka, H., Husain, S. S., and Tarnawski, A. S. (2002). von Hippel Lindau tumor suppressor and HIF-1alpha: new targets of NSAIDs inhibition of hypoxia-induced angiogenesis. *FASEB J.* 16, 264–266.

Joseph, B., Nandhu, M. S., and Paulose, C. S. (2010). Dopamine D1 and D2 receptor functional down regulation in the cerebellum of hypoxic neonatal rats: neuroprotective role of glucose and oxygen, epinephrine resuscitation. *Pharmacol. Res.* 61, 136–141. doi: 10.1016/j.phrs.2009.08.007

Judas, M., Sedmak, G., Pletikos, M., and Jovanov-Milosevic, N. (2010). Populations of subplate and interstitial neurons in fetal and adult human telencephalon. *J. Anat.* 217, 381–399. doi: 10.1111/j.1469-7580.2010.01284.x

Juul, S. E., Beyer, R. P., Bammler, T. K., McPherson, R. J., Wilkerson, J., and Farin, F. M. (2009). Microarray analysis of high-dose recombinant erythropoietin treatment of unilateral brain injury in neonatal mouse hippocampus. *Pediatr. Res.* 65, 485–492. doi: 10.1203/PDR.0b013e31819d90c8

Kali, G. T., Martinez-Biarge, M., Van Zyl, J., Smith, J., and Rutherford, M. (2015). Management of therapeutic hypothermia for neonatal hypoxic ischaemic encephalopathy in a tertiary centre in South Africa. *Arch. Dis. Child. Fetal Neonatal. Ed.* 100, F519–F523. doi: 10.1136/archdischild-2015-308398

Kaneko, K. (1985a). The effect of perinatal anoxia on amino acid metabolism in the developing brain. Part I: the effect of experimental anoxia on the free amino acid patterns in the brain of neonatal rats. *Brain Dev.* 7, 392–399.

Kaneko, K. (1985b). The effect of perinatal anoxia on amino acid metabolism in the developing brain. Part II: the effect of perinatal anoxia on the free amino acid patterns in CSF of infants and children. *Brain Dev.* 7, 400–407.

Kaneko, T., Sawada, T., Kinugawa, H., Kuriyama, Y., and Naritomi, H. (1985). A case of inverse ocular bobbing associated with cluster respiration in hypoxic encephalopathy. *Rinsho shinkeigaku* 25, 1192–1195.

Kanold, P. O. (2009). Subplate neurons: crucial regulators of cortical development and plasticity. *Front. Neuroanat.* 3:16. doi: 10.3389/neuro.05.016.2009

Kanold, P. O., Kara, P., Reid, R. C., and Shatz, C. J. (2003). Role of subplate neurons in functional maturation of visual cortical columns. *Science* 301, 521–525. doi: 10.1126/science.1084152

Kanold, P. O., and Luhmann, H. J. (2010). The subplate and early cortical circuits. *Annu. Rev. Neurosci.* 33, 23–48. doi: 10.1146/annurev-neuro-060909-153244

Kanold, P. O., and Shatz, C. J. (2006). Subplate neurons regulate maturation of cortical inhibition and outcome of ocular dominance plasticity. *Neuron* 51, 627–638. doi: 10.1016/j.neuron.2006.07.008

Karalis, F., Soubasi, V., Georgiou, T., Nakas, C. T., Simeonidou, C., Guiba-Tziampiri, O., et al. (2011). Resveratrol ameliorates hypoxia/ischemia-induced behavioral deficits and brain injury in the neonatal rat brain. *Brain Res.* 1425, 98–110. doi: 10.1016/j.brainres.2011.09.044

Kattwinkel, J., Perlman, J. M., Aziz, K., Colby, C., Fairchild, K., Gallagher, J., et al. (2010). Part 15: neonatal resuscitation: 2010 American heart association guidelines for cardiopulmonary resuscitation and emergency cardiovascular care. *Circulation* 122(18 Suppl. 3), S909–S919. doi: 10.1161/CIRCULATIONAHA.110.971119

Kaufman, S. A., Miller, S. P., Ferriero, D. M., Glidden, D. H., Barkovich, A. J., and Partridge, J. C. (2003). Encephalopathy as a predictor of magnetic resonance imaging abnormalities in asphyxiated newborns. *Pediatr. Neurol.* 28, 342–346. doi: 10.1016/S0887-8994(03)00015-8

Kaur, C., Dheen, S. T., and Ling, E. A. (2007). From blood to brain: amoeboid microglial cell, a nascent macrophage and its functions in developing brain. *Acta Pharmacol. Sin.* 28, 1087–1096. doi: 10.1111/j.1745-7254.2007.00625.x

Kaur, C., and Ling, E. A. (2009). Periventricular white matter damage in the hypoxic neonatal brain: role of microglial cells. *Prog. Neurobiol.* 87, 264–280. doi: 10.1016/j.pneurobio.2009.01.003

Kaur, C., Rathnasamy, G., and Ling, E. (2013). Roles of activated microglia in hypoxia induced neuroinflammation in the developing brain and the retina. *J. Neuroimmune Pharmacol.* 8, 66–78. doi: 10.1007/s11481-012-9347-2

Kemp, G. J., and Radda, G. K. (1994). Quantitative interpretation of bioenergetic data from 31P and 1H magnetic resonance spectroscopic studies of skeletal muscle: an analytical review. *Magn. Reson. Q.* 10, 43–63.

Kida, H., Nomura, S., Shinoyama, M., Ideguchi, M., Owada, Y., and Suzuki, M. (2013). The effect of hypothermia therapy on cortical laminar disruption following ischemic injury in neonatal mice. *PLoS ONE* 8:e68877. doi: 10.1371/journal.pone.0068877

Kim, G. S., Cho, S., Nelson, J. W., Zipfel, G. J., and Han, B. H. (2014). TrkB agonist antibody pretreatment enhances neuronal survival and long-term sensory motor function following hypoxic ischemic injury in neonatal rats. *PLoS ONE* 9:e88962. doi: 10.1371/journal.pone.0088962

Kinney, H. C., Haynes, R. L., Xu, G., Andiman, S. E., Folkerth, R. D., Sleeper, L. A., et al. (2012). Neuron deficit in the white matter and subplate in periventricular leukomalacia. *Ann. Neurol.* 71, 397–406. doi: 10.1002/ana.22612

Kletkiewicz, H., Nowakowska, A., Siejka, A., Mila-Kierzenkowska, C., Wozniak, A., Caputa, M., et al. (2016). Deferoxamine prevents cerebral glutathione and vitamin E depletions in asphyxiated neonatal rats: role of body temperature. *Int. J. Hyperthermia* 32, 211–220. doi: 10.3109/02656736.2015.1125955

Klionsky, D. J., and Emr, S. D. (2000). Autophagy as a regulated pathway of cellular degradation. *Science* 290, 1717–1721. doi: 10.1126/science.290.5497.1717

Kniesel, U., Risau, W., and Wolburg, H. (1996). Development of blood-brain barrier tight junctions in the rat cortex. *Brain Res. Dev. Brain Res.* 96, 229–240. doi: 10.1016/0165-3806(96)00117-4

Koh, S., and Jensen, F. E. (2001). Topiramate blocks perinatal hypoxia-induced seizures in rat pups. *Ann. Neurol.* 50, 366–372. doi: 10.1002/ana.1122

Koike, M., Shibata, M., Tadakoshi, M., Gotoh, K., Komatsu, M., Waguri, S., et al. (2008). Inhibition of autophagy prevents hippocampal pyramidal neuron death after hypoxic-ischemic injury. *Am. J. Pathol.* 172, 454–469. doi: 10.2353/ajpath.2008.070876

Kondo, S., Al-Hasani, H., Hoerder-Suabedissen, A., Wang, W. Z., and Molnár, Z. (2015). Secretory function in subplate neurons during cortical development. *Front. Neurosci.* 9:100. doi: 10.3389/fnins.2015.00100

Kondo, S., Hino, S. I., Saito, A., Kanemoto, S., Kawasaki, N., Asada, R., et al. (2012). Activation of OASIS family, ER stress transducers, is dependent on its stabilization. *Cell Death Differ.* 19, 1939–1949. doi: 10.1038/cdd.2012.77

Kondo, S., Murakami, T., Tatsumi, K., Ogata, M., Kanemoto, S., Otori, K., et al. (2005). OASIS, a CREB/ATF-family member, modulates UPR signalling in astrocytes. *Nat. Cell Biol.* 7, 186–194. doi: 10.1038/ncb1213

Kondo, S., Saito, A., Asada, R., Kanemoto, S., and Imaizumi, K. (2011). Physiological unfolded protein response regulated by OASIS family members, transmembrane bZIP transcription factors. *IUBMB Life* 63, 233–239. doi: 10.1002/iub.433

Kostovic, I., Jovanov-Milosevic, N., Rados, M., Sedmak, G., Benjak, V., Kostovic-Srzentic, M., et al. (2014). Perinatal and early postnatal reorganization of the subplate and related cellular compartments in the human cerebral wall as revealed by histological and MRI approaches. *Brain Struct. Funct.* 219, 231–253. doi: 10.1007/s00429-012-0496-0

Kostovic, I., and Judas, M. (2006). Prolonged coexistence of transient and permanent circuitry elements in the developing cerebral cortex of fetuses and preterm infants. *Dev. Med. Child Neurol.* 48, 388–393. doi: 10.1017/S0012162206000831

Kostovic, I., and Judas, M. (2010). The development of the subplate and thalamocortical connections in the human foetal brain. *Acta Paediatr.* 99, 1119–1127. doi: 10.1111/j.1651-2227.2010.01811.x

Kostovic, I., Judas, M., Rados, M., and Hrabac, P. (2002). Laminar organization of the human fetal cerebrum revealed by histochemical markers and magnetic resonance imaging. *Cereb. Cortex* 12, 536–544. doi: 10.1093/cercor/12.5.536

Kostovic, I., Judas, M., and Sedmak, G. (2011). Developmental history of the subplate zone, subplate neurons and interstitial white matter neurons: relevance for schizophrenia. *Int. J. Dev. Neurosci.* 29, 193–205. doi: 10.1016/j.ijdevneu.2010.09.005

Kostovic, I., and Rakic, P. (1990). Developmental history of the transient subplate zone in the visual and somatosensory cortex of the macaque monkey and human brain. *J. Comp. Neurol.* 297, 441–470. doi: 10.1002/cne.902970309

Kracer, B., Hintz, S. R., Van Meurs, K. P., and Lee, H. C. (2014). Hypothermia therapy for neonatal hypoxic ischemic encephalopathy in the state of California. *J. Pediatr.* 165, 267–273. doi: 10.1016/j.jpeds.2014.04.052

Krajnc, D., Norton, H. N., and Hadjiconstantinou, M. (1996). Glutamate, glutamine and glutamine synthetase in the neonatal rat brain following hypoxia. *Brain Res.* 707, 134–137. doi: 10.1016/0006-8993(95)01372-5

Krajnc, D., Wemlinger, T. A., Neff, N. H., and Hadjiconstantinou, M. (1994). Neonatal hypoxia: early neurotransmitter responses and the consequences of treatment with GM1 ganglioside. *J. Pharmacol. Exp. Ther.* 271, 1299–1305.

Krueger, S. R., Ghisu, G. P., Cinelli, P., Gschwend, T. P., Osterwalder, T., Wolfer, D. P., et al. (1997). Expression of neuroserpin, an inhibitor of tissue plasminogen activator, in the developing and adult nervous system of the mouse. *J. Neurosci.* 17, 8984–8996.

Krystosek, A., and Seeds, N. W. (1981a). Plasminogen activator release at the neuronal growth cone. *Science* 213, 1532–1534.

Krystosek, A., and Seeds, N. W. (1981b). Plasminogen activator secretion by granule neurons in cultures of developing cerebellum. *Proc. Natl. Acad. Sci. U.S.A.* 78, 7810–7814.

Kuan, C., Lawrence, D. A., Yang, D. E., and Adhami, F. (2010). Plasminogen Activator Inhibitor Amelioration of Newborn Hypoxic Ischemic Brain Injury. US 20100286053.

L'Abee, C., de Vries, L. S., van der Grond, J., and Groenendaal, F. (2005). Early diffusion-weighted MRI and 1H-magnetic resonance spectroscopy in asphyxiated full-term neonates. *Biol. Neonate* 88, 306–312. doi: 10.1159/000087628

Lafemina, M. J., Sheldon, R. A., and Ferriero, D. M. (2006). Acute hypoxia-ischemia results in hydrogen peroxide accumulation in neonatal but not adult mouse brain. *Pediatr. Res.* 59, 680–683. doi: 10.1203/01.pdr.0000214891.35363.6a

Lai, M. C., and Yang, S. N. (2011). Perinatal hypoxic-ischemic encephalopathy. *J. Biomed. Biotechnol.* 2011:609813. doi: 10.1155/2011/609813

Lam, J. S., Anderson, E. M., and Hao, Y. (2014). LPS quantitation procedures. *Methods Mol. Biol.* 1149, 375–402. doi: 10.1007/978-1-4939-0473-0_31

Laptook, A. R., Shankaran, S., Ambalavanan, N., Carlo, W. A., McDonald, S. A., Higgins, R. D., et al. (2009). Outcome of term infants using apgar scores at 10 minutes following hypoxic-ischemic encephalopathy. *Pediatrics* 124, 1619–1626. doi: 10.1542/peds.2009-0934

Laroia, N., McBride, L., Baggs, R., and Guillet, R. (1997). Dextromethorphan ameliorates effects of neonatal hypoxia on brain morphology and seizure threshold in rats. *Dev. Brain Res.* 100, 29–34. doi: 10.1016/S0165-3806(97)00018-7

Larroche, J. C. (1977). *Developmental Pathology of the Neonate.* Amsterdam: Excerpta Medica.

Larroque, B., Breart, G., Kaminski, M., Dehan, M., Andre, M., Burguet, A., et al. (2004). Survival of very preterm infants: epipage, a population based cohort study. *Arch. Dis. Child. Fetal Neonatal Ed.* 89, F139–F144. doi: 10.1136/adc.2002.020396

Lawn, J. E., Cousens, S., Zupan, J., and Lancet Neonatal Survival Steering Team. (2005). 4 million neonatal deaths: when? Where? Why? *Lancet* 365, 891–900.

Lebeurrier, N., Liot, G., Lopez-Atalaya, J., Fernandez-Monreal, M., Sonderegger, P., Vivien, D., et al. (2005a). Neuroprotective activity of neuroserpin against NMDA receptor-mediated excitotoxicity. *J. Cereb. Blood Flow Metab.* 25, S455.

Lebeurrier, N., Liot, G., Lopez-Atalaya, J. P., Orset, C., Fernandez-Monreal, M., Sonderegger, P., et al. (2005b). The brain-specific tissue-type plasminogen activator inhibitor, neuroserpin, protects neurons against excitotoxicity both in vitro and in vivo. *Mol. Cell. Neurosci.* 30, 552–558.

Lee, A. C., Kozuki, N., Blencowe, H., Vos, T., Bahalim, A., Darmstadt, G. L., et al. (2013). Intrapartum-related neonatal encephalopathy incidence and impairment at regional and global levels for 2010 with trends from 1990. *Pediatr. Res.* 74(Suppl. 1), 50–72. doi: 10.1038/pr.2013.206

Lee, A. S. (1987). Coordinated regulation of a set of genes by glucose and calcium ionophores in mammalian cells. *Trends Biochem. Sci.* 12, 20–23. doi: 10.1016/0968-0004(87)90011-9

Lee, A. S. (2001). The glucose-regulated proteins: stress induction and clinical applications. *Trends Biochem. Sci.* 26, 504–510. doi: 10.1016/S0968-0004(01)01908-9

Lee, A. S. (2005). The ER chaperone and signaling regulator GRP78/BiP as a monitor of endoplasmic reticulum stress. *Methods* 35, 373–381. doi: 10.1016/j.ymeth.2004.10.010

Lee, B. S., Woo, C., Kim, S., and Kim, K. (2010). Long-term neuroprotective effect of postischemic hypothermia in a neonatal rat model of severe hypoxic ischemic encephalopathy: a comparative study on the duration and depth of hypothermia. *Pediatr. Res.* 68, 303–308. doi: 10.1203/00006450-201011001-00592

Lee, T. W., Coates, L. C., and Birch, N. P. (2008). Neuroserpin regulates N-cadherin-mediated cell adhesion independently of its activity as an inhibitor of tissue plasminogen activator. *J. Neurosci. Res.* 86, 1243–1253. doi: 10.1002/jnr.21592

Lee, T. W., Tsang, V. W., and Birch, N. P. (2015a). Physiological and pathological roles of tissue plasminogen activator and its inhibitor neuroserpin in the nervous system. *Front. Cell. Neurosci.* 9:396. doi: 10.3389/fncel.2015.00396

Lee, T. W., Yang, A. S., Brittain, T., and Birch, N. P. (2015b). An analysis approach to identify specific functional sites in orthologous proteins using sequence and structural information: application to neuroserpin reveals regions that differentially regulate inhibitory activity. *Proteins* 83, 135–152. doi: 10.1002/prot.24711

Legido, A., Clancy, R. R., and Berman, P. H. (1991). Neurologic outcome after electroencephalographically proven neonatal seizures. *Pediatrics* 88, 583–596.

Lehnardt, S., Massillon, L., Follett, P., Jensen, F. E., Ratan, R., Rosenberg, P. A., et al. (2003). Activation of innate immunity in the CNS triggers neurodegeneration through a Toll-like receptor 4-dependent pathway. *Proc. Natl. Acad. Sci. U.S.A.* 100, 8514–8519. doi: 10.1073/pnas.1432609100

Lein, E. S., Finney, E. M., McQuillen, P. S., and Shatz, C. J. (1999). Subplate neuron ablation alters neurotrophin expression and ocular dominance column formation. *Proc. Natl. Acad. Sci. U.S.A.* 96, 13491–13495. doi: 10.1073/pnas.96.23.13491

Leonardo, C. C., and Pennypacker, K. R. (2009). Neuroinflammation and MMPs: potential therapeutic targets in neonatal hypoxic-ischemic injury. *J. Neuroinflammation* 6:13. doi: 10.1186/1742-2094-6-13

Levene, M., Grindulis, H., Sands, C., and Moore, J. (1986). Comparison of two methods of predicting outcome in perinatal asphyxia. *Lancet* 327, 67–69. doi: 10.1016/S0140-6736(86)90718-X

Leviton, A., and Gressens, P. (2007). Neuronal damage accompanies perinatal white-matter damage. *Trends Neurosci.* 30, 473–478. doi: 10.1016/j.tins.2007.05.009

Leviton, A., Paneth, N., Reuss, M. L., Susser, M., Allred, E. N., Dammann, O., et al. (1999). Maternal infection, fetal inflammatory response, and brain damage in very low birth weight infants. *Dev. Epidemiol. Network Invest. Pediatr. Res.* 46, 566–575. doi: 10.1203/00006450-199911000-00013

Li, A. M., Chau, V., Poskitt, K. J., Sargent, M. A., Lupton, B. A., Hill, A., et al. (2009). White matter injury in term newborns with neonatal encephalopathy. *Pediatr. Res.* 61, 85–89. doi: 10.1203/PDR.0b013e31818912d2

Li, C., and Jackson, R. M. (2002). Reactive species mechanisms of cellular hypoxia-reoxygenation injury. *Am. J. Physiol. Cell Physiol.* 282, C227–C241. doi: 10.1152/ajpcell.00112.2001

Li, M., Yu, A., Zhang, F., Dai, G., Cheng, H., Wang, X., et al. (2012). Treatment of one case of cerebral palsy combined with posterior visual pathway injury using autologous bone marrow mesenchymal stem cells. *J. Trans. Med.* 10:100. doi: 10.1186/1479-5876-10-100

Li, P., Nijhawan, D., Budihardjo, I., Srinivasula, S. M., Ahmad, M., Alnemri, E. S., et al. (1997). Cytochrome c and dATP-dependent formation of Apaf-1/caspase-9 complex initiates an apoptotic protease cascade. *Cell* 91, 479–489. doi: 10.1016/S0092-8674(00)80434-1

Liao, Y., Cotten, M., Tan, S., Kurtzberg, J., and Cairo, M. S. (2013). Rescuing the neonatal brain from hypoxic injury with autologous cord blood. *Bone Marrow Transplant.* 48, 890–900. doi: 10.1038/bmt.2012.169

Liauw, L., van Wezel-Meijler, G., Veen, S., van Buchem, M. A., and van der Grond, J. (2009). Do apparent diffusion coefficient measurements predict outcome in children with neonatal hypoxic-ischemic encephalopathy? *AJNR Am. J. Neuroradiol.* 30, 264–270. doi: 10.3174/ajnr.A1318

Lieblein-Boff, J. C., McKim, D. B., Shea, D. T., Wei, P., Deng, Z., Sawicki, C., et al. (2013). Neonatal *E. coli* infection causes neuro-behavioral deficits associated with hypomyelination and neuronal sequestration of iron. *J. Neurosci.* 33, 16334–16345. doi: 10.1523/JNEUROSCI.0708-13.2013

Lin, E. P., Miles, L., Hughes, E. A., McCann, J. C., Vorhees, C. V., McAuliffe, J. J., et al. (2014). A combination of mild hypothermia and sevoflurane affords long-term protection in a modified neonatal mouse model of cerebral hypoxia-ischemia. *Anesth. Analg.* 119, 1158–1173. doi: 10.1213/ANE.0000000000000262

Liu, Y., Silverstein, F. S., Skoff, R., and Barks, J. D. (2002). Hypoxic-ischemic oligodendroglial injury in neonatal rat brain. *Pediatr. Res.* 51, 25–33. doi: 10.1203/00006450-200201000-00007

Lochner, J. E., Honigman, L. S., Grant, W. F., Gessford, S. K., Hansen, A. B., Silverman, M. A., et al. (2006). Activity-dependent release of tissue plasminogen activator from the dendritic spines of hippocampal neurons revealed by live-cell imaging. *J. Neurobiol.* 66, 564–577. doi: 10.1002/neu.20250

Lockshin, R. A., and Zakeri, Z. (1994). Programmed cell death: early changes in metamorphosing cells. *Biochem. Cell Biol.* 72, 589–596. doi: 10.1139/o94-078

Lodish, H. F. (1988). Transport of secretory and membrane glycoproteins from the rough endoplasmic reticulum to the Golgi. A rate-limiting step in protein maturation and secretion. *J. Biol. Chem.* 263, 2107–2110.

Lorek, A., Takei, Y., Cady, E. B., Wyatt, J. S., Penrice, J., Edwards, A. D., et al. (1994). Delayed ("secondary") cerebral energy failure after acute hypoxia-ischemia in the newborn piglet: continuous 48-hour studies by phosphorus magnetic resonance spectroscopy. *Pediatr. Res.* 36, 699–706. doi: 10.1203/00006450-199412000-00003

Loron, G., Olivier, P., See, H., Le Sache, N., Angulo, L., Biran, V., et al. (2011). Ciprofloxacin prevents myelination delay in neonatal rats subjected to *E. coli* sepsis. *Ann. Neurol.* 69, 341–351. doi: 10.1002/ana.22190

Lubics, A., Reglödi, D., Tamás, A., Kiss, P., Szalai, M., Szalontay, L., et al. (2005). Neurological reflexes and early motor behavior in rats subjected to neonatal hypoxic–ischemic injury. *Behav. Brain Res.* 157, 157–165. doi: 10.1016/j.bbr.2004.06.019

Ma, J., Tong, Y., Yu, D., and Mao, M. (2012a). Tissue plasminogen activator-independent roles of neuroserpin in the central nervous system. *Neural Regen. Res.* 7, 146–151. doi: 10.3969/j.issn.1673-5374.2012.02.012

Ma, J., Yu, D., Tong, Y., and Mao, M. (2012b). Effect of neuroserpin in a neonatal hypoxic-ischemic injury model ex vivo. *Biol. Res.* 45, 357–362. doi: 10.4067/S0716-97602012000400005

Magnani, D., Hasenpusch-Theil, K., and Theil, T. (2013). Gli3 controls subplate formation and growth of cortical axons. *Cereb. Cortex* 23, 2542–2551. doi: 10.1093/cercor/bhs237

Malaeb, S. N., Davis, J. M., Pinz, I. M., Newman, J. L., Dammann, O., and Rios, M. (2014). Effect of sustained postnatal systemic inflammation on hippocampal volume and function in mice. *Pediatr. Res.* 76, 363–369. doi: 10.1038/pr.2014.106

Malik, G. K., Trivedi, R., Gupta, R. K., Hasan, K. M., Hasan, M., Gupta, A., et al. (2006). Serial quantitative diffusion tensor MRI of the term neonates with hypoxic-ischemic encephalopathy (HIE). *Neuropediatrics* 37, 337–343. doi: 10.1055/s-2007-964869

Mallard, C., Davidson, J. O., Tan, S., Green, C. R., Bennet, L., Robertson, N. J., et al. (2013). Astrocytes and microglia in acute cerebral injury underlying cerebral palsy associated with preterm birth. *Pediatr. Res.* 75, 234–240. doi: 10.1038/pr.2013.188

Mallard, C., Welin, A. K., Peebles, D., Hagberg, H., and Kjellmer, I. (2003). White matter injury following systemic endotoxemia or asphyxia in the fetal sheep. *Neurochem. Res.* 28, 215–223. doi: 10.1023/A:1022368915400

Mallard, E. C., Williams, C. E., Gunn, A. J., Gunning, M. I., and Gluckman, P. D. (1993). Frequent episodes of brief ischemia sensitize the fetal sheep brain to neuronal loss and induce striatal injury. *Pediatr. Res.* 33, 61–65. doi: 10.1203/00006450-199301000-00013

Marini, A. M., Jiang, X., Wu, X., Pan, H., Guo, Z., Mattson, M. P., et al. (2007). Preconditioning and neurotrophins: a model for brain adaptation to seizures, ischemia and other stressful stimuli. *Amino Acids* 32, 299–304. doi: 10.1007/s00726-006-0414-y

Marin-Padilla, M. (1996). Developmental neuropathology and impact of perinatal brain damage. I: hemorrhagic lesions of neocortex. *J. Neuropathol. Exp. Neurol.* 55, 758–773. doi: 10.1097/00005072-199607000-00002

Marin-Padilla, M. (1997). Developmental neuropathology and impact of perinatal brain damage. II: white matter lesions of the neocortex. *J. Neuropathol. Exp. Neurol.* 56, 219–235. doi: 10.1097/00005072-199703000-00001

Marin-Padilla, M. (1999). Developmental neuropathology and impact of perinatal brain damage. III: gray matter lesions of the neocortex. *J. Neuropathol. Exp. Neurol.* 58, 407–429. doi: 10.1097/00005072-199905000-00001

Marques-Smith, A., Lyngholm, D., Kaufmann, A. K., Stacey, J. A., Hoerder-Suabedissen, A., Becker, E. B., et al. (2016). A transient translaminar GABAergic interneuron circuit connects thalamocortical recipient layers in neonatal somatosensory cortex. *Neuron* 89, 536–549. doi: 10.1016/j.neuron.2016.01.015

Marret, S., Mukendi, R., Gadisseux, J. F., Gressens, P., and Evrard, P. (1995). Effect of ibotenate on brain development: an excitotoxic mouse model of microgyria and posthypoxic-like lesions. *J. Neuropathol. Exp. Neurol.* 54, 358–370. doi: 10.1097/00005072-199505000-00009

Martin, L. J., Brambrink, A., Koehler, R. C., and Traystman, R. J. (1997). Primary sensory and forebrain motor systems in the newborn brain are preferentially damaged by hypoxia-ischemia. *J. Compar. Neurol.* 377, 262–285. doi: 10.1002/(SICI)1096-9861(19970113)377:2<262::AID-CNE8>3.0.CO;2-1

Martin, N., Bossenmeyer-Pourie, C., Koziel, V., Jazi, R., Audonnet, S., Vert, P., et al. (2012). Non-injurious neonatal hypoxia confers resistance to brain senescence in aged male rats. *PLoS ONE* 7:e48828. doi: 10.1371/journal.pone.0048828

Martin, R., Mozet, C., Martin, H., Welt, K., Engel, C., and Fitzl, G. (2011). The effect of Ginkgo biloba extract (EGb 761) on parameters of oxidative stress in different regions of aging rat brains after acute hypoxia. *Aging Clin. Exp. Res.* 23, 255–263. doi: 10.3275/7229

Martinez-Biarge, M., Diez-Sebastian, J., Kapellou, O., Gindner, D., Allsop, J. M., Rutherford, M. A., et al. (2011). Predicting motor outcome and death in term hypoxic-ischemic encephalopathy. *Neurology* 76, 2055–2061. doi: 10.1212/WNL.0b013e31821f442d

McDonald, F. B., Dempsey, E. M., and O'Halloran, K. D. (2016). Early life exposure to chronic intermittent hypoxia primes increased susceptibility to hypoxia-induced weakness in rat sternohyoid muscle during adulthood. *Front. Physiol.* 7:69. doi: 10.3389/fphys.2016.00069

McDonald, J. W., Behrens, M. I., Chung, C., Bhattacharyya, T., and Choi, D. W. (1997). Susceptibility to apoptosis is enhanced in immature cortical neurons. *Brain Res.* 759, 228–232. doi: 10.1016/S0006-8993(97)00248-5

McDonald, J. W., and Johnston, M. V. (1992). Neuroprotective synergism of 2-amino-3-phosphonoproprionate (D,L-AP3) and MK-801 against ibotenate induced brain injury. *Neurosci. Lett.* 145, 213–216. doi: 10.1016/0304-3940(92)90025-3

McDonald, J. W., Roeser, N. F., Silverstein, F. S., and Johnston, M. V. (1989a). Quantitative assessment of neuroprotection against NMDA-induced brain injury. *Exp. Neurol.* 106, 289–296.

McDonald, J. W., Silverstein, F. S., Cardona, D., Hudson, C., Chen, R., and Johnston, M. V. (1990). Systemic administration of MK-801 protects against N-methyl-D-aspartate- and quisqualate-mediated neurotoxicity in perinatal rats. *Neuroscience* 36, 589–599. doi: 10.1016/0306-4522(90)90002-L

McDonald, J. W., Silverstein, F. S., and Johnston, M. V. (1988). Neurotoxicity of N-methyl-D-aspartate is markedly enhanced in developing rat central nervous system. *Brain Res.* 459, 200–203. doi: 10.1016/0006-8993(88)90306-X

McDonald, J. W., Silverstein, F. S., and Johnston, M. V. (1989b). Neuroprotective effects of MK-801, TCP, PCP and CPP against N-methyl-D-aspartate induced neurotoxicity in an in vivo perinatal rat model. *Brain Res.* 490, 33–40.

McDonald, J. W., Uckele, J., Silverstein, F. S., and Johnston, M. V. (1989c). HA-966 (1-hydroxy-3-aminopyrrolidone-2) selectively reduces N-methyl-D-aspartate (n.d.)-mediated brain damage. *Neurosci. Lett.* 104, 167–170.

McKinstry, R. C., Miller, J. H., Snyder, A. Z., Mathur, A., Schefft, G. L., Almli, C. R., et al. (2002). A prospective, longitudinal diffusion tensor imaging study of brain injury in newborns. *Neurology* 59, 824–833. doi: 10.1212/WNL.59.6.824

McLean, C., and Ferriero, D. (2004). Mechanisms of hypoxic-ischemic injury in the term infant. *Semin. Perinatol.* 28, 425–432. doi: 10.1053/j.semperi.2004.10.005

McPherson, R. J., and Juul, S. E. (2010). Erythropoietin for infants with hypoxic-ischemic encephalopathy. *Curr. Opin. Pediatr.* 22, 139–145. doi: 10.1097/MOP.0b013e328336eb57

McQuillen, P. S., and Ferriero, D. M. (2004). Selective vulnerability in the developing central nervous system. *Pediatr. Neurol.* 30, 227–235. doi: 10.1016/j.pediatrneurol.2003.10.001

McQuillen, P. S., and Ferriero, D. M. (2005). Perinatal subplate neuron injury: implications for cortical development and plasticity. *Brain Pathol.* 15, 250–260. doi: 10.1111/j.1750-3639.2005.tb00528.x

McQuillen, P. S., Sheldon, R. A., Shatz, C. J., and Ferriero, D. M. (2003). Selective vulnerability of subplate neurons after early neonatal hypoxia-ischemia. *J. Neurosci.* 23, 3308–3315.

McRae, A., Gilland, E., Bona, E., and Hagberg, H. (1995). Microglia activation after neonatal hypoxic-ischemia. *Dev. Brain Res.* 84, 245–252. doi: 10.1016/0165-3806(94)00177-2

Meldrum, B. (1990). Protection against ischaemic neuronal damage by drugs acting on excitatory neurotransmission. *Cerebrovasc. Brain Metab. Rev.* 2, 27–57.

Ment, L. R., Bada, H. S., Barnes, P., Grant, P. E., Hirtz, D., Papile, L. A., et al. (2002). Practice parameter: neuroimaging of the neonate: report of the quality standards subcommittee of the american academy of neurology and the practice committee of the child neurology society. *Neurology* 58, 1726–1738. doi: 10.1212/WNL.58.12.1726

Ment, L. R., Duncan, C. C., and Ehrenkranz, R. A. (1984). Perinatal cerebral infarction. *Ann. Neurol.* 16, 559–568. doi: 10.1002/ana.410160506

Ment, L. R., Stewart, W. B., Ardito, T. A., and Madri, J. A. (1991). Beagle pup germinal matrix maturation studies. *Stroke* 22, 390–395. doi: 10.1161/01.STR.22.3.390

Mercuri, E., Ricci, D., Cowan, F. M., Lessing, D., Frisone, M. F., Haataja, L., et al. (2000). Head growth in infants with hypoxic-ischemic encephalopathy: correlation with neonatal magnetic resonance imaging. *Pediatrics* 106(2 Pt 1), 235–243. doi: 10.1542/peds.106.2.235

Miguel, P. M., Schuch, C. P., Rojas, J. J., Carletti, J. V., Deckmann, I., Martinato, L. H. M., et al. (2015). Neonatal hypoxia-ischemia induces attention-deficit hyperactivity disorder-like behavior in rats. *Behav. Neurosci.* 129, 309–320. doi: 10.1037/bne0000063

Mikati, M. A., El Hokayem, J. A., and El Sabban, M. E. (2007). Effects of a single dose of erythropoietin on subsequent seizure susceptibility in rats exposed to acute hypoxia at P10. *Epilepsia* 48, 175–181. doi: 10.1111/j.1528-1167.2006.00900.x

Mikati, M. A., Zeinieh, M. P., Kurdi, R. M., Harb, S. A., El Hokayem, J. A., Daderian, R. H., et al. (2005). Long-term effects of acute and of chronic hypoxia on behavior and on hippocampal histology in the developing brain. *Dev. Brain Res.* 157, 98–102. doi: 10.1016/j.devbrainres.2005.03.007

Mikhailenko, V. A., Butkevich, I. P., Bagaeva, T. R., Makukhina, G. V., and Otellin, V. A. (2009). Short- and long-term influences of hypoxia during early postnatal period of development on behavioral and hormonal responses in rats. *Neurosci. Lett.* 464, 214–217. doi: 10.1016/j.neulet.2009.08.047

Miller, S. L., Wallace, E. M., and Walker, D. W. (2012). Antioxidant therapies: a potential role in perinatal medicine. *Neuroendocrinology* 96, 13–23. doi: 10.1159/000336378

Miller, S. P., Ramaswamy, V., Michelson, D., Barkovich, A. J., Holshouser, B., Wycliffe, N., et al. (2005). Patterns of brain injury in term neonatal encephalopathy. *J. Pediatr.* 146, 453–460. doi: 10.1016/j.jpeds.2004.12.026

Miller, S. P., Weiss, J., Barnwell, A., Ferriero, D. M., Latal-Hajnal, B., Ferrer-Rogers, A., et al. (2002). Seizure-associated brain injury in term newborns with perinatal asphyxia. *Neurology* 58, 542–548. doi: 10.1212/WNL.58.4.542

Miranda, E., and Lomas, D. (2006). Neuroserpin: a serpin to think about. *Cell. Mol. Life Sci.* 63, 709–722. doi: 10.1007/s00018-005-5077-4

Mishra, O. P., and Delivoria-Papadopoulos, M. (1989). Lipid peroxidation in developing fetal guinea pig brain during normoxia and hypoxia. *Brain Res. Dev. Brain Res.* 45, 129–135. doi: 10.1016/0165-3806(89)90014-X

Mishra, O. P., and Delivoria-Papadopoulos, M. (1999). Cellular mechanisms of hypoxic injury in the developing brain. *Brain Res. Bull.* 48, 233–238. doi: 10.1016/S0361-9230(98)00170-1

Mitha, A., Foix-L'Helias, L., Arnaud, C., Marret, S., Vieux, R., Aujard, Y., et al. (2013). Neonatal infection and 5-year neurodevelopmental outcome of very preterm infants. *Pediatrics* 132, e372-80. doi: 10.1542/peds.2012-3979

Mohsenifar, A., Lotfi, A. S., Ranjbar, B., Allameh, A., Zaker, F., Hasani, L., et al. (2007). A study of the oxidation-induced conformational and functional changes in neuroserpin. *Iran. Biomed. J.* 11, 41–46.

Molnár, Z., Adams, R., and Blakemore, C. (1998). Mechanisms underlying the early establishment of thalamocortical connections in the rat. *J. Neurosci.* 18, 5723–5745.

Moorcraft, J., Bolas, N. M., Ives, N. K., Ouwerkerk, R., Smyth, J., Rajagopalan, B., et al. (1991). Global and depth resolved phosphorus magnetic resonance spectroscopy to predict outcome after birth asphyxia. *Arch. Dis. Child* 66, 1119–1123. doi: 10.1136/adc.66.10_Spec_No.1119

Mortola, J. P. (1999). How newborn mammals cope with hypoxia. *Respir. Physiol.* 116, 95–103. doi: 10.1016/S0034-5687(99)00038-9

Mortola, J. P., and Naso, L. (1998). Thermogenesis in newborn rats after prenatal or postnatal hypoxia. *J. Appl. Physiol.* 85, 84–90.

Munuswamy-Ramanujam, G., Dai, E., Liu, L., Shnabel, M., Sun, Y. M., Bartee, M., et al. (2010). Neuroserpin, a thrombolytic serine protease inhibitor (serpin), blocks transplant vasculopathy with associated modification of T-helper cell subsets. *Thromb. Haemost.* 103, 545–555. doi: 10.1160/TH09-07-0441

Muramatsu, K., Fukuda, A., Togari, H., Wada, Y., and Nishino, H. (1997). Vulnerability to cerebral hypoxic-ischemic insult in neonatal but not in adult rats is in parallel with disruption of the blood-brain barrier. *Stroke* 28, 2281–2288; discussion 2288–2289. doi: 10.1161/01.str.28.11.2281

Murray, D. M., Bala, P., O'Connor, C. M., Ryan, C. A., Connolly, S., and Boylan, G. B. (2010). The predictive value of early neurological examination in neonatal hypoxic-ischaemic encephalopathy and neurodevelopmental outcome at 24 months. *Dev. Med. Child Neurol.* 52, e55–e59. doi: 10.1111/j.1469-8749.2009.03550.x

Murray, D. M., Boylan, G. B., Ryan, C. A., and Connolly, S. (2009). Early EEG findings in hypoxic-ischemic encephalopathy predict outcomes at 2 years. *Pediatrics* 124, e459–e467. doi: 10.1542/peds.2008-2190

Murray, D. M., O'Connor, C. M., Ryan, C. A., Korotchikova, I., and Boylan, G. B. (2016). Early EEG grade and outcome at 5 years after mild neonatal hypoxic ischemic encephalopathy. *Pediatrics* 138, e20160659. doi: 10.1542/peds.2016-0659

Myers, M. (1975). "Investigation of skin flap necrosis," in *Skin Flaps*, eds W. C. Grabb and M. B. Myers (Boston, MA: Little, Brown and Company), 3.

Nagel, S., Papadakis, M., Pfleger, K., Grond-Ginsbach, C., Buchan, A., and Wagner, S. (2012). Microarray analysis of the global gene expression profile following hypothermia and transient focal cerebral ischemia. *Neuroscience* 208, 109–122. doi: 10.1016/j.neuroscience.2012.01.048

Nakajima, W., Ishida, A., Lange, M. S., Gabrielson, K. L., Wilson, M. A., Martin, L. J., et al. (2000). Apoptosis has a prolonged role in the neurodegeneration after hypoxic ischemia in the newborn rat. *J. Neurosci.* 20, 7994–8004.

Nakajima, W., Ishida, A., and Takada, G. (1997). Magnesium attenuates a striatal dopamine increase induced by anoxia in the neonatal rat brain: an in vivo microdialysis study. *Pediatr. Res.* 41, 809–814. doi: 10.1203/00006450-199706000-00003

Nalivaeva, N. N., Fisk, L., Aviles, R. M. C., Plesneva, S. A., Zhuravin, I. A., and Turner, A. J. (2003). Effects of prenatal hypoxia on expression of amyloid precursor protein and metallopeptidases in the rat brain. *Lett. Peptide Sci.* 10, 455–462. doi: 10.1007/BF02442577

Nash, K. B., Bonifacio, S. L., Glass, H. C., Sullivan, J. E., Barkovich, A. J., Ferriero, D. M., et al. (2011). Video-EEG monitoring in newborns with hypoxic-ischemic encephalopathy treated with hypothermia. *Neurology* 76, 556–562. doi: 10.1212/WNL.0b013e31820af91a

Navarova, J., Schmidtova, M., Ujhazy, E., Dubovicky, M., and Mach, M. (2006). Selected biochemical variables in a model of neonatal anoxia in rats. *Neuro Endocrinol. Lett.* 27(Suppl. 2), 78–81.

Neil, J., Miller, J., Mukherjee, P., and Huppi, P. S. (2002). Diffusion tensor imaging of normal and injured developing human brain - a technical review. *NMR Biomed.* 15, 543–552. doi: 10.1002/nbm.784

Ness, J. K., Romanko, M. J., Rothstein, R. P., Wood, T. L., and Levison, S. W. (2001). Perinatal hypoxia-ischemia induces apoptotic and excitotoxic death of periventricular white matter oligodendrocyte progenitors. *Dev. Neurosci.* 23, 203–208. doi: 10.1159/000046144

Neufeld, M. D., Frigon, C., Graham, A. S., and Mueller, B. A. (2005). Maternal infection and risk of cerebral palsy in term and preterm infants. *J. Perinatol.* 25, 108–113. doi: 10.1038/sj.jp.7211219

Nguyen, V., and McQuillen, P. S. (2010). AMPA and metabotropic excitoxicity explain subplate neuron vulnerability. *Neurobiol. Dis.* 37, 195–207. doi: 10.1016/j.nbd.2009.10.002

Nicole, O., Docagne, F., Ali, C., Margaill, I., Carmeliet, P., MacKenzie, E. T., et al. (2001). The proteolytic activity of tissue-plasminogen activator enhances NMDA receptor-mediated signaling. *Nat. Med.* 7, 59–64. doi: 10.1038/83358

Nijboer, C. H., Groenendaal, F., Kavelaars, A., Hagberg, H. H., van Bel, F., and Heijnen, C. J. (2007). Gender-specific neuroprotection by 2-iminobiotin after hypoxia-ischemia in the neonatal rat via a nitric oxide independent pathway. *J. Cereb. Blood Flow Metab.* 27, 282–292. doi: 10.1038/sj.jcbfm.9600342

Nijboer, C. H., van der Kooij, M. A., van Bel, F., Ohl, F., Heijnen, C. J., and Kavelaars, A. (2010). Inhibition of the JNK/AP-1 pathway reduces neuronal death and improves behavioral outcome after neonatal hypoxic–ischemic brain injury. *Brain Behav. Immun.* 24, 812–821. doi: 10.1016/j.bbi.2009.09.008

Nikolov, N. M., and Cunningham, A. J. (2003). Mild therapeutic hypothermia to improve the neurologic outcome after cardiac arrest. *Surv. Anesthesiol.* 47, 219–220. doi: 10.1097/01.sa.0000087691.31092.12

Nobuta, H., Ghiani, C. A., Paez, P. M., Spreuer, V., Dong, H., Korsak, R. A., et al. (2012). STAT3-mediated astrogliosis protects myelin development in neonatal brain injury. *Ann. Neurol.* 72, 750–765. doi: 10.1002/ana.23670

Noh, M. R., Kim, S. K., Sun, W., Park, S. K., Choi, H. C., Lim, J. H., et al. (2006). Neuroprotective effect of topiramate on hypoxic ischemic brain injury in neonatal rats. *Exp. Neurol.* 201, 470–478. doi: 10.1016/j.expneurol.2006.04.038

Northington, F. J., Chavez-Valdez, R., and Martin, L. J. (2011). Neuronal cell death in neonatal hypoxia-ischemia. *Ann. Neurol.* 69, 743–758. doi: 10.1002/ana.22419

Northington, F. J., Ferriero, D. M., Graham, E. M., Traystman, R. J., and Martin, L. J. (2001). Early neurodegeneration after hypoxia-ischemia in neonatal rat is necrosis while delayed neuronal death is apoptosis. *Neurobiol. Dis.* 8, 207–219. doi: 10.1006/nbdi.2000.0371

Northington, F. J., Graham, E. M., and Martin, L. J. (2005). Apoptosis in perinatal hypoxic–ischemic brain injury: how important is it and should it be inhibited? *Brain Res. Rev.* 50, 244–257. doi: 10.1016/j.brainresrev.2005.07.003

Northington, F. J., Zelaya, M. E., O'Riordan, D. P., Blomgren, K., Flock, D. L., Hagberg, H., et al. (2007). Failure to complete apoptosis following neonatal hypoxia-ischemia manifests as "continuum" phenotype of cell death and occurs with multiple manifestations of mitochondrial dysfunction in rodent forebrain. *Neuroscience* 149, 822–833. doi: 10.1016/j.neuroscience.2007.06.060

Novikoff, A. B. (1976). The endoplasmic reticulum: a cytochemist's view (a review). *Proc. Natl. Acad. Sci. U.S.A.* 73, 2781–2787. doi: 10.1073/pnas.73.8.2781

O'Brien, J. S., and Sampson, E. L. (1965). Myelin Membrane: a molecular abnormality. *Science* 150, 1613–1614. doi: 10.1126/science.150.3703.1613

O'Connell, B., Moritz, K., Walker, D., and Dickinson, H. (2013). Treatment of pregnant spiny mice at mid gestation with a synthetic glucocorticoid has sex-dependent effects on placental glycogen stores. *Placenta* 34, 932–940. doi: 10.1016/j.placenta.2013.06.310

Oeschger, F. M., Wang, W. Z., Lee, S., Garcia-Moreno, F., Goffinet, A. M., Arbones, M. L., et al. (2012). Gene expression analysis of the embryonic subplate. *Cereb. Cortex* 22, 1343–1359. doi: 10.1093/cercor/bhr197

Oguni, H., Sugama, M., and Osawa, M. (2008). Symptomatic parieto-occipital epilepsy as sequela of perinatal asphyxia. *Pediatr. Neurol.* 38, 345–352. doi: 10.1016/j.pediatrneurol.2007.10.016

Okiyoneda, T., Harada, K., Takeya, M., Yamahira, K., Wada, I., Shuto, T., et al. (2004). Delta F508 CFTR pool in the endoplasmic reticulum is increased by calnexin overexpression. *Mol. Biol. Cell* 15, 563–574. doi: 10.1091/mbc.E03-06-0379

Okusa, C., Oeschger, F., Ginet, V., Wang, W. Z., Hoerder-Suabedissen, A., Matsuyama, T., et al. (2014). Subplate in a rat model of preterm hypoxia-ischemia. *Ann. Clin. Transl. Neurol.* 1, 679–691. doi: 10.1002/acn3.97

Omouendze, P. L., Henry, V. J., Porte, B., Dupré, N., Carmeliet, P., Gonzalez, B. J., et al. (2013). Hypoxia-ischemia or excitotoxin-induced tissue plasminogen activator-dependent gelatinase activation in mice neonate brain microvessels. *PLoS ONE* 8:e71263. doi: 10.1371/journal.pone.0071263

Osterwalder, T., Cinelli, P., Baici, A., Pennella, A., Krueger, S. R., Schrimpf, S. P., et al. (1998). The axonally secreted serine proteinase inhibitor, neuroserpin, inhibits plasminogen activators and plasmin but not thrombin. *J. Biol. Chem.* 273, 2312–2321. doi: 10.1074/jbc.273.4.2312

Osterwalder, T., Contartese, J., Stoeckli, E. T., Kuhn, T. B., and Sonderegger, P. (1996). Neuroserpin, an axonally secreted serine protease inhibitor. *EMBO J.* 15, 2944–2953.

Otoya, R. E., Seltzer, A. M., and Donoso, A. O. (1997). Acute and long-lasting effects of neonatal hypoxia on ( )-3-[125 I] MK-801 binding to NMDA brain receptors. *Exp. Neurol.* 148, 92–99. doi: 10.1006/exnr.1997.6612

Ozer, E. A., Yilmaz, O., Akhisaroglu, M., Tuna, B., Bakiler, A. R., and Ozer, E. (2002). Heat shock protein 70 expression in neonatal rats after hypoxic stress. *J. Matern Fetal Neonatal Med.* 12, 112–117. doi: 10.1080/jmf.12.2.112.117

Palmer, C., Vannucci, R. C., and Towfighi, J. (1990). Reduction of perinatal hypoxic-ischemic brain damage with allopurinol. *Pediatr. Res.* 27(4 Pt 1), 332–336. doi: 10.1203/00006450-199004000-00003

Pang, Y., Rodts-Palenik, S., Cai, Z., Bennett, W. A., and Rhodes, P. G. (2005). Suppression of glial activation is involved in the protection of IL-10 on maternal *E. coli* induced neonatal white matter injury. *Brain Res. Dev. Brain Res.* 157, 141–149. doi: 10.1016/j.devbrainres.2005.03.015

Park, D., Shin, K., Choi, E., Choi, Y., Jang, J., Kim, J., et al. (2015). Protective effects of N-acetyl-l-cysteine in human oligodendrocyte progenitor cells and restoration of motor function in neonatal rats with hypoxic-ischemic encephalopathy. *Evid. Based Complement. Alternat. Med.* 2015:764251. doi: 10.1155/2015/764251

Park, W. S., Sung, S. I., Ahn, S. Y., Yoo, H. S., Sung, D. K., Im, G. H., et al. (2015). Hypothermia augments neuroprotective activity of mesenchymal stem cells for neonatal hypoxic-ischemic encephalopathy. *PLoS ONE* 10:e0120893. doi: 10.1371/journal.pone.0120893

Parolini, O., Alviano, F., Bergwerf, I., Boraschi, D., De Bari, C., De Waele, P., et al. (2010). Toward cell therapy using placenta-derived cells: disease mechanisms, cell biology, preclinical studies, and regulatory aspects at the round table. *Stem Cells Dev.* 19, 143–154. doi: 10.1089/scd.2009.0404

Partanen, E., Kujala, T., Naatanen, R., Liitola, A., Sambeth, A., and Huotilainen, M. (2013). Learning-induced neural plasticity of speech processing before birth. *Proc. Natl. Acad. Sci. U.S.A.* 110, 15145–15150. doi: 10.1073/pnas.1302159110

Pauliah, S. S., Shankaran, S., Wade, A., Cady, E. B., and Thayyil, S. (2013). Therapeutic hypothermia for neonatal encephalopathy in low- and middle-income countries: a systematic review and meta-analysis. *PLoS ONE* 8:e58834. doi: 10.1371/journal.pone.0058834

Paulose, C. S., Chathu, F., Khan, S. R., and Krishnakumar, A. (2008). Neuroprotective role of *Bacopa monnieri* extract in epilepsy and effect of glucose supplementation during hypoxia: glutamate receptor gene expression. *Neurochem. Res.* 33, 1663–1671. doi: 10.1007/s11064-007-9513-8

Pazaiti, A., Soubasi, V., Spandou, E., Karkavelas, G., Georgiou, T., Karalis, P., et al. (2009). Evaluation of long-lasting sensorimotor consequences following neonatal hypoxic-ischemic brain injury in rats: the neuroprotective role of MgSO4. *Neonatology* 95, 33–40. doi: 10.1159/000151753

Pazos, M., Cinquina, V., Gomez, A., Layunta, R., Santos, M., Fernández-Ruiz, J., et al. (2012). Cannabidiol administration after hypoxia–ischemia to newborn rats reduces long-term brain injury and restores neurobehavioral function. *Neuropharmacology* 63, 776–783. doi: 10.1016/j.neuropharm.2012.05.034

Pedraza, M., Hoerder-Suabedissen, A., Albert-Maestro, M. A., Molnár, Z., and De Carlos, J. A. (2014). Extracortical origin of some murine subplate cell populations. *Proc. Natl. Acad. Sci. U.S.A.* 111, 8613–8618. doi: 10.1073/pnas.1323816111

Peebles, D. M., Miller, S., Newman, J. P., Scott, R., and Hanson, M. A. (2003). The effect of systemic administration of lipopolysaccharide on cerebral haemodynamics and oxygenation in the 0.65 gestation ovine fetus in utero. *BJOG* 110, 735–743. doi: 10.1111/j.1471-0528.2003.02152.x

Pelham, H. R. (1989). Heat shock and the sorting of luminal ER proteins. *EMBO J.* 8, 3171–3176.

Pellitteri, R., Catania, M. V., Bonaccorso, C. M., Ranno, E., Dell'Albani, P., and Zaccheo, D. (2014). Viability of olfactory ensheathing cells after hypoxia and serum deprivation: Implication for therapeutic transplantation. *J. Neurosci. Res.* 92, 1757–1766. doi: 10.1002/jnr.23442

Peng, Z., Li, J., Li, Y., Yang, X., Feng, S., Han, S., et al. (2013). Downregulation of miR-181b in mouse brain following ischemic stroke induces neuroprotection against ischemic injury through targeting heat shock protein A5 and ubiquitin carboxyl-terminal hydrolase isozyme L1. *J. Neurosci. Res.* 91, 1349–1362. doi: 10.1002/jnr.23255

Penrice, J., Lorek, A., Cady, E. B., Amess, P. N., Wylezinska, M., Cooper, C. E., et al. (1997). Proton magnetic resonance spectroscopy of the brain during acute hypoxia-ischemia and delayed cerebral energy failure in the newborn piglet. *Pediatr. Res.* 41, 795–802. doi: 10.1203/00006450-199706000-00001

Pereira, L. O., Arteni, N. S., Petersen, R. C., da Rocha, A. P., Achaval, M., and Netto, C. A. (2007). Effects of daily environmental enrichment on memory deficits and brain injury following neonatal hypoxia-ischemia in the rat. *Neurobiol. Learn. Mem.* 87, 101–108. doi: 10.1016/j.nlm.2006.07.003

Perera, P. N. D., Hu, Q., Tang, J., Li, L., Barnhart, M., Doycheva, D. M., et al. (2014). Delayed remote ischemic postconditioning improves long term sensory motor deficits in a neonatal hypoxic ischemic rat model. *PLoS ONE* 9:e90258. doi: 10.1371/journal.pone.0090258

Perlman, J. M. (1997). Intrapartum hypoxic-ischemic cerebral injury and subsequent cerebral palsy: medicolegal issues. *Pediatrics* 99, 851–859. doi: 10.1542/peds.99.6.851

Perlman, J. M. (2006). Summary proceedings from the neurology group on hypoxic-ischemic encephalopathy. *Pediatrics* 117(Suppl. 1), S28–S33. doi: 10.1542/peds.2005-0620E

Perlman, J. M., and Risser, R. (1993). Severe fetal acidemia: neonatal neurologic features and short-term outcome. *Pediatr. Neurol.* 9, 277–282. doi: 10.1016/0887-8994(93)90063-I

Perrin, R. G., Rutka, J. T., Drake, J. M., Meltzer, H., Hellman, J., Jay, V., et al. (1997). Management and outcomes of posterior fossa subdural hematomas in neonates. *Neurosurgery* 40, 1190-1199; discussion 1199–1200. doi: 10.1097/00006123-199706000-00016

Petersson, K. H., Pinar, H., Stopa, E. G., Faris, R. A., Sadowska, G. B., Hanumara, R. C., et al. (2002). White matter injury after cerebral ischemia in ovine fetuses. *Pediatr. Res.* 51, 768–776. doi: 10.1203/00006450-200206000-00019

Pfeffer, S. R., and Rothman, J. E. (1987). Biosynthetic protein transport and sorting by the endoplasmic reticulum and Golgi. *Annu. Rev. Biochem.* 56, 829–852. doi: 10.1146/annurev.bi.56.070187.004145

Placencia, F. X., Kong, L., and Weisman, L. E. (2009). Treatment of methicillin-resistant *Staphylococcus aureus* in neonatal mice: lysostaphin versus vancomycin. *Pediatr. Res.* 65, 420–424. doi: 10.1203/PDR.0b013e3181994a53

Poggi, S. H., Park, J., Toso, L., Abebe, D., Roberson, R., Woodard, J. E., et al. (2005). No phenotype associated with established lipopolysaccharide model for cerebral palsy. *Am. J. Obstet. Gynecol.* 192, 727–733. doi: 10.1016/j.ajog.2004.12.053

Pogledic, I., Kostovic, I., Fallet-Bianco, C., Adle-Biassette, H., Gressens, P., and Verney, C. (2014). Involvement of the subplate zone in preterm infants with periventricular white matter injury. *Brain Pathol.* 24, 128–141. doi: 10.1111/bpa.12096

Portera-Cailliau, C., Price, D. L., and Martin, L. J. (1997a). Excitotoxic neuronal death in the immature brain is an apoptosis-necrosis morphological continuum. *J. Comp. Neurol.* 378, 70–87. doi: 10.1002/(sici)1096-9861(19970203)378:1<10::aid-cne4>3.0.co;2-n

Portera-Cailliau, C., Price, D. L., and Martin, L. J. (1997b). Non-NMDA and NMDA receptor-mediated excitotoxic neuronal deaths in adult brain are morphologically distinct: further evidence for an apoptosis-necrosis continuum. *J. Comp. Neurol.* 378, 88–104.

Pourie, G., Blaise, S., Trabalon, M., Nedelec, E., Gueant, J. L., and Daval, J. L. (2006). Mild, non-lesioning transient hypoxia in the newborn rat induces delayed brain neurogenesis associated with improved memory scores. *Neuroscience* 140, 1369–1379. doi: 10.1016/j.neuroscience.2006.02.083

Price, D. J., Aslam, S., Tasker, L., and Gillies, K. (1997). Fates of the earliest generated cells in the developing murine neocortex. *J. Comp. Neurol.* 377, 414–422. doi: 10.1002/(SICI)1096-9861(19970120)377:3<414::AID-CNE8>3.0.CO;2-5

Pryds, O., Greisen, G., Lou, H., and Friis-Hansen, B. (1990). Vasoparalysis associated with brain damage in asphyxiated term infants. *J. Pediatr.* 117(1 Pt 1), 119–125. doi: 10.1016/s0022-3476(05)72459-8

Pu, Y., Garg, A., Corby, R., Gao, J. H., Zeng, C. M., Pu, Y., et al. (2008). A positive correlation between alpha-glutamate and glutamine on brain 1H-MR spectroscopy and neonatal seizures in moderate and severe hypoxic-ischemic encephalopathy. *AJNR Am. J. Neuroradiol.* 29, 216. doi: 10.3174/ajnr.A0798

Pulera, M. R., Adams, L. M., Liu, H., Santos, D. G., Nishimura, R. N., Yang, F., et al. (1998). Apoptosis in a neonatal rat model of cerebral hypoxia-ischemia. *Stroke* 29, 2622–2630. doi: 10.1161/01.STR.29.12.2622

Puyal, J., Vaslin, A., Mottier, V., and Clarke, P. G. (2009). Postischemic treatment of neonatal cerebral ischemia should target autophagy. *Ann. Neurol.* 66, 378–389. doi: 10.1002/ana.21714

Qian, Z., Gilbert, M. E., Colicos, M. A., Kandel, E. R., and Kuhl, D. (1993). Tissue-plasminogen activator is induced as an immediate–early gene during seizure, kindling and long-term potentiation. *Nature* 361, 453–457. doi: 10.1038/361453a0

Rabi, Y., Rabi, D., and Yee, W. (2007). Room air resuscitation of the depressed newborn: a systematic review and meta-analysis. *Resuscitation* 72, 353–363. doi: 10.1016/j.resuscitation.2006.06.134

Rakhade, S. N., and Jensen, F. E. (2009). Epileptogenesis in the immature brain: emerging mechanisms. *Nat. Rev. Neurol.* 5, 380–391. doi: 10.1038/nrneurol.2009.80

Rakhade, S. N., Klein, P. M., Huynh, T., Hilario-Gomez, C., Kosaras, B., Rotenberg, A., et al. (2011). Development of later life spontaneous seizures in a rodent model of hypoxia-induced neonatal seizures. *Epilepsia* 52, 753–765. doi: 10.1111/j.1528-1167.2011.02992.x

Rastogi, R. N., Prichard, J. S., and Lowden, J. A. (1968). Elevation of phosphorus levels in serum and decreased rain content of gangliosides in rats following neonatal asphyxia. *Pediatr. Res.* 2, 125–130. doi: 10.1203/00006450-196803000-00008

Raveendran, A. T., and Skaria, P. C. (2013). Learning and cognitive deficits in hypoxic neonatal rats intensified by BAX mediated apoptosis: protective role of glucose, oxygen, and epinephrine. *Int. J. Neurosci.* 123, 80–88. doi: 10.3109/00207454.2012.731457

Reddy, K., Mallard, C., Guan, J., Marks, K., Bennet, L., Gunning, M., et al. (1998). Maturational change in the cortical response to hypoperfusion injury in the fetal sheep. *Pediatr. Res.* 43, 674–682. doi: 10.1203/00006450-199805000-00017

Redline, R. W., and O'Riordan, M. A. (2000). Placental lesions associated with cerebral palsy and neurologic impairment following term birth. *Arch. Pathol. Lab. Med.* 124, 1785–1791.

Rennie, J. M., Chorley, G., Boylan, G. B., Pressler, R., Nguyen, Y., and Hooper, R. (2004). Non-expert use of the cerebral function monitor for neonatal seizure detection. *Arch. Dis. Child. Fetal Neonatal Ed.* 89, F37–F40. doi: 10.1136/fn.89.1.f37

Represa, A., Tremblay, E., and Ben-Ari, Y. (1989). Transient increase of NMDA-binding sites in human hippocampus during development. *Neurosci. Lett.* 99, 61–66. doi: 10.1016/0304-3940(89)90265-6

Ricagno, S., Caccia, S., Sorrentino, G., Antonini, G., and Bolognesi, M. (2009). Human neuroserpin: structure and time-dependent inhibition. *J. Mol. Biol.* 388, 109–121. doi: 10.1016/j.jmb.2009.02.056

Ricagno, S., Pezzullo, M., Barbiroli, A., Manno, M., Levantino, M., Santangelo, M. G., et al. (2010). Two latent and two hyperstable polymeric forms of human neuroserpin. *Biophys. J.* 99, 3402–3411. doi: 10.1016/j.bpj.2010.09.021

Rice, J. E., Vannucci, R. C., and Brierley, J. B. (1981). The influence of immaturity on hypoxic-ischemic brain damage in the rat. *Ann. Neurol.* 9, 131–141. doi: 10.1002/ana.410090206

Richardson, B., Korkola, S., Asano, H., Challis, J., Polk, D., and Fraser, M. (1996). Regional blood flow and the endocrine response to sustained hypoxemia in the preterm ovine fetus. *Pediatr. Res.* 40, 337–343. doi: 10.1203/00006450-199608000-00024

Richardson, B. S., and Bocking, A. D. (1998). Metabolic and circulatory adaptations to chronic hypoxia in the fetus. *Comp. Biochem. Physiol. A Mol. Integr. Physiol.* 119, 717–723. doi: 10.1016/S1095-6433(98)01010-1

Richardson, B. S., Carmichael, L., Homan, J., Johnston, L., and Gagnon, R. (1996). Fetal cerebral, circulatory, and metabolic responses during heart rate decelerations with umbilical cord compression. *Am. J. Obstet. Gynecol.* 175(4 Pt 1), 929–936. doi: 10.1016/S0002-9378(96)80027-5

Richer, L. P., Shevell, M. I., and Miller, S. P. (2001). Diagnostic profile of neonatal hypotonia: an 11-year study. *Pediatr. Neurol.* 25, 32–37. doi: 10.1016/S0887-8994(01)00277-6

Richetto, J., Calabrese, F., Meyer, U., and Riva, M. A. (2013). Prenatal versus postnatal maternal factors in the development of infection-induced working memory impairments in mice. *Brain Behav. Immun.* 33, 190–200. doi: 10.1016/j.bbi.2013.07.006

Riikonen, R. S., Kero, P. O., and Simell, O. G. (1992). Excitatory amino acids in cerebrospinal fluid in neonatal asphysia. *Pediatr. Neurol.* 8, 37–40. doi: 10.1016/0887-8994(92)90050-9

Rijken, D., Wijngaards, G., and Welbergen, J. (1980). Relationship between tissue plasminogen activator and the activators in blood and vascular wall. *Thromb. Res.* 18, 815–830. doi: 10.1016/0049-3848(80)90204-2

Rijken, D., Wijngaards, G., Zaal-de Jong, M., and Welbergen, J. (1979). Purification and partial characterization of plasminogen activator from human uterine tissue. *Biochim. Biophys. Acta* 580, 140–153. doi: 10.1016/0005-2795(79)90205-8

Robertson, C., and Finer, N. (1985). Term infants with hypoxic-ischemic encephalopathy: outcome at 3.5 years. *Dev. Med. Child Neurol.* 27, 473–484. doi: 10.1111/j.1469-8749.1985.tb04571.x

Robertson, C., Finer, N., and Grace, M. (1989). School performance of survivors of neonatal encephalopathy associated with birth asphyxia at term. *J. Pediatr.* 114, 753–760. doi: 10.1016/S0022-3476(89)80132-5

Robertson, J. D., Enoksson, M., Suomela, M., Zhivotovsky, B., and Orrenius, S. (2002). Caspase-2 acts upstream of mitochondria to promote cytochrome c release during etoposide-induced apoptosis. *J. Biol. Chem.* 277, 29803–29809. doi: 10.1074/jbc.M204185200

Robertson, N. J., Cowan, F. M., Cox, I. J., and Edwards, A. D. (2002). Brain alkaline intracellular pH after neonatal encephalopathy. *Ann. Neurol.* 52, 732–742. doi: 10.1002/ana.10365

Robertson, N. J., Cox, I. J., Cowan, F. M., Counsell, S. J., Azzopardi, D., and Edwards, A. D. (1999). Cerebral intracellular lactic alkalosis persisting months after neonatal encephalopathy measured by magnetic resonance spectroscopy. *Pediatr. Res.* 46, 287–296. doi: 10.1203/00006450-199909000-00007

Robertson, N. J., and Iwata, O. (2007). Bench to bedside strategies for optimizing neuroprotection following perinatal hypoxia–ischaemia in high and low resource settings. *Early Hum. Dev.* 83, 801–811. doi: 10.1016/j.earlhumdev.2007.09.015

Robinson, S., Li, Q., Dechant, A., and Cohen, M. L. (2006). Neonatal loss of gamma-aminobutyric acid pathway expression after human perinatal brain injury. *J. Neurosurg.* 104 6(Suppl.), 396–408.

Rocha-Ferreira, E., and Hristova, M. (2015). Antimicrobial peptides and complement in neonatal hypoxia-ischemia induced brain damage. *Front. Immunol.* 6:56. doi: 10.3389/fimmu.2015.00056

Rodewald, A. K., Onderdonk, A. B., Warren, H. B., and Kasper, D. L. (1992). Neonatal mouse model of group B streptococcal infection. *J. Infect. Dis.* 166, 635–639. doi: 10.1093/infdis/166.3.635

Rodriguez-Alvarez, N., Jimenez-Mateos, E. M., Dunleavy, M., Waddington, J. L., Boylan, G. B., and Henshall, D. C. (2015). Effects of hypoxia-induced neonatal seizures on acute hippocampal injury and later-life seizure susceptibility and anxiety-related behavior in mice. *Neurobiol. Dis.* 83, 100–114. doi: 10.1016/j.nbd.2015.08.023

Rodríguez-González, R., Agulla, J., Pérez-Mato, M., Sobrino, T., and Castillo, J. (2011a). Neuroprotective effect of neuroserpin in rat primary cortical cultures after oxygen and glucose deprivation and tPA. *Neurochem. Int.* 58, 337–343. doi: 10.1016/j.neuint.2010.12.006

Rodríguez-González, R., Millán, M., Sobrino, T., Miranda, E., Brea, D., de la Ossa, N. P., et al. (2011b). The natural tissue plasminogen activator inhibitor neuroserpin and acute ischaemic stroke outcome. *Thromb. Haemost.* 105, 421–429. doi: 10.1160/TH10-09-0621

Rodríguez-González, R., Sobrino, T., Rodríguez-Yáñez, M., Millán, M., Brea, D., Miranda, E., et al. (2011c). Association between neuroserpin and molecular markers of brain damage in patients with acute ischemic stroke. *J. Transl. Med.* 9:58. doi: 10.1186/1479-5876-9-58

Rodts-Palenik, S., Wyatt-Ashmead, J., Pang, Y., Thigpen, B., Cai, Z., Rhodes, P., et al. (2004). Maternal infection-induced white matter injury is reduced by treatment with interleukin-10. *Am. J. Obstet. Gynecol.* 191, 1387–1392. doi: 10.1016/j.ajog.2004.06.093

Rogalska, J., and Caputa, M. (2010). Neonatal asphyxia under hyperthermic conditions alters HPA axis function in juvenile rats. *Neurosci. Lett.* 472, 68–72. doi: 10.1016/j.neulet.2010.01.060

Rogalska, J., Caputa, M., Wentowska, K., and Nowakowska, A. (2004). Stress-induced behaviour in juvenile rats: effects of neonatal asphyxia, body temperature and chelation of iron. *Behav. Brain Res.* 154, 321–329. doi: 10.1016/j.bbr.2004.02.020

Rogalska, J., Danielisova, V., and Caputa, M. (2006). Effect of neonatal body temperature on postanoxic, potentially neurotoxic iron accumulation in the rat brain. *Neurosci. Lett.* 393, 249–254. doi: 10.1016/j.neulet.2005.09.085

Rogalska, J., Kang, P., Wotherspoon, W., Macleod, M. R., and Lai, M. (2009). Effect of hyperthermia and anoxia on glucocorticoid and mineralocorticoid receptor expression in neonatal rat hippocampus. *Neurosci. Lett.* 450, 196–200. doi: 10.1016/j.neulet.2008.11.033

Rognlien, A. G. W., Wollen, E. J., Atneosen-Åsegg, M., and Saugstad, O. D. (2014). Increased expression of inflammatory genes in the neonatal mouse brain after hyperoxic reoxygenation. *Pediatr. Res.* 77, 326–333. doi: 10.1038/pr.2014.193

Roohey, T., Raju, T. N., and Moustogiannis, A. N. (1997). Animal models for the study of perinatal hypoxic-ischemic encephalopathy: a critical analysis. *Early Hum. Dev.* 47, 115–146. doi: 10.1016/S0378-3782(96)01773-2

Rorke, L. B. (1992). Anatomical features of the developing brain implicated in pathogenesis of hypoxic-ischemic injury. *Brain Pathol.* 2, 211–221. doi: 10.1111/j.1750-3639.1992.tb00694.x

Roth, S. C., Edwards, A. D., Cady, E. B., Delpy, D. T., Wyatt, J. S., Azzopardi, D., et al. (1992). Relation between cerebral oxidative metabolism following birth asphyxia, and neurodevelopmental outcome and brain growth at one year. *Dev. Med. Child Neurol.* 34, 285–295. doi: 10.1111/j.1469-8749.1992.tb11432.x

Rotstein, M., Bassan, H., Kariv, N., Speiser, Z., Harel, S., and Gozes, I. (2006). NAP enhances neurodevelopment of newborn apolipoprotein E-deficient mice subjected to hypoxia. *J. Pharmacol. Exp. Ther.* 319, 332–339. doi: 10.1124/jpet.106.106898

Rousset, C. I., Chalon, S., Cantagrel, S., Bodard, S., Andres, C., Gressens, P., et al. (2006). Maternal exposure to LPS induces hypomyelination in the internal capsule and programmed cell death in the deep gray matter in newborn rats. *Pediatr. Res.* 59, 428–433. doi: 10.1203/01.pdr.0000199905.08848.55

Rousset, C. I., Kassem, J., Aubert, A., Planchenault, D., Gressens, P., Chalon, S., et al. (2013). Maternal exposure to lipopolysaccharide leads to transient motor dysfunction in neonatal rats. *Dev. Neurosci.* 35, 172–181. doi: 10.1159/000346579

Ruiz, C. C. U., Rosado-de-Castro, P. H., Mendez-Otero, R., and Pimentel-Coelho, P. M. (2017). "Mesenchymal stromal cell therapy for neonatal hypoxic-ischemic encephalopathy," in *Neurological Regeneration*, ed. P. Van Pham (Berlin: Springer), 105–120.

Ruiz, S., Diep, D., Gore, A., Panopoulos, A. D., Montserrat, N., Plongthongkum, N., et al. (2012). Identification of a specific reprogramming-associated epigenetic signature in human induced pluripotent stem cells. *Proc. Natl. Acad. Sci. U.S.A.* 109, 16196–16201. doi: 10.1073/pnas.1202352109

Ruth, V. J., and Raivio, K. O. (1988). Perinatal brain damage: predictive value of metabolic acidosis and the Apgar score. *BMJ* 297, 24–27. doi: 10.1136/bmj.297.6640.24

Rutherford, M., Counsell, S., Allsop, J., Boardman, J., Kapellou, O., Larkman, D., et al. (2004). Diffusion-weighted magnetic resonance imaging in term perinatal brain injury: a comparison with site of lesion and time from birth. *Pediatrics* 114, 1004–1014. doi: 10.1542/peds.2004-0222

Rutherford, M. A., Pennock, J. M., Counsell, S. J., Mercuri, E., Cowan, F. M., Dubowitz, L. M., et al. (1998). Abnormal magnetic resonance signal in the internal capsule predicts poor neurodevelopmental outcome in infants with hypoxic-ischemic encephalopathy. *Pediatrics* 102(2 Pt 1), 323–328. doi: 10.1542/peds.102.2.323

Saadani-Makki, F., Kannan, S., Lu, X., Janisse, J., Dawe, E., Edwin, S., et al. (2008). Intrauterine administration of endotoxin leads to motor deficits in a rabbit model: a link between prenatal infection and cerebral palsy. *Am. J. Obstet. Gynecol.* 199, 651.e1–651.e7. doi: 10.1016/j.ajog.2008.06.090

Sabir, H., Osredkar, D., Maes, E., Wood, T., and Thoresen, M. (2016). Xenon combined with therapeutic hypothermia is not neuroprotective after severe hypoxia-ischemia in neonatal rats. *PLoS ONE* 11:e0156759. doi: 10.1371/journal.pone.0156759

Sakurada, O., Kennedy, C., Jehle, J., Brown, J. D., Carbin, G. L., and Sokoloff, L. (1978). Measurement of local cerebral blood flow with iodo [14C] antipyrine. *Am. J. Physiol.* 234, H59–H66.

Salhab, W. A., Perlman, J. M., Silver, L., and Broyles, R. S. (2004a). Necrotizing enterocolitis and neurodevelopmental outcome in extremely low birth weight infants < 1000 g. *J. Perinatol.* 24, 534–540.

Salhab, W. A., Wyckoff, M. H., Laptook, A. R., and Perlman, J. M. (2004b). Initial hypoglycemia and neonatal brain injury in term infants with severe fetal acidemia. *Pediatrics* 114, 361–366.

Samaiya, P. K., and Krishnamurthy, S. (2015). Characterization of mitochondrial bioenergetics in neonatal anoxic model of rats. *J. Bioenerg. Biomembr.* 47, 217–222. doi: 10.1007/s10863-015-9603-2

Sampath, D., Shmueli, D., White, A. M., and Raol, Y. H. (2015). Flupirtine effectively prevents development of acute neonatal seizures in an animal model of global hypoxia. *Neurosci. Lett.* 607, 46–51. doi: 10.1016/j.neulet.2015.09.005

Sanches, E., Arteni, N., Nicola, F., Boisserand, L., Willborn, S., and Netto, C. (2013). Early hypoxia-ischemia causes hemisphere and sex-dependent cognitive impairment and histological damage. *Neuroscience* 237, 208–215. doi: 10.1016/j.neuroscience.2013.01.066

Sanches, E. F., Arteni, N. S., Spindler, C., Moysés, F., Siqueira, I. R., Perry, M. L., et al. (2012). Effects of pre-and postnatal protein malnutrition in hypoxic-ischemic rats. *Brain Res.* 1438, 85–92. doi: 10.1016/j.brainres.2011.12.024

Santiago, A. R., Baptista, F. I., Santos, P. F., Cristovao, G., Ambrosio, A. F., Cunha, R. A., et al. (2014). Role of microglia adenosine A(2A) receptors in retinal and brain neurodegenerative diseases. *Mediators Inflamm.* 2014:465694. doi: 10.1155/2014/465694

Sato, Y., Hayakawa, M., Iwata, O., Okumura, A., Kato, T., Hayakawa, F., et al. (2008). Delayed neurological signs following isolated parasagittal injury in asphyxia at term. *Eur. J. Paediatr. Neurol. Soc.* 12, 359–365. doi: 10.1016/j.ejpn.2007.10.003

Saunders, N. R., Dreifuss, J. J., Dziegielewska, K. M., Johansson, P. A., Habgood, M. D., Mollgard, K., et al. (2014). The rights and wrongs of blood-brain barrier permeability studies: a walk through 100 years of history. *Front. Neurosci.* 8:404. doi: 10.3389/fnins.2014.00404

Saunders, N. R., Habgood, M. D., and Dziegielewska, K. M. (1999). Barrier mechanisms in the brain, II. Immature brain. *Clin. Exp. Pharmacol. Physiol.* 26, 85–91. doi: 10.1046/j.1440-1681.1999.02987.x

Saunders, N. R., Liddelow, S. A., and Dziegielewska, K. M. (2012). Barrier mechanisms in the developing brain. *Front. Pharmacol.* 3:46. doi: 10.3389/fphar.2012.00046

Savman, K., Blennow, M., Gustafson, K., Tarkowski, E., and Hagberg, H. (1998). Cytokine response in cerebrospinal fluid after birth asphyxia. *Pediatr. Res.* 43, 746–751. doi: 10.1203/00006450-199806000-00006

Schanne, F. A., Kane, A. B., Young, E. E., and Farber, J. L. (1979). Calcium dependence of toxic cell death: a final common pathway. *Science* 206, 700–702. doi: 10.1126/science.386513

Scheepens, A., Wassink, G., Piersma, M. J., Van de Berg, W. D., and Blanco, C. E. (2003). A delayed increase in hippocampal proliferation following global asphyxia in the neonatal rat. *Brain Res. Dev. Brain Res.* 142, 67–76. doi: 10.1016/S0165-3806(03)00032-4

Schrimpf, S. P., Bleiker, A. J., Brecevic, L., Kozlov, S. V., Berger, P., Osterwalder, T., et al. (1997). Human neuroserpin (PI12): cDNA cloning and chromosomal localization to 3q26. *Genomics* 40, 55–62. doi: 10.1006/geno.1996.4514

Schroder, M., and Kaufman, R. J. (2005). ER stress and the unfolded protein response. *Mutat. Res.* 569, 29–63. doi: 10.1016/j.mrfmmm.2004.06.056

Schulze, C., and Firth, J. A. (1992). Interendothelial junctions during blood-brain barrier development in the rat: morphological changes at the level of individual tight junctional contacts. *Brain Res. Dev. Brain Res.* 69, 85–95. doi: 10.1016/0165-3806(92)90125-G

Seidler, F. J., and Slotkin, T. A. (1990). Effects of acute hypoxia on neonatal rat brain: regionally selective, long-term alterations in catecholamine levels and turnover. *Brain Res. Bull.* 24, 157–161. doi: 10.1016/0361-9230(90)90200-J

Semple, B. D., Blomgren, K., Gimlin, K., Ferriero, D. M., and Noble-Haeusslein, L. J. (2013). Brain development in rodents and humans: identifying benchmarks of maturation and vulnerability to injury across species. *Progress Neurobiol.* 106, 1–16. doi: 10.1016/j.pneurobio.2013.04.001

Shah, D. K., Lavery, S., Doyle, L. W., Wong, C., McDougall, P., and Inder, T. E. (2006). Use of 2-channel bedside electroencephalogram monitoring in term-born encephalopathic infants related to cerebral injury defined by magnetic resonance imaging. *Pediatrics* 118, 47–55. doi: 10.1542/peds.2005-1294

Shah, P. S. (2010). Hypothermia: a systematic review and meta-analysis of clinical trials. *Semin. Fetal Neonatal Med.* 15, 238–246. doi: 10.1016/j.siny.2010.02.003

Shah, P. S., Beyene, J., To, T., Ohlsson, A., and Perlman, M. (2006). Postasphyxial hypoxic-ischemic encephalopathy in neonates: outcome prediction rule within 4 hours of birth. *Arch. Pediatr. Adolesc. Med.* 160, 729–736. doi: 10.1001/archpedi.160.7.729

Shah, P. S., Ohlsson, A., and Perlman, M. (2007). Hypothermia to treat neonatal hypoxic ischemic encephalopathy: systematic review. *Arch. Pediatr. Adolesc. Med.* 161, 951–958. doi: 10.1001/archpedi.161.10.951

Shalak, L., and Perlman, J. M. (2004). Hypoxic–ischemic brain injury in the term infant-current concepts. *Early Hum. Dev.* 80, 125–141. doi: 10.1016/j.earlhumdev.2004.06.003

Shankaran, S., Laptook, A., Wright, L. L., Ehrenkranz, R. A., Donovan, E. F., Fanaroff, A. A., et al. (2002). Whole-body hypothermia for neonatal encephalopathy: animal observations as a basis for a randomized, controlled pilot study in term infants. *Pediatrics* 110, 377–385. doi: 10.1542/peds.110.2.377

Shankaran, S., Laptook, A. R., Ehrenkranz, R. A., Tyson, J. E., McDonald, S. A., Donovan, E. F., et al. (2005). Whole-body hypothermia for neonates with hypoxic–ischemic encephalopathy. *N. Engl. J. Med.* 353, 1574–1584. doi: 10.1056/NEJMcps050929

Shankaran, S., Pappas, A., McDonald, S. A., Vohr, B. R., Hintz, S. R., Yolton, K., et al. (2012). Childhood outcomes after hypothermia for neonatal encephalopathy. *N. Engl. J. Med.* 366, 2085–2092. doi: 10.1056/NEJMoa1112066

Shankaran, S., Woldt, E., Koepke, T., Bedard, M. P., and Nandyal, R. (1991). Acute neonatal morbidity and long-term central nervous system sequelae of perinatal asphyxia in term infants. *Early Hum. Dev.* 25, 135–148. doi: 10.1016/0378-3782(91)90191-5

Sharma, R. (2014). Prevention of Frey syndrome with superficial temporal fascia interpositioning: a retrospective study. *Int. J. Oral Maxillofac. Surg.* 43, 413–417. doi: 10.1016/j.ijom.2013.12.001

Sheldon, R. A., Sedik, C., and Ferriero, D. M. (1998). Strain-related brain injury in neonatal mice subjected to hypoxia–ischemia. *Brain Res.* 810, 114–122. doi: 10.1016/S0006-8993(98)00892-0

Shellhaas, R. A., Soaita, A. I., and Clancy, R. R. (2007). Sensitivity of amplitude-integrated electroencephalography for neonatal seizure detection. *Pediatrics* 120, 770–777. doi: 10.1542/peds.2007-0514

Shi, L., Smith, S. E., Malkova, N., Tse, D., Su, Y., and Patterson, P. H. (2009). Activation of the maternal immune system alters cerebellar development in the offspring. *Brain Behav. Immun.* 23, 116–123. doi: 10.1016/j.bbi.2008.07.012

Shimomura, C., and Ohta, H. (1988). Behavioral abnormalities and seizure susceptibility in rat after neonatal anoxia. *Brain Dev.* 10, 160–163. doi: 10.1016/S0387-7604(88)80020-2

Sidhu, R. S., Tuor, U. I., and Del Bigio, M. R. (1997). Nuclear condensation and fragmentation following cerebral hypoxia-ischemia occurs more frequently in immature than older rats. *Neurosci. Lett.* 223, 129–132. doi: 10.1016/S0304-3940(97)13426-7

Simpson, E. A., Murray, L., Paukner, A., and Ferrari, P. F. (2014). The mirror neuron system as revealed through neonatal imitation: presence from birth, predictive power and evidence of plasticity. *Philos. Trans. R. Soc. Lond. B Biol. Sci.* 369:20130289. doi: 10.1098/rstb.2013.0289

Sinclair, D. B., Campbell, M., Byrne, P., Prasertsom, W., and Robertson, C. M. (1999). EEG and long-term outcome of term infants with neonatal hypoxic-ischemic encephalopathy. *Clin. Neurophysiol.* 110, 655–659. doi: 10.1016/S1388-2457(99)00010-3

Singh, D., Kumar, P., Majumdar, S., and Narang, A. (2004). Effect of phenobarbital on free radicals in neonates with hypoxic ischemic encephalopathy–a randomized controlled trial. *J. Perinat. Med.* 32, 278–281. doi: 10.1515/JPM.2004.052

Slotkin, T., Lappi, S., McCook, E., Lorber, B., and Seidler, F. (1995). Loss of neonatal hypoxia tolerance after prenatal nicotine exposure: implications for sudden infant death syndrome. *Brain Res. Bull.* 38, 69–75. doi: 10.1016/0361-9230(95)00073-N

Slotkin, T. A., Cowdery, T. S., Orband, L., Pachman, S., and Whitmore, W. L. (1986). Effects of neonatal hypoxia on brain development in the rat: immediate and long-term biochemical alterations in discrete regions. *Brain Res.* 374, 63–74. doi: 10.1016/0006-8993(86)90395-1

Smith, P. L., Hagberg, H., Naylor, A. S., and Mallard, C. (2014). Neonatal peripheral immune challenge activates microglia and inhibits neurogenesis in the developing murine hippocampus. *Dev. Neurosci.* 36, 119–131. doi: 10.1159/000359950

Soares, D. P., and Law, M. (2009). Magnetic resonance spectroscopy of the brain: review of metabolites and clinical applications. *Clin. Radiol.* 64, 12–21. doi: 10.1016/j.crad.2008.07.002

Sokoloff, L., Reivich, M., Kennedy, C., Des Rosiers, M., Patlak, C. S., Pettigrew, K. E. A., et al. (1977). The [14C] deoxyglucose method for the measurement of local cerebral glucose utilization: theory, procedure, and normal values in the conscious and anesthetized albino rat1. *J. Neurochem.* 28, 897–916. doi: 10.1111/j.1471-4159.1977.tb10649.x

Soul, J. S., Robertson, R. L., Tzika, A. A., du Plessis, A. J., and Volpe, J. J. (2001). Time course of changes in diffusion-weighted magnetic resonance imaging in a case of neonatal encephalopathy with defined onset and duration of hypoxic-ischemic insult. *Pediatrics* 108, 1211–1214. doi: 10.1542/peds.108.5.1211

Speiser, Z., Katzir, O., Rehavi, M., Zabarski, T., and Cohen, S. (1998). Sparing by rasagiline (TVP-1012) of cholinergic functions and behavior in the postnatal anoxia rat. *Pharmacol. Biochem. Behav.* 60, 387–393. doi: 10.1016/S0091-3057(97)00603-5

Speiser, Z., Uziel, J., Defrin-Assa, R., Gitter, S., and Urca, G. (1991). Different behavioral deficits are induced by anoxia/hypoxia in neonatal and senescent rats: blockade by MK-801. *Behav. Brain Res.* 42, 181–186. doi: 10.1016/S0166-4328(05)80009-9

Spraggins, Y., Seidler, F. J., and Slotkin, T. A. (1994). Cocaine exacerbates hypoxia-Induced cell damage in the developing brain: effects on ornithine decarboxylase activity and protein synthesis. *Neonatology* 66, 254–266. doi: 10.1159/000244115

Srinivasakumar, P., Zempel, J., Wallendorf, M., Lawrence, R., Inder, T., and Mathur, A. (2013). Therapeutic hypothermia in neonatal hypoxic ischemic encephalopathy: electrographic seizures and magnetic resonance imaging evidence of injury. *J. Pediatr.* 163, 465–470. doi: 10.1016/j.jpeds.2013.01.041

Staley, K. J., Soldo, B. L., and Proctor, W. R. (1995). Ionic mechanisms of neuronal excitation by inhibitory GABAA receptors. *Science* 269, 977–981. doi: 10.1126/science.7638623

Starkov, A. A., Chinopoulos, C., and Fiskum, G. (2004). Mitochondrial calcium and oxidative stress as mediators of ischemic brain injury. *Cell Calcium* 36, 257–264. doi: 10.1016/j.ceca.2004.02.012

Steinman, K. J., Gorno-Tempini, M. L., Glidden, D. V., Kramer, J. H., Miller, S. P., Barkovich, A. J., et al. (2009). Neonatal watershed brain injury on magnetic resonance imaging correlates with verbal IQ at 4 years. *Pediatrics* 123, 1025–1030. doi: 10.1542/peds.2008-1203

Stewart, P. A., and Hayakawa, K. (1994). Early ultrastructural changes in blood-brain barrier vessels of the rat embryo. *Brain Res. Dev. Brain Res.* 78, 25–34. doi: 10.1016/0165-3806(94)90005-1

Stiller, R., von Mering, R., Konig, V., Huch, A., and Huch, R. (2002). How well does reflectance pulse oximetry reflect intrapartum fetal acidosis? *Am. J. Obst. Gynecol.* 186, 1351–1357. doi: 10.1067/mob.2002.122411

Stoll, B. J., Hansen, N. I., Adams-Chapman, I., Fanaroff, A. A., Hintz, S. R., Vohr, B., et al. (2004). Neurodevelopmental and growth impairment among extremely low-birth-weight infants with neonatal infection. *JAMA* 292, 2357–2365. doi: 10.1001/jama.292.19.2357

Stolp, H. B., Liddelow, S. A., and Saunders, N. R. (2016). Editorial: ontogeny and phylogeny of brain barrier mechanisms. *Front. Neurosci.* 10:41. doi: 10.3389/fnins.2016.00041

Stonestreet, B. S., Burgess, G. H., and Cserr, H. F. (1992). Blood-brain barrier integrity and brain water and electrolytes during hypoxia/hypercapnia and hypotension in newborn piglets. *Brain Res.* 590, 263–270. doi: 10.1016/0006-8993(92)91104-M

Stridh, L., Mottahedin, A., Johansson, M. E., Valdez, R. C., Northington, F., Wang, X., et al. (2013). Toll-like receptor-3 activation increases the vulnerability of the neonatal brain to hypoxia-ischemia. *J. Neurosci.* 33, 12041–12051. doi: 10.1523/JNEUROSCI.0673-13.2013

Stritt, C., Stern, S., Harting, K., Manke, T., Sinske, D., Schwarz, H., et al. (2009). Paracrine control of oligodendrocyte differentiation by SRF-directed neuronal gene expression. *Nat. Neurosci.* 12, 418–427. doi: 10.1038/nn.2280

Stroemer, R. P., and Rothwell, N. J. (1998). Exacerbation of ischemic brain damage by localized striatal injection of interleukin-1beta in the rat. *J. Cereb. Blood Flow Metab.* 18, 833–839. doi: 10.1097/00004647-199808000-00003

Strunk, T., Hartel, C., Temming, P., Matzke, N., Zimmer, J., and Schultz, C. (2008). Erythropoietin inhibits cytokine production of neonatal and adult leukocytes. *Acta Paediatr.* 97, 16–20. doi: 10.1111/j.1651-2227.2007.00560.x

Strunk, T., Inder, T., Wang, X., Burgner, D., Mallard, C., and Levy, O. (2014). Infection-induced inflammation and cerebral injury in preterm infants. *Lancet Infect. Dis.* 14, 751–762. doi: 10.1016/S1473-3099(14)70710-8

Suarez-Sola, M. L., Gonzalez-Delgado, F. J., Pueyo-Morlans, M., Medina-Bolivar, O. C., Hernandez-Acosta, N. C., Gonzalez-Gomez, M., et al. (2009). Neurons in the white matter of the adult human neocortex. *Front. Neuroanat.* 3:7. doi: 10.3389/neuro.05.007.2009

Svedin, P., Hagberg, H., Savman, K., Zhu, C., and Mallard, C. (2007). Matrix metalloproteinase-9 gene knock-out protects the immature brain after cerebral hypoxia-ischemia. *J. Neurosci.* 27, 1511–1518. doi: 10.1523/JNEUROSCI.4391-06.2007

Svedin, P., Kjellmer, I., Welin, A. K., Blad, S., and Mallard, C. (2005). Maturational effects of lipopolysaccharide on white-matter injury in fetal sheep. *J. Child Neurol.* 20, 960–964. doi: 10.1177/08830738050200120501

Tagin, M. A., Woolcott, C. G., Vincer, M. J., Whyte, R. K., and Stinson, D. A. (2012). Hypothermia for neonatal hypoxic ischemic encephalopathy: an updated systematic review and meta-analysis. *Arch. Pediatr. Adolesc. Med.* 166, 558–566. doi: 10.1001/archpediatrics.2011.1772

Tahraoui, S. L., Marret, S., Bodenant, C., Leroux, P., Dommergues, M. A., Evrard, P., et al. (2001). Central role of microglia in neonatal excitotoxic lesions of the murine periventricular white matter. *Brain Pathol.* 11, 56–71. doi: 10.1111/j.1750-3639.2001.tb00381.x

Tajiri, N., Kaneko, Y., Shinozuka, K., Ishikawa, H., Yankee, E., McGrogan, M., et al. (2013). Stem cell recruitment of newly formed host cells via a successful seduction? Filling the gap between neurogenic niche and injured brain site. *PLoS ONE* 8:e74857. doi: 10.1371/journal.pone.0074857

Takada, S., dos Santos Haemmerle, C., Motta-Teixeira, L., Machado-Nils, A., Lee, V., Takase, L., et al. (2015). Neonatal anoxia in rats: hippocampal cellular and subcellular changes related to cell death and spatial memory. *Neuroscience* 284, 247–259. doi: 10.1016/j.neuroscience.2014.08.054

Takada, S. H., Motta-Teixeira, L. C., Machado-Nils, A. V., Lee, V. Y., Sampaio, C. A., Polli, R. S., et al. (2016). Impact of neonatal anoxia on adult rat hippocampal volume, neurogenesis and behavior. *Behav. Brain Res.* 296, 331–338. doi: 10.1016/j.bbr.2015.08.039

Takada, T., Takata, K., and Ashihara, E. (2016). Inhibition of monocarboxylate transporter 1 suppresses the proliferation of glioblastoma stem cells. *J. Physiol. Sci.* 66, 387–396. doi: 10.1007/s12576-016-0435-6

Takahashi, S., Tanaka, H., and Oki, J. (1999). Development of spinal motoneurons in rats after a neonatal hypoxic insult. *Pediatr. Neurol.* 21, 715–720. doi: 10.1016/S0887-8994(99)00080-6

Takao, K., and Miyakawa, T. (2015). Genomic responses in mouse models greatly mimic human inflammatory diseases. *Proc. Natl. Acad. Sci. U.S.A.* 112, 1167–1172. doi: 10.1073/pnas.1401965111

Takeoka, M., Soman, T. B., Yoshii, A., Caviness, V. S. Jr., Gonzalez, R. G., Grant, P. E., et al. (2002). Diffusion-weighted images in neonatal cerebral hypoxic-ischemic injury. *Pediatr. Neurol.* 26, 274–281. doi: 10.1016/S0887-8994(01)00403-9

Talos, D. M., Fishman, R. E., Park, H., Folkerth, R. D., Follett, P. L., Volpe, J. J., et al. (2006). Developmental regulation of alpha-amino-3-hydroxy-5-methyl-4-isoxazole-propionic acid receptor subunit expression in forebrain and relationship to regional susceptibility to hypoxic/ischemic injury. I. Rodent cerebral white matter and cortex. *J. Comp. Neurol.* 497, 42–60. doi: 10.1002/cne.20972

Tanaka, H., Takahashi, S., Miyamoto, A., Oki, J., Cho, K., and Okuno, A. (1995). Effects of neonatal hypoxia on brainstem cholinergic neurons-pedunculopontine nucleus and laterodorsal tegmental nucleus. *Brain Dev.* 17, 264–270. doi: 10.1016/0387-7604(95)00043-B

Tang, Y., Pacary, E., Freret, T., Divoux, D., Petit, E., Schumann-Bard, P., et al. (2006). Effect of hypoxic preconditioning on brain genomic response before and following ischemia in the adult mouse: identification of potential neuroprotective candidates for stroke. *Neurobiol. Dis.* 21, 18–28. doi: 10.1016/j.nbd.2005.06.002

Tao, F., Lu, S. D., Zhang, L. M., Huang, Y. L., and Sun, F. Y. (2001). Role of excitatory amino acid transporter 1 in neonatal rat neuronal damage induced by hypoxia-ischemia. *Neuroscience* 102, 503–513. doi: 10.1016/S0306-4522(00)00485-1

Teesalu, T., Kulla, A., Simisker, A., Sirén, V., Lawrence, D. A., Asser, T., et al. (2004). Tissue plasminogen activator and neuroserpin are widely expressed in the human central nervous system. *Thromb. Haemost.* 92, 358–368. doi: 10.1160/th02-12-0310

Thompson, C., Puterman, A., Linley, L., Hann, F., Elst, C. V. D., Molteno, C., et al. (1997). The value of a scoring system for hypoxic ischaemic encephalopathy in predicting neurodevelopmental outcome. *Acta Paediatr.* 86, 757–761. doi: 10.1111/j.1651-2227.1997.tb08581.x

Thompson, D. K., Warfield, S. K., Carlin, J. B., Pavlovic, M., Wang, H. X., Bear, M., et al. (2007). Perinatal risk factors altering regional brain structure in the preterm infant. *Brain* 130(Pt 3), 667–677. doi: 10.1093/brain/awl277

Thoresen, M., Hobbs, C. E., Wood, T., Chakkarapani, E., and Dingley, J. (2009). Cooling combined with immediate or delayed xenon inhalation provides equivalent long-term neuroprotection after neonatal hypoxia-ischemia. *J. Cereb. Blood Flow Metab.* 29, 707–714. doi: 10.1038/jcbfm.2008.163

Ting, P., Yamaguchi, S., Bacher, J. D., Killens, R. H., and Myers, R. E. (1983). Hypoxic-ischemic cerebral necrosis in midgestational sheep fetuses: physiopathologic correlations. *Exp. Neurol.* 80, 227–245. doi: 10.1016/0014-4886(83)90019-5

Tjärnlund-Wolf, A., Olsson, S., Jood, K., Blomstrand, C., and Jern, C. (2011). No evidence for an association between genetic variation at the SERPINI1 locus and ischemic stroke. *J. Neurol.* 258, 1885. doi: 10.1007/s00415-011-6022-0

Toet, M. C., Hellstrom-Westas, L., Groenendaal, F., Eken, P., and de Vries, L. S. (1999). Amplitude integrated EEG 3 and 6 hours after birth in full term neonates with hypoxic-ischaemic encephalopathy. *Arch. Dis. Child. Fetal Neonatal Ed.* 81, F19–F23. doi: 10.1136/fn.81.1.f19

Toet, M. C., van der Meij, W., de Vries, L. S., Uiterwaal, C. S., and van Huffelen, K. C. (2002). Comparison between simultaneously recorded amplitude integrated electroencephalogram (cerebral function monitor) and standard electroencephalogram in neonates. *Pediatrics* 109, 772–779. doi: 10.1542/peds.109.5.772

Tolner, E. A., Hochman, D. W., Hassinen, P., Otahal, J., Gaily, E., Haglund, M. M., et al. (2011). Five percent CO(2) is a potent, fast-acting inhalation anticonvulsant. *Epilepsia* 52, 104–114. doi: 10.1111/j.1528-1167.2010.02731.x

Tomimatsu, T., Fukuda, H., Endoh, M., Mu, J., Watanabe, N., Kohzuki, M., et al. (2002). Effects of neonatal hypoxic–ischemic brain injury on skilled motor tasks and brainstem function in adult rats. *Brain Res.* 926, 108–117. doi: 10.1016/S0006-8993(01)03311-X

Toso, L., Poggi, S., Park, J., Einat, H., Roberson, R., Dunlap, V., et al. (2005). Inflammatory-mediated model of cerebral palsy with developmental sequelae. *Am. J. Obstet. Gynecol.* 193(3 Pt 2), 933–941. doi: 10.1016/j.ajog.2005.05.072

Towfighi, J., Yager, J., Housman, C., and Vannucci, R. (1991). Neuropathology of remote hypoxic-ischemic damage in the immature rat. *Acta Neuropathol.* 81, 578–587. doi: 10.1007/BF00310141

Towfighi, J., Zec, N., Yager, J., Housman, C., and Vannucci, R. C. (1995). Temporal evolution of neuropathologic changes in an immature rat model of cerebral hypoxia: a light microscopic study. *Acta Neuropathol.* 90, 375–386. doi: 10.1007/BF00315011

Tran, T. V., and Weisman, L. E. (2004). Dexamethasone effects on group B streptococcal infection in newborn rats. *Pediatr. Infect. Dis. J.* 23, 47–52. doi: 10.1097/01.inf.0000105107.76541.ee

Tremblay, E., Roisin, M. P., Represa, A., Charriaut-Marlangue, C., and Ben-Ari, Y. (1988). Transient increased density of NMDA binding sites in the developing rat hippocampus. *Brain Res.* 461, 393–396. doi: 10.1016/0006-8993(88)90275-2

Triulzi, F., Parazzini, C., and Righini, A. (2006). Patterns of damage in the mature neonatal brain. *Pediatr. Radiol.* 36, 608–620. doi: 10.1007/s00247-006-0203-5

Trommer, B. L., Groothuis, D. R., and Pasternak, J. F. (1987). Quantitative analysis of cerebral vessels in the newborn puppy: the structure of germinal matrix vessels may predispose to hemorrhage. *Pediatr. Res.* 22, 23–28. doi: 10.1203/00006450-198707000-00007

Tu, Y. F., Tsai, Y. S., Wang, L. W., Wu, H. C., Huang, C. C., and Ho, C. J. (2011). Overweight worsens apoptosis, neuroinflammation and blood-brain barrier damage after hypoxic ischemia in neonatal brain through JNK hyperactivation. *J. Neuroinflammation* 8:40. doi: 10.1186/1742-2094-8-40

Tuor, U., Chumas, P., and Del Bigio, M. (1995). Prevention of hypoxic-ischemic damage with dexamethasone is dependent on age and not influenced by fasting. *Exp. Neurol.* 132, 116–122. doi: 10.1016/0014-4886(95)90065-9

Tuor, U. I., and Grewal, D. (1994). Autoregulation of cerebral blood flow: influence of local brain development and postnatal age. *Am. J. Physiol.* 267(6 Pt 2), H2220–H2228.

Uehara, T., Tabuchi, M., and Mori, E. (1999). Risk factors for silent cerebral infarcts in subcortical white matter and basal ganglia. *Stroke* 30, 378–382. doi: 10.1161/01.STR.30.2.378

Ujhazy, E., Schmidtova, M., Dubovicky, M., Navarova, J., Brucknerova, I., and Mach, M. (2006). Neurobehavioural changes in rats after neonatal anoxia: effect of antioxidant stobadine pretreatment. *Neuro Endocrinol. Lett.* 27(Suppl. 2), 82–85.

Valiente, M., Obenauf, A. C., Jin, X., Chen, Q., Zhang, X. H., Lee, D. J., et al. (2014). Serpins promote cancer cell survival and vascular co-option in brain metastasis. *Cell* 156, 1002–1016. doi: 10.1016/j.cell.2014.01.040

van der Worp, H. B., Sena, E. S., Donnan, G. A., Howells, D. W., and Macleod, M. R. (2007). Hypothermia in animal models of acute ischaemic stroke: a systematic review and meta-analysis. *Brain* 130(Pt 12), 3063–3074. doi: 10.1093/brain/awm083 van Laerhoven, H., de Haan, T. R., Offringa, M., Post, B., and van der Lee, J. H. (2013). Prognostic tests in term neonates with hypoxic-ischemic encephalopathy: a systematic review. *Pediatrics* 131, 88–98. doi: 10.1542/peds.2012-1297

Vandenberg, R. J., and Ryan, R. M. (2013). Mechanisms of glutamate transport. *Physiol. Rev.* 93, 1621–1657. doi: 10.1152/physrev.00007.2013

Vannucci, R., Connor, J., Mauger, D., Palmer, C., Smith, M., Towfighi, J., et al. (1999). Rat model of perinatal hypoxic-ischemic brain damage. *J. Neurosci. Res.* 55, 158–163. doi: 10.1002/(SICI)1097-4547(19990115)55:2<158::AID-JNR3>3.0.CO;2-1

Vannucci, R. C., Brucklacher, R. M., and Vannucci, S. J. (2005). Glycolysis and perinatal hypoxic-ischemic brain damage. *Dev. Neurosci.* 27, 185–190. doi: 10.1159/000085991

Vannucci, R. C., Christensen, M. A., and Stein, D. T. (1989). Regional cerebral glucose utilization in the immature rat: effect of hypoxia-ischemia. *Pediatr. Res.* 26, 208–214. doi: 10.1203/00006450-198909000-00011

Vannucci, R. C., Christensen, M. A., and Yager, J. Y. (1993). Nature, time-course, and extent of cerebral edema in perinatal hypoxic-ischemic brain damage. *Pediatr. Neurol.* 9, 29–34. doi: 10.1016/0887-8994(93)90006-X

Vannucci, R. C., and Duffy, T. E. (1976). Carbohydrate metabolism in fetal and neonatal rat brain during anoxia and recovery. *Am. J. Physiol.* 230, 1269–1275.

Vannucci, R. C., Lyons, D. T., and Vasta, F. (1988). Regional cerebral blood flow during hypoxia-ischemia in immature rats. *Stroke* 19, 245–250. doi: 10.1161/01.STR.19.2.245

Vannucci, R. C., and Vannucci, S. J. (2005). Perinatal hypoxic-ischemic brain damage: evolution of an animal model. *Dev. Neurosci.* 27, 81–86. doi: 10.1159/000085978

Vannucci, R. C., and Yager, J. Y. (1992). Glucose, lactic acid, and perinatal hypoxic-ischemic brain damage. *Pediatr. Neurol.* 8, 3–12. doi: 10.1016/0887-8994(92)90045-Z

Vannucci, S. J., and Hagberg, H. (2004). Hypoxia-ischemia in the immature brain. *J. Exp. Biol.* 207(Pt 18), 3149–3154. doi: 10.1242/jeb.01064

Vannucci, S. J., and Vannucci, R. C. (1980). Glycogen metabolism in neonatal rat brain during anoxia and recovery. *J. Neurochem.* 34, 1100–1105. doi: 10.1111/j.1471-4159.1980.tb09946.x

Vargas-Origel, A., Espinosa-Garcia, J. O., Muniz-Quezada, E., Vargas-Nieto, M. A., and Aguilar-Garcia, G. (2004). Prevention of hypoxic-ischemic encephalopathy with high-dose, early phenobarbital therapy. *Gac. Med. Mex.* 140, 147–153.

Venerosi, A., Cutuli, D., Chiarotti, F., and Calamandrei, G. (2006). C-section birth per se or followed by acute global asphyxia altered emotional behaviour in neonate and adult rats. *Behav. Brain Res.* 168, 56–63. doi: 10.1016/j.bbr.2005.10.010

Vento, M., Asensi, M., Sastre, J., Garcia-Sala, F., Pallardo, F. V., and Vina, J. (2001a). Resuscitation with room air instead of 100% oxygen prevents oxidative stress in moderately asphyxiated term neonates. *Pediatrics* 107, 642–647.

Vento, M., Asensi, M., Sastre, J., Garcia-Sala, F., and Vina, J. (2001b). Six years of experience with the use of room air for the resuscitation of asphyxiated newly born term infants. *Biol. Neonate* 79, 261–267.

Verma, P. K., Panerai, R. B., Rennie, J. M., and Evans, D. H. (2000). Grading of cerebral autoregulation in preterm and term neonates. *Pediatr. Neurol.* 23, 236–242. doi: 10.1016/S0887-8994(00)00184-3

Vermeulen, R. J., Fetter, W. P., Hendrikx, L., Van Schie, P. E., van der Knaap, M. S., and Barkhof, F. (2003). Diffusion-weighted MRI in severe neonatal hypoxic ischaemia: the white cerebrum. *Neuropediatrics* 34, 72–76. doi: 10.1055/s-2003-39599

Vincer, M. J., Allen, A. C., Joseph, K. S., Stinson, D. A., Scott, H., and Wood, E. (2006). Increasing prevalence of cerebral palsy among very preterm infants: a population-based study. *Pediatrics* 118, e1621–e1626. doi: 10.1542/peds.2006-1522

Vohr, B. R., Wright, L. L., Dusick, A. M., Mele, L., Verter, J., Steichen, J. J., et al. (2000). Neurodevelopmental and functional outcomes of extremely low birth weight infants in the National Institute of Child Health and Human Development Neonatal Research Network, 1993-1994. *Pediatrics* 105, 1216–1226. doi: 10.1542/peds.105.6.1216

Volpe, A. R., Petrone, M. E., De Vizio, W., Davies, R. M., and Proskin, H. M. (1996). A review of plaque, gingivitis, calculus and caries clinical efficacy studies with a fluoride dentifrice containing triclosan and PVM/MA copolymer. *J. Clin. Den.* 7(Suppl.), S1–S14.

Volpe, J. (ed.). (1995). "Hypoxic-ischemic encephalopathy: neuropathology and pathogenesis," in *Neurology of the Newborn*, (London: W B Saunders), 279–313.

Volpe, J. (2001). *Hypoxic-Ischemic Encephalopathy in Neurology of the Newborn.* Philadelphia, PA: WB Saunders.

Volpe, J. J. (1977). Neonatal seizures. *Clin. Perinatol.* 4, 43–63.

Volpe, J. J. (1989). Intraventricular hemorrhage in the premature infant–current concepts. Part I. *Ann. Neurol.* 25, 3–11. doi: 10.1002/ana.410250103

Volpe, J. J. (2008). *Neurology of the Newborn.* Philadelphia, PA: Elsevier Health Sciences.

Volpe, J. J. (2009). The encephalopathy of prematurity–brain injury and impaired brain development inextricably intertwined. *Semin. Pediatr. Neurol.* 16, 167–178. doi: 10.1016/j.spen.2009.09.005

Volpe, J. J. (2012). Neonatal encephalopathy: an inadequate term for hypoxic–ischemic encephalopathy. *Ann. Neurol.* 72, 156–166. doi: 10.1002/ana.23647

Waddell, J., Hanscom, M., Shalon Edwards, N., McKenna, M. C., and McCarthy, M. M. (2016). Sex differences in cell genesis, hippocampal volume and behavioral outcomes in a rat model of neonatal HI. *Exp. Neurol.* 275(Pt 2), 285–295. doi: 10.1016/j.expneurol.2015.09.003

Walsh, B. H., Murray, D. M., and Boylan, G. B. (2011). The use of conventional EEG for the assessment of hypoxic ischaemic encephalopathy in the newborn: a review. *Clin. Neurophysiol.* 122, 1284–1294. doi: 10.1016/j.clinph.2011.03.032

Wang, C. T., Lin, H. J., Cheng, B. C., Lin, M. T., and Chang, C. P. (2015). Attenuating systemic inflammatory markers in simulated high-altitude exposure by heat shock protein 70-mediated hypobaric hypoxia preconditioning in rats. *J. Formos. Med. Assoc.* 114, 328–338. doi: 10.1016/j.jfma.2012.11.015

Wang, L., Goldstein, F. C., Veledar, E., Levey, A. I., Lah, J. J., Meltzer, C. C., et al. (2009). Alterations in cortical thickness and white matter integrity in mild cognitive impairment measured by whole-brain cortical thickness mapping and diffusion tensor imaging. *Am. J. Neuroradiol.* 30, 893–899. doi: 10.3174/ajnr.A1484

Wang, L. S., Zhou, J., Shao, X. M., and Tang, X. C. (2002). Huperzine A attenuates cognitive deficits and brain injury in neonatal rats after hypoxia–ischemia. *Brain Res.* 949, 162–170. doi: 10.1016/S0006-8993(02)02977-3

Wang, S., Zhang, X. Q., Song, C. G., Xiao, T., Zhao, M., Zhu, G., et al. (2015). In vivo effects of bumetanide at brain concentrations incompatible with NKCC1 inhibition on newborn DGC structure and spontaneous EEG seizures following hypoxia-induced neonatal seizures. *Neurosci.* 286, 203–215. doi: 10.1016/j.neuroscience.2014.11.031

Wang, X., Hagberg, H., Nie, C., Zhu, C., Ikeda, T., and Mallard, C. (2007a). Dual role of intrauterine immune challenge on neonatal and adult brain vulnerability to hypoxia-ischemia. *J. Neuropathol. Exp. Neurol.* 66, 552–561.

Wang, X., Hagberg, H., Zhu, C., Jacobsson, B., and Mallard, C. (2007b). Effects of intrauterine inflammation on the developing mouse brain. *Brain Res.* 1144, 180–185. doi: 10.1016/j.brainres.2007.01.083

Wang, X., Rousset, C. I., Hagberg, H., and Mallard, C. (2006). Lipopolysaccharide-induced inflammation and perinatal brain injury. *Semin. Fetal Neonatal Med.* 11, 343–353. doi: 10.1016/j.siny.2006.04.002

Wang, X., Zhu, C., Qiu, L., Hagberg, H., Sandberg, M., and Blomgren, K. (2003). Activation of ERK1/2 after neonatal rat cerebral hypoxia-ischaemia. *J. Neurochem.* 86, 351–362. doi: 10.1046/j.1471-4159.2003.01838.x

Wannier-Morino, P., Rager, G., Sonderegger, P., and Grabs, D. (2003). Expression of neuroserpin in the visual cortex of the mouse during the developmental critical period. *Eur. J. Neurosci.* 17, 1853–1860. doi: 10.1046/j.1460-9568.2003.02628.x

Ward, P., Counsell, S., Allsop, J., Cowan, F., Shen, Y., Edwards, D., et al. (2006). Reduced fractional anisotropy on diffusion tensor magnetic resonance imaging after hypoxic-ischemic encephalopathy. *Pediatrics* 117, e619–e630. doi: 10.1542/peds.2005-0545

Wasterlain, C. G. (1979). Does anoxemia play a role in the effects of neonatal seizures on brain growth? An experimental study in the rat. *Eur. Neurol.* 18, 222–229. doi: 10.1159/000115080

Watanabe, S., Fukuda, T., and Ueko, S. (1980). Changes in electroencephalogram of the rat following olfactory bulbectomy. *Tohoku J. Exp. Med.* 130, 41–48. doi: 10.1620/tjem.130.41

Weeke, L. C., Boylan, G. B., Pressler, R. M., Hallberg, B., Blennow, M., Toet, M. C., et al. (2016). Role of EEG background activity, seizure burden and

MRI in predicting neurodevelopmental outcome in full-term infants with hypoxic-ischaemic encephalopathy in the era of therapeutic hypothermia. *Eur. J. Paediatr. Neurol.* 20, 855–864. doi: 10.1016/j.ejpn.2016.06.003

Welsh, F. A., O'Connor, M. J., Marcy, V. R., Spatacco, A. J., and Johns, R. L. (1982). Factors limiting regeneration of ATP following temporary ischemia in cat brain. *Stroke* 13, 234–242. doi: 10.1161/01.STR.13.2.234

Westphal, O. (1965). Bacterial lipopolysaccharide-extraction with phenol water and further application of procedure. *Methods Carbohydr. Chem.* 1, 83–91.

White, A. R., and Cappai, R. (2003). Neurotoxicity from glutathione depletion is dependent on extracellular trace copper. *J. Neurosci. Res.* 71, 889–897. doi: 10.1002/jnr.10537

Wigglesworth, J. S., and Pape, K. E. (1978). An integrated model for haemorrhagic and ischaemic lesions in the newborn brain. *Early Hum. Dev.* 2, 179–199. doi: 10.1016/0378-3782(78)90010-5

Williams, C. E., Gunn, A. J., Mallard, C., and Gluckman, P. D. (1992). Outcome after ischemia in the developing sheep brain: an electroencephalographic and histological study. *Ann. Neurol.* 31, 14–21. doi: 10.1002/ana.410310104

Wilson-Costello, D., Friedman, H., Minich, N., Siner, B., Taylor, G., Schluchter, M., et al. (2007). Improved neurodevelopmental outcomes for extremely low birth weight infants in 2000-2002. *Pediatrics* 119, 37–45. doi: 10.1542/peds.2006-1416

Woo, T. U., Beale, J. M., and Finlay, B. L. (1991). Dual fate of subplate neurons in a rodent. *Cereb. Cortex* 1, 433–443. doi: 10.1093/cercor/1.5.433

Wood, P. L. (1995). Microglia as a unique cellular target in the treatment of stroke: potential neurotoxic mediators produced by activated microglia. *Neurol. Res.* 17, 242–248. doi: 10.1080/01616412.1995.11740321

Wu, J., Echeverry, R., Guzman, J., and Yepes, M. (2010). Neuroserpin protects neurons from ischemia-induced plasmin-mediated cell death independently of tissue-type plasminogen activator inhibition. *Am. J. Pathol.* 177, 2576–2584. doi: 10.2353/ajpath.2010.100466

Wu, J., and Kaufman, R. J. (2006). From acute ER stress to physiological roles of the Unfolded Protein Response. *Cell Death Differ.* 13, 374–384. doi: 10.1038/sj.cdd.4401840

Wyatt, J. S., Edwards, A. D., Azzopardi, D., and Reynolds, E. O. (1989). Magnetic resonance and near infrared spectroscopy for investigation of perinatal hypoxic-ischaemic brain injury. *Arch. Dis. Child.* 64, 953–963. doi: 10.1136/adc.64.7_Spec_No.953

Xiong, M., Li, J., Ma, S., Yang, Y., and Zhou, W. (2013). Effects of hypothermia on oligodendrocyte precursor cell proliferation, differentiation and maturation following hypoxia ischemia in vivo and in vitro. *Exp. Neurol.* 247, 720–729. doi: 10.1016/j.expneurol.2013.03.015

Yager, J., Towfighi, J., and Vannucci, R. (1993). Influence of mild hypothermia on hypoxic-ischemic brain damage in the immature rat. *Pediatr. Res.* 34, 525–529. doi: 10.1203/00006450-199310000-00029

Yager, J. Y., and Ashwal, S. (2009). Animal models of perinatal hypoxic-ischemic brain damage. *Pediatr. Neurol.* 40, 156–167. doi: 10.1016/j.pediatrneurol.2008.10.025

Yager, J. Y., Brucklacher, R. M., and Vannucci, R. C. (1991). Cerebral oxidative metabolism and redox state during hypoxia-ischemia and early recovery in immature rats. *Am. J. Physiol.* 261(4 Pt 2), H1102–H1108.

Yager, J. Y., Brucklacher, R. M., and Vannucci, R. C. (1996). Paradoxical mitochondrial oxidation in perinatal hypoxic-ischemic brain damage. *Brain Res.* 712, 230–238. doi: 10.1016/0006-8993(95)01423-3

Yager, J. Y., Heitjan, D. F., Towfighi, J., and Vannucci, R. C. (1992). Effect of insulin-induced and fasting hypoglycemia on perinatal hypoxic-ischemic brain damage. *Pediatr. Res.* 31, 138–142. doi: 10.1203/00006450-199202000-00009

Yamamoto, H., Inaba, S., Nishiura, Y., Kishi, F., and Kawakami, Y. (1985). Acute inhalation of cigarette smoke augments hypoxic chemosensitivity in humans. *J. Appl. Physiol.* 58, 717–723.

Yamamoto, H., and Kato, T. (1986). The effect of neonatal anoxia on brain cholecystokinin-8-like immunoreactivity and monoamine levels of mature rats. *Brain Res.* 391, 285–288. doi: 10.1016/0165-3806(86)90294-4

Yamamoto, K., Yamamoto, Y., Fujimiya, T., and Okae, M. (1986). Effects of ethanol on the blood gas and acid-base state in hypoxic rats. *Jpn. J. Legal Med.* 40, 357–360.

Yang, D., and Kuan, C. (2015). Anti-tissue Plasminogen Activator (tPA) as an Effective Therapy of Neonatal Hypoxia–Ischemia with and without Inflammation. *CNS Neurosci. Ther.* 21, 367–373. doi: 10.1111/cns.12365

Yang, D., Li, S. Y., Yeung, C. M., Chang, R. C. C., So, K. F., Wong, D., et al. (2012). *Lycium barbarum* extracts protect the brain from blood-brain barrier disruption and cerebral edema in experimental stroke. *PLoS ONE* 7:e33596. doi: 10.1371/journal.pone.0033596

Yang, D., Sun, Y. Y., Lin, X., Baumann, J. M., Warnock, M., Lawrence, D. A., et al. (2013a). Taming neonatal hypoxic-ischemic brain injury by intranasal delivery of plasminogen activator inhibitor-1. *Stroke* 44, 2623–2627. doi: 10.1161/STROKEAHA.113.001233

Yang, D., Sun, Y. Y., Nemkul, N., Baumann, J. M., Shereen, A., Dunn, R. S., et al. (2013b). Plasminogen activator inhibitor-1 mitigates brain injury in a rat model of infection-sensitized neonatal hypoxia-ischemia. *Cereb. Cortex* 23, 1218–1229. doi: 10.1093/cercor/bhs115

Yao, L., Kan, E. M., Kaur, C., Dheen, S. T., Hao, A., Lu, J., et al. (2013). Notch-1 signaling regulates microglia activation via NF-kappaB pathway after hypoxic exposure in vivo and in vitro. *PLoS ONE* 8:e78439. doi: 10.1371/journal.pone.0078439

Yazaki, M., Liepnieks, J. J., Murrell, J. R., Takao, M., Guenther, B., Piccardo, P., et al. (2001). Biochemical characterization of a neuroserpin variant associated with hereditary dementia. *Am. J. Pathol.* 158, 227–233. doi: 10.1016/S0002-9440(10)63961-2

Yepes, M. (2015). Tissue-type plasminogen activator is a neuroprotectant in the central nervous system. *Front. Cell. Neurosci.* 9:304. doi: 10.3389/fncel.2015.00304

Yepes, M., and Lawrence, D. A. (2004a). Neuroserpin: a selective inhibitor of tissue-type plasminogen activator in the central nervous system. *Thromb. Haemost.* 91, 457–464. doi: 10.1160/th03-12-0766

Yepes, M., and Lawrence, D. A. (2004b). New functions for an old enzyme: nonhemostatic roles for tissue-type plasminogen activator in the central nervous system. *Exp. Biol. Med.* 229, 1097–1104.

Yepes, M., and Lawrence, D. A. (2004c). Tissue-type plasminogen activator and neuroserpin: a well-balanced act in the nervous system? *Trends Cardiovasc. Med.* 14, 173–180.

Yepes, M., Sandkvist, M., Coleman, T. A., Moore, E., Wu, J. Y., Mitola, D., et al. (2002). Regulation of seizure spreading by neuroserpin and tissue-type plasminogen activator is plasminogen-independent. *J. Clin. Invest.* 109, 1571–1578. doi: 10.1172/JCI0214308

Yepes, M., Sandkvist, M., Wong, M. K., Coleman, T. A., Smith, E., Cohan, S. L., et al. (2000). Neuroserpin reduces cerebral infarct volume and protects neurons from ischemia-induced apoptosis. *Blood* 96, 569–576.

Yoon, B. H., Kim, C. J., Romero, R., Jun, J. K., Park, K. H., Choi, S. T., et al. (1997). Experimentally induced intrauterine infection causes fetal brain white matter lesions in rabbits. *Am. J. Obstet. Gynecol.* 177, 797–802. doi: 10.1016/S0002-9378(97)70271-0

You, Y., and Kaur, C. (2000). Expression of induced nitric oxide synthase in amoeboid microglia in postnatal rats following an exposure to hypoxia. *Neurosci. Lett.* 279, 101–104. doi: 10.1016/S0304-3940(99)00967-2

Yuan, T. M., Yu, H. M., Gu, W. Z., and Li, J. P. (2005). White matter damage and chemokine induction in developing rat brain after intrauterine infection. *J. Perinatal Med.* 33, 415–422. doi: 10.1515/JPM.2005.074

Zanelli, S., Goodkin, H. P., Kowalski, S., and Kapur, J. (2014). Impact of transient acute hypoxia on the developing mouse EEG. *Neurobiol. Dis.* 68, 37–46. doi: 10.1016/j.nbd.2014.03.005

Zeinieh, M. P., Talhouk, R. S., El-Sabban, M. E., and Mikati, M. A. (2010). Differential expression of hippocampal connexins after acute hypoxia in the developing brain. *Brain Dev.* 32, 810–817. doi: 10.1016/j.braindev.2009.11.003

Zeinstra, E., Fock, J. M., Begeer, J. H., van Weerden, T. W., Maurits, N. M., and Zweens, M. J. (2001). The prognostic value of serial EEG recordings following acute neonatal asphyxia in full-term infants. *Eur. J. Paediatr. Neurol.* 5, 155–160. doi: 10.1053/ejpn.2001.0496

Zhang, C. P., Zhu, L. L., Zhao, T., Zhao, H., Huang, X., Ma, X., et al. (2006). Characteristics of neural stem cells expanded in lowered oxygen and the potential role of hypoxia-inducible factor-1Alpha. *Neurosignals* 15, 259–265. doi: 10.1159/000103385

Zhang, Q., Ding, Y., Yao, Y., Yu, Y., Yang, L., and Cui, H. (2013). Creating rat model for hypoxic brain damage in neonates by oxygen deprivation. *PLoS ONE* 8:e83589. doi: 10.1371/journal.pone.0083589

Zhang, Q., Yuan, L., Liu, D., Wang, J., Wang, S., Zhang, Q., et al. (2014). Hydrogen sulfide attenuates hypoxia-induced neurotoxicity through inhibiting microglial activation. *Pharmacol. Res.* 84, 32–44. doi: 10.1016/j.phrs.2014.04.009

Zhang, X., Zhang, Q., Li, W., Nie, D., Chen, W., Xu, C., et al. (2014). Therapeutic effect of human umbilical cord mesenchymal stem cells on neonatal rat hypoxic–ischemic encephalopathy. *J. Neurosci. Res.* 92, 35–45. doi: 10.1002/jnr.23304

Zhang, Y., He, K., Wang, F., Li, X., and Liu, D. (2015). Notch-1 signaling regulates astrocytic proliferation and activation after hypoxia exposure. *Neurosci. Lett.* 603, 12–18. doi: 10.1016/j.neulet.2015.07.009

Zhang, Z., Zhang, L., Yepes, M., Jiang, Q., Li, Q., Arniego, P., et al. (2002). Adjuvant treatment with neuroserpin increases the therapeutic window for tissue-type plasminogen activator administration in a rat model of embolic stroke. *Circulation* 106, 740–745. doi: 10.1161/01.CIR.0000023942.10849.41

Zhao, B. Q., Tejima, E., and Lo, E. H. (2007). Neurovascular proteases in brain injury, hemorrhage and remodeling after stroke. *Stroke* 38(Suppl. 2), 748–752. doi: 10.1161/01.STR.0000253500.32979.d1

Zheng, T., and Weiss, M. D. (2013). Neonatal transplant in hypoxic injury. *Methods Mol. Biol.* 1059, 147–156. doi: 10.1007/978-1-62703-574-3_13

Zheng, X. R., Zhang, S. S., Yin, F., Tang, J. L., Yang, Y. J., Wang, X., et al. (2012). Neuroprotection of VEGF-expression neural stem cells in neonatal cerebral palsy rats. *Behav. Brain Res.* 230, 108–115. doi: 10.1016/j.bbr.2012.01.026

Zhou, C., Lippman, J. J., Sun, H., and Jensen, F. E. (2011). Hypoxia-induced neonatal seizures diminish silent synapses and long-term potentiation in hippocampal CA1 neurons. *J. Neurosci.* 31, 18211–18222. doi: 10.1523/JNEUROSCI.4838-11.2011

Zhu, C., Kang, W., Xu, F., Cheng, X., Zhang, Z., Jia, L., et al. (2009). Erythropoietin improved neurologic outcomes in newborns with hypoxic-ischemic encephalopathy. *Pediatrics* 124, e218–e226. doi: 10.1542/peds.2008-3553

Zhu, C., Xu, F., Wang, X., Shibata, M., Uchiyama, Y., Blomgren, K., et al. (2006). Different apoptotic mechanisms are activated in male and female brains after neonatal hypoxia-ischaemia. *J. Neurochem.* 96, 1016–1027. doi: 10.1111/j.1471-4159.2005.03639.x

3

Changes in the Transcriptome of Human Astrocytes Accompanying Oxidative Stress-Induced Senescence

*Elizabeth P. Crowe[1], Ferit Tuzer[1], Brian D. Gregory[2], Greg Donahue[3], Sager J. Gosai[2], Justin Cohen[1], Yuk Y. Leung[4], Emre Yetkin[1], Raffaella Nativio[3], Li-San Wang[4], Christian Sell[1], Nancy M. Bonini[2], Shelley L. Berger[3], F. Brad Johnson[4] and Claudio Torres[1]**

[1] Department of Pathology and Laboratory Medicine, Drexel University College of Medicine, Philadelphia, PA, USA, [2] Department of Biology, Penn Genome Frontiers Institute, University of Pennsylvania, Philadelphia, PA, USA, [3] Epigenetics Program, Department of Cell and Developmental Biology, Perelman School of Medicine, University of Pennsylvania, Philadelphia, PA, USA, [4] Department of Pathology and Laboratory Medicine, Perelman School of Medicine, University of Pennsylvania, Philadelphia, PA, USA

Edited by:
Daniela Tropea,
Trinity College, Dublin, Ireland

Reviewed by:
James C. Vickers,
University of Tasmania, Australia
David Morgan,
University of South Florida, USA

***Correspondence:**
Claudio Torres
claudio.torres@drexelmed.edu

Aging is a major risk factor for many neurodegenerative disorders. A key feature of aging biology that may underlie these diseases is cellular senescence. Senescent cells accumulate in tissues with age, undergo widespread changes in gene expression, and typically demonstrate altered, pro-inflammatory profiles. Astrocyte senescence has been implicated in neurodegenerative disease, and to better understand senescence-associated changes in astrocytes, we investigated changes in their transcriptome using RNA sequencing. Senescence was induced in human fetal astrocytes by transient oxidative stress. Brain-expressed genes, including those involved in neuronal development and differentiation, were downregulated in senescent astrocytes. Remarkably, several genes indicative of astrocytic responses to injury were also downregulated, including glial fibrillary acidic protein and genes involved in the processing and presentation of antigens by major histocompatibility complex class II proteins, while pro-inflammatory genes were upregulated. Overall, our findings suggest that senescence-related changes in the function of astrocytes may impact the pathogenesis of age-related brain disorders.

Keywords: astrocyte senescence, astrocyte function, brain aging, RNA sequencing, brain oxidative stress

INTRODUCTION

Astrocytes are the most abundant population of cells within the central nervous system (CNS) and the structural diversity and functional complexity of cortical astrocytes is a distinguishing feature of the primate brain (Oberheim et al., 2006). Astrocytes form a functionally coupled network through a series of gap junctions and have pleiotropic roles in maintaining the blood–brain barrier and controlling cerebral blood flow (Abbott et al., 2006); regulating ion, water and neurotransmitter homeostasis (Simard and Nedergaard, 2004); and modulating synaptic transmission as part of the tripartite synapse (Perea et al., 2009). Astrocytes can respond to CNS insults through the acquisition of immune cell features (Jensen et al., 2013), and during repair, astrocytes undergo a spectrum of molecular and functional changes termed reactive astrogliosis (Sofroniew, 2009).

Recently, there has been a paradigm shift toward recognizing the integral role of glial cells in the pathogenesis of age-related cognitive decline and neurodegeneration (Nagelhus et al., 2013; Phatnani and Maniatis, 2015; Pekny et al., 2016). Secreted factors from astrocytes exacerbate the neurotoxicity of amyloid beta (Aβ) in primary culture (Garwood et al., 2011), and contribute to the decline in hippocampal neurogenesis in aged brains (Miranda et al., 2012). Altered astrocyte physiology has also been linked to aging and to the most common age-related neurodegenerative disorder, Alzheimer's disease (AD), by transcriptome profiling of gene expression changes in astrocytes from aged mouse cortex (Orre et al., 2014) and in glial fibrillary acidic protein (GFAP)-positive cells isolated by laser-capture microdissection from postmortem tissues of subjects with AD (Simpson et al., 2011; Sekar et al., 2015). Therefore, a greater understanding of how aging impacts astrocytes should provide new insight into age-related diseases of the brain.

Aging is the greatest risk factor for cognitive decline and neurodegenerative disease, and a key feature of aging biology that may underlie age-related diseases is cellular senescence. In support of this idea, senescent cells accumulate in tissues with age, including the brain, and at sites of aging-related pathology (Price et al., 2002; Krishnamurthy et al., 2004; Herbig et al., 2006; Bhat et al., 2012; Jurk et al., 2012, 2014; Zhu et al., 2014), undergo widespread changes in gene expression, and demonstrate a pro-inflammatory secretion pattern (Coppé et al., 2008). The induction of senescence in astrocytes has been implicated in neurodegenerative disease (Bhat et al., 2012; Chinta et al., 2013). Either a cell-intrinsic loss of function or the acquisition of detrimental neuroinflammatory function in astrocytes could have profound consequences for the aging CNS. While senescence-associated gene expression changes have been described in cell-types from the periphery that were senescent *in situ* or induced to senesce *in vitro* (Shelton et al., 1999; Gruber et al., 2010), they remain largely understudied in the context of the CNS.

Treatment with sublethal concentrations of hydrogen peroxide (H_2O_2) induces senescence in a variety of cell types (Chen et al., 1998; Kim et al., 2011). Our previous studies characterized this type of stress-induced senescence in human astrocytes as determined by changes in cell morphology (enlarged and flattened shape), cessation of division, increased senescence-associated β-galactosidase activity (85% of positive cells compared to 5% of controls), increased expression of p53 and the cyclin-dependent kinase inhibitors p21 and $p16^{INK4a}$, and a p38MAPK-dependent increase in interleukin-6 secretion (Bitto et al., 2010; Bhat et al., 2012). Astrocytes are sensitive to oxidative stress and low doses of H_2O_2 are enough to induce the senescence program compared to other cell types (Bitto et al., 2010; Bhat et al., 2012; Aravinthan et al., 2014). This is physiologically relevant because the CNS is particularly exposed to elevated levels of oxidative stress due to several factors including a high metabolic rate with an elevated oxygen consumption compared to its relatively small weight, low antioxidant capacity, and high concentration of lipids and pro-oxidant metals. The generation of this robust oxidative environment disturbs cells and results in oxidative damage to macromolecules, which is a common underlying feature of both aging and diseased brains (Smith et al., 1991; Esiri, 2007; Radak et al., 2011). Levels of mitochondrial H_2O_2 and defects in protective mechanisms that reduce it are implicated in cognitive defects in AD mouse models and also in inflammation (Yin et al., 2016).

In order to better understand how astrocyte senescence relates to changes in astrocyte physiology during aging, we investigated global changes in the astrocyte transcriptome using RNA Sequencing (RNA-Seq) following the induction of oxidative stress-induced senescence using H_2O_2. From this analysis, we confirmed that senescent astrocytes acquire an inflammatory phenotype indicative of the senescence-associated secretory phenotype (SASP) and downregulate the expression of brain-expressed genes. In keeping with the myriad of complex functions that astrocytes perform in the healthy brain, senescent astrocytes could affect tissue dysfunction during aging and neurodegenerative disease via multiple mechanisms.

MATERIALS AND METHODS

Cell Culture and Senescence Induction

Human fetal astrocytes (passage 1) were obtained from ScienCell Research Laboratories (Carlsbad, CA, USA) and cultured in ambient O_2 and 5% CO_2 as previously described (Bitto et al., 2010; Bhat et al., 2012). In order to induce premature senescence via oxidative stress, cells were seeded at standard density (1×10^4 cells/cm^2) and the following day treated with 200 μM hydrogen peroxide (H_2O_2) for 2 h. Cells were considered senescent at least 5 days after the initiation of treatment, as verified previously, (Bitto et al., 2010) and in subsequent quantitative real-time PCR (qRT-PCR) experiments by increases in senescence marker p21, flattened and enlarged morphology, and cessation of division, and were harvested 7 days after treatment. Viability of senescent astrocytes was not significantly different than the controls (92% ± 1 vs. 95% ± 2.7; $p = 0.08$) as measured by the Guava ViaCount assay (EMD Millipore).

RNA Preparation and Sequencing

Total RNA was isolated using the RNeasy Mini Kit (Qiagen; Valencia, CA, USA) according to the manufacturer's instructions and the concentration was determined using a NanoDrop ND-1000 spectrophotometer (NanoDrop; Rockland, DE, USA). RNA-Seq libraries were prepared as previously described (Elliott et al., 2013). RNA-Seq libraries were prepared from two replicate cDNA libraries per condition. We used two biological replicates from one donor, where a biological replicate is defined as an independent growth of cells and subsequent analysis, based on the "Standards, Guidelines and Best Practices for RNA-Seq" published by The ENCODE consortium[1] recommending

[1] genome.ucsc.edu/ENCODE/protocols/dataStandards/ENCODE_RNAseq_Standards_V1.0.pdf

the use of a minimum of two biological replicates in RNA-Seq experiments, where a biological replicate is defined as an independent growth of cells and subsequent analysis. The two replicate cDNA libraries per condition (four libraries in total) were submitted to the Next Generation Sequencing Core (NGSC) at the Perelman School of Medicine, University of Pennsylvania, for sequencing. The Illumina HiSeq sequencing platform was used to generate 50 bp single-end sequencing reads. Analysis of RNA-Seq data, including read mapping and differential gene expression analysis using the DESeq package with a Benjamini–Hochberg correction, was performed as previously described by Elliott et al. (2013). The RNA-Seq dataset was deposited in the Gene Expression Omnibus (GEO) at the National Center for Biotechnology under the accession number GSE58910.

Gene Ontology and Gene Set Intersection Analysis

Gene Ontology (GO) analysis was performed on transcripts that were significantly differentially expressed in senescent astrocytes with a greater than 1.5-fold change and a p-value ≤ 0.05 (Benjamini–Hochberg adjusted). The functional annotation clustering tool of the online bioinformatics resource Database for Annotation, Visualization and Integrated Discovery (DAVID) version 6.7 (Huang da et al., 2009) was used to perform GO analysis limited to biological process terms (BP_FAT). By satisfying a false discovery rate (FDR) of 10%, GO terms were considered to be enriched. In addition, all GO categories have a gene count of 10 or greater and a fold-enrichment of 2 or greater. Enriched GO biological process terms were collapsed if they shared 25 or more differentially expressed transcripts and thus considered functionally synonymous. Enrichment (N, B, n, b) is defined as (b/n)/(B/N) where N is the total number of transcripts in the experiment, B is the total number of transcripts within a GO term, n is the number of total transcripts in the intersection of the two gene sets in comparison, b is the number of transcripts in the intersection that belong to that GO term. "Count" is the number of genes in the single or collapsed GO term. "Weight" is the summed weight of all genes in the GO term, where each gene is given a weight inversely proportional to the total number of GO terms it appears in. "FDR," i.e., false discovery rate is the percent likelihood of that GO term coming up by the same number of random genes by chance, as calculated by Benjamini–Yekutieli correction of the p-value obtained by Fisher's Exact test. "Genes" represents the genes constituting the GO term. GO analysis on the intersection of senescence and AD downregulated transcripts was done similarly. The enrichment and statistical significance of gene set overlaps between astrocyte and hepatocyte senescence was performed on http://nemates.org/MA/progs/overlap_stats.html, with the number of detected transcripts from the RNA-Seq, 19580, as the total number of genes. In comparison of gene expression in senescent astrocytes to those from AD patient brains, we only compared genes with expression levels in our control set matching those in the Stanford Brain database (Zhang et al., 2014). This criterion was expression level of greater than or less than 100 in both datasets. For this comparison, "Percentage" is "Count" as a percentage of the total number of input genes. P-value is a modified Fisher's exact p-value corrected for the representation of the gene set in the whole genome. List total is the total number of genes in the input that are part of any ontology.

Identification of Transcription Factor Motifs on Differentially Expressed Genes

The chromosomal coordinates of all promoter regions 1000 bp upstream of the transcription start site were obtained using the RefSeq genes track, refGene table and the hg19 human genome assembly on UCSC Genome Browser – Table Browser tool[2]. For all genes up- or downregulated 1.5 fold or more which enriched GO categories, promoter coordinates were submitted to the Cistrome Analysis Pipeline[3] SeqPos tool. Public motif databases Transfac and JASPAR were searched for motifs enriched in the promoter sequences. Additionally, a *de novo* motif analysis was performed to find motifs with no correlate in the public databases. Results were filtered by human and mouse species-specificity, using a 1000 bp scan length.

qRT-PCR Validation

Candidate genes were chosen based upon pathways of interest for validation by qRT-PCR. Total RNA was independently isolated as described. Primers were designed using the PrimerQuest design tool to span an exon–exon junction and were supplied by Integrated DNA Technologies (IDT, Coralville, IA, USA). The NCBI Basic Local Alignment Search Tool (BLAST) was used to confirm the specificity of primer sequences. The primers used in qRT-PCR assays are listed in Supplementary Table S1. SYBR Green-based RT-PCR was performed with Verso 1-Step RT-qPCR reagents (Thermo Fisher Scientific; Pittsburgh, PA, USA) on an Applied Biosystems 7500 Real-Time PCR System (Life Technologies, Grand Island, NY, USA). Dissociation curve analysis was performed to verify single products for each reaction. The absence of product in reactions without reverse transcriptase (no RT) was also verified. Data analysis was performed using DataAssist software v3.01 (Life Technologies, Grand Island, NY, USA). The data were glyceraldehyde-3-phosphate dehydrogenase (GAPDH)-normalized and expressed as fold change (RQ) relative to pre-senescent astrocytes.

Cell Cycle Analysis

Pre-senescent astrocytes (60–70% confluent) and astrocytes treated with H_2O_2 to undergo stress-induced premature senescence were grown in complete Astrocyte Medium (AM, ScienCell) as described (Bitto et al., 2010; Bhat et al., 2012), harvested by trypsinization, washed in phosphate buffered saline (PBS), and fixed with ice cold 70% ethanol overnight at 4°C. Fixed cells were centrifuged to remove ethanol, washed with PBS, and stained with Guava Cell Cycle reagent (EMD Millipore; Billerica,

[2]https://genome.ucsc.edu/

[3]http://cistrome.org/ap/root

MA, USA) containing the nuclear DNA stain propidium iodide (PI) for 30 min at room temperature in the dark. Guava Cell Cycle data were acquired using Guava EasyCyte Mini flow cytometer using the Guava Cell Cycle program (Guava Technologies, Hayward, CA, USA). The percentage of cells in cell debris, G1-, S-, and G2/M-phase of the cell cycle was determined using the ModFit LT curve fitting algorithm, version 4.0.5 (Verity Software House, Topsham, ME, USA).

Bromodeoxyuridine (BrdU) Incorporation Assay

Pre-senescent astrocytes in log phase of growth and astrocytes that were treated with H_2O_2 to undergo stress-induced premature senescence 7 days prior were treated with 10 μM BrdU (5-bromo-2′-deoxyuridine; BD Pharmingen; San Diego, CA, USA) in complete astrocyte medium for 30 min. After this incubation, cells were harvested by trypsinization, washed in PBS, and fixed with ice cold 70% ethanol. Fixed cells were centrifuged to remove ethanol, resuspended in 2N HCl and incubated for 30 min at room temperature for DNA denaturation, neutralized with 0.1 M $Na_2B_4O_7$ (pH 8.5), and washed two times in PBS containing 5% fetal bovine serum (FBS). Anti-BrdU monoclonal antibody (eBioscience; San Diego, CA, USA) diluted 1:100 in PBS containing 0.5% Tween-20 was applied for 30 min at room temperature, after which cells were washed, and resuspended in goat anti-mouse-Alexa Fluor 488 (Molecular Probes, Life Technologies; Grand Island, NY, USA) diluted 1:100 in 1x PBS containing 0.5% Tween-20 for 20 min at room temperature in the dark and then washed twice with PBS-5% FBS. Cells were stained with Guava Cell Cycle solution as described previously and analyzed using the Guava EasyCyte Mini flow cytometer using the Guava ExpressPlus program and the percent of cells labeled with BrdU was quantified. The percent of BrdU positive cells was quantified using FlowJo software v10 (Tree Star; Ashland, OR, USA).

Immunofluorescence

Cells were seeded on coverslips and fixed with 4% paraformaldehyde in PBS, permeabilized with PBS containing 0.1% Triton-X-100, and blocked in PBS containing 0.1% bovine serum albumin (BSA) and 5% normal donkey serum for 2 h at room temperature. Coverslips were incubated with rabbit anti-phosphorylated histone H3 (Ser10) (Upstate Biotechnology; Lake Placid, NY, USA) diluted 1:500 in PBS containing 0.1% BSA overnight at room temperature. Following washes with PBS, coverslips were incubated with Alexa-Fluor Donkey 555 anti-Rabbit (Life Technologies; Carlsbad, CA, USA) diluted 1:500 in PBS 0.1% BSA for 1 h at room temperature protected from light. Coverslips were then washed, stained with DAPI, and mounted on slides with Vectashield fluorescence mounting medium (Vector Laboratories; Burlingame, CA, USA). Cells were visualized using an Olympus BX61 fluorescence microscope coupled with a Hamamatsu ORCA-ER camera and using SlideBook software (Intelligent Innovations, Inc., Denver, CO, USA). The percent of cells positive for phosphorylated histone H3 was quantified.

RESULTS

RNA-Seq Broad Picture of Differentially-Expressed (DE) Genes

We sequenced two biological replicates each of pre-senescent astrocytes and astrocytes induced to senesce by oxidative stress, and obtained approximately 12 to 35 million reads per sample. From these datasets, ~97.5% of all reads mapped to the reference human genome (hg 19; see Supplementary Table S2 for all mapped transcripts). We also found by a principle component analysis (PCA) that these samples were tightly clustered based on cellular treatment (**Figure 1A**). Expression levels of genes between the pre-senescent and senescent repeats were highly correlated, with r^2-values of 0.986 and 0.998, respectively. In total, these results suggest that these high-throughput sequencing libraries were highly reproducible and were differentiated from one another based on the biological differences of pre- and post-senescent astrocytes.

We then performed a differential expression analysis that revealed significant senescence-associated changes in the transcriptome. Overall, there were 3569 significantly differentially expressed transcripts ($p_{adj} < 0.05$), which represents 18.3% of the total number of detected transcripts, with 1772 transcripts being downregulated in senescence and 1797 transcripts upregulated in senescence (**Figure 1B**). These results demonstrate that there are significant changes to the astrocyte transcriptome during oxidative stress-induced senescence.

Gene Ontology Term Enrichment Analysis and Tissue Expression of DE Genes

To identify functional categories of differentially expressed transcripts in senescent astrocytes, we performed GO enrichment analysis using biological process terms with the functional annotation-clustering tool in the DAVID, using a cut-off of 1.5-fold differential expression to define up- or downregulated genes. 1510 downregulated and 1258 upregulated transcripts satisfied this criterion with $p_{adj} < 0.05$, (Supplementary Table S2). Genes involved in cell division, major histocompatibility complex (MHC) class II antigen processing and presentation, metabolism, and CNS development and differentiation were enriched among the downregulated transcripts in senescent astrocytes (**Figures 2A,B**; Supplementary Table S3). MHC Class II presentation and gliogenesis were the two most enriched non-cell division related processes formed by the senescence downregulated transcripts, with enrichment scores of 4 and 3.5, respectively. Among the upregulated gene GO categories, several have known associations with senescence (**Figures 2C,D**; Supplementary Table S4). Inflammation, modification of the extracellular matrix and resistance to apoptosis are known senescence-associated changes (Yoon et al., 2004; Hampel et al., 2006; Freund et al., 2010; Childs et al., 2014) and are represented by the GO terms regulation of I-kappaB kinase/NF-kappaB cascade, positive regulation of cytokine production, extracellular structure organization, vasculature development, and resistance to apoptosis. Cellular adhesion (regulation of cell adhesion,

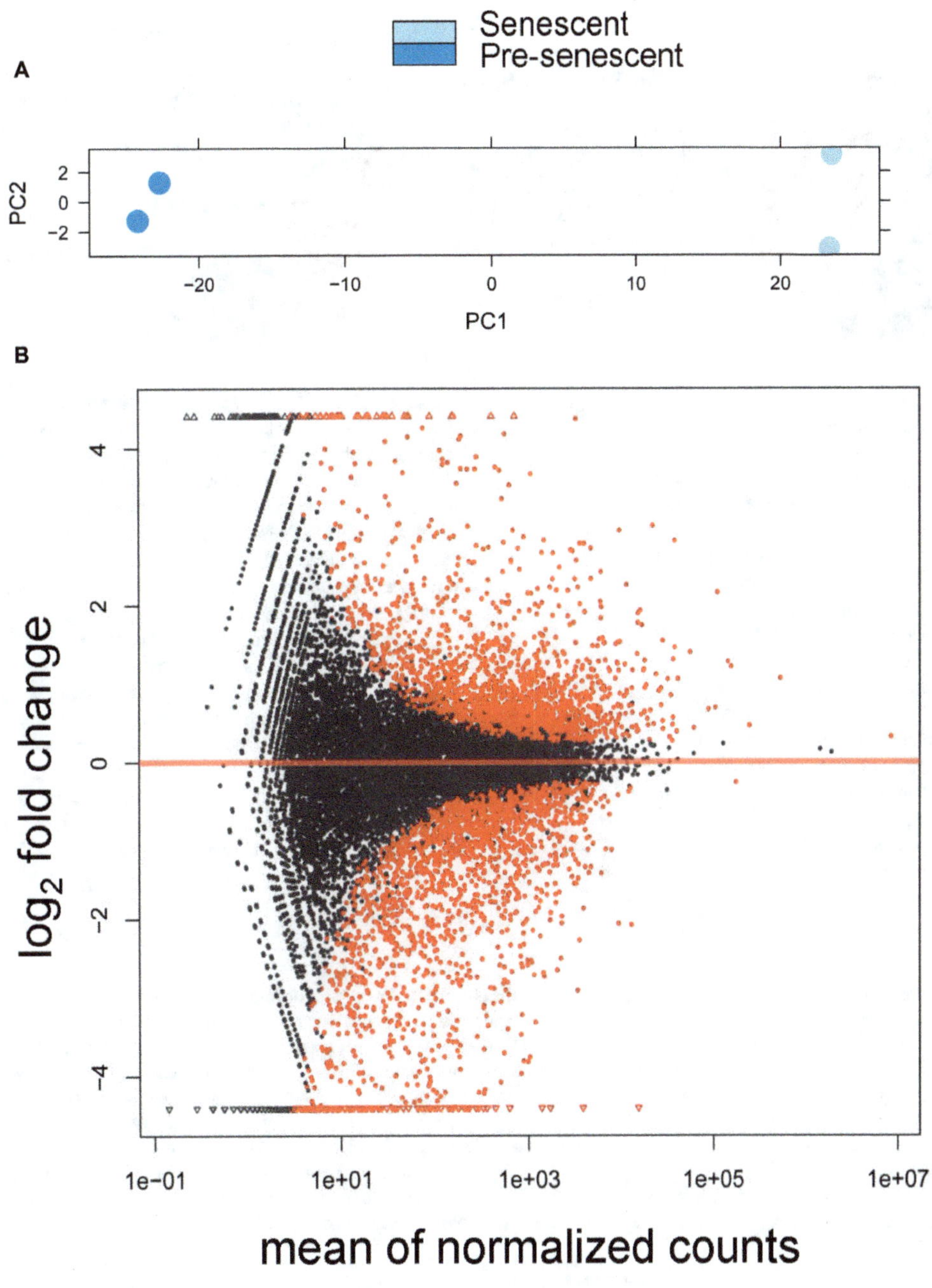

FIGURE 1 | Differential expression analysis of pre-senescent vs. senescent astrocyte transcriptomes. (A) Principle component analysis (PCA) revealed the greatest variability in the RNA-Seq data was due to the treatment condition (PC = principle component). **(B)** DESeq Plot showing the expression fold changes compared to pre-senescent and the expression levels of 19520 transcripts (gray) out of which 3569 are differentially expressed transcripts with each symbol representing a single transcript (red symbols are statistically significant at $p < 0.05$ Benjamini–Hochberg adjusted). A positive $\log_2$ fold change indicates transcripts that are upregulated in senescent cells, whereas a negative $\log_2$ fold change represents transcripts significantly downregulated in pre-senescent astrocytes. "Mean normalized counts" are the raw read counts, normalized by the total library size, and averaged for each group.

regulation of cell motion, positive regulation of binding) and cytoskeleton (actin cytoskeleton organization) related genes were also previously seen to be upregulated in *in vitro* senescence of human dermal fibroblasts (Yoon et al., 2004). The upregulation of inflammatory genes suggests a mechanism by which astrocyte senescence may be causing further damage in the brain.

In order to identify possible regulators of the senescence-associated genes, we analyzed the promoter regions of differentially regulated genes for over-represented transcription factor binding motifs. GO categories formed by downregulated genes yielded a total of 13 motifs, while those formed by upregulated genes yielded only 1 motif, that for p53, formed

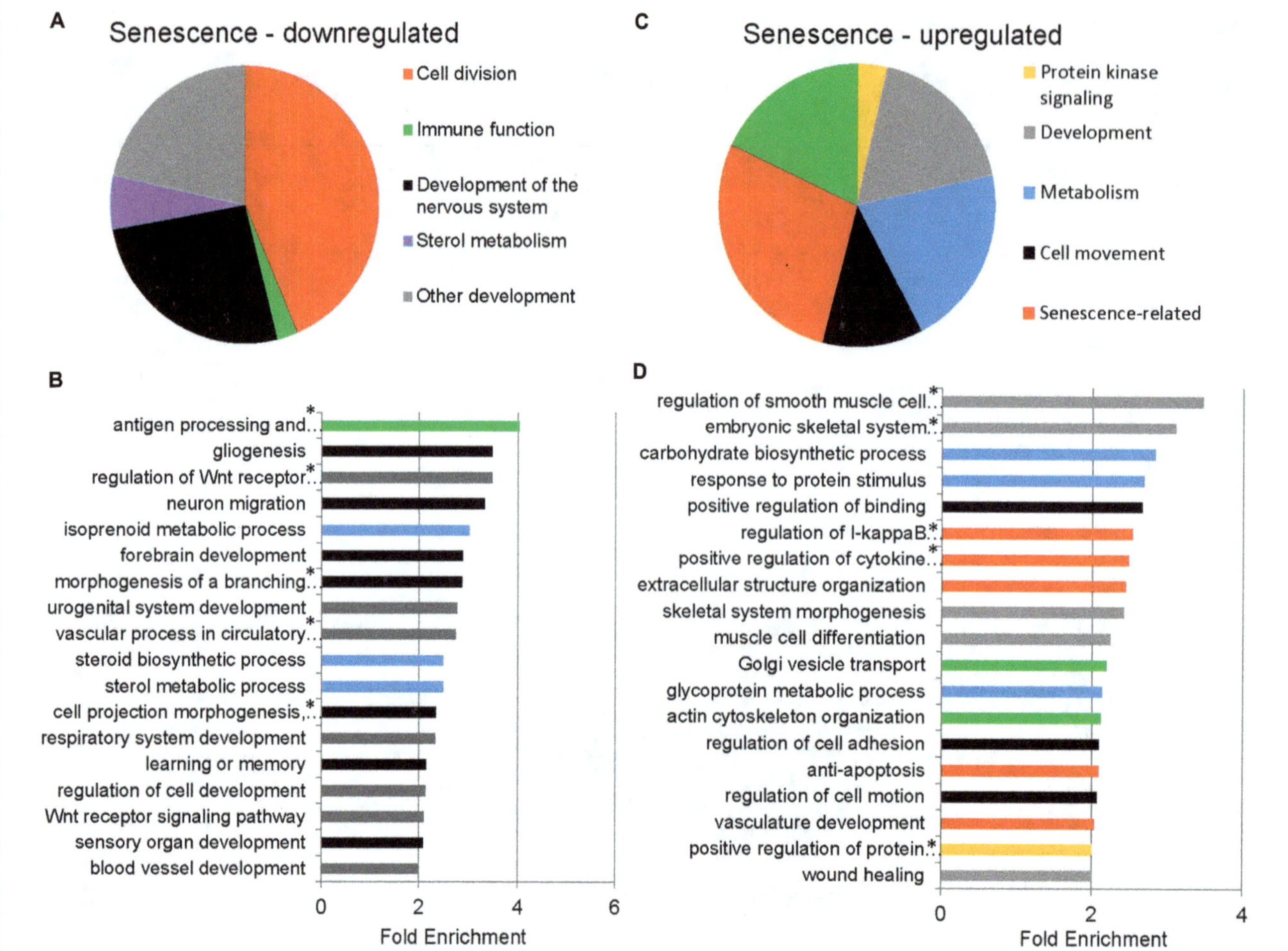

FIGURE 2 | Gene Ontology (GO) term enrichment analysis for senescent astrocyte down- and upregulated transcripts. (A) The top overrepresented GO biological process classes in astrocyte downregulated transcripts (p_{adj} < 0.05 and fold change of 1.5 or greater; Supplementary Table S3) are shown in the pie chart. The weighted number of genes in each category corresponds to the width of the wedges in the pie chart. **(B)** GO terms that are not cell division related are expanded below in a bar graph. Developmental categories are coded in gray, immune function is in green, sterol metabolism in blue, and development of the nervous system is in black. **(C)** The top overrepresented GO biological process classes by fold enrichment within astrocyte upregulated transcripts (p_{adj} < 0.05 and fold change of 1.5 or greater; Supplementary Table S4). **(D)** All GO terms overrepresented by the senescence upregulated genes, ranked by fold enrichment, color coded as in **(C)**. *Full names of GO terms: antigen processing and presentation of peptide or polysaccharide antigen via major histocompatibility complex (MHC) class II, regulation of Wnt receptor signaling pathway, morphogenesis of a branching structure, the combined term of "cell projection morphogenesis, cell morphogenesis involved in differentiation, neuron differentiation," regulation of smooth muscle cell proliferation, embryonic skeletal system development, regulation of I-kappaB kinase/NF-kappaB cascade, positive regulation of cytokine production, positive regulation of protein kinase cascade.

by the genes in the 'extracellular structure organization' GO category (Supplementary Table S5).

To determine whether genes with differential expression in oxidative stress-induced astrocyte senescence are brain-expressed, we analyzed differentially expressed transcripts (p_{adj} < 0.05) that also had a ≥1.5-fold change, for tissue expression using the UniProt tissue expression database (DAVID:UP_TISSUE). Of all the non-exclusive expression sites found (FDR <10%) for downregulated transcripts, genes belonging to CNS sites comprise the vast majority (762 transcripts or 94.8%), with expressed tissue definition of brain and hippocampus (**Figure 3A**). Therefore, upon the induction of senescence in astrocytes, we see a loss of brain-expressed genes. In contrast, none of the genes upregulated in senescence was CNS-enriched (not shown). CNS enrichment for all detected transcripts was 27%, which is the ratio of the total size of the CNS expression gene sets (7858) to all the defined tissue expression gene sets (29348, FDR <10%, **Figure 3B**). Thus, H_2O_2 induced astrocyte senescence specifically downregulates genes that are CNS-enriched.

Validation of RNA-Seq by qRT-PCR

Astrocyte-Enriched Genes

To determine whether our astrocyte transcriptome data is similar to previously published astrocyte gene expression data, we compared our list of differentially expressed transcripts with cell-type specific markers of astrocytes as described in a previous microarray study (Cahoy et al., 2008). The expression levels

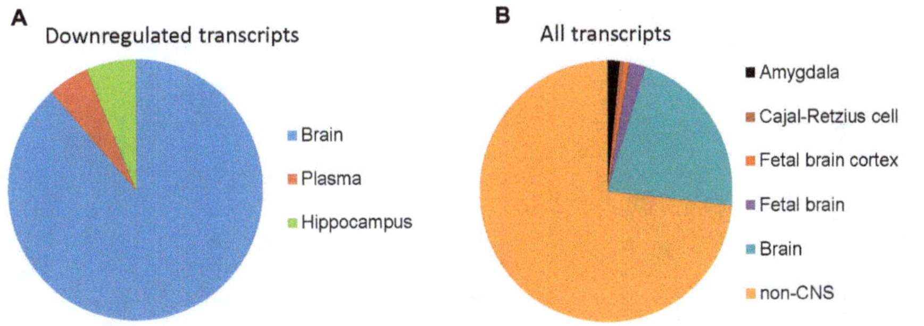

FIGURE 3 | Tissue expression of detected transcripts in senescent astrocytes. **(A)** Tissue annotation expression for astrocyte 1.5-fold or more downregulated transcripts using DAVID (controlling for an FDR at 10%). The width of wedges corresponds to the number of astrocyte downregulated transcripts with tissue expression annotation information that are expressed in the indicated tissues. **(B)** Tissue expression annotation for all transcripts detected in astrocytes.

of selected astrocyte-enriched genes GFAP, S100B, ALDH1L1, FGFR3, CNS enriched Synapse Differentiation Induced Gene 1 (SynDIG1) and a non-CNS enriched gene, KLF3 were validated by qRT-PCR. The expression of astrocyte and CNS enriched genes was lost or diminished in senescent astrocytes, while that of KLF3 did not change (**Figure 4B**). We verified the association of this decrease in GFAP with senescence by measuring the levels of this protein in pre-senescent astrocytes [cumulative population doubling (cPD) 8.1] and astrocytes that reached replicative senescence, as verified by cessation of growth (cPD 12.2). The GFAP expression in pre-senescent astrocytes was greatly reduced in replicative senescence, confirming our findings with oxidative stress-induced senescence (Supplementary Figure S1). When comparing the $\log_2$-fold changes in transcript levels between pre-senescent and senescent astrocytes using qRT-PCR and RNA-Seq, we observed a significant positive correlation ($r^2 = 0.656$, $n = 17$) between the results from the two distinct methodologies (**Figure 4A**; Supplementary Table S6). Thus, the loss of astrocyte-enriched genes, combined with the GO analysis demonstrating reduced expression of genes involved in glial and neuronal development suggests loss of normal function in these cells upon undergoing oxidative stress-induced senescence.

Senescence-Enriched Genes

We validated by qRT-PCR the levels of senescence-related transcripts that were differentially expressed by RNA-Seq. The levels of senescence-related transcripts *CCND1* (Cyclin D1), *IL8*, *IGFBP5*, and *ICAM-1* were significantly increased (**Figure 4C**) and correlated with changes observed with RNA-Seq (**Figure 4A**; Supplementary Table S6).

Treatment with H_2O_2 to induce senescence robustly induces p21 expression in human diploid fibroblasts (Chen et al., 1998). Surprisingly, the expression of *CDKN1A*, which encodes for the cyclin-dependent kinase inhibitor p21, was not called as significantly differentially expressed in our dataset, although a trend toward increased expression in senescent astrocytes was apparent (RNA-Seq, fold change = 5.84, $p_{adj} = 0.11$). One potential reason for this is low levels of read coverage for this transcript; therefore, we determined the mRNA expression level of p21 using qRT-PCR (**Figure 4C**). We confirmed an almost fourfold increase in p21 mRNA in senescent astrocytes compared with pre-senescent controls.

Cell Cycle Analysis

Gene Ontology analysis revealed that genes involved in cell cycle, cell division, and mitosis were over-represented among the downregulated genes in senescent astrocytes consistent with the lost proliferative potential of these cells ("cell division" category, **Figure 2A**). In order to examine the cell cycle distribution of senescent astrocytes, cells were stained for DNA content 7 days after H_2O_2 treatment and flow cytometric analysis was performed. Pre-senescent astrocytes that were serum-starved for 24 h arrested predominantly in G0/G1, while in senescent astrocyte cultures, we observed an increase in the fraction of cells with 4N DNA content and a concomitant loss of cells in G0/G1 compared with pre-senescent controls cultured in complete growth medium (**Figures 5A,B**).

The proliferative arrest associated with the onset of cellular senescence has often been presumed to occur solely in G1; however, replicatively senescent cells retain the capacity to synthesize DNA under certain conditions and accumulate in both G1 and G2/M (Mao et al., 2012). A multi-phase cell cycle arrest is also a feature of many cell types exposed to oxidative stress and DNA damage (Baus et al., 2003; Oyama et al., 2011). In order to address the possibility that senescent cells with G2 DNA content are progressing to mitosis, we stained astrocytes for phosphorylated histone H3 (Ser10), which is a marker of mitotic chromosome condensation (Hendzel et al., 1997). Compared with pre-senescent controls, H_2O_2-treated astrocytes exhibited few phospho-H3-positive cells (**Figure 5D**). In pre-senescent and senescent astrocyte cultures, we observed a similar proportion of cells with DNA content between 2N and 4N; therefore, we pulsed the cells with BrdU to determine whether they were actively synthesizing DNA. The BrdU-positive population was significantly reduced in senescent astrocytes compared with pre-senescent controls (**Figure 5C**). Overall, these results support a multi-phase cell cycle arrest in H_2O_2-induced senescence in human astrocytes.

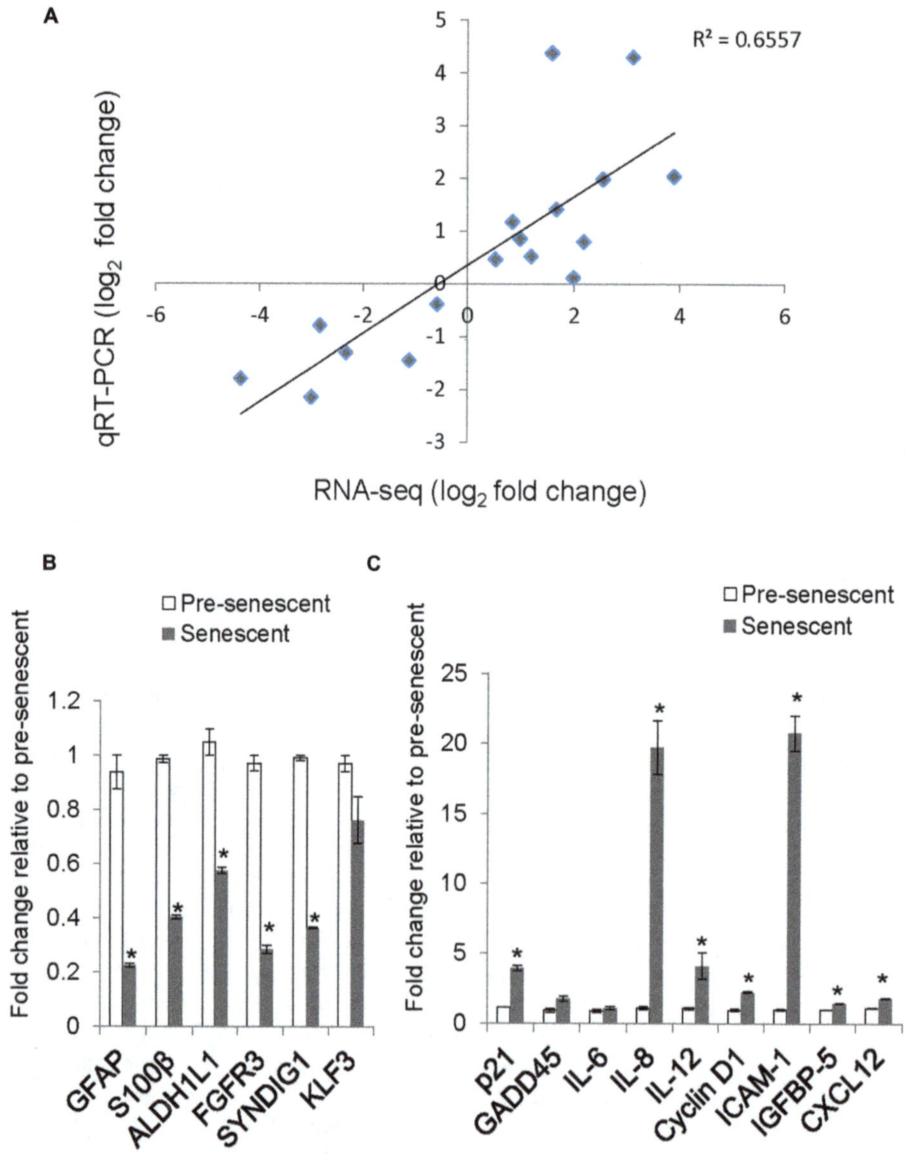

FIGURE 4 | Validation of selected genes by quantitative real-time PCR (qRT-PCR) and comparison with RNA-Seq $\log_2$ fold change. (A) A scatter plot of pre-senescence to senescence $\log_2$-fold changes obtained by RNA-Seq and qRT-PCR for selected transcripts. Each symbol represents a single transcript, $n = 17$, Pearson $r = 0.809$, ($p < 0.001$ 95% CI 0.659 to 0.939). **(B)** Relative levels of astrocyte/brain enriched-genes. Error bars indicate SEM of two independent samples. **(C)** Relative levels of senescence or SASP-related transcripts. Error bars indicate SEM of two independent samples. *indicates $p < 0.05$, student's *t*-test.

DISCUSSION

In order to better understand how astrocyte senescence is linked to aging-related decline in cognition and neurodegeneration, an unbiased interrogation of the changes that occur at the molecular level is essential. Here, we report a comprehensive analysis of the astrocyte transcriptome following the induction of senescence by oxidative stress. Although gene expression changes have been profiled extensively in brain tissue homogenates from different brain regions during aging (Wood et al., 2013) and in Alzheimer's disease (Twine et al., 2011), fewer studies have addressed cell-type specific changes in these contexts (Simpson et al., 2011; Orre et al., 2014; Sekar et al., 2015). To our knowledge, this is the first report of senescence-associated gene expression changes in a CNS-derived cell type using a whole transcriptome sequencing method (RNA-Seq), which is an accurate and quantitative measurement of transcript abundance.

As expected from the cessation of cell cycle in senescence, the majority of genes downregulated in astrocyte senescence following oxidative stress were related to the cell cycle. Several upregulated genes were also related to senescence-associated phenotypes, such as chronic inflammation (comprising *NFkB activation* and *cytokine production*), extracellular remodeling, and changes in cell morphology (actin cytoskeleton organization).

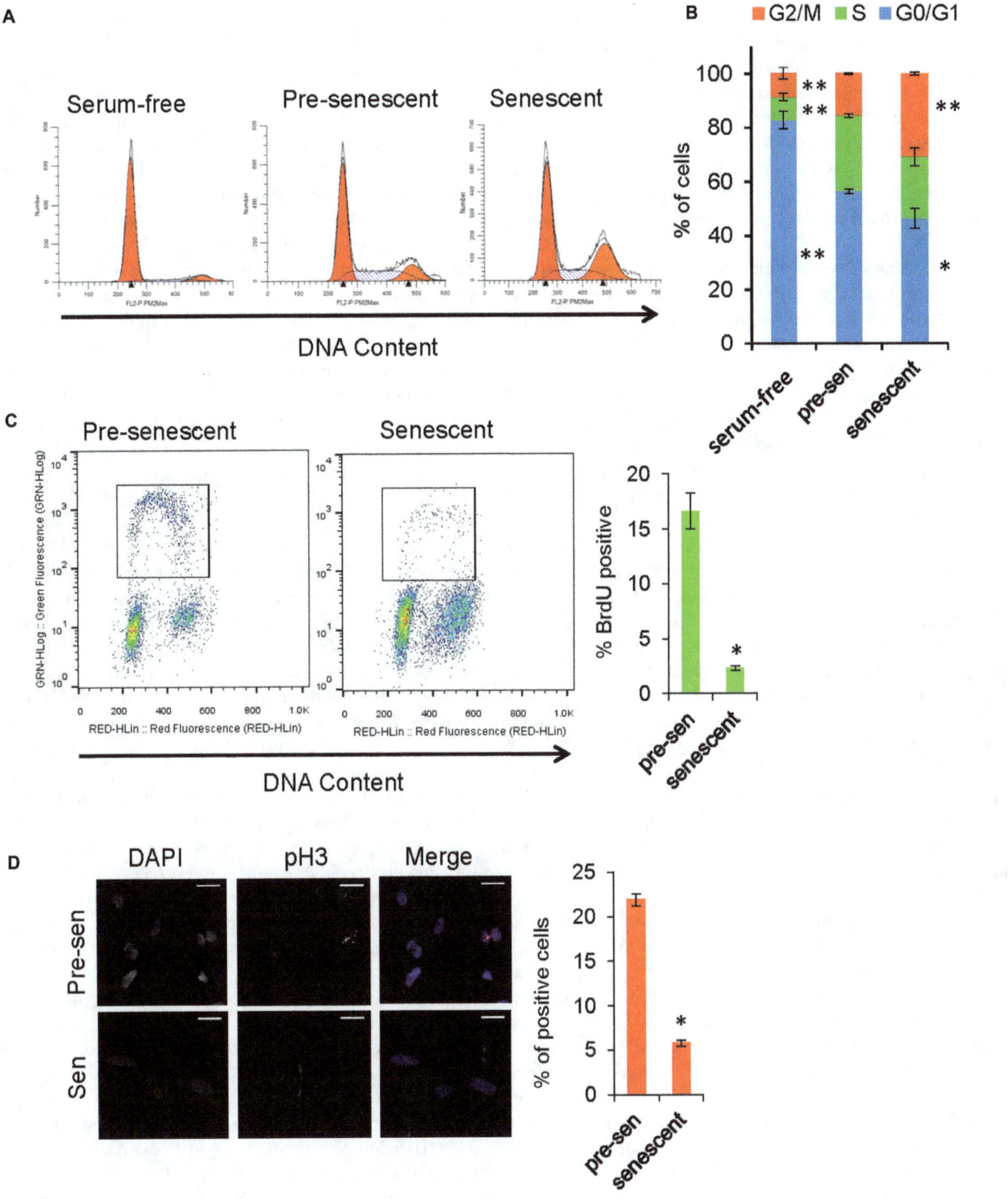

FIGURE 5 | Cell cycle analysis of senescent astrocytes. (A) Representative cell cycle profiles of subconfluent pre-senescent astrocytes that were serum-starved, kept in complete growth media, or kept in complete growth media and treated with H_2O_2 (200 μM) to induce senescence 7 days prior to staining for DNA content and flow cytometric analysis. Arrowheads indicate, left: Diploid (2N), right: tetraploid (4N) DNA content. **(B)** Graph for percentage of cells in G0/G1 (blue), S (green), or G2/M (red) phases of the cell cycle, that is representative of at least four independent experiments. $^*p < 0.02$, $^{**}p < 0.001$ vs. pre-senescent in growth medium using one-way ANOVA followed by Bonferroni *post hoc* testing. **(C)** Pre-senescent and senescent astrocytes were stained for DNA content and BrdU incorporation. The BrdU-positive population was significantly reduced in senescent astrocytes compared with pre-senescent controls $^*p < 0.01$, Student's *t*-test. **(D)** Representative images of immunofluorescence staining for mitosis marker phosphorylated histone H3 (pH3) (red) and DAPI (blue), with percent of cells staining positive for pH3 shown in the bar graph. $^*p < 0.01$, student's *t*-test.

We found that oxidative stress-induced astrocyte senescence is accompanied by a loss of brain-expressed transcripts involved in neuronal and glial differentiation and development, axonogenesis, and axon guidance. These results are supported by studies of *in vitro* aging in astrocytes where prolonged culture of astrocytes results in a decline in their functional properties including a loss of neuroprotective capacity (Pertusa et al., 2007); and in impaired synaptic transmission in co-culture with neurons (Kawano et al., 2012). The loss of differentiated function upon senescence is also a feature of human ocular keratocytes (Kipling et al., 2009).

The expression of classical markers of astrocyte reactivity — glial fibrillary acidic protein (GFAP) and S100β— is down-regulated with oxidative stress-induced astrocyte senescence in our study. Interestingly, this finding correlates with recent transcriptome analyses showing a decrease in GFAP expression in astrocytes isolated from the brains of aged mice (Orre et al., 2014) and in aged rat cortical tissue homogenates (Wood et al., 2013). Although aging in astrocytes has traditionally been synonymous with an increase in GFAP expression (Pertusa et al., 2007), recent studies have highlighted the heterogeneity of astrocyte expression of stereotypical markers, including GFAP and S100β, in different brain regions during aging (Rodríguez et al., 2014). Furthermore, the response of astrocytes to different CNS insults, in a process termed reactive astrogliosis, is also more heterogeneous than was once thought (Anderson et al., 2014). Although astrocyte senescence shares some features of reactive astrogliosis including cell hypertrophy and the production of inflammatory mediators, whether astrocyte senescence and reactive astrogliosis are distinct phenomena or part of a continuum of changes will require a more comprehensive analysis of these two phenotypes. It is possible that downregulation of certain markers of astrogliosis helps limit the damaging effects of gliosis, or, alternatively, the downregulation may reflect an inability of senescent astrocytes to respond properly to injury. The upregulation of several cytokines and pro-inflammatory genes, on the other hand, suggests that while astrocyte function is decreased in oxidative stress-induced senescence, the cells may be inducing a more general pro-inflammatory environment. The upregulation of Golgi vesicle transport related genes in senescence (**Figure 2**) suggests an increase in the rate of vesicle secretion, which, together with the above categories, would contribute to the SASP. Ablation of reactive astrocytes with upregulated GFAP and vimentin expression, or deletion of these proteins in knockout models have resulted in increased neurodegeneration and immune cell infiltration in models of spinal cord injury and infantile neuronal ceroid lipofuscinosis, respectively (Faulkner et al., 2004; Macauley et al., 2011), supporting a protective role for reactive astrocytes. The decreased GFAP and S100β expression seen in senescent astrocytes may be a contributing factor to neurodegenerative conditions that arise with age.

Astrocyte senescence may be downregulating certain astrocyte immune functions, and in this sense it would be different from astrogliosis. Senescence induced by oxidative stress in astrocytes downregulates the expression of genes involved in antigen processing and presentation on MHC class II proteins. These results are in concordance with a recent RNA-Seq dataset from rat cerebral cortex, which demonstrates a significant downregulation of MHC class II genes (*Cd74*, RT1-ba, *RT1-Da*, and *RT1-Db1*) during aging (Wood et al., 2013). Human homologs of these genes were also downregulated significantly in oxidative stress-induced astrocyte senescence (Supplementary Figure S2). In contrast, mRNA levels of MHC class II genes are elevated in the rat hippocampus with normal aging, suggesting regional differences (Frank et al., 2006). MHC class I and II genes are upregulated in astrocytes isolated from aged mouse cortex (Orre et al., 2014), however, this trend is reversed for MHC class II in the microglial population, suggesting that overall gene expression changes seen in whole brain regions may not be representative of every cell type. In the human brain, a decrease in both GFAP and MHC class II receptors was also observed by immunostaining in the temporal cortex of aged AD subjects (>80 years) compared with younger AD subjects (<80 years; Hoozemans et al., 2010). Furthermore, SNPs in the MHC class II region have been strongly associated with AD in a recent meta-analysis of GWAS studies (Alperovitch et al., 2013), suggesting potentially important functional links to AD pathology.

Although human astrocytes undergo inducible expression of MHC class II antigens, their role as functional antigen presenting cells is controversial (Jensen et al., 2013); therefore, the functional significance of a loss of MHC class II gene expression in senescent astrocytes is unclear. In professional antigen-presenting cells, activation of p38MAPK has been shown to negatively regulate *CIITA*, the master regulator of MHC class II gene expression (Yao et al., 2006). Because p38 MAPK activation is a key pathway driving senescence, this suggests a possible convergence between the senescence program (Iwasa et al., 2003; Bhat et al., 2012) and dysregulation of immune function during aging or immunosenescence. Consistent with this idea, inducible MHC class II expression is impaired during aging in murine macrophages (Herrero et al., 2001).

There are also parallels between gene expression changes in astrocytes with AD and our senescence RNA-Seq data, as expected from the increase of senescent astrocytes in AD brain (Bhat et al., 2012). We compared senescence gene expression changes *in vitro* to those in astrocytes captured by laser capture microdissection from brains of deceased subjects with early or late stage AD, as analyzed by microarray in a previously published study (Simpson et al., 2011). Thirty-one genes showed a decrease greater than 1.5-fold in both astrocyte senescence *in vitro* and in astrocytes in AD (Supplementary Table S7). Seven GO terms were significantly represented (FDR < 10%) by the genes downregulated in senescence and AD, out of which four were related to development of non-CNS organs. The remaining three GO categories were *neuron development*, *cell-cell signaling*, and *neuron differentiation* (Supplementary Table S8). The fold changes for the genes in these GO categories are shown in Supplementary Figure S3.

We thus observe that genes involved in generation and differentiation of neural cell types were commonly down-regulated in astrocytes in oxidative stress induced senescence and in Alzheimer's disease. Among these genes, the neurotrophic tyrosine kinase 2 receptor (NTRK2) gene codes for the tyrosine kinase B receptor (TrkB). TrkB's primary ligand is brain-derived neurotrophic factor (BDNF) and its phosphorylation activates pathways involved in neuronal survival, growth, differentiation, transmission, and synaptic plasticity (Boulle et al., 2012). Expression of NRTK2 was also lower in neurons from the anterior cingulate cortex of brains from patients with autism spectrum disorder (Chandley et al., 2015). Another gene with known CNS function that is represented in these GO terms is FGF9. Knockdown of FGF9 downregulates astrogenesis in the developing rat brain and when added to *ex vivo* cultures, FGF9 upregulates this process (Falcone et al., 2015). FGF9 conditional knockdown caused movement and growth defects in mice, with defects in Bergmann glia formation and Purkinje cell alignment possibly due to a lack of signals from the Bergmann glia. Moreover, extracellular FGF9 was shown to be necessary for glia to form radial morphology. (Lin et al., 2009). Other genes related to neural regeneration and development that are not included in these GO terms were also commonly downregulated between oxidative stress-induced astrocyte senescence and AD (Supplementary Table S7). One such gene, teneurin transmembrane protein 4 (TENM4), encodes for the teneurin-4 (Ten-4) transmembrane protein. An insertion into this gene was responsible for tremors in mice and caused defects in myelination of small diameter axons. The cause was shown to be inhibited oligodendrocyte differentiation, growth and process formation, due to defective FAK signaling by Ten-4 (Suzuki et al., 2012). Ten-4 overexpression and knockdown experiments have shown that this protein is necessary for filopodia formation and neurite outgrowth in neurons via FAK and N-WASP signaling (Suzuki et al., 2014). An intronic variant of this gene was also significantly overrepresented in genomes of bipolar disorder patients (Witt et al., 2014). The protein product (γ-1-syntrophin) of another gene downregulated in senescence and AD, SNTG1, binds and localizes the neurotrophic peptide γ-enolase to the plasma membrane and neurite growth cones of neuroblastoma cells. Knockdown of γ-1-syntrophin disrupts this localization and inhibits the neurite outgrowth and cell proliferation induced by exogenous γ-enolase peptide (Hafner et al., 2010; Falcone et al., 2015). Furthermore, numerous observations of senescence markers in mammalian development may explain the abundance of GO terms related to development of other tissues in the senescence up- and downregulated genes (Meisler and Paigen, 1972; Barral et al., 2014). These gene classes are also an important part of the total down regulated transcriptome in oxidative stress-induced astrocyte senescence. These findings suggest that senescence may be contributing to AD through slowing down of regeneration and differentiation of astrocytes and neurons. Changes in neurogenesis rates were indeed observed in multiple animal and *in vitro* models of AD (Winner and Winkler, 2015).

We define the transcriptional response of human astrocytes to H_2O_2 induced senescence, which has unique characteristics compared to that of other cell types. Whereas H_2O_2 induced senescence led to three times as many upregulated genes as downregulated genes in a human hepatocyte cell line (Aravinthan et al., 2014), the number of downregulated genes was slightly higher for astrocyte senescence (Supplementary Figure S4). There were significantly more genes regulated in the same direction by senescence in both cell types than would be expected by chance, however, the differentially regulated gene sets from the two cell types are clearly distinct. These findings suggest cell-type specific responses to oxidative stress induced senescence, with shared mechanisms.

Aging is a major risk factor for chronic diseases in a host of organ systems. The clearance of senescent cells alleviates several signs of pathology associated with aging (Baker et al., 2011, 2016), suggesting that the presence of senescent cells may be deleterious for tissue and organism homeostasis. There is now strong evidence that senescent cells accumulate in tissues, including brain, during aging and in the setting of pathology. We propose that oxidative stress-induced astrocyte senescence is a model for understanding how the basic processes of aging may lead to a decline in cognition and neurodegeneration, and for identification of potential targets for therapeutic intervention.

AUTHOR CONTRIBUTIONS

Conceived and designed experiments EC, FT, BG, GD, SG, CS, FJ, and CT. Perform the experiments EC, FT, BG, SG, and CS. Analyzed the data EC, FT, BG, GD, SG, YL, EY, JC, RN, L-SW, NB, SB, FJ, and CT. Contributed reagents/materials/analysis tools BG, GD, SG, YL, EY, JC, RN, L-SW, CS, NB, SB, FJ, and CT. Wrote the manuscript EC, FT, BG, GD, YL, FJ, and CT.

FUNDING

Research reported in this publication was supported by grants NIH/NINDS 1RO1NS078283, NIH/NIA F30AG043307, and NIH/NIA R21AG046943.

ACKNOWLEDGMENTS

The authors thank Dr. Gregg Johannes for providing assistance with qRT-PCR assays. We would like to thank Drs. Elizabeth Powell and Katharine Irvine for their guidance about hepatocyte datasets and generosity in sharing their data.

REFERENCES

Abbott, N., Rönnbäck, L., and Hansson, E. (2006). Astrocyte-endothelial interactions at the blood-brain barrier. *Nat. Rev. Neurosci.* 7, 41–53. doi: 10.1038/nrn1824

Alperovitch, A., Boland, A., Delepoine, M., Dubois, B., Duron, E., Epelbaum, J., et al. (2013). Meta-analysis of 74,046 individuals identifies 11 new susceptibility loci for Alzheimer's disease. *Nat. Genet.* 45, 1452–1458. doi: 10.1038/ng.2802

Anderson, M., Ao, Y., and Sofroniew, M. (2014). Heterogeneity of reactive astrocytes. *Neurosci. Lett.* 565, 23–29. doi: 10.1016/j.neulet.2013.12.030

Aravinthan, A., Shannon, N., Heaney, J., Hoare, M., Marshall, A., and Alexander, G. J. (2014). The senescent hepatocyte gene signature in chronic liver disease. *Exp. Gerontol.* 60, 37–45. doi: 10.1016/j.exger.2014.09.011

Baker, D., Wijshake, T., Tchkonia, T., LeBrasseur, N., Childs, B., van de Sluis, B., et al. (2011). Clearance of p16Ink4a-positive senescent cells delays ageing-associated disorders. *Nature* 479, 232–236. doi: 10.1038/nature10600

Baker, D. J., Childs, B. G., Durik, M., Wijers, M. E., Sieben, C. J., Zhong, J., et al. (2016). Naturally occurring p16(Ink4a)-positive cells shorten healthy lifespan. *Nature* 530, 184–189. doi: 10.1038/nature16932

Barral, S., Beltramo, R., Salio, C., Aimar, P., Lossi, L., and Merighi, A. (2014). Phosphorylation of histone H2AX in the mouse brain from development to senescence. *Int. J. Mol. Sci.* 15, 1554–1573. doi: 10.3390/ijms15011554

Baus, F., Gire, V., Fisher, D., Piette, J., and Dulić, V. (2003). Permanent cell cycle exit in G2 phase after DNA damage in normal human fibroblasts. *EMBO J.* 22, 3992–4002. doi: 10.1093/emboj/cdg387

Bhat, R., Crowe, E. P., Bitto, A., Moh, M., Katsetos, C. D., Garcia, F. U., et al. (2012). Astrocyte senescence as a component of Alzheimer's disease. *PLoS ONE* 7:e45069. doi: 10.1371/journal.pone.0045069

Bitto, A., Sell, C., Crowe, E., Lorenzini, A., Malaguti, M., Hrelia, S., et al. (2010). Stress-induced senescence in human and rodent astrocytes. *Exp. Cell Res.* 316, 2961–2968. doi: 10.1016/j.yexcr.2010.06.021

Boulle, F., Kenis, G., Cazorla, M., Hamon, M., Steinbusch, H. W., Lanfumey, L., et al. (2012). TrkB inhibition as a therapeutic target for CNS-related disorders. *Prog. Neurobiol.* 98, 197–206. doi: 10.1016/j.pneurobio.2012.06.002

Cahoy, J., Emery, B., Kaushal, A., Foo, L., Zamanian, J., Christopherson, K., et al. (2008). A transcriptome database for astrocytes, neurons, and oligodendrocytes: a new resource for understanding brain development and function. *J. Neurosci.* 28, 264–278. doi: 10.1523/jneurosci.4178-07.2008

Chandley, M. J., Crawford, J. D., Szebeni, A., Szebeni, K., and Ordway, G. A. (2015). NTRK2 expression levels are reduced in laser captured pyramidal neurons from the anterior cingulate cortex in males with autism spectrum disorder. *Mol. Autism* 6, 28. doi: 10.1186/s13229-015-0023-2

Chen, Q., Bartholomew, J., Campisi, J., Acosta, M., Reagan, J., and Ames, B. (1998). Molecular analysis of H_2O_2-induced senescent-like growth arrest in normal human fibroblasts: p53 and Rb control G1 arrest but not cell replication. *Biochem. J.* 332(Pt. 1), 43–50. doi: 10.1042/bj3320043

Childs, B. G., Baker, D. J., Kirkland, J. L., Campisi, J., and van Deursen, J. M. (2014). Senescence and apoptosis: dueling or complementary cell fates? *EMBO Rep.* 15, 1139–1153. doi: 10.15252/embr.201439245

Chinta, S., Lieu, C., Demaria, M., Laberge, R. M., Campisi, J., and Andersen, J. (2013). Environmental stress, ageing and glial cell senescence: a novel mechanistic link to Parkinson's disease? *J. Intern. Med.* 273, 429–436. doi: 10.1111/joim.12029

Coppé, J.-P., Patil, C., Rodier, F., Sun, Y., Muñoz, D., Goldstein, J., et al. (2008). Senescence-associated secretory phenotypes reveal cell-nonautonomous functions of oncogenic RAS and the p53 tumor suppressor. *PLoS Biol.* 6:2853–2868. doi: 10.1371/journal.pbio.0060301

Elliott, R., Li, F., Dragomir, I., Chua, M., Gregory, B., and Weiss, S. (2013). Analysis of the host transcriptome from demyelinating spinal cord of murine coronavirus-infected mice. *PLoS ONE* 8:e75346. doi: 10.1371/journal.pone.0075346

Esiri, M. M. (2007). Ageing and the brain. *J. Pathol.* 211, 181–187. doi: 10.1002/path.2089

Falcone, C., Filippis, C., Granzotto, M., and Mallamaci, A. (2015). Emx2 expression levels in NSCs modulate astrogenesis rates by regulating EgfR and Fgf9. *Glia* 63, 412–422. doi: 10.1002/glia.22761

Faulkner, J. R., Herrmann, J. E., Woo, M. J., Tansey, K. E., Doan, N. B., and Sofroniew, M. V. (2004). Reactive astrocytes protect tissue and preserve function after spinal cord injury. *J. Neurosci.* 24, 2143–2155. doi: 10.1523/JNEUROSCI.3547-03.2004

Frank, M., Barrientos, R., Biedenkapp, J., Rudy, J., Watkins, L., and Maier, S. (2006). mRNA up-regulation of MHC II and pivotal pro-inflammatory genes in normal brain aging. *Neurobiol. Aging* 27, 717–722. doi: 10.1016/j.neurobiolaging.2005.03.013

Freund, A., Orjalo, A. V., Desprez, P. Y., and Campisi, J. (2010). Inflammatory networks during cellular senescence: causes and consequences. *Trends Mol. Med.* 16, 238–246. doi: 10.1016/j.molmed.2010.03.003

Garwood, C., Pooler, A., Atherton, J., Hanger, D., and Noble, W. (2011). Astrocytes are important mediators of Aβ-induced neurotoxicity and tau phosphorylation in primary culture. *Cell Death Dis.* 2, e167. doi: 10.1038/cddis.2011.50

Gruber, H., Hoelscher, G., Ingram, J., Zinchenko, N., and Hanley, E. (2010). Senescent vs. non-senescent cells in the human annulus in vivo: cell harvest with laser capture microdissection and gene expression studies with microarray analysis. *BMC Biotechnol.* 10:5. doi: 10.1186/1472-6750-10-5

Hafner, A., Obermajer, N., and Kos, J. (2010). gamma-1-syntrophin mediates trafficking of gamma-enolase towards the plasma membrane and enhances its neurotrophic activity. *Neurosignals* 18, 246–258. doi: 10.1159/000324292

Hampel, B., Fortschegger, K., Ressler, S., Chang, M. W., Unterluggauer, H., Breitwieser, A., et al. (2006). Increased expression of extracellular proteins as a hallmark of human endothelial cell in vitro senescence. *Exp. Gerontol.* 41, 474–481. doi: 10.1016/j.exger.2006.03.001

Hendzel, M. J., Wei, Y., Mancini, M. A., Van Hooser, A., Ranalli, T., Brinkley, B. R., et al. (1997). Mitosis-specific phosphorylation of histone H3 initiates primarily within pericentromeric heterochromatin during G2 and spreads in an ordered fashion coincident with mitotic chromosome condensation. *Chromosoma* 106, 348–360. doi: 10.1007/s004120050256

Herbig, U., Ferreira, M., Condel, L., Carey, D., and Sedivy, J. M. (2006). Cellular senescence in aging primates. *Science* 311:1257. doi: 10.1126/science.1122446

Herrero, C., Marqués, L., Lloberas, J., and Celada, A. (2001). IFN-gamma-dependent transcription of MHC class II IA is impaired in macrophages from aged mice. *J. Clin. Invest.* 107, 485–493. doi: 10.1172/jci11696

Hoozemans, J. J., Rozemuller, A. J., van Haastert, E. S., Eikelenboom, P., and van Gool, W. A. (2010). Neuroinflammation in Alzheimer's disease wanes with age. *J. Neuroinflammation* 8, 171. doi: 10.1186/1742-2094-8-171

Huang da, W., Sherman, B. T., and Lempicki, R. A. (2009). Systematic and integrative analysis of large gene lists using DAVID bioinformatics resources. *Nat. Protoc.* 4, 44–57. doi: 10.1038/nprot.2008.211

Iwasa, H., Han, J., and Ishikawa, F. (2003). Mitogen-activated protein kinase p38 defines the common senescence-signalling pathway. *Genes Cells* 8, 131–144. doi: 10.1046/j.1365-2443.2003.00620.x

Jensen, C., Massie, A., and De Keyser, J. (2013). Immune players in the CNS: the astrocyte. *J. Neuroimmune Pharmacol.* 8, 824–839. doi: 10.1007/s11481-013-9480-6

Jurk, D., Wang, C., Miwa, S., Maddick, M., Korolchuk, V., Tsolou, A., et al. (2012). Postmitotic neurons develop a p21-dependent senescence-like phenotype driven by a DNA damage response. *Aging Cell* 11, 996–1004. doi: 10.1111/j.1474-9726.2012.00870.x

Jurk, D., Wilson, C., Passos, J. F., Oakley, F., Correia-Melo, C., Greaves, L., et al. (2014). Chronic inflammation induces telomere dysfunction and accelerates ageing in mice. *Nat. Commun.* 2, 4172. doi: 10.1038/ncomms5172

Kawano, H., Katsurabayashi, S., Kakazu, Y., Yamashita, Y., Kubo, N., Kubo, M., et al. (2012). Long-term culture of astrocytes attenuates the readily releasable pool of synaptic vesicles. *PLoS ONE* 7:e48034. doi: 10.1371/journal.pone.0048034

Kim, J.-S., Kim, E.-J., Kim, H.-J., Yang, J.-Y., Hwang, G.-S., and Kim, C.-W. (2011). Proteomic and metabolomic analysis of H2O2-induced premature senescent human mesenchymal stem cells. *Exp. Gerontol.* 46, 500–510. doi: 10.1016/j.exger.2011.02.012

Kipling, D., Jones, D., Smith, S., Giles, P., Jennert-Burston, K., Ibrahim, B., et al. (2009). A transcriptomic analysis of the EK1.Br strain of human fibroblastoid keratocytes: the effects of growth, quiescence and senescence. *Exp. Eye Res.* 88, 277–285. doi: 10.1016/j.exer.2008.11.030

Krishnamurthy, J., Torrice, C., Ramsey, M., Kovalev, G., Al-Regaiey, K., Su, L., et al. (2004). Ink4a/Arf expression is a biomarker of aging. *J. Clin. Invest.* 114, 1299–1307. doi: 10.1172/jci22475

Lin, Y., Chen, L., Lin, C., Luo, Y., Tsai, R. Y., and Wang, F. (2009). Neuron-derived FGF9 is essential for scaffold formation of Bergmann radial fibers and migration of granule neurons in the cerebellum. *Dev. Biol.* 329, 44–54. doi: 10.1016/j.ydbio.2009.02.011

Macauley, S. L., Pekny, M., and Sands, M. S. (2011). The role of attenuated astrocyte activation in infantile neuronal ceroid lipofuscinosis. *J. Neurosci.* 31, 15575–15585. doi: 10.1523/JNEUROSCI.3579-11.2011

Mao, Z., Ke, Z., Gorbunova, V., and Seluanov, A. (2012). Replicatively senescent cells are arrested in G1 and G2 phases. *Aging (Albany NY)* 4, 431–435. doi: 10.18632/aging.100467

Meisler, M., and Paigen, K. (1972). Coordinated development of - glucuronidase and -galactosidase in mouse organs. *Science* 177, 894–896. doi: 10.1126/science.177.4052.894

Miranda, C., Braun, L., Jiang, Y., Hester, M., Zhang, L., Riolo, M., et al. (2012). Aging brain microenvironment decreases hippocampal neurogenesis through Wnt-mediated survivin signaling. *Aging Cell* 11, 542–552. doi: 10.1111/j.1474-9726.2012.00816.x

Nagelhus, E. A., Amiry-Moghaddam, M., Bergersen, L. H., Bjaalie, J. G., Eriksson, J., Gundersen, V., et al. (2013). The glia doctrine: addressing the role of glial cells in healthy brain ageing. *Mech. Ageing Dev.* 134, 449–459. doi: 10.1016/j.mad.2013.10.001

Oberheim, N., Wang, X., Goldman, S., and Nedergaard, M. (2006). Astrocytic complexity distinguishes the human brain. *Trends Neurosci.* 29, 547–553. doi: 10.1016/j.tins.2006.08.004

Orre, M., Kamphuis, W., Osborn, L., Melief, J., Kooijman, L., Huitinga, I., et al. (2014). Acute isolation and transcriptome characterization of cortical astrocytes and microglia from young and aged mice. *Neurobiol. Aging* 35, 1–14. doi: 10.1016/j.neurobiolaging.2013.07.008

Oyama, K., Takahashi, K., and Sakurai, K. (2011). Hydrogen peroxide induces cell cycle arrest in cardiomyoblast H9c2 cells, which is related to hypertrophy. *Biol. Pharm. Bull.* 34, 501–506. doi: 10.1248/bpb.34.501

Pekny, M., Pekna, M., Messing, A., Steinhauser, C., Lee, J. M., Parpura, V., et al. (2016). Astrocytes: a central element in neurological diseases. *Acta Neuropathol.* 131, 323–345. doi: 10.1007/s00401-015-1513-1

Perea, G., Navarrete, M., and Araque, A. (2009). Tripartite synapses: astrocytes process and control synaptic information. *Trends Neurosci.* 32, 421–431. doi: 10.1016/j.tins.2009.05.001

Pertusa, M., García-Matas, S., Rodríguez-Farré, E., Sanfeliu, C., and Cristòfol, R. (2007). Astrocytes aged in vitro show a decreased neuroprotective capacity. *J. Neurochem.* 101, 794–805. doi: 10.1111/j.1471-4159.2006.04369.x

Phatnani, H., and Maniatis, T. (2015). Astrocytes in neurodegenerative disease. *Cold Spring Harb. Perspect. Biol* 7, a020628. doi: 10.1101/cshperspect.a020628

Price, J., Waters, J., Darrah, C., Pennington, C., Edwards, D., Donell, S., et al. (2002). The role of chondrocyte senescence in osteoarthritis. *Aging Cell* 1, 57–65. doi: 10.1046/j.1474-9728.2002.00008.x

Radak, Z., Zhao, Z., Goto, S., and Koltai, E. (2011). Age-associated neurodegeneration and oxidative damage to lipids, proteins and DNA. *Mol. Aspects Med.* 32, 305–315. doi: 10.1016/j.mam.2011.10.010

Rodríguez, J., Yeh, C.-Y., Terzieva, S., Olabarria, M., Kulijewicz-Nawrot, M., and Verkhratsky, A. (2014). Complex and region-specific changes in astroglial markers in the aging brain. *Neurobiol. Aging* 35, 15–23. doi: 10.1016/j.neurobiolaging.2013.07.002

Sekar, S., McDonald, J., Cuyugan, L., Aldrich, J., Kurdoglu, A., Adkins, J., et al. (2015). Alzheimer's disease is associated with altered expression of genes involved in immune response and mitochondrial processes in astrocytes. *Neurobiol. Aging* 36, 583–591. doi: 10.1016/j.neurobiolaging.2014.09.027

Shelton, D., Chang, E., Whittier, P., Choi, D., and Funk, W. (1999). Microarray analysis of replicative senescence. *Curr. Biol.* 9, 939–945. doi: 10.1016/s0960-9822(99)80420-5

Simard, M., and Nedergaard, M. (2004). The neurobiology of glia in the context of water and ion homeostasis. *Neuroscience* 129, 877–896. doi: 10.1016/j.neuroscience.2004.09.053

Simpson, J., Ince, P., Shaw, P., Heath, P., Raman, R., Garwood, C., et al. (2011). Microarray analysis of the astrocyte transcriptome in the aging brain: relationship to Alzheimer's pathology and APOE genotype. *Neurobiol. Aging* 32, 1795–1807. doi: 10.1016/j.neurobiolaging.2011.04.013

Smith, C., Carney, J., Starke-Reed, P., Oliver, C., Stadtman, E., Floyd, R., et al. (1991). Excess brain protein oxidation and enzyme dysfunction in normal aging and in Alzheimer disease. *Proc. Natl. Acad. Sci. U.S.A.* 88, 10540–10543. doi: 10.1073/pnas.88.23.10540

Sofroniew, M. (2009). Molecular dissection of reactive astrogliosis and glial scar formation. *Trends Neurosci.* 32, 638–647. doi: 10.1016/j.tins.2009.08.002

Suzuki, N., Fukushi, M., Kosaki, K., Doyle, A. D., de Vega, S., Yoshizaki, K., et al. (2012). Teneurin-4 is a novel regulator of oligodendrocyte differentiation and myelination of small-diameter axons in the CNS. *J. Neurosci.* 32, 11586–11599. doi: 10.1523/JNEUROSCI.2045-11.2012

Suzuki, N., Numakawa, T., Chou, J., de Vega, S., Mizuniwa, C., Sekimoto, K., et al. (2014). Teneurin-4 promotes cellular protrusion formation and neurite outgrowth through focal adhesion kinase signaling. *FASEB J.* 28, 1386–1397. doi: 10.1096/fj.13-241034

Twine, N., Janitz, K., Wilkins, M., and Janitz, M. (2011). Whole transcriptome sequencing reveals gene expression and splicing differences in brain regions affected by Alzheimer's disease. *PLoS ONE* 6:e16266. doi: 10.1371/journal.pone.0016266

Winner, B., and Winkler, J. (2015). Adult neurogenesis in neurodegenerative diseases. *Cold Spring Harb. Perspect. Biol.* 7, a021287. doi: 10.1101/cshperspect.a021287

Witt, S. H., Kleindienst, N., Frank, J., Treutlein, J., Muhleisen, T., Degenhardt, F., et al. (2014). Analysis of genome-wide significant bipolar disorder genes in borderline personality disorder. *Psychiatr Genet.* 24, 262–265. doi: 10.1097/YPG.0000000000000060

Wood, S., Craig, T., Li, Y., Merry, B., and de Magalhães, J. (2013). Whole transcriptome sequencing of the aging rat brain reveals dynamic RNA changes in the dark matter of the genome. *Age (Dordr).* 35, 763–776. doi: 10.1007/s11357-012-9410-1

Yao, Y., Xu, Q., Kwon, M.-J., Matta, R., Liu, Y., Hong, S.-C., et al. (2006). ERK and p38 MAPK signaling pathways negatively regulate CIITA gene expression in dendritic cells and macrophages. *J. Immunol.* 177, 70–76. doi: 10.4049/jimmunol.177.1.70

Yin, F., Sancheti, H., Patil, I., and Cadenas, E. (2016). Energy metabolism and inflammation in brain aging and Alzheimer's disease. *Free Radic Biol. Med.* doi: 10.1016/j.freeradbiomed.2016.04.200 [Epub ahead of print].

Yoon, I. K., Kim, H. K., Kim, Y. K., Song, I. H., Kim, W., Kim, S., et al. (2004). Exploration of replicative senescence-associated genes in human dermal fibroblasts by cDNA microarray technology. *Exp. Gerontol.* 39, 1369–1378. doi: 10.1016/j.exger.2004.07.002

Zhang, Y., Chen, K., Sloan, S. A., Bennett, M. L., Scholze, A. R., O'Keeffe, S., et al. (2014). An RNA-sequencing transcriptome and splicing database of glia, neurons, and vascular cells of the cerebral cortex. *J. Neurosci.* 34, 11929–11947. doi: 10.1523/JNEUROSCI.1860-14.2014

Zhu, Y., Armstrong, J. L., Tchkonia, T., and Kirkland, J. L. (2014). Cellular senescence and the senescent secretory phenotype in age-related chronic diseases. *Curr. Opin. Clin. Nutr. Metab. Care* 17, 324–328. doi: 10.1097/MCO.0000000000000065

4

Calpastatin Overexpression Preserves Cognitive Function Following Seizures, While Maintaining Post-Injury Neurogenesis

Vanessa M. Machado[1,2,3], *Ana Sofia Lourenço*[1,2,3], *Cláudia Florindo*[2,3], *Raquel Fernandes*[3], *Caetana M. Carvalho*[1] and *Inês M. Araújo*[2,3,4]*

Center for Neuroscience and Cell Biology, University of Coimbra, Coimbra, Portugal, [2]Center for Biomedical Research, CBMR, University of Algarve, Faro, Portugal, [3]Regenerative Medicine Program, Department of Biomedical Sciences and Medicine, University of Algarve, Faro, Portugal, [4]Algarve Biomedical Center, University of Algarve, Faro, Portugal

Edited by:
Andrew Harkin,
Trinity College, Dublin, Ireland

Reviewed by:
Daniela Tropea,
Trinity College, Dublin, Ireland
Xiaochu Lou,
University of Wisconsin-Madison, USA

***Correspondence:**
Inês M. Araújo
imaraujo@ualg.pt

In the adult mammalian brain, new neurons continue to be produced throughout life in two main regions in the brain, the subgranular zone (SGZ) in the hippocampus and the subventricular zone in the walls of the lateral ventricles. Neural stem cells (NSCs) proliferate in these niches, and migrate as neuroblasts, to further differentiate in locations where new neurons are needed, either in normal or pathological conditions. However, the endogenous attempt of brain repair is not very efficient. Calpains are proteases known to be involved in neuronal damage and in cell proliferation, migration and differentiation of several cell types, though their effects on neurogenesis are not well known. Previous work by our group has shown that the absence of calpastatin (CAST), the endogenous inhibitor of calpains, impairs early stages of neurogenesis. Since the hippocampus is highly associated with learning and memory, we aimed to evaluate whether calpain inhibition would help improve cognitive recovery after lesion and efficiency of post-injury neurogenesis in this region. For that purpose, we used the kainic acid (KA) model of seizure-induced hippocampal lesion and mice overexpressing CAST. Selected cognitive tests were performed on the 3rd and 8th week after KA-induced lesion, and cell proliferation, migration and differentiation in the dentate gyrus (DG) of the hippocampus of adult mice were analyzed using specific markers. Cognitive recovery was evaluated by testing the animals for recognition, spatial and associative learning and memory. Cognitive function was preserved by CAST overexpression following seizures, while modulation of post-injury neurogenesis was similar to wild type (WT) mice. Calpain inhibition could still be potentially able to prevent the impairment in the formation of new neurons, given that the levels of calpain activity could be reduced under a certain threshold and other harmful effects from the pathological environment could also be controlled.

Keywords: calpains, calpastatin, cognition, hippocampus, post-injury neurogenesis

---

Abbreviations: BrdU, 5-bromo-2′-deoxyuridine; CAST, calpastatin; DCX, doublecortin; DG, dentate gyrus; EdU, 5-ethynyl-2′-deoxyuridine; FC, fear conditioning; GZ, granular zone; hCAST, mice overexpressing calpastatin; KA, kainic acid; NeuN, neuronal nuclei; NSC, neural stem cell; OR, object recognition; SAL, saline; SGZ, subgranular zone; WM, water maze; WT, wild type.

INTRODUCTION

New neurons in the adult mammalian brain are known to originate from mainly two regions, the subventricular zone, in the walls of the lateral ventricles, and the subgranular zone (SGZ), in the dentate gyrus (DG) of the hippocampus (Bond et al., 2015). Neural stem cells (NSCs) from the subventricular zone migrate long distances, through a rostral migratory stream, into the olfactory bulb, differentiating into interneurons. NSCs from the SGZ, in turn, migrate shorter distances into the granular zone (GZ), where they fully mature into granule neurons after 2 months (Aimone et al., 2014; Jin, 2016). Functions of these newborn cells from both regions have been consistently associated with learning and memory (Deng et al., 2010; Lazarini and Lledo, 2011).

When a brain lesion occurs, behavioral traits and adult neurogenesis can become altered. In neurodegenerative diseases, neurogenesis is mostly hampered, but in acute disorders, such as temporal lobe epilepsy, NSC proliferation can increase, in a possible attempt to repair the damage. However, this repair is limited by impaired cell migration or decreased survival of new neurons (Kaneko and Sawamoto, 2009; Ma et al., 2009).

Another feature of brain damage is excitotoxicity, which leads to an increase of cellular levels of calcium, activating several proteases, including calpains (Neumar et al., 2001). Calpains are ubiquitously expressed calcium-activated proteases, with only one known natural endogenous inhibitor, a protein called calpastatin (CAST; Murachi, 1984). In the CNS, calpain inhibition has been shown to afford neuroprotection, showing improved neuronal function and limiting neuronal damage in several brain disorders (Saez et al., 2006). Although little is known about their contribution to neurogenesis, calpains were seen to be involved in cell proliferation, migration and differentiation in other systems (Rock et al., 2000; Yajima and Kawashima, 2002; Lokuta et al., 2003; Parnaud et al., 2005; Qiu et al., 2006; Shimada et al., 2008; Kashiwagi et al., 2010; Kuchay et al., 2012).

Previous studies by our group show that increased calpain activity, through lack of CAST, can impair early stages of neurogenesis in the hippocampus, the main structure involved in learning and memory (Machado et al., 2015). Moreover, the kainic acid (KA) model of seizure-induced hippocampal lesion presents excitotoxic damage mediated by calpains (Araújo et al., 2008) and is characterized by pathologic alterations in hippocampal neurogenesis (Carreira et al., 2010). With this work, we proposed to assess whether overexpression of CAST (hCAST mice) could improve cognitive recovery and neurogenesis after KA-induced hippocampal lesion.

MATERIALS AND METHODS

Animals

Three-month old male and female hCAST mice (Rao et al., 2008), in a C57BL/6 background, and their wild type (WT) littermates, were used in this study. hCAST mice present CAST overexpression, due to the cloning of a human CAST construct (Hitomi et al., 1998) into a Thymocyte differentiation antigen 1.1 expression cassette (Thy1). The animals were kept in our animal facilities, in a room with controlled temperature (21 ± 1°C) and humidity (55%), with food and water *ad libitum* in a 12-h dark:light cycle. All experiments were performed in accordance with institutional and European guidelines (2010/63/EU) for the care and use of laboratory animals. The procedures performed in mice described in this work have been reviewed and approved by the Animal Welfare Body of the Center for Neuroscience and Cell Biology and have been approved by the Direcção Geral de Alimentação e Veterinária (reference 0421/000/000/2013).

KA Treatment

Hippocampal damage was induced by administering KA subcutaneously (25 mg/kg, in a concentration of 5 mg/ml, in a saline (SAL) solution of 0.9% NaCl), as previously described by our group (Carreira et al., 2010). After KA administration, the animals went through several stages, according to a well-defined scale (Schauwecker and Steward, 1997): immobility (I), tail/forelimb extension/rigid posture (II), repetitive movements/head bobbing (III), rearing and falling (IV), continuous rearing and falling (V), severe tonic-clonic seizures (VI). Only mice that reached stage V or higher were used in this study. SAL-treated animals were used as controls.

Behavior Analysis and Neuronal Differentiation

For the studies of short-term behavioral recovery, three different behavioral tests were performed in WT and hCAST mice, on the 3rd week after KA or SAL treatment (**Figure 1A**): object recognition (OR; **Figure 1C**), water maze (WM; **Figure 1D**) and fear conditioning (FC; **Figure 1E**), as explained further in more detail. To assess long-term behavioral recovery and neuronal differentiation after lesion, WT and hCAST mice were treated as shown in **Figure 1B**. The thymidine analog 5-ethynyl-2′-deoxyuridine (EdU) was intraperitoneally administered to WT and hCAST mice on days 3, 4 and 5 after KA or SAL treatment, and the animals were sacrificed by transcardial perfusion after 8 weeks, when new neurons are fully mature (Aimone et al., 2014). Behavioral analysis was performed during the last week.

Object Recognition

For the study of recognition memory, the OR test (Bevins and Besheer, 2006) was used. Mice were presented to two similar objects, following habituation to the apparatus ($40 \times 40 \times 40$ cm^3 acrylic box), after which one of the objects was replaced by a novel one. Each stage of the test had the duration of 5 min, 2 h apart, and the apparatus and objects were cleaned with 10% ethanol between animals. In the presence of the objects, the percentage of time spent with each object (totalizing 100%) was measured. The analysis was done in videos acquired with a GoPro Hero (GoPro, Inc., San Mateo, CA, USA) during testing of 3–5 animals per group (for short-term recovery) and 12–15 animals per group (for long-term recovery), using the Any-maze software (version 4.99, Stoelting Co., Wood Dale, IL, USA).

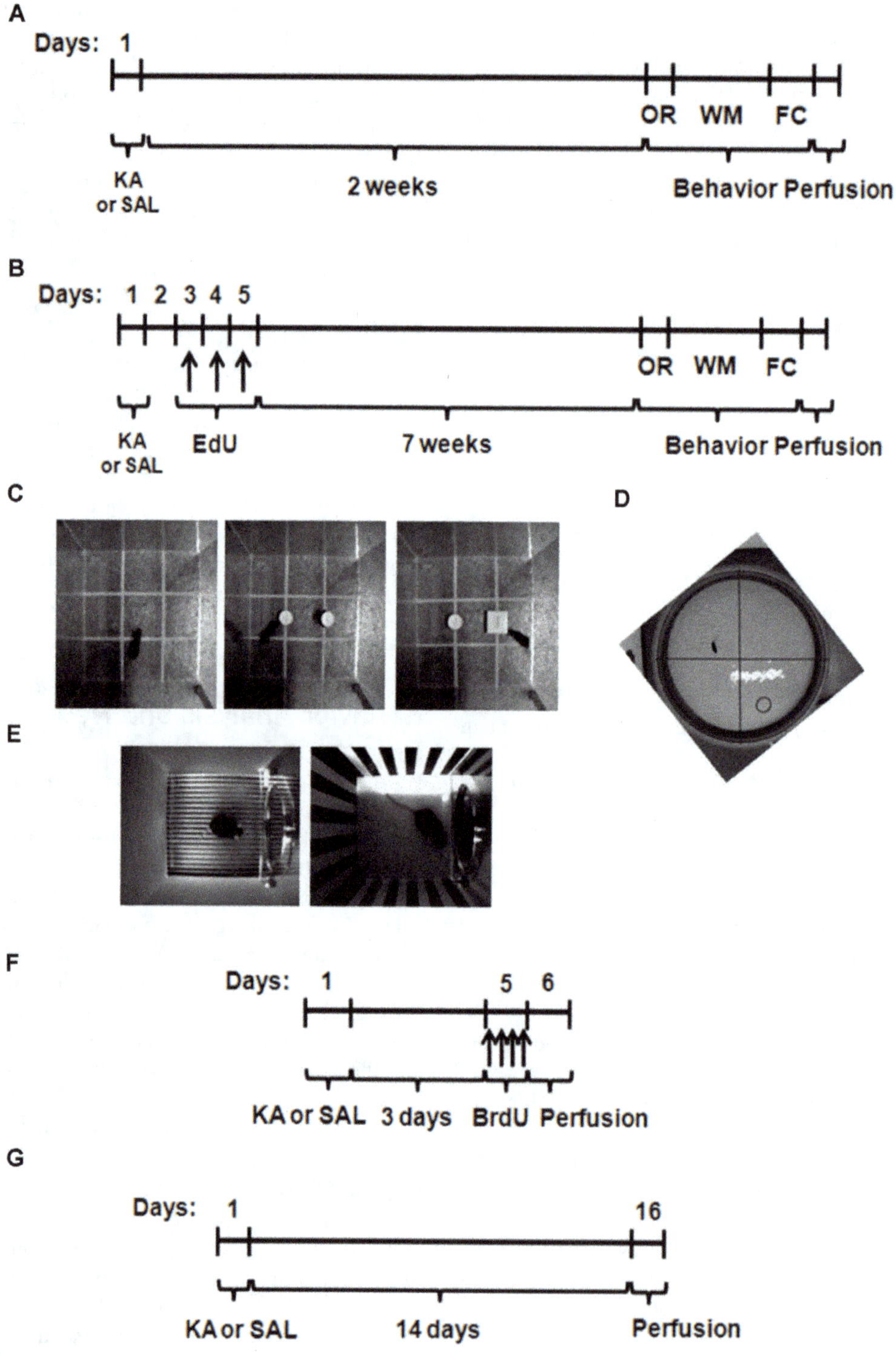

FIGURE 1 | Experimental procedures for the study of behavioral recovery and neurogenesis after kainic acid (KA) or saline (SAL) treatment. Wild type (WT) and hCAST mice were treated with either SAL or KA (25 mg/kg, s.c.). **(A)** To study behavioral recovery in the short-term group, the cognitive behavior of the animals was tested on the 3rd week after treatment. **(B)** For the behavioral recovery in the long-term group and the study of neuronal differentiation, mice were given 5-ethynyl-2′-deoxyuridine (EdU; 50 mg/kg, i.p.) on days 3, 4 and 5, 8 weeks before sacrifice, and the cognitive behavior was tested during the last week. **(C)** On the first day, object recognition (OR) was tested. **(D)** Water maze (WM) trials were performed on the next 3 days and the final test, without the platform, was on day 4. **(E)** On the next day, fear conditioning (FC) trials were performed. One day later, the animals were at first left on the same context and, after 3 h, the context was completely modified and the cued test performed. The animals were sacrificed on the next day. **(F)** To study neural stem cell (NSC) proliferation, mice were given 5-bromo-2′-deoxyuridine (BrdU; four doses of 50 mg/kg, i.p.) on day 5, up to 12 h before sacrifice. **(G)** To study neuroblast migration, mice were sacrificed 14 days after treatment.

Morris Water Maze

To evaluate spatial learning and memory, the WM test (Morris et al., 1982) was performed. During the first 3 days, the animals were trained to find a platform (10 cm diameter, carved to increase grip) hidden 0.5 cm below the water surface level in a circular pool (1.52 m diameter), in a fixed location. Visual cues on the walls around the pool were provided to help the mice locating the platform and the water temperature was maintained at 22°C ± 1°C. The pool was divided into four quadrants and, on each day of training, the animals were placed in a different quadrant, always facing the border of the pool, under the course of four 60 s trials, 30 min apart. The latency to escape was measured as the time each animal took to find and climb onto the platform. If the animal did not reach the platform within the course of the trial, the latency to escape was considered 60 s and the animal was left on the platform for 10 s, in order to learn the platform location. On the last day of testing, the platform was removed and the mice were placed in the quadrant opposite to the target quadrant (where the platform was previously located), facing the border of the pool. The time spent on each quadrant and the number of crossings over the previous platform location were measured for 60 s, to evaluate if the animals remembered where the platform was located during training. All animals were dried under an infrared light after each trial. The analysis was done in videos acquired with a GoPro Hero (GoPro, Inc., San Mateo, CA, USA) during testing of 4–5 animals per group (for short-term recovery) and 11–16 animals per group (for long-term recovery), using the Any-maze software (version 4.99, Stoelting Co., Wood Dale, IL, USA).

Fear Conditioning

Associative learning and memory were tested by performing the FC test (Wehner and Radcliffe, 2004). The first day of testing consisted of learning to associate a cue tone (80 dB) with a footshock (0.7 mA). For this part of the test, mice were placed in a chamber (17 × 17 × 25 cm^3) with a grid floor inside a soundproof box (Stoelting Co., Wood Dale, IL, USA), with a background white noise, 70% ethanol scent and 100% lux lighting (context A). After 2 min (acquisition/habituation), the tone was played for 30 s and the footshock given during the last 2 s of tone. This was repeated two more times, after a 60 s rest. On the next day, the association of the context with the footshock was tested (context test), by placing the mice inside the chamber in the same conditions as during learning for 5 min, without presentation of tone or footshock. After 3 h, the association of the footshock with the tone (cued test) was tested, by placing the animals in a completely different environment for 3 min (habituation to new context) and then playing the tone for the last 3 min. The new context consisted of a background fan noise, vanilla scent, 10% lux lighting, and the previously used chamber was altered by using striped black and white walls and a white floor covering the grid (context B). During the whole FC testing, the chamber was cleaned with 10% ethanol between animals, and the fear behavior measured by calculating the percentage of freezing time, for 3–5 animals per group (for short-term recovery) and 9–16 animals per group (for long-term recovery), using the Any-maze software (version 4.99, Stoelting Co., Wood Dale, IL, USA).

NSC Proliferation

Cell proliferation after KA or SAL treatment was assessed by the incorporation of the thymidine analog 5-bromo-2′-deoxyuridine (BrdU), as shown in **Figure 1F**. WT and hCAST mice were given either KA or SAL (9–14 animals per group) and BrdU was administered intraperitoneally (four doses of 50 mg/kg, 2 h apart) on day 5, when a peak of proliferation is known to occur in the DG after KA treatment (Carreira et al., 2010). The animals were sacrificed after at least 12 h, by transcardial perfusion.

Neuroblast Migration

In order to investigate neuroblast migration after lesion, WT and hCAST mice were given either KA or SAL (6–9 animals per group) and sacrificed by transcardial perfusion, after 14 days (**Figure 1G**), when an increase in cell migration is known to occur in the DG after KA treatment (Carreira et al., 2015). Cell migration in the DG was then assessed by analyzing neuroblast staining with doublecortin (DCX), as described further in more detail.

EdU Detection and Immunohistochemistry

Brains used for immunohistochemistry and EdU detection were obtained after transcardial perfusion of the mice with 0.9% NaCl and 4% paraformaldehyde. The brains were removed and kept in 4% paraformaldehyde overnight for further fixation and then dehydrated in 20% sucrose in phosphate buffer for at least one day, at 4°C. Coronal sections from the hippocampal region were cryosectioned (30 μm thick, in 6-series) using a CryoStar NX50 cryostat (Thermo Fisher Scientific, Waltham, MA, USA) and stored in an antifreeze solution (30% ethylene glycol and 30% glycerol in phosphate buffer), at 4°C. Free-floating brain sections from one of the series were labeled against BrdU, DCX, EdU or EdU/NeuN (neuronal nuclei), as previously described (Morte et al., 2013; Machado et al., 2015). EdU labeling was performed using a commercially available kit (Click-iT® EdU Alexa Fluor® 488 HCS Assay, Thermo Fisher Scientific, Waltham, MA, USA). After rinsing with 3% bovine serum albumin, the sections were permeabilized with 0.5% triton X-100 for 45 min, rinsed again and then incubated with a reaction cocktail (reaction buffer, CuSO4, Alexa Fluor 488 and reaction buffer additive) for 1 h, protected from light, at room temperature. For immunohistochemistry, sections were rinsed with PBS and then blocked for 1 h, at room temperature, in 5% blocking solution in 0.25% triton X-100, using normal horse serum. After blocking, the sections were kept with the primary antibodies—rat anti-BrdU 1:50 (AbD Serotec, Oxford, UK), goat anti-DCX 1:400 (Santa Cruz Biotechnology, Inc., Dallas, TX, USA), mouse anti-NeuN 1:200 (Merck Millipore, Billerica, MA, USA)—for 48 h, at 4°C. Sections were then rinsed in 2% blocking solution and incubated for 2 h, at room temperature and protected from light, with the correspondent Alexa Fluor-conjugated secondary antibodies—donkey anti-rat

488, donkey anti-goat 594 and donkey anti-mouse 594; 1:200 (Thermo Fisher Scientific, Waltham, MA, USA). For the labeling of BrdU, a DNA denaturation step with 1 M HCl for 20 min, at 65°C, was performed in the beginning. In the cases where NeuN was not labeled, nuclei were stained with 2 μg/ml Hoechst 33342 for 10 min, at room temperature. For the combination of EdU and NeuN, EdU labeling was performed, followed by the immunohistochemistry, starting with the blocking step. The entire procedure was done using an orbital shaker. After a final rinsing step, the sections were mounted in gelatin-coated slides, with DAKO fluorescence mounting medium.

Analysis of Incorporation of BrdU and EdU

For the analysis of incorportation of the thymidine analogs, BrdU-positive and EdU-positive cells in the SGZ, the first layer of cells adjacent to the hilus, in the GZ or in the hilus of five central coronal sections of the hippocampal region were counted for each animal (Salazar-Colocho et al., 2008; Machado et al., 2015), directly under an epifluorescence microscope (Axio Imager Z2 microscope, Zeiss, Oberkochen, Germany). Cell counting was carried out in both upper and lower blades of the DG.

DCX Immunoreactivity

DCX immunoreactivity in the DG was determined in images acquired in a laser scanning microscope (LSM710, Zeiss, Jena, Germany). The quantification of the DCX-positive area was performed in ImageJ (version 1.47v, National Institutes of Health, Bethesda, MD, USA), using a threshold analysis in five central coronal sections of the hippocampal region of each animal. This consisted in defining the optimal staining threshold and calculating the area labeled with DCX (Komitova et al., 2005; Machado et al., 2015).

Neuronal Differentiation Analysis

For the quantification of newborn neurons, the percentage of cells labeled for both EdU and NeuN was determined in a total of up to 50 EdU-positive cells (Carreira et al., 2015) in the DG of eight animals per group, in images (orthogonal reconstructions of projections from 0.73 μm z-stacks) acquired in a LSM710 (Zeiss, Jena, Germany).

FluoroJade C Staining

For FluoroJade C staining, coronal sections from the hippocampal region of WT and hCAST mice (3–4 animals per group) treated with KA for 24 h were mounted in gelatin-coated slides. After air-drying for at least 24 h, the sections were rinsed twice in distilled water, and then immersed for 5 min in 0.1% sodium hydroxide prepared in 80% ethanol, 1 min in 70% ethanol and rinsed twice for 2 min in distilled water. The slides with the sections were then transferred to a 0.06% potassium permanganate solution and left in an orbital shaker for 10 min. After another rinsing step, the slides were left with agitation and protected from light for 10 min in 0.0001% FluoroJade C prepared in 0.1% acetic acid. The sections were rinsed three more times for 1 min in distilled water and dried for 15 min at 60°C, after which they were immersed in xylene and coverslipped with DPX mounting medium. Images were acquired in an epifluorescence microscope (Axio Imager Z2 microscope, Zeiss, Oberkochen, Germany) and the percentage of staining in the GZ and the hilus measured using a threshold analysis in ImageJ (version 1.47v, National Institutes of Health, Bethesda, MD, USA; Carreira et al., 2010; Machado et al., 2015).

Statistical Analysis

Data are expressed as means ± SEM. Statistical significance was determined using the Kruskal-Wallis test, with Dunn's post-test, or the Mann-Whitney test, as indicated in the figure legends, using the GraphPad Prism 5 software (GraphPad Software, Inc., La Jolla, CA, USA). Differences were considered significant when $p < 0.05$.

RESULTS

Short-Term Impairment in Novel Object Exploration after KA Treatment Is Prevented in Mice Overexpressing CAST

To evaluate whether CAST overexpression would allow for a better and/or faster recovery after brain injury, we performed several cognitive behavioral tests on WT and hCAST mice, on the 3rd (short-term) or 8th (long-term) week after treatment with either KA or SAL. We first tested the animals for OR memory (3–5 animals per group for short-term recovery and 12–15 animals per group for long-term recovery). We observed that, for both time periods, WT mice treated with SAL spent significantly more time exploring the novel object (short-term recovery: 58.3 ± 3.7%, long-term recovery: 62.9 ± 3.3%) than the familiar object, that they had already explored previously (short-term recovery: 41.7 ± 3.7%, $p < 0.05$, long-term recovery: 37.1 ± 3.3%, $p < 0.001$). However, after KA treatment, only WT mice from the long-term recovery group were able to distinguish the novel object (58.9 ± 4.5%), from the familiar object (41.1 ± 4.5%, $p < 0.05$; **Figure 2**, left panels), indicating impairment in recognition memory in the short-term group. On the other hand, all mice overexpressing CAST spent more time exploring the novel object, in both short-term recovery (SAL, novel object: 61.5 ± 5.0%, familiar object: 38.5 ± 5.0%, $p > 0.05$; KA, novel object: 61.1 ± 1.3%, familiar object: 34.9 ± 1.3%, $p < 0.01$) and long-term recovery (SAL, novel object: 62.9 ± 3.8%, familiar object: 37.1 ± 3.8%, $p < 0.001$; KA, novel object: 59.7 ± 3.6%, familiar object: 40.3 ± 3.6%, $p < 0.001$; **Figure 2**, right panels).

Long-Term Impairment in Spatial Memory for an Exact Location during the Water Maze Test after KA Treatment Is Prevented in Mice Overexpressing CAST

In order to study spatial learning and memory, the Morris WM test was performed (4–5 animals per group for short-term recovery and 11–16 animals per group for long-term recovery). During trials (**Figure 3A**), we observed that KA-treated mice

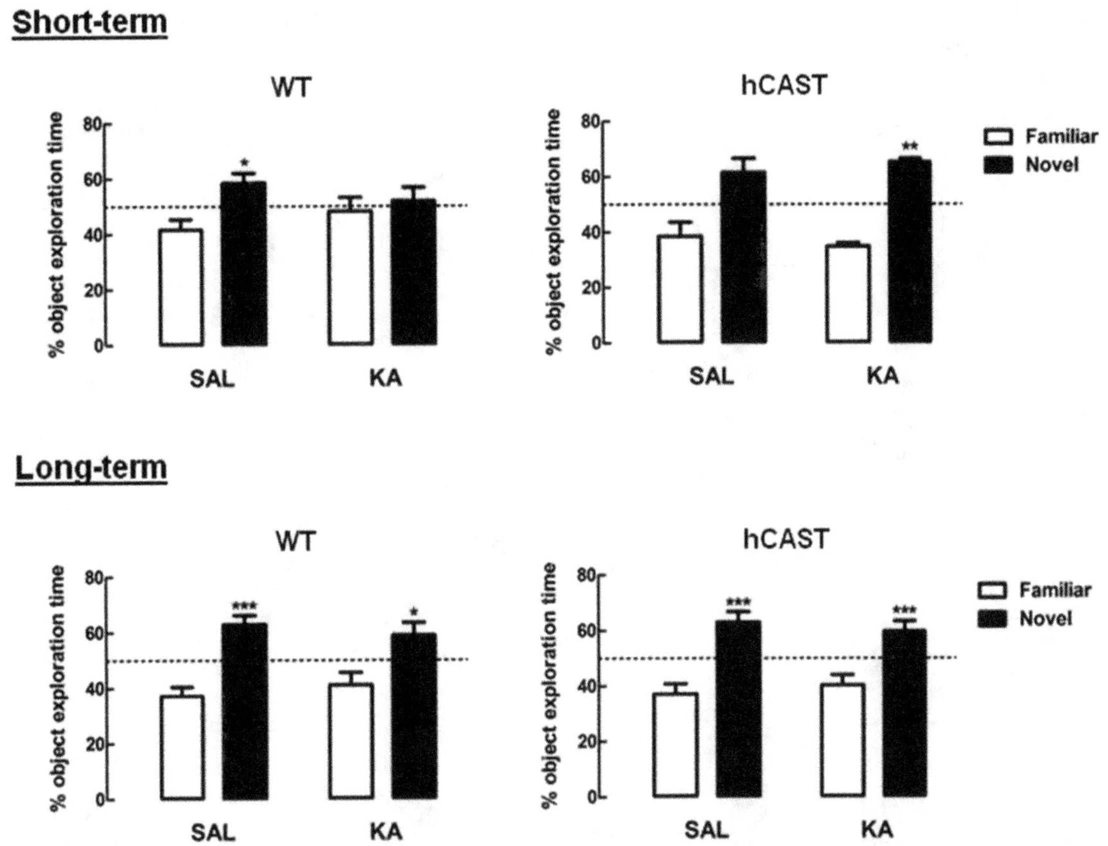

FIGURE 2 | KA-treated WT mice present short-term impairment in novel object exploration, but not KA-treated hCAST mice. WT and hCAST mice behavior was tested on the 3rd (short-term) or 8th week (long-term) after treatment with either SAL or KA. Recognition memory was assessed by measuring the percentage of exploration time during the presentation of a novel object, in the OR test. Data are presented as means ± SEM of 3–5 animals per group (for short-term recovery) and 12–15 animals per group (for long-term recovery). Statistical significance was determined using the Kruskal-Wallis test (Dunn's post-test), $*p < 0.05$, $**p < 0.01$ and $***p < 0.001$, significantly different from familiar object.

in the short-term recovery period learned the platform location similarly to SAL on all days (Day 1, WT: 49.3 ± 7.3 s, hCAST: 39.4 ± 4.1 s; Day 2, WT: 36.3 ± 10.0 s, hCAST: 15.5 ± 3.6 s; Day 3, WT: 24.2 ± 10.9 s, hCAST: 14.2 ± 4.7 s, $p > 0.05$), as well as all KA-treated mice in the long-term recovery period (Day 1, WT: 38.4 ± 2.7 s, hCAST: 47.9 ± 2.7 s; Day 2, WT: 26.4 ± 3.9 s, hCAST: 30.9 ± 5.3 s; Day 3, WT: 17.4 ± 4.9 s, hCAST: 20.7 ± 2.1 s, $p > 0.05$). All mice showed improved spatial learning over the course of the trials.

After learning the platform location, the platform was removed and the spatial memory evaluated by calculating the percentage of time spent in the target quadrant (where the platform previously was) and by counting the number of crossings through the exact previous platform location. Time spent in the target quadrant was maintained with KA treatment in both time periods, by comparison with SAL (short-term recovery, WT: 60.4 ± 3.7%, hCAST: 49.0 ± 5.7%, $p > 0.05$; long-term recovery, WT: 56.4 ± 4.1%, hCAST: 49.0 ± 4.3%, $p > 0.05$; **Figure 3B**, left panels), indicating that all animals remembered the relative position of the platform. The number of platform crossings (**Figure 3B**, right panels), in turn, also seemed to be maintained with KA treatment in the short-term recovery period when comparing to SAL (WT: 4.3 ± 1.6, hCAST: 3.8 ± 0.9, $p > 0.05$). However, in the long-term recovery period, the number of platform crossings was significantly impaired in KA-treated WT mice (2.4 ± 0.4) by comparison with SAL treatment (4.5 ± 0.7, $p < 0.05$), indicating increased difficulty in remembering the exact platform location, which is not observed in mice overexpressing CAST (SAL: 3.0 ± 0.6, $p > 0.05$).

Associative Fear Memory Is Preserved after KA Treatment

Lastly, associative learning and memory was evaluated, by performing the FC test (3–5 animals per group for short-term recovery and 9–16 animals per group for long-term recovery). By the end of the trials, on the first day, the animals successfully learned to associate the cue tone with a footshock. All animals spent nearly half the time of the last hearing of the tone freezing, both in the short-term recovery (WT SAL: 42.7 ± 5.4%, hCAST SAL: 51.5 ± 5.3%, $p > 0.05$) and in the long-term recovery (WT SAL: 48.9 ± 6.8%, hCAST SAL: 47.1 ± 4.5%, $p > 0.05$; **Figure 4A**).

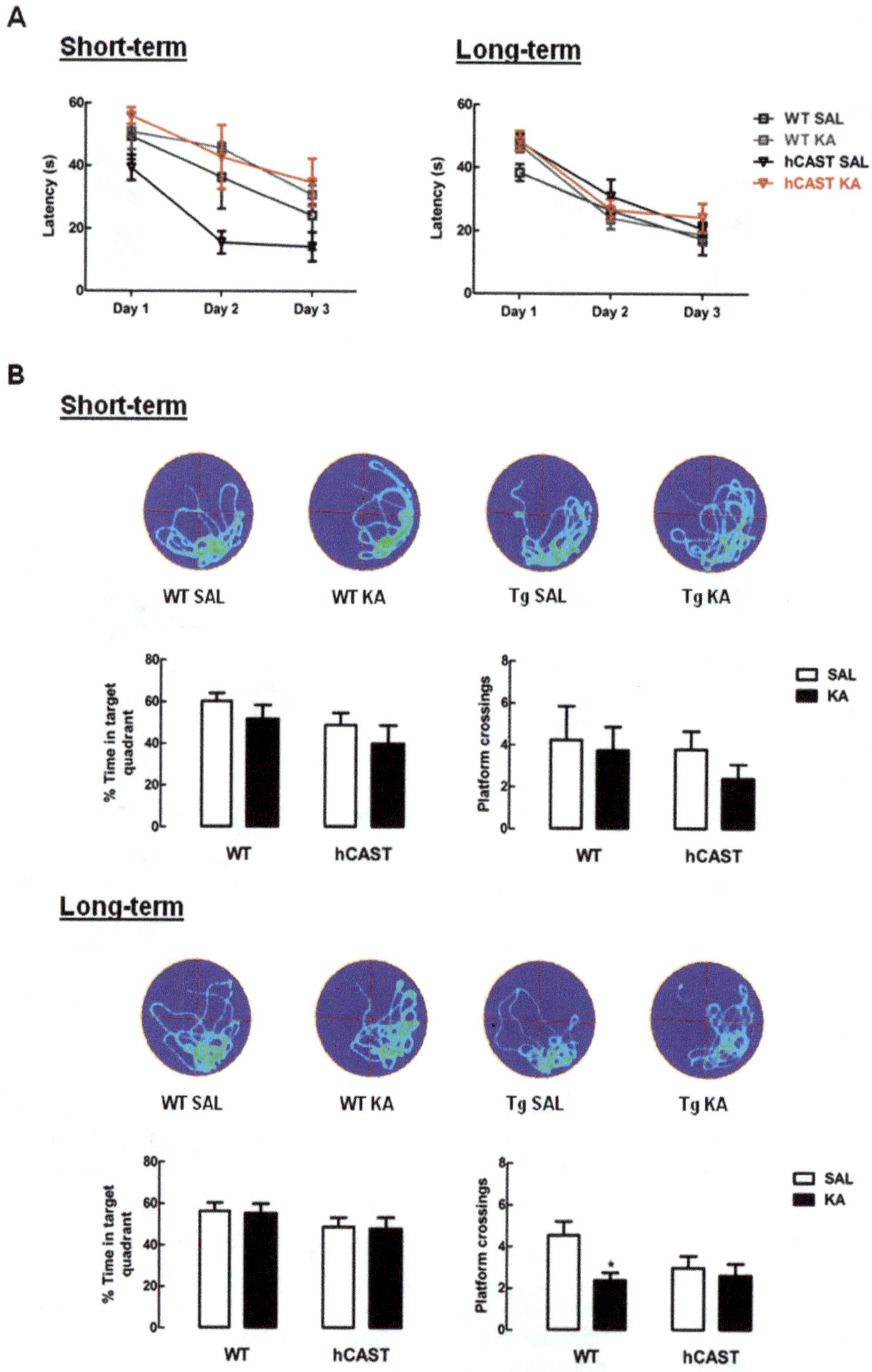

FIGURE 3 | Spatial memory for the exact platform location is impaired in KA-treated WT mice from the long-term recovery period. WT and hCAST mice behavior was tested on the 3rd (short-term) or 8th (long-term) week after treatment with either SAL or KA. **(A)** Spatial learning was assessed by measuring the escape latency on the first 3 days of WM (four trials per day, latency of 60 s if the platform was not reached). **(B)** Spatial memory was assessed by measuring the percentage of time spent on the target quadrant and the number of crossings in the exact location the platform was during trials, on the last day of WM. Representative images of occupancy track plots for each group are shown in the top panels. Data are presented as means ± SEM of 4–5 animals per group (for short-term recovery) and 11–16 animals per group (for long-term recovery). Statistical significance was determined using the Kruskal-Wallis test (Dunn's post-test), $^{*}p < 0.05$, significantly different from SAL.

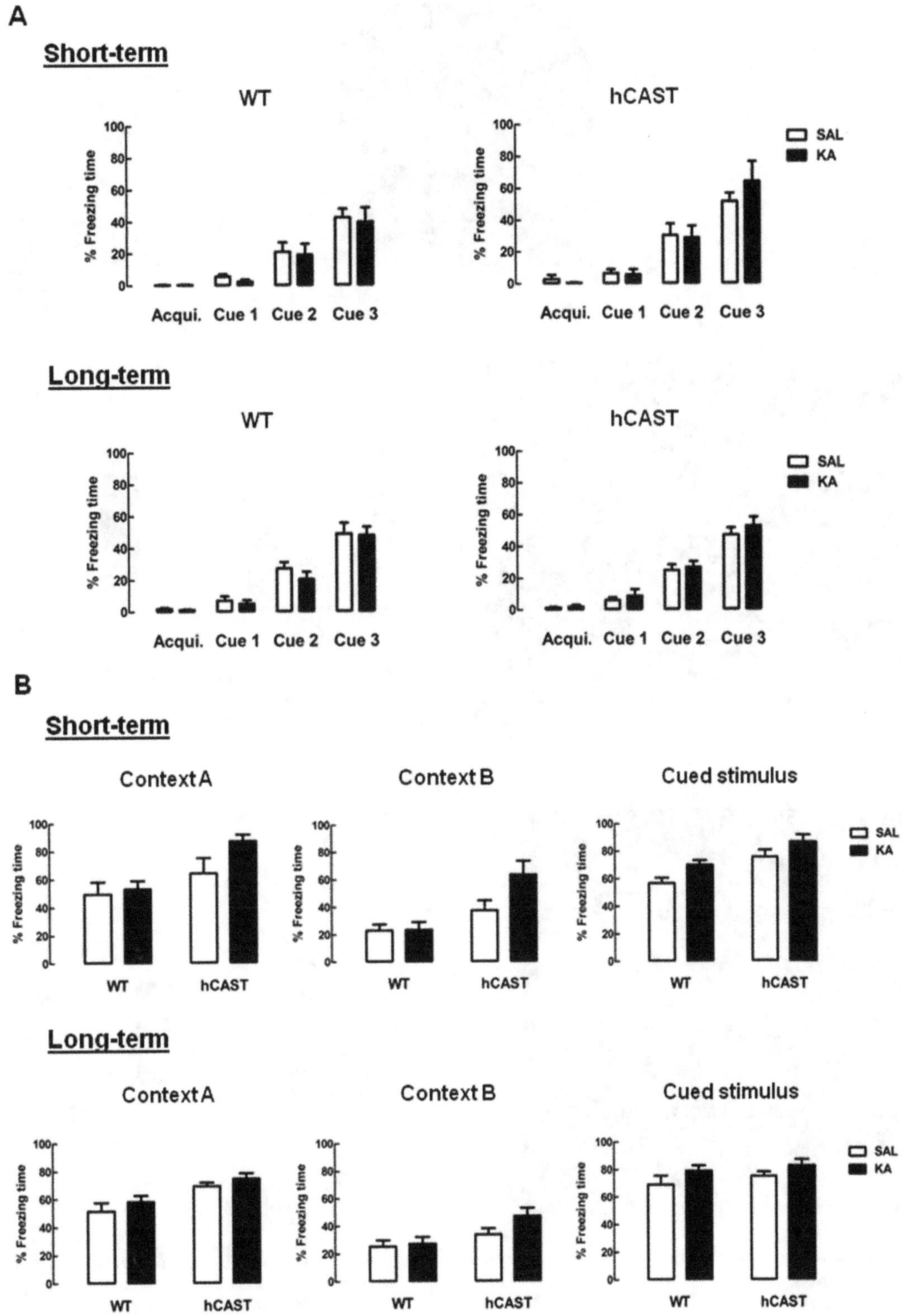

FIGURE 4 | Associative fear memory is preserved after KA treatment. WT and hCAST mice behavior was tested on the 3rd (short-term) or 8th (long-term) week after treatment with either SAL or KA. **(A)** Associative learning was assessed by measuring the percentage of freezing time during FC trials, with the delivery of a footshock by the end of each cue tone. Acqui. (acquisition). **(B)** Associative memory to the context and cue tone were assessed by measuring the percentage of freezing time during the FC context test (context A) and cued test (cued stimulus), in a new context (context B). Data are presented as means ± SEM of 3–5 animals per group (for short-term recovery) and 9–16 animals per group (for long-term recovery). Statistical significance was determined using the Kruskal-Wallis test (Dunn's post-test), $p > 0.05$ between treatments.

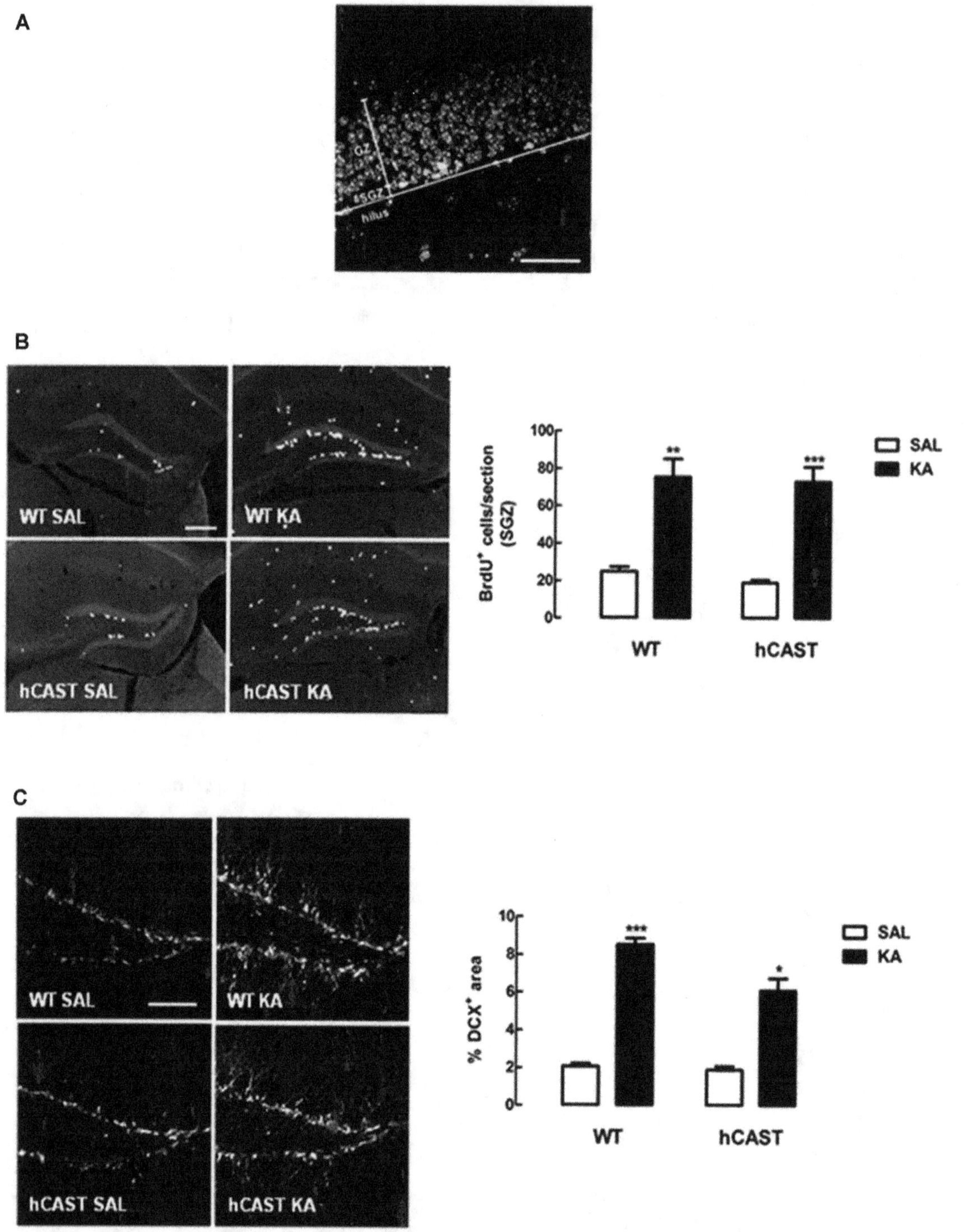

FIGURE 5 | KA treatment enhances NSC proliferation and neuroblast migration in the dentate gyrus (DG). (A) Representative image of a section of the DG, showing the division into granular zone (GZ), subgranular zone (SGZ) and hilus. EdU in green and nuclei, stained for Hoechst 33342, in gray. Scale bar: 50 μm. **(B)** WT and hCAST mice were treated with either SAL or KA and were given BrdU on the day before sacrifice, to assess cell proliferation. Representative images from hippocampal brain sections for each group (left panels), showing BrdU-positive cells in white. Scale bar: 200 μm. BrdU-positive cells were counted in the SGZ of five central coronal sections of the hippocampal region for each animal (right panel). **(C)** WT and hCAST mice were treated with either SAL or KA and sacrificed after 14 days, to assess cell migration. Representative images from hippocampal brain sections for each group (left panels), showing migrating neuroblasts, labeled for doublecortin (DCX), in white. Scale bar: 100 μm. Percentage of DCX-positive area was determined in the DG of five central coronal sections of the hippocampal region for each animal (right panel). Data are presented as means ± SEM of 9–14 animals per group (for cell proliferation) and 6–9 animals per group (for cell migration). Statistical significance was determined using the Kruskal-Wallis test (Dunn's post-test), *$p < 0.05$, **$p < 0.01$ and ***$p < 0.001$, significantly different from SAL.

When tested for associative memory to context (context A; **Figure 4B**, left panels), all KA-treated mice seemed to recognize the context similarly to SAL, both in the short-term recovery (WT: 48.9 ± 6.8%, hCAST: 64.2 ± 10.8%, $p > 0.05$) and in the long-term recovery (WT: 51.5 ± 6.0%, hCAST: 69.4 ± 2.6%, $p > 0.05$). When in the context meant for the cued test (context B; **Figure 4B**, middle panels), all hCAST mice from the short-term recovery group treated with KA spent over half the time freezing (SAL: 37.4 ± 7.2%, KA: 63.4 ± 9.8%, $p > 0.05$), while the percentage of freezing time was maintained low in WT mice (SAL: 23.1 ± 4.5%, KA: 23.5 ± 5.7%, $p > 0.05$). In the long-term recovery group, the percentage of freezing time was more similar to SAL in both WT and hCAST mice (WT: 25.4 ± 4.4%, hCAST: 33.8 ± 4.4%, $p > 0.05$). Moreover, all KA-treated mice seemed to maintain the associative memory to the cued stimulus by comparison with SAL, both in the short-term recovery (WT: 56.7 ± 3.9%, hCAST: 75.5 ± 5.2%, $p > 0.05$) and in the long-term recovery (WT: 69.1 ± 6.5%, hCAST: 75.1 ± 3.2%, $p > 0.05$; **Figure 4B**, right panels).

CAST Overexpression Maintains Enhancement of Early Hippocampal Neurogenesis after KA Treatment

In order to study the effects of CAST overexpression on the early stages of hippocampal neurogenesis after a brain insult, NSC proliferation and neuroblast migration were analyzed in the DG of adult mice (**Figure 5A**), after treatment with either SAL or KA (9–14 animals per group for cell proliferation and 6–9 animals per group for cell migration). Cell proliferation was assessed by incorporation of the thymidine analog BrdU into the DNA of dividing NSCs from the SGZ of the hippocampus. We observed that cell proliferation was greatly enhanced in mice overexpressing CAST after KA treatment (73.1 ± 8.0 cells/section), when compared to SAL-treated mice (19.2 ± 1.5 cells/section, $p < 0.001$), similarly to what was seen in WT mice (KA: 75.6 ± 9.7 cells/section, SAL: 25.0 ± 2.5 cells/section, $p < 0.01$; **Figure 5B**).

With regard to neuroblast migration, as assessed by DCX staining in the DG, we also observed a significant increase in KA-treated mice overexpressing CAST (6.1 ± 0.6%), when compared to SAL-treated mice (1.9 ± 0.2%, $p < 0.05$). Although cell migration in the DG of KA-treated WT mice (8.5 ± 0.3%) was also enhanced in comparison with SAL (2.1 ± 0.2%, $p < 0.001$), CAST overexpression seemed to attenuate this effect (**Figure 5C**).

To evaluate whether differences in neuronal death after lesion could be observed, WT and hCAST mice (3–4 animals per group) were sacrificed 24 h after KA treatment and FluoroJade C staining was performed. We observed that hCAST mice presented an amount of dying neurons similar to WT mice in the DG, both in the GZ (WT: 0.1 ± 0.1%, hCAST: 0.2 ± 0.0%, $p > 0.05$) and in the hilus (WT: 0.3 ± 0.2%, hCAST: 0.5 ± 0.1%, $p > 0.05$; Supplementary Figure 1).

CAST Overexpression Affects Cell Differentiation in the DG Similarly to WT after KA Treatment

Besides cell proliferation and migration, we were also interested in investigating differentiation of newborn cells after treatment with KA. For that purpose, mice were treated with the thymidine analog EdU (eight animals per group), and the number of EdU-positive cells remaining in the DG after 8 weeks was counted. We observed that the number of newborn cells still surviving in the DG was generally enhanced with KA-treatment in WT (SGZ + GZ: 9.7 ± 1.8 cells/section, hilus: 1.6 ± 0.3 cells/section) and hCAST (SGZ + GZ: 9.2 ± 1.1 cells/section, hilus: 1.6 ± 0.3 cells/section) mice, when compared to SAL treatment (SGZ + GZ, WT: 1.8 ± 0.1 cells/section, $p < 0.01$, hCAST: 1.6 ± 0.3 cells/section, $p < 0.001$; hilus, WT: 0.3 ± 0.1 cells/section, $p < 0.01$, hCAST: 0.6 ± 0.2 cells/section, $p > 0.05$; **Figure 6A**). When assessing neuronal differentiation specifically, by determining the percentage of those cells that colocalized with a neuronal marker (NeuN), we observed that treatment with KA seemed to reduce the amount of new neurons in the DG in WT mice (52.5 ± 8.0%) and in mice overexpressing CAST (47.0 ± 4.1%), when compared to SAL-treated animals (WT: 71.6 ± 4.4%, $p > 0.05$; hCAST: 67.2 ± 4.2%, $p < 0.05$; **Figure 6B**), suggesting decreased neuronal survival.

DISCUSSION

The realization that the adult mammalian brain is not an immutable organ and that new neurons are able to form and thrive in the neuronal circuitry has opened new doors for the putative treatment of neurodegenerative disorders and brain lesions. NSCs not only give origin to new neurons in the healthy brain, but are also known to increase the formation of new cells after lesion. NSCs can travel as neuroblasts into regions where neurons were lost as a consequence of brain damage, in what seems like an endogenous attempt to replace those lost neurons. However, this process is not very efficient, as most of the new cells die, fail to integrate the networks, or do it erroneously (Kaneko and Sawamoto, 2009; Ma et al., 2009). While cell transplantation into the sites of injury, for example, also seems promising, modulating endogenous neurogenesis would offer a less invasive approach for the treatment of brain damage. Calpains are proteases involved in neurodegeneration and their inhibition has been shown to be neuroprotective in several diseases (Saez et al., 2006), though their influence in neurogenesis is still not very clear. One of the approaches for the study of calpains is the modulation of their selective endogenous inhibitor, CAST. We had previously seen that the absence of CAST impairs NSC proliferation and neuroblast migration in the adult mouse brain (Machado et al., 2015), namely hippocampal neurogenesis, which has been implicated in learning and memory. Thus, we were interested in investigating whether overexpressing CAST would improve cognitive recovery after hippocampal injury, induced with KA, and its effects on post-injury neurogenesis. Finding a way to modulate calpain

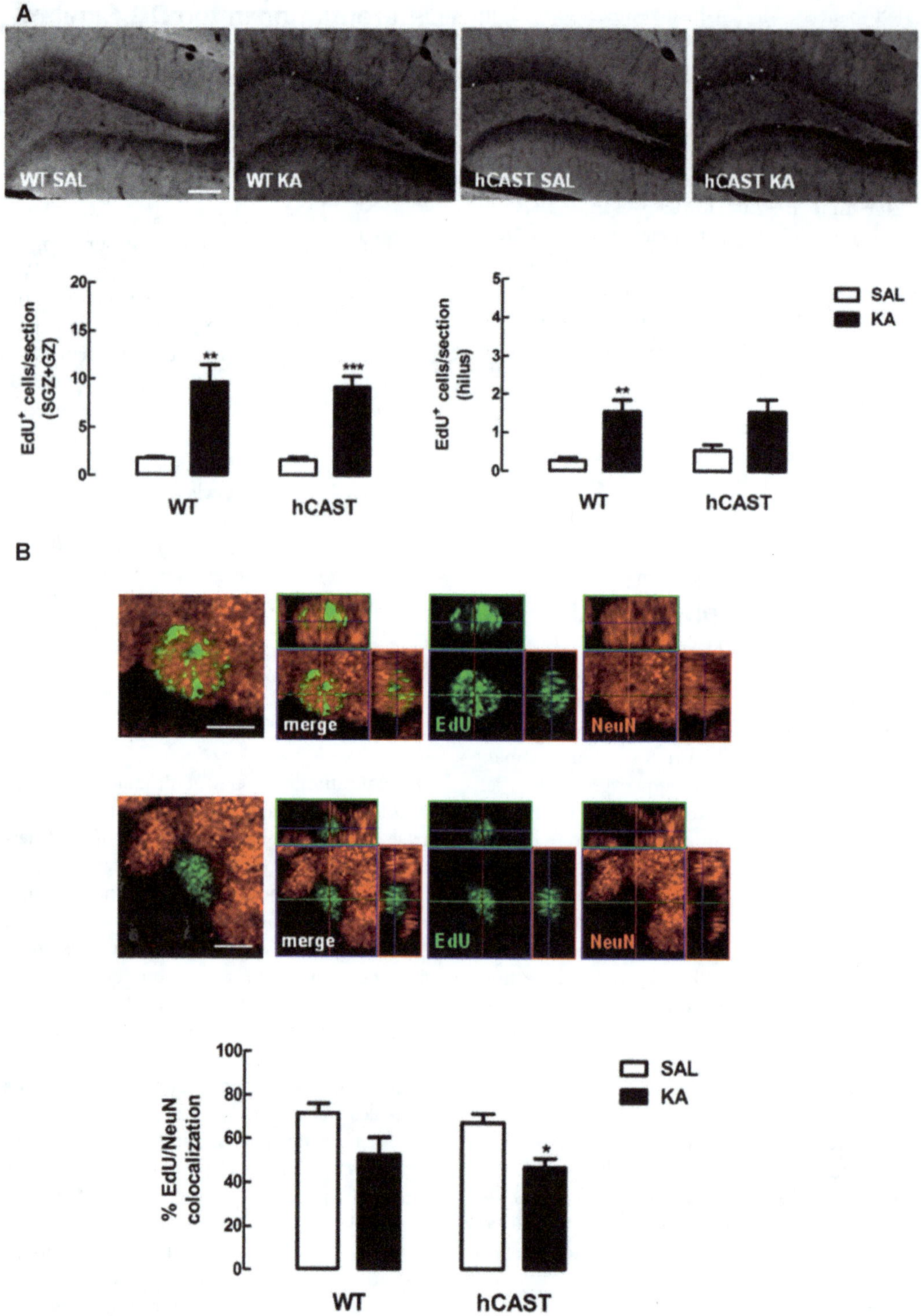

FIGURE 6 | CAST overexpression affects cell differentiation in the DG similarly to WT after KA treatment. WT and hCAST mice were treated with either SAL or KA and sacrificed 8 weeks after EdU administration, to assess neuronal differentiation. **(A)** Representative images from hippocampal brain sections for each group (top panels), showing EdU-positive cells in white. Scale bar: 200 μm. EdU-positive cells were counted in the SGZ, GZ and hilus of five central coronal sections of the hippocampal region for each animal (bottom panels). **(B)** Representative images from hippocampal brain sections of EdU-positive/neuronal nuclei (NeuN)-positive and EdU-positive/NeuN-negative cells in the DG (top panels), showing cells labeled for EdU in green and cells labeled for NeuN in red. Scale bar: 5 μm. The percentage of cells labeled for both EdU and NeuN in the DG (bottom panel) was determined in a total of up to 50 EdU-positive cells. Data are presented as means ± SEM of eight animals per group. Statistical significance was determined using the Kruskal-Wallis test (Dunn's post-test), $^{*}p < 0.05$, $^{**}p < 0.01$ and $^{***}p < 0.001$, significantly different from SAL.

activity in order to help improve the outcome of brain injury would highly benefit patients with neurodegenerative diseases or other types of brain insults.

KA induces excitotoxicity and consequent cell death, by activating ionotropic receptors highly abundant in the hippocampus (Wang et al., 2005; Carta et al., 2014). The KA model of brain lesion is thus often used for research involving hippocampal damage, especially in studies of temporal lobe epilepsy (Levesque and Avoli, 2013). It is also a good model for investigating hippocampal injury and its consequences (Araújo et al., 2008; Carreira et al., 2010, 2015). Since the hippocampus is the main structure involved in learning and memory, it is not surprising that treatment with KA in rodents can induce cognitive impairment (Stubley-Weatherly et al., 1996), which has also been reported in patients with temporal lobe epilepsy (Hattiangady and Shetty, 2008). With this in mind, we were especially interested in verifying whether mice overexpressing CAST would show differences in cognitive recovery on the 3rd (short-term) or 8th week (long-term) after KA treatment. In the short-term group, neurons born a few days after the brain insult are still immature, while in the long-term group those neurons are already fully mature and integrated (Deng et al., 2010). We tested the mice for three different types of cognitive behavior: recognition memory (OR), spatial learning and memory (WM) and associative learning and memory (FC).

The OR test makes use of the natural exploratory behavior of rodents. In the presence of a familiar and a novel object, rats and mice will normally spend relatively more time exploring the novel one, in a process shown by several studies to implicate the hippocampus (Cohen and Stackman, 2015). It was thus not a surprise that KA treatment impaired recognition of the previously explored object in WT mice from the short-term recovery group. In the long-term group, however, this impairment seemed to be overcome, suggesting that the newly formed cells ultimately succeeded in restoring the networks necessary for OR. Interestingly, CAST overexpression prevented impairment after KA treatment even in the short-term group. Having in mind that in this group the newly formed neurons are still immature, it is unlikely that they were already able to restore lost connections. This might thus mean that the regions involved in recognition memory were less affected when CAST was overexpressed.

Spatial memory, in turn, has long been known to require the hippocampus, being one of the most affected by hippocampal lesions (Best et al., 2001; Martin and Clark, 2007). In a fundamental work by Richard Morris (Morris et al., 1982), for example, rats with hippocampi removed took longer to learn to reach an escape platform hidden in a pool, but not a visible platform, and also had more difficulty in distinguishing the exact previous escape location when the platform was removed from the pool. This indicates the importance of the hippocampal integrity in navigating through space using only distal environmental cues. In our study, we used this Morris WM test to investigate whether impairment in spatial memory was also seen in our model and if CAST overexpression could be beneficial. By the end of the trials, all animals were able to learn to reach the platform, and also spent a high percentage of time in the target quadrant when platform was removed. Moreover, in the short-term group, there seemed to be no differences in the number of crossings over the exact previous platform location. In the long-term group, however, the number of crossings was impaired in KA-treated WT mice in comparison with SAL, which was not seen in mice overexpressing CAST. Interestingly, certain neurons in the hippocampus, the place cells, have the peculiarity of firing only when the animal enters a specific position in space. Different place cells respond to different locations of the same environment, allowing the brain to create a spatial map of that particular environment (O'Keefe and Dostrovsky, 1971). Additionally, a study on the pattern of place-cell activity during a WM test in rats has shown that the percentage of place cells firing maximally was more than doubled near the platform when compared to other locations in the pool (Hollup et al., 2001). This indicates a great contribution of these cells to the correct mental positioning of the platform in this particular task. Our results may suggest a loss of place cells or correct place-cell activity in WT mice treated with KA, since they seemed to have only a general idea of the platform whereabouts, but failed to determine exactly where it was, as compared to SAL-treated mice. This notion is further corroborated by a study showing that seizure-induced hippocampal lesion can indeed affect the activity of place cells several weeks later, making them less precise and less stable (Liu et al., 2003). The existing place cells in mice overexpressing CAST seem therefore to be less affected by KA treatment, suggesting that calpain inhibition may also limit the seizure-induced damage of these cells.

The FC test was the last to be performed, since it was the most stressful for the animals. This test is based on the association of an aversive stimulus with a tone and with the context where it occurred, which is measured by the time the animal spends freezing, i.e., when the only observed movement is from breathing, a known indicative of fear in rodents (Blanchard and Blanchard, 1969; Wehner and Radcliffe, 2004). As with the other performed cognitive tests, the FC test also has the involvement of the hippocampus, but only in relation to context, being the response to the cued stimulus dependent on the integrity of the amygdala (Phillips and LeDoux, 1992). For that reason, during learning, we were expecting all mice to associate the cued tone with the aversive stimulus, with progressively more time spent freezing with further tone presentations. Indeed, by the last time the tone was played, all animals spent around half of the time freezing, in contrast with virtually no freezing that was observed when they were first placed in the chamber. On the following day, the animals were placed in the exact same context, without presentation of tone or footshock, and SAL-treated animals presented associative memory to this context, by presenting freezing behavior for most of the time spent inside the chamber, as expected. However, KA-treatment failed to impair the time spent freezing, which may be linked with the relative resistance of the used strain to KA-induced cell death (McKhann et al., 2003). Even though differences in associative memory might be too subtle for detection, freezing to the modified context seemed to be increased in KA-treated mice overexpressing CAST from the short-term recovery group, since they spent over half the time freezing. Unlike the other mice, that seemed to understand the context was different, these mice seemed to assimilate that they were in a similar situation as before. One interesting feature of the aforementioned place cells is that they can be involved in the mechanisms of pattern separation, the ability to discriminate between very similar memories, and pattern completion, the ability to recall a previous memory in full based only on some of the components that composed that memory (Sahay et al., 2011). If these mechanisms are not balanced, there is an alteration in the perception of the environment. For instance, if pattern completion is relatively enhanced, there is generalization of the current environment, which means that several contexts may be linked together, even if they present reduced similarities (Sahay et al., 2011). This imbalance may thus be what caused the tendency of KA-treated hCAST mice from the short-term group to present higher freezing in the modified context, since the small similarities between both contexts could have been enough for them to recall the aversive stimulus. A possible explanation for this may relate to the findings that young granule cells (immature neurons) seem to be involved with pattern separation and older granule cells with pattern completion (Nakashiba et al., 2012). Assuming that old neurons can be more resistant, and that this might be the case in KA-treated mice overexpressing CAST, relatively more younger ones would die (Spalding et al., 2013). Since KA enhances the early stages of neurogenesis, an increased number of younger granule cells is expected to exist in the hippocampus of mice from the short-term group. At first, the new cells do not appear to be enough to compensate for the relative higher number of older cells, though later on they seem to regain balance, since the differential behavioral response to the new context of hCAST mice treated with KA from the short-term recovery group is lost in the long-term group. On the other hand, assuming that in WT mice younger and older neurons are lost more or less equally in KA-treated WT mice, and since the balance between younger and older granule cells seems to be maintained, by observation of memory association to the new context, we suggest that the new young neurons may not be fully functional. Electrophysiology studies would help to evaluate if this is in fact the case. Lastly, like with learning, we were expecting, and observed, associative memory to the cue tone to be maintained in all animals, since the hippocampus does not seem to be involved in this process.

Furthermore, we wanted to evaluate whether CAST overexpression affected the modulation of post-injury hippocampal neurogenesis. Like with other types of brain damage, an enhancement of endogenous neurogenesis has also been reported after seizures. Independently of the model chosen to induce seizures in rodents, NSC proliferation is specially shown to be largely increased in the DG after just a few days (Parent et al., 1997; Gray and Sundstrom, 1998; Nakagawa et al., 2000; Hüttmann et al., 2003; Mohapel et al., 2004; Jessberger et al., 2007; Sierra et al., 2015). Interestingly, evidence of increased cell proliferation has also been observed in the hippocampus of patients with temporal lobe epilepsy (Blümcke et al., 2001; Crespel et al., 2005). In the model used by our group, the peak of cell proliferation in the DG was shown to occur on day 5 after seizure induction, with a significant increase in neuroblast migration after 14 days (Carreira et al., 2015), results that we were able to replicate in the present work. This heavy enhancement of early neurogenesis indicates that the microenvironment in the hippocampus not long after seizures is extremely pro-neurogenic, which makes it difficult for changes due to altered levels of calpain activity to be observed. Nonetheless, since increased calpain activity can impair NSC proliferation and migration of neuroblasts, it is important to exclude whether, in this case, calpain inhibition, by overexpression of CAST, increases cell proliferation and migration to alarming levels. An even more extreme rise in cell proliferation could originate unwanted cellular masses of undifferentiated cells, and more migrating cells could also mean more cells migrating into ectopic regions, interfering with the normal neuronal networks (Parent et al., 2006).

Regarding cell proliferation, the enhancement observed after KA treatment was similar in WT mice and in mice overexpressing CAST. Curiously, however, while the increase in neuroblast migration in KA-treated WT mice was around 4-fold, it dropped to 3-fold with the overexpression of CAST. Brain damage is closely associated with an increase in calpain activity, and it is known that calpain inhibition can be neuroprotective (Saez et al., 2006). This means that the fact that CAST was already overexpressed when seizures were induced may have attenuated the damage. Even though the amount of dying neurons in the DG 24 h after KA treatment seems similar to WT in a preliminary study by our group, the surrounding circuitry may still be more preserved with CAST overexpression, or different types of neurons may be affected. Less damage could therefore also mean a less dramatic increase in neurogenesis. In the long term this could be favorable, proven that more cells would integrate correctly in the existing networks. Cell proliferation in the DG was shown by another group to substantially rise even after less severe seizures, with no further increase with seizure severity (Mohapel et al., 2004). This might explain why we observed a similar increase in cell proliferation even with the overexpression of CAST.

This increase in neurogenesis after lesion, however, is only efficient if the new cells ultimately differentiate, survive and integrate the neuronal circuitry correctly. After seizures, this is usually not the case. Despite the enhancement in the early stages of neurogenesis, most of the new cells end up differentiating into astrocytes, with relatively less neurons surviving 1–2 months after seizures (Hattiangady and Shetty, 2010; Carreira et al., 2015; Sierra et al., 2015). Moreover, several newly formed neurons resembling granule cells are found ectopically in the hilus, and have also been reported to occur in patients with temporal lobe epilepsy (Parent et al., 1997, 2006). These ectopic granule-like hilar cells are hyperexcitable, contributing to a disruption of the existing neuronal networks and possibly aggravating the outcome of the disease (Dashtipour et al., 2001; Cameron et al., 2011). Our findings with WT mice are consistent with what has been reported. After a 2-month period, there were significantly more new cells found in the hilus, SGZ and GZ of the DG of mice treated with KA. Though not significant, the percentage of new neurons seemed to be decreased in these mice, which is in accordance with the aforementioned reduced survival of new neurons after seizures. The overall increase in the number of new cells may thus be justifiable by the increased differentiation into astrocytes that occurs after seizures. The results obtained with hCAST mice were very similar, indicating that suppression of calpain activity provided by CAST overexpression is not enough to compensate for the impairment of neuronal differentiation in the DG. Although calpain inhibition was shown to increase neuronal differentiation *in vitro*, in a cell line from fetal NSCs (Santos et al., 2012), we cannot exclude that *in vivo* and in the developed brain other mechanisms may compensate for the decrease in calpain activity under a certain threshold, or even help in maintaining levels of calpain activity too elevated, especially in a pathologic environment. In this case, additional factors, such as nitric oxide from inflammatory origin, may also contribute for neuronal impairment (Carreira et al., 2015). This multifactorial feature of brain pathology must thus be taken into account when developing new strategies for brain repair. Nonetheless, even though the percentage of neurons formed after seizures is not ameliorated by CAST overexpression, the ones that thrive may still be more functional and better integrated in the hippocampal neuronal networks.

Overall, the fact that CAST was already overexpressed prior to lesion may have masked potential benefits of calpain inhibition on post-injury neurogenesis. Moreover, the fact that the absence of CAST and, consequently, increased calpain activity, can impair hippocampal neurogenesis, does not necessarily mean that reduced or lack of calpain activity can enhance it. In conclusion, even though reduced calpain activity does not seem to be able to enhance hippocampal neurogenesis, it could potentially be able to prevent the impairment in the formation of new neurons after injury, given that the levels of calpain activity could be reduced under a certain threshold. Strategies to reduce the harmful effects of the pathologic environment, such as controlling neuroinflammation, could also help boost the outcome of calpain inhibition in the survival of new neurons. Moreover, these observations are in regard to hippocampal neurogenesis. Cells derived from the subventricular zone may hold more promise for the enhancement of endogenous neurogenesis with calpain inhibition, encouraging further research involving these cells and calpain activity in the field of brain damage.

AUTHOR CONTRIBUTIONS

VMM: conception and design of the work, acquisition, analysis, interpretation of data, drafting of manuscript; ASL: design and acquisition; CF and RF: acquisition; CMC: conception and design of the work; IMA: conception and design of the work, interpretation of data, drafting of manuscript. All authors revised and approved the final version of the manuscript.

FUNDING

This work was supported by the Foundation for Science and Technology (FCT, Portugal), COMPETE and FEDER (grants PTDC/SAU-NMC/112183/2009, UID/NEU/04539/2013 and UID/BIM/04773/2013). VMM and ASL were supported by FCT (fellowships SFRH/BD/78050/2011 and SFRH/BD/79308/2011).

ACKNOWLEDGMENTS

We thank Dr. Ralph Nixon and Dr. Mala Rao for providing us the animals used in this study. VMM and ASL are PhD students of the PhD program in Biomedical Sciences of the University of Algarve.

REFERENCES

Aimone, J. B., Li, Y., Lee, S. W., Clemenson, G. D., Deng, W., and Gage, F. H. (2014). Regulation and function of adult neurogenesis: from genes to cognition. *Physiol. Rev.* 94, 991–1026. doi: 10.1152/physrev.00004.2014

Araújo, I. M., Gil, J. M., Carreira, B. P., Mohapel, P., Petersen, Å., Pinheiro, P. S., et al. (2008). Calpain activation is involved in early caspase-independent neurodegeneration in the hippocampus following status epilepticus. *J. Neurochem.* 105, 666–676. doi: 10.1111/j.1471-4159.2007.05181.x

Best, P. J., White, A. M., and Minai, A. (2001). Spatial processing in the brain: the activity of hippocampal place cells. *Annu. Rev. Neurosci.* 24, 459–486. doi: 10.1146/annurev.neuro.24.1.459

Bevins, R. A., and Besheer, J. (2006). Object recognition in rats and mice: a one-trial non-matching-to-sample learning task to study 'recognition memory'. *Nat. Protoc.* 1, 1306–1311. doi: 10.1038/nprot.2006.205

Blanchard, R. J., and Blanchard, D. C. (1969). Crouching as an index of fear. *J. Comp. Physiol. Psychol.* 67, 370–375. doi: 10.1037/h0026779

Blümcke, I., Schewe, J.-C., Normann, S., Brüstle, O., Schramm, J., Elger, C. E., et al. (2001). Increase of nestin-immunoreactive neural precursor cells in the dentate gyrus of pediatric patients with early-onset temporal lobe epilepsy. *Hippocampus* 11, 311–321. doi: 10.1002/hipo.1045

Bond, A. M., Ming, G. L., and Song, H. (2015). Adult mammalian neural stem cells and neurogenesis: five decades later. *Cell Stem Cell* 17, 385–395. doi: 10.1016/j.stem.2015.09.003

Cameron, M. C., Zhan, R.-Z., and Nadler, J. V. (2011). Morphologic integration of hilar ectopic granule cells into dentate gyrus circuitry in the pilocarpine model of temporal lobe epilepsy. *J. Comp. Neurol.* 519, 2175–2192. doi: 10.1002/cne.22623

Carreira, B. P., Morte, M. I., Inácio, A., Costa, G., Rosmaninho-Salgado, J., Agasse, F., et al. (2010). Nitric oxide stimulates the proliferation of neural stem cells bypassing the epidermal growth factor receptor. *Stem Cells* 28, 1219–1230. doi: 10.1002/stem.444

Carreira, B. P., Santos, D. F., Santos, A. I., Carvalho, C. M., and Araújo, I. M. (2015). Nitric oxide regulates neurogenesis in the hippocampus following seizures. *Oxid. Med. Cell. Longev.* 2015:451512. doi: 10.1155/2015/451512

Carta, M., Fièvre, S., Gorlewicz, A., and Mulle, C. (2014). Kainate receptors in the hippocampus. *Eur. J. Neurosci.* 39, 1835–1844. doi: 10.1111/ejn.12590

Cohen, S. J., and Stackman, R. W. Jr. (2015). Assessing rodent hippocampal involvement in the novel object recognition task. A review. *Behav. Brain Res.* 285, 105–117. doi: 10.1016/j.bbr.2014.08.002

Crespel, A., Rigau, V., Coubes, P., Rousset, M. C., de Bock, F., Okano, H., et al. (2005). Increased number of neural progenitors in human temporal lobe epilepsy. *Neurobiol. Dis.* 19, 436–450. doi: 10.1016/j.nbd.2005.01.020

Dashtipour, K., Tran, P. H., Okazaki, M. M., Nadler, J. V., and Ribak, C. E. (2001). Ultrastructural features and synaptic connections of hilar ectopic granule cells in the rat dentate gyrus are different from those of granule cells in the granule cell layer. *Brain Res.* 890, 261–271. doi: 10.1016/s0006-8993(00) 03119-x

Deng, W., Aimone, J. B., and Gage, F. H. (2010). New neurons and new memories: how does adult hippocampal neurogenesis affect learning and memory? *Nat. Rev. Neurosci.* 11, 339–350. doi: 10.1038/nrn2822

Gray, W. P., and Sundstrom, L. E. (1998). Kainic acid increases the proliferation of granule cell progenitors in the dentate gyrus of the adult rat. *Brain Res.* 790, 52–59. doi: 10.1016/s0006-8993(98)00030-4

Hattiangady, B., and Shetty, A. K. (2008). Implications of decreased hippocampal neurogenesis in chronic temporal lobe epilepsy. *Epilepsia* 49, 26–41. doi: 10.1111/j.1528-1167.2008.01635.x

Hattiangady, B., and Shetty, A. K. (2010). Decreased neuronal differentiation of newly generated cells underlies reduced hippocampal neurogenesis in chronic temporal lobe epilepsy. *Hippocampus* 20, 97–112. doi: 10.1002/hipo.20594

Hitomi, K., Yokoyama, A., and Maki, M. (1998). Expression of biologically active human calpastatin in baculovirus-infected insect cells and in Escherichia coli. *Biosci. Biotechnol. Biochem.* 62, 136–141. doi: 10.1271/bbb.62.136

Hollup, S. A., Molden, S., Donnett, J. G., Moser, M. B., and Moser, E. I. (2001). Accumulation of hippocampal place fields at the goal location in an annular watermaze task. *J. Neurosci.* 21, 1635–1644.

Hüttmann, K., Sadgrove, M., Wallraff, A., Hinterkeuser, S., Kirchhoff, F., Steinhauser, C., et al. (2003). Seizures preferentially stimulate proliferation of radial glia-like astrocytes in the adult dentate gyrus: functional and immunocytochemical analysis. *Eur. J. Neurosci.* 18, 2769–2778. doi: 10.1111/j. 1460-9568.2003.03002.x

Jessberger, S., Nakashima, K., Clemenson, G. D. Jr., Mejia, E., Mathews, E., Ure, K., et al. (2007). Epigenetic modulation of seizure-induced neurogenesis and cognitive decline. *J. Neurosci.* 27, 5967–5975. doi: 10.1523/JNEUROSCI. 0110-07.2007

Jin, X. (2016). The role of neurogenesis during development and in the adult brain. *Eur. J. Neurosci.* 44, 2291–2299. doi: 10.1111/ejn.13251

Kaneko, N., and Sawamoto, K. (2009). Adult neurogenesis and its alteration under pathological conditions. *Neurosci. Res.* 63, 155–164. doi: 10.1016/j.neures.2008. 12.001

Kashiwagi, A., Schipani, E., Fein, M. J., Greer, P. A., and Shimada, M. (2010). Targeted deletion of Capn4 in cells of the chondrocyte lineage impairs chondrocyte proliferation and differentiation. *Mol. Cell. Biol.* 30, 2799–2810. doi: 10.1128/MCB.00157-10

Komitova, M., Mattsson, B., Johansson, B. B., and Eriksson, P. S. (2005). Enriched environment increases neural stem/progenitor cell proliferation and neurogenesis in the subventricular zone of stroke-lesioned adult rats. *Stroke* 36, 1278–1282. doi: 10.1161/01.str.0000166197.94147.59

Kuchay, S. M., Wieschhaus, A. J., Marinkovic, M., Herman, I. M., and Chishti, A. H. (2012). Targeted gene inactivation reveals a functional role of calpain-1 in platelet spreading. *J. Thromb. Haemost.* 10, 1120–1132. doi: 10.1111/j.1538-7836.2012.04715.x

Lazarini, F., and Lledo, P. M. (2011). Is adult neurogenesis essential for olfaction? *Trends Neurosci.* 34, 20–30. doi: 10.1016/j.tins.2010.09.006

Levesque, M., and Avoli, M. (2013). The kainic acid model of temporal lobe epilepsy. *Neurosci. Biobehav. Rev.* 37, 2887–2899. doi: 10.1016/j.neubiorev. 2013.10.011

Liu, X., Muller, R. U., Huang, L. T., Kubie, J. L., Rotenberg, A., Rivard, B., et al. (2003). Seizure-induced changes in place cell physiology: relationship to spatial memory. *J. Neurosci.* 23, 11505–11515.

Lokuta, M. A., Nuzzi, P. A., and Huttenlocher, A. (2003). Calpain regulates neutrophil chemotaxis. *Proc. Natl. Acad. Sci. U S A* 100, 4006–4011. doi: 10.1073/pnas.0636533100

Ma, D. K., Bonaguidi, M. A., Ming, G. L., and Song, H. (2009). Adult neural stem cells in the mammalian central nervous system. *Cell Res.* 19, 672–682. doi: 10.1038/cr.2009.56

Machado, V. M., Morte, M. I., Carreira, B. P., Azevedo, M. M., Takano, J., Iwata, N., et al. (2015). Involvement of calpains in adult neurogenesis: implications for stroke. *Front. Cell. Neurosci.* 9:22. doi: 10.3389/fncel.2015. 00022

Martin, S. J., and Clark, R. E. (2007). The rodent hippocampus and spatial memory: from synapses to systems. *Cell. Mol. Life Sci.* 64, 401–431. doi: 10.1007/s00018-007-6336-3

McKhann, G. M. II, Wenzel, H. J., Robbins, C. A., Sosunov, A. A., and Schwartzkroin, P. A. (2003). Mouse strain differences in kainic acid sensitivity, seizure behavior, mortality and hippocampal pathology. *Neuroscience* 122, 551–561. doi: 10.1016/s0306-4522(03)00562-1

Mohapel, P., Ekdahl, C. T., and Lindvall, O. (2004). Status epilepticus severity influences the long-term outcome of neurogenesis in the adult dentate gyrus. *Neurobiol. Dis.* 15, 196–205. doi: 10.1016/j.nbd.2003.11.010

Morris, R. G., Garrud, P., Rawlins, J. N., and O'Keefe, J. (1982). Place navigation impaired in rats with hippocampal lesions. *Nature* 297, 681–683. doi: 10.1038/297681a0

Morte, M. I., Carreira, B. P., Machado, V., Carmo, A., Nunes-Correia, I., Carvalho, C. M., et al. (2013). Evaluation of proliferation of neural stem cells *in vitro* and *in vivo*. *Curr. Protoc. Stem Cell Biol.* Chapter 2:Unit 2D.14. doi: 10.1002/9780470151808.sc02d14s24

Murachi, T. (1984). Calcium-dependent proteinases and specific inhibitors: calpain and calpastatin. *Biochem. Soc. Symp.* 49, 149–167.

Nakagawa, E., Aimi, Y., Yasuhara, O., Tooyama, I., Shimada, M., McGeer, P. L., et al. (2000). Enhancement of progenitor cell division in the dentate gyrus triggered by initial limbic seizures in rat models of epilepsy. *Epilepsia* 41, 10–18. doi: 10.1111/j.1528-1157.2000. tb01498.x

Nakashiba, T., Cushman, J. D., Pelkey, K. A., Renaudineau, S., Buhl, D. L., McHugh, T. J., et al. (2012). Young dentate granule cells mediate pattern separation, whereas old granule cells facilitate pattern completion. *Cell* 149, 188–201. doi: 10.1016/j.cell.2012.01.046

Neumar, R. W., Meng, F. H., Mills, A. M., Xu, Y. A., Zhang, C., Welsh, F. A., et al. (2001). Calpain activity in the rat brain after transient forebrain ischemia. *Exp. Neurol.* 170, 27–35. doi: 10.1006/exnr.2001.7708

O'Keefe, J., and Dostrovsky, J. (1971). The hippocampus as a spatial map. Preliminary evidence from unit activity in the freely-moving rat. *Brain Res.* 34, 171–175. doi: 10.1016/0006-8993(71)90358-1

Parent, J. M., Elliott, R. C., Pleasure, S. J., Barbaro, N. M., and Lowenstein, D. H. (2006). Aberrant seizure-induced neurogenesis in experimental temporal lobe epilepsy. *Ann. Neurol.* 59, 81–91. doi: 10.1002/ana.20699

Parent, J. M., Yu, T. W., Leibowitz, R. T., Geschwind, D. H., Sloviter, R. S., and Lowenstein, D. H. (1997). Dentate granule cell neurogenesis is increased by seizures and contributes to aberrant network reorganization in the adult rat hippocampus. *J. Neurosci.* 17, 3727–3738.

Parnaud, G., Hammar, E., Rouiller, D. G., and Bosco, D. (2005). Inhibition of calpain blocks pancreatic beta-cell spreading and insulin secretion. *Am. J. Physiol. Endocrinol. Metab.* 289, E313–E321. doi: 10.1152/ajpendo. 00006.2005

Phillips, R. G., and LeDoux, J. E. (1992). Differential contribution of amygdala and hippocampus to cued and contextual fear conditioning. *Behav. Neurosci.* 106, 274–285. doi: 10.1037/0735-7044.106.2.274

Qiu, K., Su, Y., and Block, E. R. (2006). Use of recombinant calpain-2 siRNA adenovirus to assess calpain-2 modulation of lung endothelial cell migration and proliferation. *Mol. Cell. Biochem.* 292, 69–78. doi: 10.1007/s11010-006-9219-2

Rao, M. V., Mohan, P. S., Peterhoff, C. M., Yang, D. S., Schmidt, S. D., Stavrides, P. H., et al. (2008). Marked calpastatin (CAST) depletion in Alzheimer's disease accelerates cytoskeleton disruption and neurodegeneration: neuroprotection by CAST overexpression. *J. Neurosci.* 28, 12241–12254. doi: 10.1523/JNEUROSCI.4119-08.2008

Rock, M. T., Dix, A. R., Brooks, W. H., and Roszman, T. L. (2000). α1 integrin-mediated T cell adhesion and cell spreading are regulated by calpain. *Exp. Cell Res.* 261, 260–270. doi: 10.1006/excr.2000.5048

Saez, M. E., Ramirez-Lorca, R., Moron, F. J., and Ruiz, A. (2006). The therapeutic potential of the calpain family: new aspects. *Drug Discov. Today* 11, 917–923. doi: 10.1016/j.drudis.2006.08.009

Sahay, A., Wilson, D. A., and Hen, R. (2011). Pattern separation: a common function for new neurons in hippocampus and olfactory bulb. *Neuron* 70, 582–588. doi: 10.1016/j.neuron.2011.05.012

Salazar-Colocho, P., Lanciego, J. L., Del Rio, J., and Frechilla, D. (2008). Ischemia induces cell proliferation and neurogenesis in the gerbil hippocampus in response to neuronal death. *Neurosci. Res.* 61, 27–37. doi: 10.1016/j.neures.2008.01.008

Santos, D. M., Xavier, J. M., Morgado, A. L., Solá, S., and Rodrigues, C. M. (2012). Distinct regulatory functions of calpain 1 and 2 during neural stem cell self-renewal and differentiation. *PLoS One* 7:e33468. doi: 10.1371/journal.pone.0033468

Schauwecker, P. E., and Steward, O. (1997). Genetic determinants of susceptibility to excitotoxic cell death: implications for gene targeting approaches. *Proc. Natl. Acad. Sci. U S A* 94, 4103–4108. doi: 10.1073/pnas.94.8.4103

Shimada, M., Greer, P. A., McMahon, A. P., Bouxsein, M. L., and Schipani, E. (2008). *In vivo* targeted deletion of calpain small subunit, Capn4, in cells of the osteoblast lineage impairs cell proliferation, differentiation and bone formation. *J. Biol. Chem.* 283, 21002–21010. doi: 10.1074/jbc.M710354200

Sierra, A., Martín-Suárez, S., Valcárcel-Martín, R., Pascual-Brazo, J., Aelvoet, S. A., Abiega, O., et al. (2015). Neuronal hyperactivity accelerates depletion of neural stem cells and impairs hippocampal neurogenesis. *Cell Stem Cell* 16, 488–503. doi: 10.1016/j.stem.2015.04.003

Spalding, K. L., Bergmann, O., Alkass, K., Bernard, S., Salehpour, M., Huttner, H. B., et al. (2013). Dynamics of hippocampal neurogenesis in adult humans. *Cell* 153, 1219–1227. doi: 10.1016/j.cell.2013.05.002

Stubley-Weatherly, L., Harding, J. W., and Wright, J. W. (1996). Effects of discrete kainic acid-induced hippocampal lesions on spatial and contextual learning and memory in rats. *Brain Res.* 716, 29–38. doi: 10.1016/0006-8993(95)01589-2

Wang, Q., Yu, S., Simonyi, A., Sun, G. Y., and Sun, A. Y. (2005). Kainic acid-mediated excitotoxicity as a model for neurodegeneration. *Mol. Neurobiol.* 31, 3–16. doi: 10.1385/mn:31:1-3:003

Wehner, J. M., and Radcliffe, R. A. (2004). Cued and contextual fear conditioning in mice. *Curr. Protoc. Neurosci.* Chapter 8:Unit 8.5C. doi: 10.1002/0471142301.ns0805cs27

Yajima, Y., and Kawashima, S. (2002). Calpain function in the differentiation of mesenchymal stem cells. *Biol. Chem.* 383, 757–764. doi: 10.1515/bc.2002.079

5

The Many Faces of Elongator in Neurodevelopment and Disease

Marija Kojic and Brandon Wainwright*

Genomics of Development and Disease Division, Institute for Molecular Bioscience, The University of Queensland, Brisbane, QLD, Australia

Edited by:
Daniela Tropea,
Trinity College Dublin, Ireland

Reviewed by:
Gregg Stanwood,
Florida State University, USA
Hansen Wang,
University of Toronto, Canada

***Correspondence:**
Marija Kojic
m.kojic@imb.uq.edu.au

Development of the nervous system requires a variety of cellular activities, such as proliferation, migration, axonal outgrowth and guidance and synapse formation during the differentiation of neural precursors into mature neurons. Malfunction of these highly regulated and coordinated events results in various neurological diseases. The Elongator complex is a multi-subunit complex highly conserved in eukaryotes whose function has been implicated in the majority of cellular activities underlying neurodevelopment. These activities include cell motility, actin cytoskeleton organization, exocytosis, polarized secretion, intracellular trafficking and the maintenance of neural function. Several studies have associated mutations in Elongator subunits with the neurological disorders familial dysautonomia (FD), intellectual disability (ID), amyotrophic lateral sclerosis (ALS) and rolandic epilepsy (RE). Here, we review the various cellular activities assigned to this complex and discuss the implications for neural development and disease. Further research in this area has the potential to generate new diagnostic tools, better prevention strategies and more effective treatment options for a wide variety of neurological disorders.

Keywords: Elongator complex, neurodevelopment, neurological disorders, tRNA modifications, translation

INTRODUCTION

There are over 600 known neurological disorders and we are still far from fully understanding and finding treatment options for the majority of them. Many neurological disorders are inherited diseases, arising from defects in the development of the nervous system. Neurodevelopment is a complex dynamic process regulated by various genetic and environmental factors. The process is comprised of a series of intricate and coordinated events, required for converting neural precursor cells into functional neurons. Deregulation of these complex processes leads to abnormal neurodevelopment and profound neurological dysfunction. Genetic analysis of various neurodevelopmental disorders, including familial dysautonomia (FD; Anderson et al., 2001; Slaugenhaupt et al., 2001; Cuajungco et al., 2003), intellectual disability (ID; Najmabadi et al., 2011; Cohen et al., 2015), amyotrophic lateral sclerosis (ALS; Simpson et al., 2009) and rolandic epilepsy (RE; Strug et al., 2009), have identified mutations in Elongator complex subunits, suggesting that this highly evolutionarily conserved complex plays an important role in regulating neurodevelopment. In eukaryotes, Elongator is associated with diverse cellular activities including transcriptional elongation (Hawkes et al., 2002; Kim et al., 2002), cytoplasmic kinase signaling (Holmberg et al., 2002; Close et al., 2006), exocytosis (Rahl et al., 2005), cytoskeletal organization (Johansen et al., 2008), tubulin acetylation (Creppe et al., 2009) and translation (Huang et al., 2005; Esberg et al., 2006; Johansson et al., 2008; Bauer et al., 2012). In this review, we discuss the growing experimental evidence supporting the importance of Elongator in cellular processes known to be crucially important for neurodevelopment and nervous system function.

THE ELONGATOR COMPLEX

The Elongator complex consists of six subunits (Elp1–Elp6), which are organized into two three-subunit sub-complexes: the core sub-complex Elp123 (Elp1–Elp3), and the accessory sub-complex Elp456 (Elp4–Elp6; Otero et al., 1999; Li et al., 2001; Winkler et al., 2001). Each Elongator subunit is structurally well characterized in yeast (**Figure 1A**). Elp1 is the largest of the six subunits and acts as a scaffold for other Elongator proteins. This subunit harbors several WD40 repeats within two WD40 propeller domains, and one tetratricopeptide repeat (TRP) domain that binds specific peptide ligands and mediates protein–protein interactions (Cortajarena and Regan, 2006). An additional Elp1 domain has been recently identified: the C-terminus-localized dimerization domain (Xu et al., 2015; **Figure 1B**). Elp2 is the second largest subunit of Elongator complex with two WD40 propeller domains (**Figure 1C**; Fellows et al., 2000). Together with Elp1, Elp2 contributes to the stability of Elp123 sub-complex and integrates signals from different factors that regulate Elongator activity. Elp3 functions as the enzymatic core of Elongator, harboring two domains essential for Elongator function. These include: the S-adenosyl-L-methionine (SAM) binding domain required to catalyze a variety of radical reactions (Paraskevopoulou et al., 2006), and the histone acetyl-transferase (HAT) domain (**Figure 1D**; Wittschieben et al., 1999). Elongator subunits Elp4–6 share a RecA-like fold (**Figure 1E**) and assemble into a heterohexameric, ring-like structure. Glatt et al. (2012) showed that Elp4, 5 and 6 specifically bind to the anti-codon loop of transfer RNAs (tRNAs) and preserve ATPase activity, likely as means to control tRNA binding and release. The interaction of Elongator subunits and complex assembly has been reported by two separate studies, both proposing that the Elp456 heterohexamer bridges two peripherally attached Elp123 sub-complexes. These data indicate that Elongator is a dodecameric complex containing two copies of each of the six Elongator subunits (**Figure 1F**; Glatt et al., 2012; Lin et al., 2012). Elongator subunits are evolutionarily highly conserved from yeast to humans both in their sequence and interaction with other subunits. Conserved function across all species has been clearly demonstrated using a variety of different cross-species rescue experiments (Li et al., 2005; Chen et al., 2006, 2009). Deletion of any of the genes encoding the six subunits confers almost identical biochemical phenotypes in yeast (Fellows et al., 2000; Winkler et al., 2001; Frohloff et al., 2003), suggesting that there is a tight functional association between the proteins comprising the Elongator complex, and that the functional integrity of Elongator is compromised in the absence of any of its subunits.

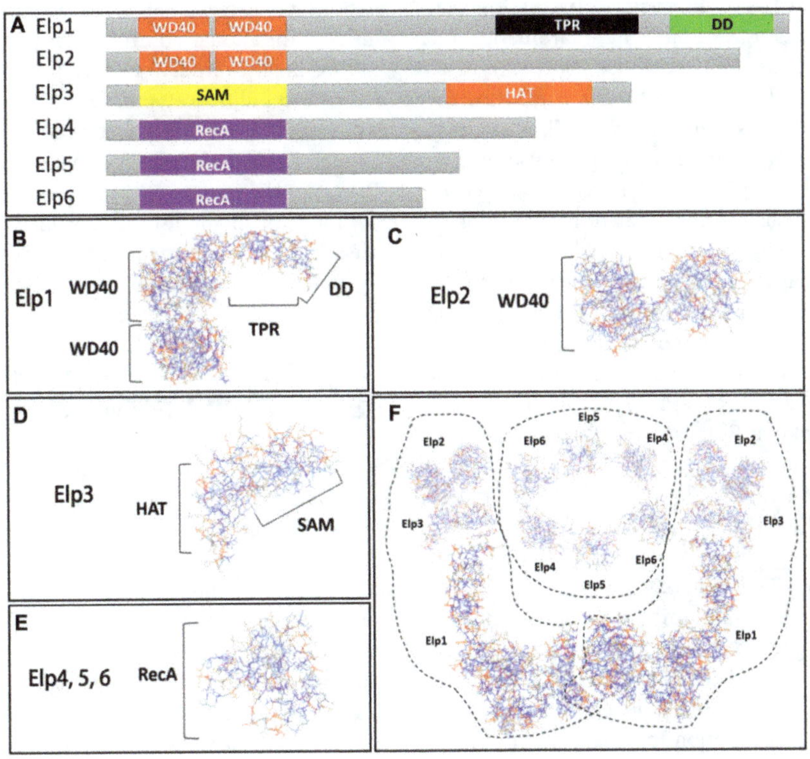

FIGURE 1 | The Elongator complex architecture. **(A)** Schematic view of Elongator subunits (Elp1–6) and their domain structure highlighted by different colors. Structural model of: **(B)** Elp1 harboring two WD40 propeller domains, tetratricopeptide repeat (TRP) and DD domain; **(C)** Elp2 containing two WD40 propeller domains; **(D)** Elp3 with histone acetyl-transferase (HAT) and S-adenosyl-L-methionine (SAM) domain **(E)** and Elp4, 5 and 6 subunits that share a RecA fold. **(F)** The Elongator complex assembly in dodecamer with two Elp123 trimeric sub-complexes peripherally attached to the ring-like hexameric Elp456 sub-complex. Structural models of Elp1–6 were prepared using program Phyre2 (Kelley and Sternberg, 2009).

The Elongator complex has been reported to orchestrate multiple functions across diverse organisms. Several loss-of-function studies have illustrated a key role for this complex in development by regulating a variety of different cellular activities. For example, yeast Elp mutants are hypersensitive to high temperature and osmotic conditions, presenting with defects in exocytosis, telomeric gene silencing, DNA damage response and adaption to new growth medium (Wittschieben et al., 1999; Rahl et al., 2005; Li et al., 2009; Chen et al., 2011). In *Arabidopsis thaliana*, mutations in Elp subunits resulted in impaired root growth (Nelissen et al., 2005), whilst deletion of Elp3 in *Drosophila melanogaster* was shown to be lethal at the larval stage (Walker et al., 2011). Elongator-deficient *Caenorhabditis elegans* exhibit defects in neurodevelopment (Solinger et al., 2010). In mice, a transgenic Elp1 knockout resulted in embryonic lethality due to failed neurulation and vascular system formation (Chen et al., 2009). Furthermore, several human neurological disorders have been linked to a deficiency of the Elongator, which will be discussed in more detail below.

The substrate specificity of Elongator remains controversial, and the definite number of roles this complex plays in different cellular activities is still to be confirmed (also reviewed in Svejstrup, 2007; Versées et al., 2010; Glatt and Müller, 2013). The complex was initially identified in yeast as the major component of RNA polymerase II (RNAPII) holo-enzyme (Otero et al., 1999; Wittschieben et al., 1999). *In vitro* studies using the HeLa cell line further confirmed that Elongator directly interacts with RNAPII and facilitates transcription in a chromatin- and acetyl-CoA-dependent manner (Hawkes et al., 2002; Kim et al., 2002). The Elongator complex has also been reported to play two other distinct nuclear roles. Knockdown of Elp3 has been shown to impair paternal DNA demethylation in mouse zygotes, a process that requires the Elp3 SAM domain (Okada et al., 2010). The complex was also demonstrated to be involved in microRNA (miRNA) biogenesis in *Arabidopsis*, whereby Elongator is believed to play a role in coupling the transcription of primary miRNAs and their subsequent processing (Fang et al., 2015). The majority of Elongator has been found to be located in the cytoplasm, consistent with the various cellular processes assigned to this complex that take place in the cytosol. Two studies have reported that Elongator regulates cytoplasmic kinase signaling through its interaction with c-Jun N-terminal kinase (JNK; Holmberg et al., 2002; Close et al., 2006). Holmberg et al. (2002) showed that Elongator is involved in the assembly of JNK-MAPK module through the association of Elp1 with JNK, resulting in JNK activation. Rahl et al. (2005) proposed an active requirement for the Elongator complex in the establishment and maintenance of yeast cell polarity, and in exocytosis, through its interaction with Rab GTPase Sec2p. As suggested by the authors, Elongator negatively regulates Sec2p-dependent, polarized secretion through a transcription-independent pathway. Johansen et al. (2008) proposed a model in which Elp1-assisted localization of filamin A into membrane ruffles regulates neuron migration in rats. Another study linked Elongator to the process of cytoskeletal organization and cell motility by demonstrating acetylation of α-tubulin by this complex in murine cortical neurons (Creppe et al., 2009). Although the Elongator complex has been implicated in the various cellular processes described here thus far, there is accumulating evidence in the last decade to indicate that the main role of this complex is to maintain translational fidelity via regulation of tRNA modifications. In eukaryotes, U_{34} in the anticodons of $tRNA^{Lys}{}_{UUU}$, $tRNA^{Glu}{}_{UUC}$ and $tRNA^{Gln}{}_{UUG}$ are modified to 5-carbamoyl-methyl-uridine (ncm^5U), 5-methoxy-carbonyl-methyl-uridine (mcm^5U), or 5-methoxy-carbonyl-methyl-2-thio-uridine (mcm^5s^2U). A number of studies have reported that these modifications require the Elongator complex (Huang et al., 2005; Esberg et al., 2006; Johansson et al., 2008; Bauer et al., 2012). The methyl-group transfer to tRNA U_{34} by Elongator likely involves a SAM-mediated mechanism in conjunction with an electron transfer from a cofactor complex Kti11/Kti13 (Boal et al., 2011; Kolaj-Robin et al., 2015). However, the precise molecular mechanism that underlies the tRNA modification by this complex is yet to be elucidated.

It is still unclear whether Elongator has many distinct functions in a cell or it regulates one process that leads to different downstream effects, via altered translation. Interestingly, Esberg et al. (2006) found that elevated levels of two tRNA species bypass all the *in vivo* requirements of Elongator in transcription and exocytosis. All the phenotypes of Elongator-deficient yeast cells can be suppressed by overexpression of $tRNA^{Lys}{}_{UUU}$ and $tRNA^{Glu}{}_{UUC}$ (Esberg et al., 2006). A recent study by Bauer et al. (2012) demonstrated that translation of a large number of proteins is regulated by Elongator and that cell division is under translational control of this complex. The most recent finding in *Caenorhabditis elegans* shows that Elongator is not a direct tubulin acetytransferase, but it rather regulates the expression of α-tubulin acetyltransferase at translational level, through its elevated AAA codon content and tRNA modification (Bauer and Hermand, 2012). The other cell activities regulated by Elongator might also be explained by its tRNA modification role and codon-dependent regulation of translation, which future experiments will elucidate.

ROLE OF ELONGATOR IN NEURODEVELOPMENT

Neural development is a complex process that requires neural induction, migration, differentiation, axon guidance and synapse formation. Both cell motility and the actin cytoskeleton play a central role in regulating how neuronal precursors proliferate and migrate to different parts of the developing brain. Once neural precursors have reached their final destination they undergo the process of differentiation, which involves the production and extension of axons and dendrites to form synapses, resulting in the establishment of functional neural circuits. Synapses are specialized sites of cell–cell contact where electrical signals trigger the release of neurotransmitters, which in turn activates postsynaptic receptors (Haucke et al., 2011). This highly regulated process is based on cytoskeletal organization, vesicular trafficking and polarized exocytosis. Here, we review the roles of Elongator during neurodevelopment, from transcription to translation (**Figure 2**).

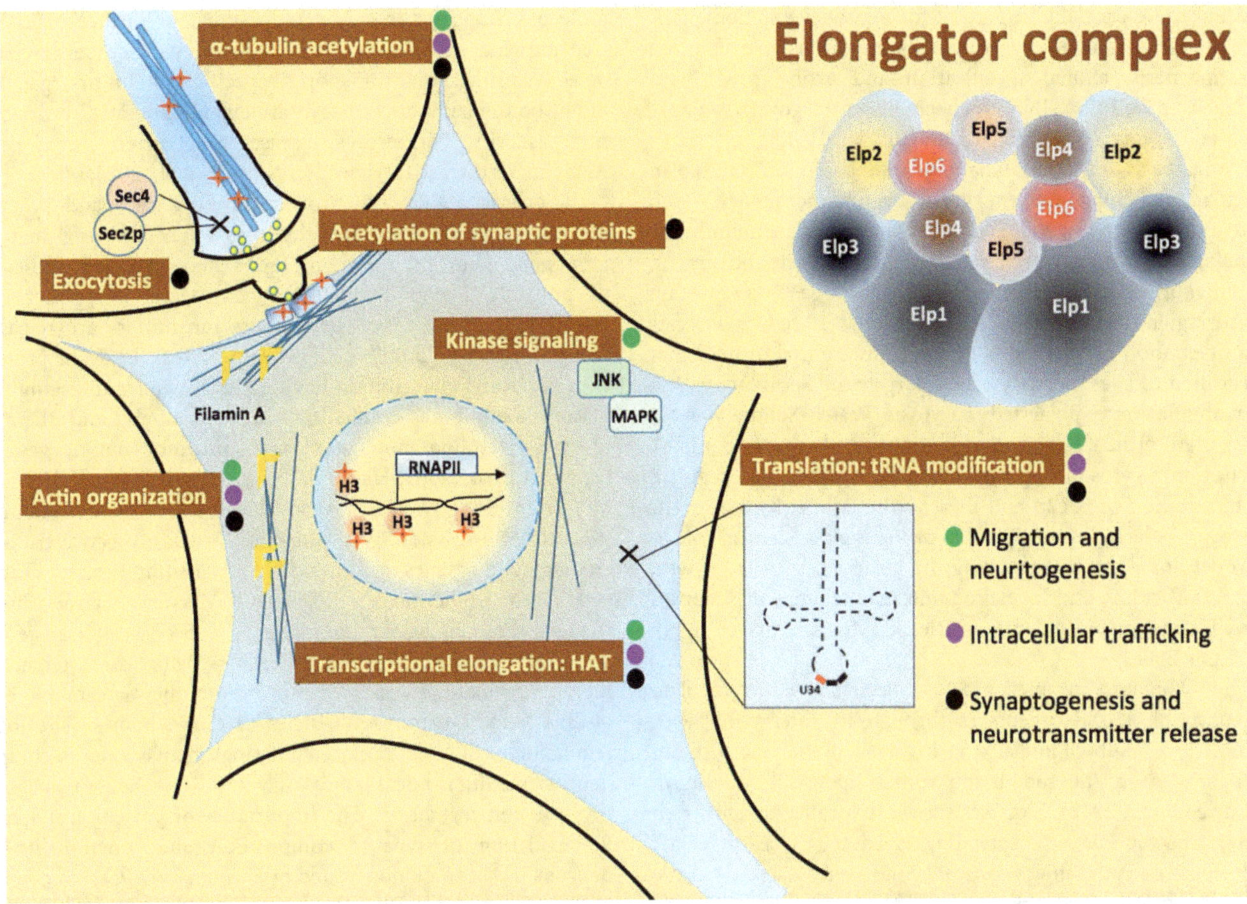

FIGURE 2 | Multiple roles of the Elongator complex in neurons. The six-subunit Elongator complex is proposed to play multiple roles in cell: a role of histone-acetyl transferase (HAT) required for transcriptional elongation, it assists c-Jun N-terminal kinase (JNK)-MAPK module assembly, negatively regulates exocytosis through Sec2p-Sec4 interaction, regulates actin organization via Filamin A, promotes α-tubulin and synaptic proteins acetylation, and modifies transfer RNA (tRNA) U_{34}. Elongator functions can be associated to cell activities critical for development and maintenance of the nervous system: migration and branching of neurons, intracellular trafficking and synapse formation, marked with green, purple and black circle in the figure, respectively.

Neurodevelopmental processes are dependent upon a broad number of factors regulating the expression of hundreds of genes controlling the terminal differentiation of neurons. The majority of genes activated during developmental processes are regulated at the level of transcriptional elongation (Muse et al., 2007). Elongator has been linked to the transcriptional regulation of several genes critical to various neurodevelopmental processes. Studies in human 293T (Han et al., 2007) and HeLa (Li et al., 2011) cell lines clearly demonstrate a role for the Elongator complex in the transcriptional elongation of heat shock protein 70 (HSP70), a gene that plays an important role in protecting of cells from apoptotic stimuli and in the stabilization of protein structures (Jäättelä et al., 1992; Mosser et al., 1997; Han et al., 2007). HSPs are developmentally regulated in the nervous system. HSP70 has been suggested to play an important role in both developing and adult mammalian brain and its expression within the nervous system is significantly higher compared to non-neuronal tissue (Manzerra et al., 1997). HSP70 has a neuroprotective role (attenuation of toxicity in a variety of neurodegenerative disease models (Arawaka et al., 2010)), and plays a role in axonal transport and neuronal signaling (de Waegh and Brady, 1989; Houenou et al., 1996; Thekkuveettil and Lakhotia, 1996). Elongator is also required for the activation of several genes involved in cell migration, such as those coding for the integrin receptor CD61, tenascin-C, and actin cytoskeleton modulators (Close et al., 2006). Integrins and tenascin-C are widely expressed in neuronal extracellular matrix during CNS development and they are shown to enhance neuronal precursors proliferation, migration and differentiation (Garcion et al., 2001; Flanagan et al., 2006). Taken together, these data show that the Elongator complex is responsible for the transcriptional regulation of a number of proteins that each plays a crucial role in various steps of development and maintenance of the nervous system.

The Elongator complex regulates a broad number of neurodevelopmental transcription-independent processes. Elongator activates JNK (Holmberg et al., 2002; Close et al., 2006), a stress-activated protein kinase that modulates the activity of a vast number of pathways. JNK signaling has been reported to be crucially important for neurodevelopment. JNK knockout studies in mice revealed its important role in brain morphogenesis, axonal specification and axon growth and guidance. In addition, JNK has been shown to govern synapse and memory formation (reviewed in Coffey, 2014).

Elongator is linked to synaptogenesis based on its role in vesicular trafficking and exocytosis via interacting with Rab proteins (Rahl et al., 2005). Rab proteins regulate membrane trafficking, which include vesicle formation, vesicle movement, and membrane fusion (Pfeffer, 2001). The yeast Rab protein Sec4p regulates exocytosis of post-Golgi secretory vesicles (Salminen and Novick, 1987). Sec2p is an essential protein that is recruited to sites of exocytosis, it targets the Sec4p activation event and facilitates polarized exocytosis (Walch-Solimena et al., 1997). Rahl et al. (2005) propose that the Elongator complex function in a cytosolic signal transduction pathway to regulate the localization of Sec2p and thereby the Rab activation event critical for polarized secretion. Rab proteins play a central role in neurodevelopment, by regulating the polarized neurite growth, axonal trafficking, and formation and maintenance of synapses (specific functions in synaptic vesicle exocytosis, reviewed in Ng and Tang, 2008).

The Elongator complex has also been shown to regulate migration of neural precursors through its interaction with filamin A, whereby Elongator is involved in the recruitment of filamin A in the membrane ruffles upon cell migration (Johansen et al., 2008). Elp3 was shown to localize to actin-rich domains at the edges of spreading HeLa cells (Barton et al., 2009). Filamin A organizes cortical actin filaments and dynamic three-dimensional networks in the leading edges of migrating cells and is essential for regulating the polarity of neocortical neurons during radial migration through the subventricular zone (SVZ) and intermediate zone (IZ) of the cerebrum (Nagano et al., 2004). Loss-of-function mutations in filamin A give rise to human periventricular heterotopia, a neurodevelopmental disorder caused by a failure of neurons to migrate to the cortex (Fox et al., 1998).

Acetylation of α-tubulin by the Elongator complex is yet another Elongator function that may play role in neural migration and branching (Creppe et al., 2009). In neurons the majority of cellular α-tubulin is acetylated. Creppe et al. (2009) demonstrated that lowering α-tubulin acetylation levels in microtubules through expression of α-tubulin K40A (a dominant-negative α-tubulin form that cannot be acetylated) recapitulated the migratory defects induced by Elp1/Elp3 silencing. The reduced acetylated α-tubulin levels seen upon Elongator deficiency in this study, suggest that this complex does not exclusively regulate cell motility via its association with filamin A, as migratory defects did not affect cell transition through neocortical SVZ and IZ or promote the formation of periventricular nodular heterotopia, nor via transcriptional elongation of key genes coding for proteins involved in cell migration, as the identity of these genes was cell-specific. The relationship between α-tubulin acetylation, neuron migration and branching is not yet clear but could rely on intracellular trafficking as α-tubulin acetylation is known to increase binding of motor proteins that regulate bidirectional molecular transport in axons and dendrites (Reed et al., 2006). The growing experimental and clinical evidence suggest that defective intracellular transport of specific proteins or organelles might be the hallmarks of several neurodegenerative processes, such as ALS, Parkinson's disease, Huntington disease and Alzheimer's disease (reviewed in Nguyen et al., 2010).

Elongator regulates neurotransmitter release and synapse formation, as demonstrated by one study showing that in *Drosophila* neurons, this complex is necessary and sufficient to acetylate Bruchpilot (BRP), an integral component of the presynaptic density where neurotransmitters are released (Miśkiewicz et al., 2011). BRP is a large cytoskeletal-like protein with its individual strands having their N termini facing the plasma membrane, contacting Ca^{2+} channels, and their C termini extending into cytoplasm capturing synaptic vesicles (Fouquet et al., 2009; Hallermann et al., 2010). Thus, BRP acts by concentrating synaptic vesicles at active zones, and facilitating synaptic transmission by establishing proximity between Ca^{2+} channels and vesicles to allow efficient transmitter release (Kittel et al., 2006; Hallermann et al., 2010). Miśkiewicz et al. (2011) suggest a model where Elongator is a BRP acetyltransferase and acetylation of BRP reorganizes its cytoplasmic tentacles, thereby regulating vesicle capturing by the C-terminal end of BRP and transport of vesicles at dense bodies. The local regulation of Elongator may enable single active zones to control neurotransmitter release and may hold the key to synaptic transmission regulation. The importance of protein acetylation in regulation of synapse composition and functionality in neurons has been demonstrated by recent study (Catarino et al., 2013). The possible role of Elongator in vesicular trafficking, exocytosis and synaptic transmission using above mentioned mechanisms remains to be tested in humans, yet evolutionary conservation of Elongator implies that it may play a similar role.

Recent studies have focused largely upon the pivotal role of Elongator in tRNA modification and these can be related to neurodevelopment in multiple ways. One recent report shows that Elongator is indeed linked to the translation of a variety of cell proteins, including those implicated in cell division (Bauer and Hermand, 2012). tRNA are more than simple adaptor molecules and have a surprising range of functions in the cell, such as tuning translation and protein expression in a tissue-specific manner and stress signaling, whereby these functions are all dependent on its modifications (Giegé, 2008; Thompson and Parker, 2009; Kirchner and Ignatova, 2015). Klassen et al. (2015) recently showed that the loss of wobble uridine modifications in the Elongator deficient yeast strain affects $tRNA^{Lys}_{UUU}$ function and results in a reduced total protein level. Moreover, the loss of these modifications in a subset of tRNAs was shown to lead to ribosome pausing at their cognate codons in both, yeast and *C. elegans* (Nedialkova and Leidel, 2015). Hence, upon Elongator malfunction, the kinetics of translation is perturbed, leading to the disruption of protein homeostasis in a cell and aggregate formation, as suggested by Nedialkova and associates. Neurons are particularly sensitive to the toxicity of misfolded proteins, hence, this could be the basis of neurodegenerative pathologies. In accordance with this, it can be postulated that Elongator-dependent tRNA modification regulate critical steps in biosynthesis and homeostasis of proteins required for the development and survival of specific neurons.

ELONGATOR DEFECTS IN NEUROLOGICAL DISORDERS

Mutations in Elongator complex subunits have been linked to different neuronal diseases (**Table 1**). *Elp1* mutations have been linked to an autosomal recessive disorder, FD (Anderson et al., 2001; Slaugenhaupt et al., 2001; Cuajungco et al., 2003). FD is among the most frequent hereditary sensory and autonomic neuropathies (Axelrod and Abularrage, 1982; Axelrod, 2002). The progressive degeneration of the sensory and autonomic nervous system in FD patients results in the following symptoms: cardiovascular dysfunction, pain insensitivity, gastrointestinal dysfunction, scoliosis, vomiting, defective lacrimation, extensive sweating and postural hypotension (Aguayo et al., 1971; Axelrod and Abularrage, 1982). Mortality in FD patients is high, and only 40% of patients survive beyond age 20 (Axelrod, 2004). FD patients have a mutation in the donor splice site of intron 20 of the *Elp1* gene, resulting in aberrant splicing (Anderson et al., 2001; Slaugenhaupt et al., 2001; Cuajungco et al., 2003). This mis-splicing results in tissue-specific exon skipping and consequently reduced levels of the Elp1 full-length protein. The FD mutation is incompletely penetrant, since the full length Elp1 is still synthesized albeit at lower levels in other cell types, whereas, in the central and peripheral nervous system only the truncated product is made (Slaugenhaupt et al., 2001; Cuajungco et al., 2003). This Elp1 truncated form cannot be detected in patients due to its degradation by the nonsense-mediated decay pathway (Cuajungco et al., 2003; Slaugenhaupt et al., 2004). Hence, Elp1 levels are very low in neuronal tissue from FD patients and unchanged in lymphoblasts for instance (Slaugenhaupt et al., 2001; Cuajungco et al., 2003). Heterozygous carriers also show reduced Elp1 expression but do not develop FD, suggesting the existence of an Elp1 tissue-specific threshold for the appropriate nervous system development and functioning. Experiments in HeLa, neuronal derived Elp1 RNAi cells and FD fibroblasts, showed that the Elp1-deficient cells exhibit defects in cell motility *in vitro* (Close et al., 2006). More recently, one group demonstrated that the cerebrum and fibroblasts from FD patients have reduced levels of mcm^5s^2 modifications at tRNA U_{34} (Karlsborn et al., 2014), which was further confirmed by Yoshida et al. (2015). This suggests that reduced levels of Elp1 due to aberrant splicing result in inefficient translation in FD, once again supporting the hypothesis that the predominant role of Elongator is the regulation of the rate of translation.

ID is a disorder characterized by incomplete mental development, which results in limitations in both intellectual functioning and adaptive behavior (Schalock et al., 2010). A large-scale sequencing study identified missense mutations in the *Elp2* gene to be associated with ID or related neurological disabilities. Homozygous mutations in the *Elp2* gene were found in two families, each with three children suffering from moderate or severe IDs (Najmabadi et al., 2011). Cohen et al. (2015) recently reported on one more family with two brothers being affected by severe ID, spastic diplegia and self-injury. In both brothers, sequencing analysis found *Elp2* missense mutations to be linked with the inheritance of this disorder. One of the two *Elp2* gene mutations identified in this family was shown to have the same amino acid position as the recessive missense mutation in one of the two previously reported families (Najmabadi et al., 2011). The mechanism of this neurodevelopmental dysfunction may be related to the compromised function of the Elongator complex, due to the presence of a dysfunctional Elp2 subunit that normally acts as a signal-transducing platform. Thus, *Elp2* is likely to be a novel gene that has an important role in the development of recessive cognitive disorders, such as ID.

ALS, commonly called motor neuron disease, has been associated to allelic variants of *Elp3* gene (Simpson et al., 2009). ALS is a neurodegenerative disease characterized by progressive muscle weakness and atrophy due to degeneration of motor neurones in the primary motor cortex, corticospinal tracts, brainstem and spinal cord (Rowland and Shneider, 2001). Within 3 years of onset of the disease, respiratory muscle weakness generally results in death. The causative molecular pathway underlying ALS remains unknown and it is considered to be a complex disease caused by interplay between multiple mechanisms (Rowland and Shneider, 2001). Two independent studies performed by Simpson et al. (2009): a microsatellite-based genetic association study of ALS in humans and a mutagenesis screen in *Drosophila melanogaster*, identified allelic variants of *Elp3* gene as crucial for axonal biology. In the genetic association study, *Elp3* allelic variants were associated with ALS in three different populations. A mutagenesis screen in *Drosophila* identified *Elp3* mutations that conferred abnormal photoreceptor axonal targeting and neurodegeneration. In addition to this, Elp3 knockdown in zebrafish via morpholino technology resulted in dose-dependent shortening and abnormal branching of motor neurons. Therefore, understanding

TABLE 1 | Elongator defects in neurological disorders.

Neurological disorder	Affected Elp	Mutation	Reference
Familial dysautonomia	Elpl	Mutation in the donor splice site of intron 20	Anderson et al. (2001), Slaugenhaupt et al. (2001) and Cuajungco et al. (2003)
Intellectual disability	Elp2	Missense mutations	Najmabadi et al. (2011) and Cohen et al. (2015)
Amyotrophic lateral sclerosis	Elp3	Association with specific haplotype	Simpson et al. (2009)
Rolandic epilepsy	Elp4	Non-coding mutations	Strug et al. (2009)

Elongator function is a promising route whereby we might gain insights into the mechanism of motor neuron degeneration in ALS.

Elp4 mutations have been linked to RE, the most common human epilepsy, with onset at 7–10 years of age (Gomez and Klass, 1983). A neurodevelopmental disorder with epileptic focus typically located in the lower motor and/or somatosensory cortex (rolandic area; Koutroumanidis, 2007), RE is characterized by centro-temporal spikes (CTS) on an electroencephalogram. The common form of RE appears to have complex genetic inheritance, where the genetic contribution to the disease is yet to be elucidated. A recent study suggests that *Elp4* mutations are associated with CTS in RE families (Strug et al., 2009). A genome-wide association study in RE was conducted and fine mapping evidence pointed to the association of CTS with SNP markers in *Elp4* in both, discovery and replication data sets. Beside RE, there are other neurodevelopmental disorders associated with the CTS trait, such as speech disorder (Echenne et al., 1992) developmental coordination disorder (Scabar et al., 2006) and attention deficit-hyperactivity disorder (Holtmann et al., 2003) that could be also linked to *Elp4*, as in the case of RE. Strug et al. (2009) hypothesized that a non-coding mutation in *Elp4* gene impairs Elongator-mediated interaction of genes important for brain development, which leads to the susceptibility to seizures in neurodevelopmental disorders.

Given that Elongator has been shown to be involved in a variety of neurodevelopmental processes, this complex might be associated with a broad range of neurological disorders. Neurodegenerative diseases are mostly accompanied by transcriptional dysfunction, leading to neuronal death and in many of these cases, chromatin acetylation status is impaired by a mechanism related to the loss of HAT activity (Selvi et al., 2010). On the other hand, the Elongator association with neurological disorders could be through its tRNA modification role. Growing experimental evidence supports the link between tRNAs and neurological disorders (Kirchner and Ignatova, 2015). Several reports have associated ID and mutations in genes that encode for tRNA modification enzymes (Torres et al., 2014). A defect in Elongator complex-dependent tRNA modification could perturb translation in two different ways, by reducing the protein synthesis due to general slow-down of translation of lysine rich proteins that are found predominantly in the ribosomal machinery, or by leading to translational inaccuracy and protein misfolding. Neurons are known to be vulnerable to misfolded proteins, and the prion-like spread of pathogenic misfolded proteins probably holds a key as a general mechanism underlying neurodegeneration (Raj et al., 2012; Zhou et al., 2012). Warren et al. (2013) proposed the term "molecular nexopathy" to link accumulation of toxic protein aggregates with neural network disintegration, and argued that this can be a new paradigm of neurodegenerative diseases. Elongator-dependent regulation of translation could be an important factor contributing to this new paradigm.

CONCLUDING REMARKS

The Elongator complex is a dodecamer composed of six subunits (Elp1–6) with two Elp123 trimeric sub-complexes peripherally attached to the ring-like hexameric Elp456 sub-complex (Glatt et al., 2012). It is a highly conserved complex among eukaryotes and its function is dependent on the integrity of all its subunits. Although a large number of cellular functions have been attributed to this complex, the predominant role of Elongator is in regulating tRNA modification. Yet a large amount of data exists to support a possibility that Elongator acts as a transcriptional regulator. Future high-resolution structural and functional studies aimed to identifying Elongator interactors, regulators, the molecular mechanism underlying its activity and substrate specificity will shed light on the true nature of this multi-subunit complex.

Elongator activity has been linked to a host of cellular processes crucial for neurodevelopment, including cytoskeletal organization, neuritogenesis, axon growth, axonal transport, neuronal signaling and cell motility. A role for Elongator in a number of distinct neurological disorders is emerging yet. The mechanism by which the perturbation of the complex leads to the specific neuropathogenic effects is yet to be defined. Once this is elucidated, exploration of methods to complement for Elongator dysfunction offers an approach to developing effective therapies for a variety of neurological disorders.

AUTHOR CONTRIBUTIONS

MK: main conception and design of the work, drafting the manuscript. BW: substantial contribution to the conception and design of the manuscript, critical revision of the work presented here. Both authors approve this manuscript to be published.

ACKNOWLEDGMENTS

We thank Dr. Laura Genovesi and Dr. Christelle Adolphe for critical reading of the manuscript.

REFERENCES

Aguayo, A. J., Nair, C. P., and Bray, G. M. (1971). Peripheral nerve abnormalities in the riley-day syndrome. Findings in a sural nerve biopsy. *Arch. Neurol.* 24, 106–116. doi: 10.1001/archneur.1971.00480320034003

Anderson, S. L., Coli, R., Daly, I. W., Kichula, E. A., Rork, M. J., Volpi, S. A., et al. (2001). Familial dysautonomia is caused by mutations of the IKAP gene. *Am. J. Hum. Genet.* 68, 753–758. doi: 10.1086/318808

Arawaka, S., Machiya, Y., and Kato, T. (2010). Heat shock proteins as suppressors of accumulation of toxic prefibrillar intermediates and misfolded proteins in neurodegenerative diseases. *Curr. Pharm. Biotechnol.* 11, 158–166. doi: 10.2174/138920110790909713

Axelrod, F. B. (2002). Hereditary sensory and autonomic neuropathies. Familial dysautonomia and other HSANs. *Clin. Auton. Res.* 12, I2–I14. doi: 10.1007/s102860200014

Axelrod, F. B. (2004). Familial dysautonomia. *Muscle Nerve* 29, 352–363. doi: 10.1002/mus.10499

Axelrod, F. B., and Abularrage, J. J. (1982). Familial dysautonomia: a prospective study of survival. *J. Pediatr.* 101, 234–236. doi: 10.1016/s0022-3476(82)80130-3

Barton, D., Braet, F., Marc, J., Overall, R., and Gardiner, J. (2009). ELP3 localises to mitochondria and actin-rich domains at edges of HeLa cells. *Neurosci. Lett.* 455, 60–64. doi: 10.1016/j.neulet.2009.03.006

Bauer, F., and Hermand, D. (2012). A coordinated codon-dependent regulation of translation by Elongator. *Cell Cycle* 11, 4524–4529. doi: 10.4161/cc.22689

Bauer, F., Matsuyama, A., Candiracci, J., Dieu, M., Scheliga, J., Wolf, D. A., et al. (2012). Translational control of cell division by Elongator. *Cell Rep.* 1, 424–433. doi: 10.1016/j.celrep.2012.04.001

Boal, A. K., Grove, T. L., McLaughlin, M. I., Yennawar, N. H., Booker, S. J., and Rosenzweig, A. C. (2011). Structural basis for methyl transfer by a radical SAM enzyme. *Science* 332, 1089–1092. doi: 10.1126/science.1205358

Catarino, T., Ribeiro, L., Santos, S. D., and Carvalho, A. L. (2013). Regulation of synapse composition by protein acetylation: the role of acetylated cortactin. *J. Cell Sci.* 126, 149–162. doi: 10.1242/jcs.110742

Chen, Y.-T., Hims, M. M., Shetty, R. S., Mull, J., Liu, L., Leyne, M., et al. (2009). Loss of mouse Ikbkap, a subunit of elongator, leads to transcriptional deficits and embryonic lethality that can be rescued by human IKBKAP. *Mol. Cell. Biol.* 29, 736–744. doi: 10.1128/MCB.01313-08

Chen, C., Huang, B., Eliasson, M., Rydén, P., and Byström, A. S. (2011). Elongator complex influences telomeric gene silencing and DNA damage response by its role in wobble uridine tRNA modification. *PLoS Genet.* 7:e1002258. doi: 10.1371/journal.pgen.1002258

Chen, Z., Zhang, H., Jablonowski, D., Zhou, X., Ren, X., Hong, X., et al. (2006). Mutations in ABO1/ELO2, a subunit of holo-Elongator, increase abscisic acid sensitivity and drought tolerance in *Arabidopsis thaliana*. *Mol. Cell. Biol.* 26, 6902–6912. doi: 10.1128/mcb.00433-06

Close, P., Hawkes, N., Cornez, I., Creppe, C., Lambert, C. A., Rogister, B., et al. (2006). Transcription impairment and cell migration defects in elongator-depleted cells: implication for familial dysautonomia. *Mol. Cell* 22, 521–531. doi: 10.1016/j.molcel.2006.04.017

Coffey, E. T. (2014). Nuclear and cytosolic JNK signalling in neurons. *Nat. Rev. Neurosci.* 15, 285–299. doi: 10.1038/nrn3729

Cohen, J. S., Srivastava, S., Farwell, K. D., Lu, H. M., Zeng, W., Lu, H., et al. (2015). ELP2 is a novel gene implicated in neurodevelopmental disabilities. *Am. J. Med. Genet. A* 167, 1391–1395. doi: 10.1002/ajmg.a.36935

Cortajarena, A. L., and Regan, L. (2006). Ligand binding by TPR domains. *Protein Sci.* 15, 1193–1198. doi: 10.1110/ps.062092506

Creppe, C., Malinouskaya, L., Volvert, M. L., Gillard, M., Close, P., Malaise, O., et al. (2009). Elongator controls the migration and differentiation of cortical neurons through acetylation of α-tubulin. *Cell* 136, 551–564. doi: 10.1016/j.cell.2008.11.043

Cuajungco, M. P., Leyne, M., Mull, J., Gill, S. P., Lu, W., Zagzag, D., et al. (2003). Tissue-specific reduction in splicing efficiency of *IKBKAP* due to the major mutation associated with familial dysautonomia. *Am. J. Hum. Genet.* 72, 749–758. doi: 10.1086/368263

de Waegh, S., and Brady, S. T. (1989). Axonal transport of a clathrin uncoating atpase (HSC70): a role for hsc70 in the modulation of coated vesicle assembly *in vivo*. *J. Neurosci. Res.* 23, 433–440. doi: 10.1002/jnr.490230409

Echenne, B., Cheminai, R., Rivier, F., Negre, C., Touchon, J., and Billiard, M. (1992). Epileptic electroencephalographic abnormalities and developmental dysphasias: a study of 32 patients. *Brain Dev.* 14, 216–225. doi: 10.1016/s0387-7604(12)80233-6

Esberg, A., Huang, B., Johansson, M. J. O., and Byström, A. S. (2006). Elevated levels of two tRNA species bypass the requirement for elongator complex in transcription and exocytosis. *Mol. Cell* 24, 139–148. doi: 10.1016/j.molcel.2006.07.031

Fang, X., Cui, Y., Li, Y., and Qi, Y. (2015). Transcription and processing of primary microRNAs are coupled by Elongator complex in Arabidopsis. *Nat. Plants* 1:15075. doi: 10.1038/nplants.2015.75

Fellows, J., Erdjument-Bromage, H., Tempst, P., and Svejstrup, J. Q. (2000). The Elp2 subunit of elongator and elongating RNA polymerase II holoenzyme is a WD40 repeat protein. *J. Biol. Chem.* 275, 12896–12899. doi: 10.1074/jbc.275.17.12896

Flanagan, L. A., Rebaza, L. M., Derzic, S., Schwartz, P. H., and Monuki, E. S. (2006). Regulation of human neural precursor cells by laminin and integrins. *J. Neurosci. Res.* 83, 845–856. doi: 10.1002/jnr.20778

Fouquet, W., Owald, D., Wichmann, C., Mertel, S., Depner, H., Dyba, M., et al. (2009). Maturation of active zone assembly by *Drosophila* Bruchpilot. *J. Cell Biol.* 186, 129–145. doi: 10.1083/jcb.200812150

Fox, J. W., Lamperti, E. D., Ekşioğlu, Y. Z., Hong, S. E., Feng, Y., Graham, D. A., et al. (1998). Mutations in filamin 1 prevent migration of cerebral cortical neurons in human periventricular heterotopia. *Neuron* 21, 1315–1325. doi: 10.1016/s0896-6273(00)80651-0

Frohloff, F., Jablonowski, D., Fichtner, L., and Schaffrath, R. (2003). Subunit communications crucial for the functional integrity of the yeast RNA polymerase II elongator (γ-toxin target (TOT)) complex. *J. Biol. Chem.* 278, 956–961. doi: 10.1074/jbc.m210060200

Garcion, E., Faissner, A., and ffrench-Constant, C. (2001). Knockout mice reveal a contribution of the extracellular matrix molecule tenascin-C to neural precursor proliferation and migration. *Development* 128, 2485–2496.

Giegé, R. (2008). Toward a more complete view of tRNA biology. *Nat. Struct. Mol. Biol.* 15, 1007–1014. doi: 10.1038/nsmb.1498

Glatt, S., Létoquart, J., Faux, C., Taylor, N. M. I., Séraphin, B., and Müller, C. W. (2012). The Elongator subcomplex Elp456 is a hexameric RecA-like ATPase. *Nat. Struct. Mol. Biol.* 19, 314–320. doi: 10.1038/nsmb.2234

Glatt, S., and Müller, C. W. (2013). Structural insights into Elongator function. *Curr. Opin. Struct. Biol.* 23, 235–242. doi: 10.1016/j.sbi.2013.02.009

Gomez, M. R., and Klass, D. W. (1983). Epilepsies of infancy and childhood. *Ann. Neurol.* 13, 113–124. doi: 10.1002/ana.410130202

Hallermann, S., Kittel, R. J., Wichmann, C., Weyhersmüller, A., Fouquet, W., Mertel, S., et al. (2010). Naked dense bodies provoke depression. *J. Neurosci.* 30, 14340–14345. doi: 10.1523/JNEUROSCI.2495-10.2010

Han, Q., Hou, X., Su, D., Pan, L., Duan, J., Cui, L., et al. (2007). hELP3 Subunit of the Elongator complex regulates the transcription of *HSP70* gene in human cells. *Acta Biochim. Biophys. Sin. (Shanghai)* 39, 453–461. doi: 10.1111/j.1745-7270.2007.00293.x

Haucke, V., Neher, E., and Sigrist, S. J. (2011). Protein scaffolds in the coupling of synaptic exocytosis and endocytosis. *Nat. Rev. Neurosci.* 12, 127–138. doi: 10.1038/nrn2948

Hawkes, N. A., Otero, G., Winkler, G. S., Marshall, N., Dahmus, M. E., Krappmann, D., et al. (2002). Purification and characterization of the human elongator complex. *J. Biol. Chem.* 277, 3047–3052. doi: 10.1074/jbc.m110445200

Holmberg, C., Katz, S., Lerdrup, M., Herdegen, T., Jäättelä, M., Aronheim, A., et al. (2002). A novel specific role for IκB kinase complex-associated protein in cytosolic stress signaling. *J. Biol. Chem.* 277, 31918–31928. doi: 10.1074/jbc.M200719200

Holtmann, M., Becker, K., Kentner-Figura, B., and Schmidt, M. H. (2003). Increased frequency of rolandic spikes in ADHD children. *Epilepsia* 44, 1241–1244. doi: 10.1046/j.1528-1157.2003.13403.x

Houenou, L. J., Li, L., Lei, M., Kent, C. R., and Tytell, M. (1996). Exogenous heat shock cognate protein Hsc70 prevents axotomy-induced death of spinal sensory neurons. *Cell Stress Chaperones* 1, 161–166. doi: 10.1379/1466-1268(1996)001<0161:EHSCPH>2.3.CO;2

Huang, B. O., Johansson, M. J., and Byström, A. S. (2005). An early step in wobble uridine tRNA modification requires the Elongator complex. *RNA* 11, 424–436. doi: 10.1261/rna.7247705

Jäättelä, M., Wissing, D., Bauer, P. A., and Li, G. C. (1992). Major heat shock protein hsp70 protects tumor cells from tumor necrosis factor cytotoxicity. *EMBO J.* 11, 3507–3512.

Johansen, L. D., Naumanen, T., Knudsen, A., Westerlund, N., Gromova, I., Junttila, M., et al. (2008). IKAP localizes to membrane ruffles with filamin A and regulates actin cytoskeleton organization and cell migration. *J. Cell Sci.* 121, 854–864. doi: 10.1242/jcs.013722

Johansson, M. J. O., Esberg, A., Huang, B., Björk, G. R., and Byström, A. S. (2008). Eukaryotic wobble uridine modifications promote a functionally redundant decoding system. *Mol. Cell. Biol.* 28, 3301–3312. doi: 10.1128/MCB.01542-07

Karlsborn, T., Tükenmez, H., Chen, C., and Byström, A. S. (2014). Familial dysautonomia (FD) patients have reduced levels of the modified wobble nucleoside mcm^5s^2U in tRNA. *Biochem. Biophys. Res. Commun.* 454, 441–445. doi: 10.1016/j.bbrc.2014.10.116

Kelley, L. A., and Sternberg, M. J. (2009). Protein structure prediction on the Web: a case study using the Phyre server. *Nat. Protoc.* 4, 363–371. doi: 10.1038/nprot.2009.2

Kim, J.-H., Lane, W. S., and Reinberg, D. (2002). Human Elongator facilitates RNA polymerase II transcription through chromatin. *Proc. Natl. Acad. Sci. U S A* 99, 1241–1246. doi: 10.1073/pnas.251672198

Kirchner, S., and Ignatova, Z. (2015). Emerging roles of tRNA in adaptive translation, signalling dynamics and disease. *Nat. Rev. Genet.* 16, 98–112. doi: 10.1038/nrg3861

Kittel, R. J., Wichmann, C., Rasse, T. M., Fouquet, W., Schmidt, M., Schmid, A., et al. (2006). Bruchpilot promotes active zone assembly, Ca^{2+} channel clustering and vesicle release. *Science* 312, 1051–1054. doi: 10.1126/science.1126308

Klassen, R., Grunewald, P., Thüring, K. L., Eichler, C., Helm, M., and Schaffrath, R. (2015). Loss of anticodon wobble uridine modifications affects $tRNA^{Lys}$ function and protein levels in *Saccharomyces cerevisiae*. *PLoS One* 10:e0119261. doi: 10.1371/journal.pone.0119261

Kolaj-Robin, O., McEwen, A. G., Cavarelli, J., and Séraphin, B. (2015). Structure of the Elongator cofactor complex Kti11/Kti13 provides insight into the role of Kti13 in Elongator-dependent tRNA modification. *FEBS J.* 282, 819–833. doi: 10.1111/febs.13199

Koutroumanidis, M. (2007). Panayiotopoulos syndrome: an important electroclinical example of benign childhood system epilepsy. *Epilepsia* 48, 1044–1053. doi: 10.1111/j.1528-1167.2007.01096.x

Li, Q., Fazly, A. M., Zhou, H., Huang, S., Zhang, Z., and Stillman, B. (2009). The elongator complex interacts with PCNA and modulates transcriptional silencing and sensitivity to DNA damage agents. *PLoS Genet.* 5:e1000684. doi: 10.1371/journal.pgen.1000684

Li, F., Lu, J., Han, Q., Zhang, G., and Huang, B. (2005). The Elp3 subunit of human Elongator complex is functionally similar to its counterpart in yeast. *Mol. Genet. Genomics* 273, 264–272. doi: 10.1007/s00438-005-1120-2

Li, F., Ma, J., Ma, Y., Hu, Y., Tian, S., White, R. E., et al. (2011). hElp3 directly modulates the expression of HSP70 gene in HeLa cells via HAT activity. *PLoS One* 6:e29303. doi: 10.1371/journal.pone.0029303

Li, Y., Takagi, Y., Jiang, Y., Tokunaga, M., Erdjument-Bromage, H., Tempst, P., et al. (2001). A multiprotein complex that interacts with RNA polymerase II elongator. *J. Biol. Chem.* 276, 29628–29631. doi: 10.1074/jbc.c100274200

Lin, Z., Zhao, W., Diao, W., Xie, X., Wang, Z., Zhang, J., et al. (2012). Crystal structure of elongator subcomplex Elp4–6. *J. Biol. Chem.* 287, 21501–21508. doi: 10.1074/jbc.M112.341560

Manzerra, P., Rush, S. J., and Brown, I. R. (1997). Tissue-specific differences in heat shock protein hsc70 and hsp70 in the control and hyperthermic rabbit. *J. Cell. Physiol.* 170, 130–137. doi: 10.1002/(SICI)1097-4652(199702)170:2<130::AID-JCP4>3.0.CO;2-P

Miśkiewicz, K., Jose, L. E., Bento-Abreu, A., Fislage, M., Taes, I., Kasprowicz, J., et al. (2011). ELP3 controls active zone morphology by acetylating the ELKS family member bruchpilot. *Neuron* 72, 776–788. doi: 10.1016/j.neuron.2011.10.010

Mosser, D. D., Caron, A. W., Bourget, L., Denis-Larose, C., and Massie, B. (1997). Role of the human heat shock protein hsp70 in protection against stress-induced apoptosis. *Mol. Cell. Biol.* 17, 5317–5327. doi: 10.1128/mcb.17.9.5317

Muse, G. W., Gilchrist, D. A., Nechaev, S., Shah, R., Parker, J. S., Grissom, S. F., et al. (2007). RNA polymerase is poised for activation across the genome. *Nat. Genet.* 39, 1507–1511. doi: 10.1038/ng.2007.21

Nagano, T., Morikubo, S., and Sato, M. (2004). Filamin a and FILIP (filamin A-interacting protein) regulate cell polarity and motility in neocortical subventricular and intermediate zones during radial migration. *J. Neurosci.* 24, 9648–9657. doi: 10.1523/JNEUROSCI.2363-04.2004

Najmabadi, H., Hu, H., Garshasbi, M., Zemojtel, T., Abedini, S. S., Chen, W., et al. (2011). Deep sequencing reveals 50 novel genes for recessive cognitive disorders. *Nature* 478, 57–63. doi: 10.1038/nature10423

Nedialkova, D. D., and Leidel, S. A. (2015). Optimization of codon translation rates via tRNA modifications maintains proteome integrity. *Cell* 161, 1606–1618. doi: 10.1016/j.cell.2015.05.022

Nelissen, H., Fleury, D., Bruno, L., Robles, P., De Veylder, L., Traas, J., et al. (2005). The elongata mutants identify a functional Elongator complex in plants with a role in cell proliferation during organ growth. *Proc. Natl. Acad. Sci. U S A* 102, 7754–7759. doi: 10.1073/pnas.0502600102

Ng, E. L., and Tang, B. L. (2008). Rab GTPases and their roles in brain neurons and glia. *Brain Res. Rev.* 58, 236–246. doi: 10.1016/j.brainresrev.2008.04.006

Nguyen, L., Humbert, S., Saudou, F., and Chariot, A. (2010). Elongator–an emerging role in neurological disorders. *Trends Mol. Med.* 16, 1–6. doi: 10.1016/j.molmed.2009.11.002

Okada, Y., Yamagata, K., Hong, K., Wakayama, T., and Zhang, Y. (2010). A role for elongator in zygotic paternal genome demethylation. *Nature* 463, 554–558. doi: 10.1038/nature08732

Otero, G., Fellows, J., Li, Y., de Bizemont, T., Dirac, A. M. G., Gustafsson, C. M., et al. (1999). Elongator, a multisubunit component of a novel RNA polymerase II holoenzyme for transcriptional elongation. *Mol. Cell* 3, 109–118. doi: 10.1016/s1097-2765(00)80179-3

Paraskevopoulou, C., Fairhurst, S. A., Lowe, D. J., Brick, P., and Onesti, S. (2006). The Elongator subunit Elp3 contains a Fe4S4 cluster and binds S-adenosylmethionine. *Mol. Microbiol.* 59, 795–806. doi: 10.1111/j.1365-2958.2005.04989.x

Pfeffer, S. R. (2001). Rab GTPases: specifying and deciphering organelle identity and function. *Trends Cell Biol.* 11, 487–491. doi: 10.1016/s0962-8924(01)02147-x

Rahl, P. B., Chen, C. Z., and Collins, R. N. (2005). Elp1p, the yeast homolog of the FD disease syndrome protein, negatively regulates exocytosis independently of transcriptional elongation. *Mol. Cell* 17, 841–853. doi: 10.1016/j.molcel.2005.02.018

Raj, A., Kuceyeski, A., and Weiner, M. (2012). A network diffusion model of disease progression in dementia. *Neuron* 73, 1204–1215. doi: 10.1016/j.neuron.2011.12.040

Reed, N. A., Cai, D., Blasius, T. L., Jih, G. T., Meyhofer, E., Gaertig, J., et al. (2006). Microtubule acetylation promotes kinesin-1 binding and transport. *Curr. Biol.* 16, 2166–2172. doi: 10.1016/j.cub.2006.09.014

Rowland, L. P., and Shneider, N. A. (2001). Amyotrophic lateral sclerosis. *N. Engl. J. Med.* 344, 1688–1700. doi: 10.1056/NEJM200105313442207

Salminen, A., and Novick, P. J. (1987). A ras-like protein is required for a post-Golgi event in yeast secretion. *Cell* 49, 527–538. doi: 10.1016/0092-8674(87)90455-7

Scabar, A., Devescovi, R., Blason, L., Bravar, L., and Carrozzi, M. (2006). Comorbidity of DCD and SLI: significance of epileptiform activity during sleep. *Child Care Health Dev.* 32, 733–739. doi: 10.1111/j.1365-2214.2006.00705.x

Schalock, R. L., Borthwick-Duffy, S. A., Bradley, V. J., Buntinx, W. H. E., Coulter, D. L., Craig, E. M., et al. (2010). *Intellectual Disability: Definition, Classification and Systems of Supports ERIC.* Washington, DC: American Association on Intellectual and Developmental Disabilities..

Selvi, B. R., Cassel, J.-C., Kundu, T. K., and Boutillier, A.-L. (2010). Tuning acetylation levels with HAT activators: therapeutic strategy in neurodegenerative diseases. *Biochim. Biophys. Acta* 1799, 840–853. doi: 10.1016/j.bbagrm.2010.08.012

Simpson, C. L., Lemmens, R., Miskiewicz, K., Broom, W. J., Hansen, V. K., van Vught, P. W. J., et al. (2009). Variants of the *elongator protein 3 (ELP3)* gene are associated with motor neuron degeneration. *Hum. Mol. Genet.* 18, 472–481. doi: 10.1093/hmg/ddn375

Slaugenhaupt, S. A., Blumenfeld, A., Gill, S. P., Leyne, M., Mull, J., Cuajungco, M. P., et al. (2001). Tissue-specific expression of a splicing mutation in the *IKBKAP* gene causes familial dysautonomia. *Am. J. Hum. Genet.* 68, 598–605. doi: 10.1086/318810

Slaugenhaupt, S. A., Mull, J., Leyne, M., Cuajungco, M. P., Gill, S. P., Hims, M. M., et al. (2004). Rescue of a human mRNA splicing defect by the plant cytokinin kinetin. *Hum. Mol. Genet.* 13, 429–436. doi: 10.1093/hmg/ddh046

Solinger, J. A., Paolinelli, R., Klöss, H., Scorza, F. B., Marchesi, S., Sauder, U., et al. (2010). The Caenorhabditis elegans Elongator complex regulates neuronal alpha-tubulin acetylation. *PLoS Genet.* 6:e1000820. doi: 10.1371/journal.pgen.1000820

Strug, L. J., Clarke, T., Chiang, T., Chien, M., Baskurt, Z., Li, W., et al. (2009). Centrotemporal sharp wave EEG trait in rolandic epilepsy maps to Elongator Protein Complex 4 (ELP4). *Eur. J. Hum. Genet.* 17, 1171–1181. doi: 10.1038/ejhg.2008.267

Svejstrup, J. Q. (2007). Elongator complex: how many roles does it play? *Curr. Opin. Cell Biol.* 19, 331–336. doi: 10.1016/j.ceb.2007.04.005

Thekkuveettil, A., and Lakhotia, S. C. (1996). Regulation of HSP70 in excitatory neurons: possible implications for neuronal functioning. *J. Biosci.* 21, 631–639. doi: 10.1007/bf02703141

Thompson, D. M., and Parker, R. (2009). Stressing Out over tRNA Cleavage. *Cell* 138, 215–219. doi: 10.1016/j.cell.2009.07.001

Torres, A. G., Batlle, E., and Ribas de Pouplana, L. (2014). Role of tRNA modifications in human diseases. *Trends Mol. Med.* 20, 306–314. doi: 10.1016/j.molmed.2014.01.008

Versées, W., De Groeve, S., and Van Lijsebettens, M. (2010). Elongator, a conserved multitasking complex? *Mol. Microbiol.* 76, 1065–1069. doi: 10.1111/j.1365-2958.2010.07162.x

Walch-Solimena, C., Collins, R. N., and Novick, P. J. (1997). Sec2p mediates nucleotide exchange on Sec4p and is involved in polarized delivery of post-golgi vesicles. *J. Cell Biol.* 137, 1495–1509. doi: 10.1083/jcb.137.7.1495

Walker, J., Kwon, S. Y., Badenhorst, P., East, P., McNeill, H., and Svejstrup, J. Q. (2011). Role of elongator subunit Elp3 in *Drosophila melanogaster* larval development and immunity. *Genetics* 187, 1067–1075. doi: 10.1534/genetics.110.123893

Warren, J. D., Rohrer, J. D., Schott, J. M., Fox, N. C., Hardy, J., and Rossor, M. N. (2013). Molecular nexopathies: a new paradigm of neurodegenerative disease. *Trends Neurosci.* 36, 561–569. doi: 10.1016/j.tins.2013.06.007

Winkler, G. S., Petrakis, T. G., Ethelberg, S., Tokunaga, M., Erdjument-Bromage, H., Tempst, P., et al. (2001). RNA polymerase II elongator holoenzyme is composed of two discrete subcomplexes. *J. Biol. Chem.* 276, 32743–32749. doi: 10.1074/jbc.m105303200

Wittschieben, B. Ø., Otero, G., de Bizemont, T., Fellows, J., Erdjument-Bromage, H., Ohba, R., et al. (1999). A novel histone acetyltransferase is an integral subunit of elongating RNA polymerase II holoenzyme. *Mol. Cell* 4, 123–128. doi: 10.1016/s1097-2765(00)80194-x

Xu, H., Lin, Z., Li, F., Diao, W., Dong, C., Zhou, H., et al. (2015). Dimerization of elongator protein 1 is essential for Elongator complex assembly. *Proc. Natl. Acad. Sci. U S A* 112, 10697–10702. doi: 10.1073/pnas.1502597112

Yoshida, M., Kataoka, N., Miyauchi, K., Ohe, K., Iida, K., Yoshida, S., et al. (2015). Rectifier of aberrant mRNA splicing recovers tRNA modification in familial dysautonomia. *Proc. Natl. Acad. Sci. U S A* 112, 2764–2769. doi: 10.1073/pnas.1415525112

Zhou, J., Gennatas, E. D., Kramer, J. H., Miller, B. L., and Seeley, W. W. (2012). Predicting regional neurodegeneration from the healthy brain functional connectome. *Neuron* 73, 1216–1227. doi: 10.1016/j.neuron.2012.03.004

6

Intracellular Fibroblast Growth Factor 14: Emerging Risk Factor for Brain Disorders

Jessica Di Re[1,2], *Paul A. Wadsworth*[3] *and Fernanda Laezza*[2,4,5]*

[1]Neuroscience Graduate Program, University of Texas Medical Branch, Galveston, TX, USA, [2]Department of Pharmacology and Toxicology, University of Texas Medical Branch, Galveston, TX, USA, [3]Biochemistry and Molecular Biology Graduate Program, The University of Texas Medical Branch, Galveston, TX, USA, [4]Mitchell Center for Neurodegenerative Diseases, The University of Texas Medical Branch, Galveston, TX, USA, [5]Center for Addiction Research, The University of Texas Medical Branch, Galveston, TX, USA

Edited by:
Daniela Tropea, Trinity College, Dublin, Ireland

Reviewed by:
Alexander Dityatev, German Center for Neurodegenerative Diseases (DZNE), Germany
Elsa Fabbretti, University of Nova Gorica, Slovenia

***Correspondence:**
Fernanda Laezza
felaezza@utmb.edu

The finely tuned regulation of neuronal firing relies on the integrity of ion channel macromolecular complexes. Minimal disturbances of these tightly regulated networks can lead to persistent maladaptive plasticity of brain circuitry. The intracellular fibroblast growth factor 14 (FGF14) belongs to the nexus of proteins interacting with voltage-gated Na+ (Na_V) channels at the axonal initial segment. Through isoform-specific interactions with the intracellular C-terminal tail of neuronal Na_V channels ($Na_V1.1$, $Na_V1.2$, $Na_V1.6$), FGF14 controls channel gating, axonal targeting and phosphorylation in neurons effecting excitability. FGF14 has been also involved in synaptic transmission, plasticity and neurogenesis in the cortico-mesolimbic circuit with cognitive and affective behavioral outcomes. In translational studies, interest in FGF14 continues to rise with a growing list of associative links to diseases of the cognitive and affective domains such as neurodegeneration, depression, anxiety, addictive behaviors and recently schizophrenia, suggesting its role as a converging node in the etiology of complex brain disorders. Yet, a full understanding of FGF14 function in neurons is far from being complete and likely to involve other functions unrelated to the direct regulation of Na_V channels. The goal of this Mini Review article is to provide a summary of studies on the emerging role of FGF14 in complex brain disorders.

Keywords: neuronal excitability, intracellular signaling, protein-protein interactions, biological psychiatry

INTRODUCTION

In 2014, nearly one in four adults in the United States was diagnosed with a mental illness (National Institutes of Mental Health[1]). Treatment for many of these illnesses is hampered by limited efficacy of the medications and patient noncompliance due to intolerable side effects. To address this need, the National Institutes of Mental Health has launched an initiative to research these illnesses from all levels, ranging from genomic to behavioral. Dubbed the Research Domain Criteria (RDoC), this initiative proposes to complement top-down understanding of these diseases, beginning with human behavior, with bottom-up research by understanding the molecular and cellular causes of these disorders.

[1]https://www.nimh.nih.gov/health/statistics/index.shtml

Because many neuropsychiatric disorders are associated with maladaptive plasticity and excitability, one area of importance within neurons is the axon initial segment (AIS), which serves as the action potential initiation site (Palmer and Stuart, 2006). This highly complex subcellular region contains a nexus of scaffolding and regulatory proteins that ensure proper targeting, clustering and function of the ion channels underlying the action potential (Ogawa and Rasband, 2008; Hsu et al., 2014). Neuropsychiatric disorders have been associated with many of these proteins, including ankyrin-G, α-spectrins, β-spectrins, neurofascin, contactin and intracellular fibroblast growth factors (iFGFs; Hsu et al., 2014). One such protein, fibroblast growth factor 14 (FGF14, also known as fibroblast homologous factor 4 or FHF4), is an iFGF that binds to voltage-gated Na^+ (Na_V) channels and promotes their localization to the proximal region of the axon, providing the fine-tuned regulation necessary for normal functioning (Lou et al., 2005; Laezza et al., 2007, 2009; Goetz et al., 2009; Wang et al., 2011, 2012; Wildburger et al., 2015; Ali et al., 2016; Bosch et al., 2016; Hsu et al., 2016; Pablo et al., 2016). Loss of functional FGF14 may change the biophysical properties of Na_V channels or alter their localization to the AIS, leading to changes in neuronal excitability (Goldfarb et al., 2007; Shakkottai et al., 2009; Bosch et al., 2015; Hsu et al., 2016). Recent findings also show that FGF14 regulates the function of voltage-gated K^+ and Ca^{2+} channels, however none of these interactions are direct, and therefore might represent a different type of regulation from what has been described for Na_V channels (Yan et al., 2013; Pablo and Pitt, 2017).

Initially cloned on the basis of sequence similarity with other FGF members, FGF14 was first associated to a human disease with the F145S mutation causing spinocerebellar ataxia 27 (SCA27), a naturally occurring complex neurodegenerative disorder characterized by onset of ataxia in early adulthood and deficits in cognition, memory and behavior (Smallwood et al., 1996; van Swieten et al., 2003; Brusse et al., 2006). Genetic deletion of FGF14 in mice recapitulates some of these symptoms at the behavior and circuitry level (Wang et al., 2002; Wozniak et al., 2007).

Since then, FGF14 has been indicated by several linkage and genome wide association studies (GWAS) to be a putative risk factor for other neuropsychiatric diseases including depression, addiction and schizophrenia, as well as neurodegenerative diseases, such as Alzheimer's Disease (Detera-Wadleigh et al., 1999; Park et al., 2004; Mulle et al., 2005; Need et al., 2009; Johnson et al., 2011; Verbeek et al., 2012; Singh and Rajeswari, 2015; Yang et al., 2015). These recent associations clearly indicate that the role of this gene in the CNS is yet to be fully understood. In the next paragraphs, we will summarize some of the most recent studies on FGF14 in animal models and human tissue.

HISTORICAL PROSPECTIVE: FGF14 AS VOLTAGE-GATED Na^+ (Na_V) CHANNEL INTERACTING PROTEIN

While iFGFs share a conserved core β-trefoil region with other FGFs their functions and distributions are distinct from canonical FGFs (Itoh and Ornitz, 2008). Canonical FGFs are normally secreted to activate FGF receptors on the cell surface, however iFGFs lack a secretory sequence, fail to activate or antagonize FGF receptors and are primarily found in the cytoplasm, nucleus or the AIS (Smallwood et al., 1996; Olsen et al., 2003; Ornitz and Itoh, 2015; Pablo et al., 2016). Initial discoveries using yeast-two-hybrid screening identified

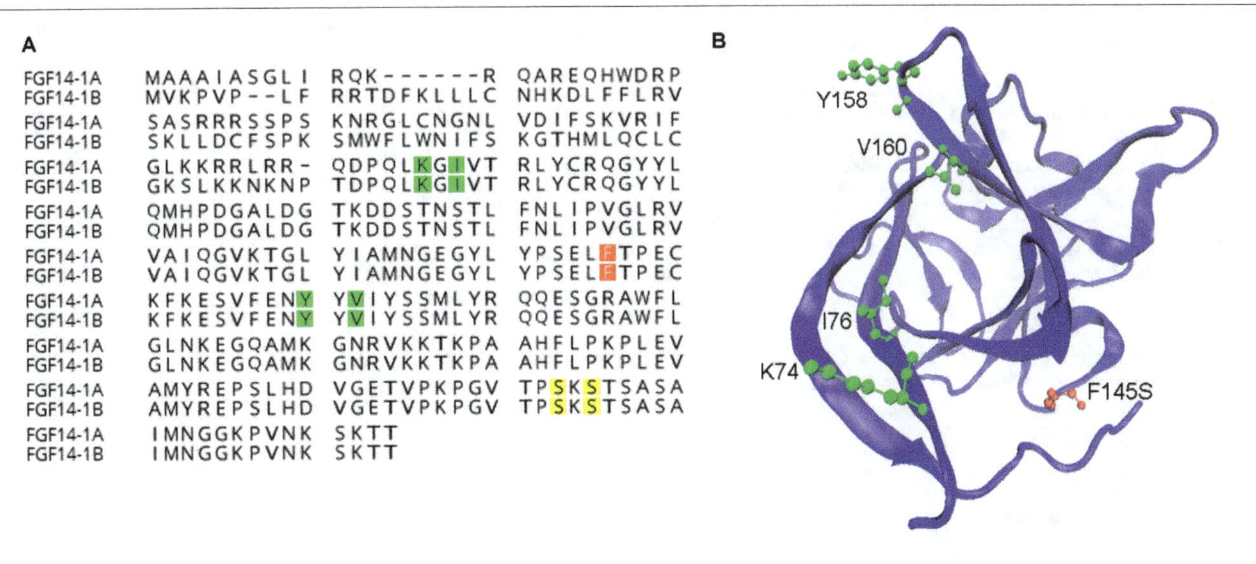

FIGURE 1 | Known functions of amino acids in fibroblast 14 (FGF14). (A) Alignment of wild-type FGF14-1a and FGF14-1b protein sequences with highlighted residues representing surface hot-spots for FGF14:Na_V1.6 interactions (green, Ali et al., 2016), casein kinase II (CK-2) phosphorylation sites (yellow, Hsu et al., 2016), and the spinocerebellar ataxia 27 (SCA27) F145S mutation site (red, Laezza et al., 2007). **(B)** An FGF14 homology model generated using the FGF13:Na_V1.5 crystal structure (Protein Data Bank ID: 4DCK) as template, visualized using the visual molecular dynamic (VMD) software package (Humphrey et al., 1996). Surface hot-spots important for protein:protein interactions (green) and the SCA27 F145S mutation (red) are shown.

FGF12 and FGF13 as direct interactors of Na_V channels (Liu et al., 2003; Wittmack et al., 2004; Rush et al., 2006) and subsequent studies resulted in similar discoveries for the two isoforms of FGF14 (Lou et al., 2005; Laezza et al., 2007, 2009), aligned in the illustration of **Figure 1A**. To date, the evidence for direct interaction and functional modulation of Na_V channels by FGF14 ranges from crystal structure to biochemical in cell assays to animal models and includes recent identification of critical amino acid residues at the FGF14: Na_V1.6 channel complex illustrated in **Figure 1B** (Lou et al., 2005; Laezza et al., 2007, 2009; Goetz et al., 2009; Ali et al., 2014, 2016; Hsu et al., 2016; Pablo et al., 2016).

The N-terminus of FGF14 is alternatively spliced into two isoforms: FGF14-1a and FGF14-1b. FGF14-1a shares sequence homology with FGF12-1a and FGF13-1a, while the amino terminus of FGF14-1b contains a unique 69 amino-acid sequence and is the more prevalent isoform in the CNS (Munoz-Sanjuan et al., 2000). Importantly, the interaction of FGF14 in cells that heterologously express individual Na_V isoforms shows that FGF14 is unique, as it results in very distinct isoform-specific Na+ current phenotypes that are dictated by the two FGF14 splice variants (Lou et al., 2005; Laezza et al., 2009; Ali et al., 2016). In primary hippocampal neurons, overexpression of FGF14-1b increases Na+ current density, causes a hyperpolarizing shift in the voltage-dependence of activation and a depolarizing shift in the voltage-dependence of inactivation, while the F145S, SCA27 dominant negative loss-of-function mutation causes opposite phenotypes, possibly by disrupting the function of wild-type FGF14 (Laezza et al., 2007). Neurons from *Fgf14*$^{-/-}$ mice exhibit impaired excitability in both the hippocampus and cerebellum (Goldfarb et al., 2007; Shakkottai et al., 2009; Bosch et al., 2015; Hsu et al., 2016). The effect of FGF14 on Na_V channels and excitability is summarized in **Table 1**.

FGF14 AS SCAFFOLD FOR KINASES

Recent studies have added a new dimension to FGF14, showing that its interaction with the Na_V channel is controlled by selective kinases (Shavkunov et al., 2012, 2013; Hsu et al., 2015, 2016). Initial studies using the luciferase complementation assay demonstrated that the FGF14:Na_V1.6 complex formation is controlled by glycogen synthase kinase 3 (GSK; Shavkunov et al., 2013) and more recently by the GSK3 priming kinase, casein kinase II (CK2) which phosphorylates FGF14 at S228 and S230 (Hsu et al., 2016; **Figure 1B**). Inhibition of either GSK3 or CK2 is sufficient to disrupt the FGF14:Na_V channel complex formation with consequences for targeting of the two proteins to the AIS and for intrinsic excitability (Shavkunov et al., 2013; Hsu et al., 2016). It is possible that phosphorylation at these kinase specific sites that confers functional specificity to FGF14 contributing to regulation of other ion channels (i.e., voltage-gated K^+ and Ca^{2+} channels).

More is known about the specific phosphorylation of FGF14 by GSK3 and CK2, however other kinases have been shown to affect FGF14:Na_V1.6 interactions (Shavkunov et al., 2012; Hsu et al., 2015). Importantly, many

TABLE 1 | Effect of splice variants in heterologous systems and knockout animals.

Isoforms	FGF14-1a (HEK-293)	FGF14-1b (HEK-cells)	FGF14-1b (Neuronal cell line)	FGF14-1b (Hippocampal neurons)	FGF14 Knockout (Granule neurons and CA1 hippocampal) neurons)
Na_V1.1	Depolarizing shift in voltage dependence of activation, depolarizing shift in voltage dependence of inactivation (Lou et al., 2005)	Decreases in current density, depolarizing shift in voltage dependence of inactivation (Lou et al., 2005)	Decreases current density (Laezza et al., 2009)	-	-
Na_V1.2	Depolarizing shift in steady state inactivation (Laezza et al., 2009)	-	Decreases current density, small depolarizing shift in steady-state inactivation (Laezza et al., 2009)	-	-
Na_V1.5	Decreases current density, depolarizing shift in voltage dependence of inactivation (Lou et al., 2005)	Decreases current density, hyperpolarizing shift in inactivation (Lou et al., 2005)	-	-	-
Na_V1.6	Depolarizing shift in steady-state inactivation, slower recovery from inactivation (Laezza et al., 2009)	-	Decreases current density, depolarizing shift in steady-state inactivation (Laezza et al., 2009)	-	-
Native Na_V channels	-	-	-	Increases current density, hyperpolarizing shift in voltage-dependence of activation, depolarizing shift in steady-state inactivation (Laezza et al., 2007)	Reduces evoked repetitive firing (Goldfarb et al., 2007; Hsu et al., 2016)

kinases involved in tyrosine receptor kinase signaling are implicated in this regulation, including the mitogen activated protein kinase (MAPK), C-Jun N-terminal kinase (JNK; Hsu et al., 2015). JNK signaling is disrupted in insulin resistance associated with type-II diabetes and Alzheimer's disease (Najem et al., 2016). Functional enrichment of single nucleotide polymorphisms (SNPs) in patients with type-II diabetes and Alzheimer's disease shows that FGF14 is significantly overrepresented in these two diseases because of its phosphorylation by JNK (Hao et al., 2015). Changes in the mRNA expression of MAPK/JNK signaling proteins, including FGF14, are also significantly overrepresented in early-onset Alzheimer's disease patients (Antonell et al., 2013). Taken together, these results indicate that the interaction between JNK and FGF14 might be an important area for future research in Alzheimer's disease.

FGF14 AS REGULATOR OF EXCITATORY AND INHIBITORY SYNAPTIC TRANSMISSION

Numerous are the reports of the effect of genetic deletion of *Fgf14* on synaptic transmission. Studies in the cerebellum of *Fgf14*$^{-/-}$ mice revealed decreased excitatory transmission from granule cells to Purkinje cells (parallel fibers, PF), a phenotype that is accompanied by reduced AMPA receptor-mediated excitatory postsynaptic currents and decreased expression of vesicular glutamate transporter 1, a specific presynaptic marker at PF-Purkinje neuron synapses (Tempia et al., 2015). Presynaptic changes in neurotransmitter release have been also reported at the Schaffer's collaterals to CA1 synapses where deletion of *Fgf14* results in reduction in the ready-releasable pool of presynaptic glutamate and diminished expression of synaptobrevin, synaptophysin, syntaxin I (Xiao et al., 2007). Other changes in presynaptic function have been reported at inhibitory GABAergic terminals onto CA1 pyramidal cells of *Fgf14*$^{-/-}$ mice, which exhibit reduced expression of glutamic acid decarboxylase 67 (GAD67) and vesicular GABA transporter (vGAT), presumably deriving from fast-spiking parvalbumin (PV) interneurons synapses (Alshammari T. K. et al., 2016). Additional studies in the same animal model identified selective loss of PV interneurons, reduced γ frequency oscillations and deficits in working memory (Alshammari T. K. et al., 2016). Collectively, these results recapitulate some endophenotypes of schizophrenia and are supported by human studies finding significant reduction and co-variation of *FGF14*, *PV*, *vGAT* and *GAD67* in post-mortem samples from schizophrenic patients compared to healthy control individuals (Alshammari T. K. et al., 2016). Whether all these changes at presynaptic glutamatergic and GABAergic terminals result from neuroadaptive responses to impaired firing or represent disruption of a separate function of the FGF14 protein remains to be determined. However, the evidence for genetic links between *vGAT*, *GAD67* and *FGF14* might argue for a "separate function" hypothesis of FGF14 that results from a control at the gene level.

FGF14 IS REQUIRED FOR SYNAPTIC PLASTICITY

Studies have also supported a role of FGF14 in synaptic plasticity in the hippocampus. *Fgf14*$^{-/-}$ mice show impaired long-term potentiation (LTP) at the Schaffer's collaterals to CA1 synapses, which is accompanied by decreased expression of synaptic vesicles docked at the active zone, and fewer miniature excitatory postsynaptic currents in primary hippocampal neurons (Xiao et al., 2007). Short-term plasticity is also impaired at these *Fgf14*$^{-/-}$ terminals, at which repetitive stimuli causes significant synaptic fatigue, consistent with impaired presynaptic function (Xiao et al., 2007).

FGF14 AS FACTOR REQUIRED FOR NEUROGENESIS

Adult neurogenesis, or the proliferation, differentiation and integration of new neurons into existing brain circuitry has become an area of research interest in part due to its implication in the cognitive pathophysiology of several neuropsychiatric disorders, including Alzheimer's disease, depression and schizophrenia (Ming and Song, 2005; Taupin, 2005, 2008; Reif et al., 2007; Johnson et al., 2009; Sun et al., 2011; Jun et al., 2012; Walton et al., 2012; Ouchi et al., 2013). It was recently found that FGF14 is required for the maturation of progenitor cells in the dentate gyrus of the hippocampus. *Fgf14*$^{-/-}$ mice show impaired transition from late immature neuronal progenitor cells to mature neurons, which is accompanied by reduced paired-pulse facilitation at the perforant path to granule neurons in the dentate gyrus (Alshammari M. A. et al., 2016). Overall, deletion of FGF14 results in an immature dentate gyrus, an endophenotype that corroborates a link between the gene and schizophrenia (Hagihara et al., 2013).

TABLE 2 | Single nucleotide polymorphisms (SNPs) in FGF14 introns associated with neuropsychiatric disease.

Intronic SNP ID	Associated disease	Citation
rs636674	Major depressive disorder	Verbeek et al. (2012)
rs1457315	Major depressive disorder	Verbeek et al. (2012)
rs4772439	Major depressive disorder	Verbeek et al. (2012)
rs7992504	Major depressive disorder	Verbeek et al. (2012)
rs9518615	Major depressive disorder	Verbeek et al. (2012)
rs9518638	Major depressive disorder	Verbeek et al. (2012)
rs9557792	Major depressive disorder	Verbeek et al. (2012)
rs128655694	Major depressive disorder	Verbeek et al. (2012)
rs17688345	Major depressive disorder	Verbeek et al. (2012)
rs35700852	Major depressive disorder	Verbeek et al. (2012)
rs4772445	Schizophrenia	Need et al. (2009)
rs9554852	Substance dependence	Drgon et al. (2011)
rs16959573	Substance dependence	Johnson et al. (2011)
rs17502818	Substance use	Johnson et al. (2011)
rs2476230	Antidepressant response	Hunter et al. (2013)
rs17502999	Entorhinal cortex volume change in Alzheimer's disease	Yang et al. (2015)

FGF14 AS AN ASSOCIATED FACTOR FOR NEUROPSYCHIATRIC DISEASE

As many neuropsychiatric disorders are heterogeneous and complex, GWAS have become an important tool for sorting relevant genetic information from large patient populations. Numerous GWAS have reported SNPs in *FGF14* in the context of neuropsychiatric disorders (**Table 2**). Although all these SNPs are in the *FGF14* intronic region and thus their role on the protein expression and function are unclear, they might provide guidance for future investigations. A Brazilian pilot study on early onset/familial schizophrenia found a link between early-onset schizophrenia and *FGF14* (Gadelha et al., 2012). GWAS in German cohort found an association between *FGF14* and schizophrenia, which is corroborated by a linkage study of familial schizophrenia in Canadian families of Celtic or German descent (Brzustowicz et al., 1999; Need et al., 2009). Additionally, SNPs in *FGF14* have been associated with dependence on alcohol and illegal substances in humans, and a fine-mapping study found several SNPs to be associated with major depressive disorder in a study of Dutch twins (Drgon et al., 2011; Johnson et al., 2011; Verbeek et al., 2012). Furthermore, an *FGF14* SNP is associated with volumetric changes in the entorhinal cortex in AD patients (Yang et al., 2015). Overall, genetic variations in *FGF14* are linked to the pathophysiology of several neuropsychiatric disorders, a promising area for further research that is supported by studies in *Fgf14*$^{-/-}$ preclinical models (Alshammari T. K. et al., 2016; Alshammari M. A. et al., 2016).

CONCLUSION

FGF14 plays a role in all fundamental properties of neurons: intrinsic firing, synaptic transmission of excitatory and inhibitory neurons and plasticity, while deletion of the gene leads to disruptive motor and cognitive behaviors. The role of FGF14 in humans is yet to be fully understood, but the emerging technologies for genome sequencing and protein characterization will provide potential opportunities for identifying new disease signatures associated with FGF14.

AUTHOR CONTRIBUTIONS

All of the authors have contributed substantially to the work. JDR and FL contributed to writing and editing the manuscript. PAW created the image and legend for **Figure 1**.

FUNDING

This research was funded by National Institute of Mental Health: grant no. 1R01MH111107-01A1, R01 MH095995-A1 and the National Institutes of Health: grant no 5T32AG051131-02.

REFERENCES

Ali, S. R., Singh, A. K., and Laezza, F. (2016). Identification of amino acid residues in fibroblast growth factor 14 (FGF14) required for structure-function interactions with voltage-gated sodium channel Nav1.6. *J. Biol. Chem.* 291, 11268–11284. doi: 10.1074/jbc.m115.703868

Ali, S., Shavkunov, A., Panova, N., Stoilova-McPhie, S., and Laezza, F. (2014). Modulation of the FGF14:FGF14 homodimer interaction through short peptide fragments. *CNS. Neurol. Disord. Drug. Targets* 13, 1559–15570. doi: 10.2174/1871527313666141126103309

Alshammari, T. K., Alshammari, M. A., Nenov, M. N., Hoxha, E., Cambiaghi, M., Marcinno, A., et al. (2016). Genetic deletion of fibroblast growth factor 14 recapitulates phenotypic alterations underlying cognitive impairment associated with schizophrenia. *Transl. Psychiatry* 6:e806. doi: 10.1038/tp.2016.66

Alshammari, M. A., Alshammari, T. K., Nenov, M. N., Scala, F., and Laezza, F. (2016). Fibroblast growth factor 14 modulates the neurogenesis of granule neurons in the adult dentate gyrus. *Mol. Neurobiol.* 53, 7254–7270. doi: 10.1007/s12035-015-9568-5

Antonell, A., Lladó, A., Altirriba, J., Botta-Orfila, T., Balasa, M., Fernández, M., et al. (2013). A preliminary study of the whole-genome expression profile of sporadic and monogenic early-onset alzheimer's disease. *Neurobiol. Aging* 34, 1772–1778. doi: 10.1016/j.neurobiolaging.2012.12.026

Bosch, M. K., Carrasquillo, Y., Ransdell, J. L., Kanakamedala, A., Ornitz, D. M., and Nerbonne, J. M. (2015). Intracellular FGF14 (iFGF14) is required for spontaneous and evoked firing in cerebellar purkinje neurons and for motor coordination and balance. *J. Neurosci.* 35, 6752–6769. doi: 10.1523/JNEUROSCI.2663-14.2015

Bosch, M. K., Nerbonne, J. M., Townsend, R. R., Miyazaki, H., Nukina, N., Ornitz, D. M., et al. (2016). Proteomic analysis of native cerebellar iFGF14 complexes. *Channels (Austin)* 10, 297–312. doi: 10.1080/19336950.2016.1153203

Brusse, E., de Koning, I., Maat-Kievit, A., Oostra, B. A., Heutink, P., and van Swieten, J. C. (2006). Spinocerebellar ataxia associated with a mutation in the *fibroblast growth factor 14* gene (SCA27): a new phenotype. *Mov. Disord.* 21, 396–401. doi: 10.1002/mds.20708

Brzustowicz, L. M., Honer, W. G., Chow, E. W., Little, D., Hogan, J., Hodgkinson, K., et al. (1999). Linkage of familial schizophrenia to chromosome 13q32. *Am. J. Hum. Genet.* 65, 1096–1103. doi: 10.1086/302579

Detera-Wadleigh, S. D., Badner, J. A., Berrettini, W. H., Yoshikawa, T., Goldin, L. R., Turner, G., et al. (1999). A high-density genome scan detects evidence for a bipolar-disorder susceptibility locus on 13q32 and other potential loci on 1q32 and 18p11.2. *Proc. Natl. Acad. Sci. U S A* 96, 5604–5609. doi: 10.1073/pnas.96.10.5604

Drgon, T., Johnson, C. A., Nino, M., Drgonova, J., Walther, D. M., and Uhl, G. R. (2011). "Replicated" genome wide association for dependence on illegal substances: genomic regions identified by overlapping clusters of nominally positive SNPs. *Am. J. Med. Genet. B Neuropsychiatr. Genet.* 156, 125–138. doi: 10.1002/ajmg.b.31143

Gadelha, A., Ota, V. K., Cano, J. P., Melaragno, M. I., Smith, M. A., de Jesus Mari, J., et al. (2012). Linkage replication for chromosomal region 13q32 in schizophrenia: evidence from a Brazilian pilot study on early onset schizophrenia families. *PLoS One* 7:e52262. doi: 10.1371/journal.pone.0052262

Goetz, R., Dover, K., Laezza, F., Shtraizent, N., Huang, X., Tchetchik, D., et al. (2009). Crystal structure of a fibroblast growth factor homologous factor (FHF) defines a conserved surface on FHFs for binding and modulation of voltage-gated sodium channels. *J. Biol. Chem.* 284, 17883–17896. doi: 10.1074/jbc.m109.001842

Goldfarb, M., Schoorlemmer, J., Williams, A., Diwakar, S., Wang, Q., Huang, X., et al. (2007). Fibroblast growth factor homologous factors control neuronal excitability through modulation of voltage-gated sodium channels. *Neuron* 55, 449–463. doi: 10.1016/j.neuron.2007.07.006

Hagihara, H., Takao, K., Walton, N. M., Matsumoto, M., and Miyakawa, T. (2013). Immature dentate gyrus: an endophenotype of neuropsychiatric disorders. *Neural Plast.* 2013:318596. doi: 10.1155/2013/318596

Hao, K., Di Narzo, A. F., Ho, L., Luo, W., Li, S., Chen, R., et al. (2015). Shared genetic etiology underlying Alzheimer's disease and type 2 diabetes. *Mol. Aspects Med.* 43–44, 66–76. doi: 10.1016/j.mam.2015.06.006

Hsu, W. C., Nenov, M. N., Shavkunov, A., Panova, N., Zhan, M., and Laezza, F. (2015). Identifying a kinase network regulating FGF14:Nav1.6 complex assembly using split-luciferase complementation. *PLoS One* 10:e0117246. doi: 10.1371/journal.pone.0117246

Hsu, W.-C. J., Nilsson, C. L., and Laezza, F. (2014). Role of the axonal initial segment in psychiatric disorders: function, dysfunction, and intervention. *Front. Psychiatry* 5:109. doi: 10.3389/fpsyt.2014.00109

Hsu, W.-C. J., Scala, F., Nenov, M. N., Wildburger, N. C., Elferink, H., Singh, A. K., et al. (2016). CK2 activity is required for the interaction of FGF14 with voltage-gated sodium channels and neuronal excitability. *FASEB J.* 30, 2171–2186. doi: 10.1096/fj.201500161

Humphrey, W., Dalke, A., and Schulten, K. (1996). VMD: visual molecular dynamics. *J. Mol. Graph.* 14, 33–38. doi: 10.1016/0263-7855(96)00018-5

Hunter, A. M., Leuchter, A. F., Power, R. A., Muthén, B., McGrath, P. J., Lewis, C. M., et al. (2013). A genome-wide association study of a sustained pattern of antidepressant response. *J. Psychiatr. Res.* 47, 1157–1165. doi: 10.1016/j.jpsychires.2013.05.002

Itoh, N., and Ornitz, D. M. (2008). Functional evolutionary history of the mouse Fgf gene family. *Dev. Dyn.* 237, 18–27. doi: 10.1002/dvdy.21388

Johnson, M. A., Ables, J. L., and Eisch, A. J. (2009). Cell-intrinsic signals that regulate adult neurogenesis *in vivo*: insights from inducible approaches. *BMB Rep.* 42, 245–259. doi: 10.5483/bmbrep.2009.42.5.245

Johnson, C., Drgon, T., Walther, D., and Uhl, G. R. (2011). Genomic regions identified by overlapping clusters of nominally-positive SNPs from genome-wide studies of alcohol and illegal substance dependence. *PLoS One* 6:e19210. doi: 10.1371/journal.pone.0019210

Jun, H., Mohammed Qasim Hussaini, S., Rigby, M. J., and Jang, M. H. (2012). Functional role of adult hippocampal neurogenesis as a therapeutic strategy for mental disorders. *Neural Plast.* 2012:854285. doi: 10.1155/2012/854285

Laezza, F., Gerber, B. R., Lou, J. Y., Kozel, M. A., Hartman, H., Craig, A. M., et al. (2007). The FGF14(F145S) mutation disrupts the interaction of FGF14 with voltage-gated Na+ channels and impairs neuronal excitability. *J. Neurosci.* 27, 12033–12044. doi: 10.1523/JNEUROSCI.2282-07.2007

Laezza, F., Lampert, A., Kozel, M. A., Gerber, B. R., Rush, A. M., Nerbonne, J. M., et al. (2009). FGF14 N-terminal splice variants differentially modulate Nav1.2 and Nav1.6-encoded sodium channels. *Mol. Cell. Neurosci.* 42, 90–101. doi: 10.1016/j.mcn.2009.05.007

Liu, C. J., Dib-Hajj, S. D., Renganathan, M., Cummins, T. R., and Waxman, S. G. (2003). Modulation of the cardiac sodium channel Nav1.5 by fibroblast growth factor homologous factor 1B. *J. Biol. Chem.* 278, 1029–1036. doi: 10.1074/jbc.M207074200

Lou, J. Y., Laezza, F., Gerber, B. R., Xiao, M., Yamada, K. A., Hartmann, H., et al. (2005). Fibroblast growth factor 14 is an intracellular modulator of voltage-gated sodium channels. *J. Physiol.* 569, 179–193. doi: 10.1113/jphysiol.2005.097220

Ming, G. L., and Song, H. (2005). Adult neurogenesis in the mammalian central nervous system. *Annu. Rev. Neurosci.* 28, 223–250. doi: 10.1146/annurev.neuro.28.051804.101459

Mulle, J. G., McDonough, J. A., Chowdari, K. V., Nimgaonkar, V., and Chakravarti, A. (2005). Evidence for linkage to chromosome 13q32 in an independent sample of schizophrenia families. *Mol. Psychiatry* 10, 429–431. doi: 10.1038/sj.mp.4001639

Munoz-Sanjuan, I., Smallwood, P. M., and Nathans, J. (2000). Isoform diversity among fibroblast growth factor homologous factors is generated by alternative promoter usage and differential splicing. *J. Biol. Chem.* 275, 2589–2597. doi: 10.1074/jbc.275.4.2589

Najem, D., Bamji-Mirza, M., Yang, Z., and Zhang, Z. (2016). Aβ-induced insulin resistance and the effects of insulin on the cholesterol synthesis pathway and Aβ secretion in neural cells. *Neurosci. Bull.* 32, 227–238. doi: 10.1007/s12264-016-0034-9

Need, A. C., Ge, D., Weale, M. E., Maia, J., Feng, S., Heinzen, E. L., et al. (2009). A genome-wide investigation of SNPs and CNVs in schizophrenia. *PLoS Genet.* 5:e1000373. doi: 10.1371/journal.pgen.1000373

Ogawa, Y., and Rasband, M. N. (2008). The functional organization and assembly of the axon initial segment. *Curr. Opin. Neurobiol.* 18, 307–313. doi: 10.1016/j.conb.2008.08.008

Olsen, S. K., Garbi, M., Zampieri, N., Eliseenkova, A. V., Ornitz, D. M., Goldfarb, M., et al. (2003). Fibroblast growth factor (FGF) homologous factors share structural but not functional homology with FGFs. *J. Biol. Chem.* 278, 34226–34236. doi: 10.1074/jbc.M303183200

Ornitz, D. M., and Itoh, N. (2015). The fibroblast growth factor signaling pathway. *Wiley Interdiscip. Rev. Dev. Biol.* 4, 215–266. doi: 10.1002/wdev.176

Ouchi, Y., Banno, Y., Shimizu, Y., Ando, S., Hasegawa, H., Adachi, K., et al. (2013). Reduced adult hippocampal neurogenesis and working memory deficits in the Dgcr8-deficient mouse model of 22q11.2 deletion-associated schizophrenia can be rescued by IGF2. *J. Neurosci.* 33, 9408–9419. doi: 10.1523/JNEUROSCI.2700-12.2013

Pablo, J. L., and Pitt, G. S. (2017). FGF14 is a regulator of KCNQ2/3 channels. *Proc. Natl. Acad. Sci. U S A* 114, 154–159. doi: 10.1073/pnas.1610158114

Pablo, J. L., Wang, C., Presby, M. M., and Pitt, G. S. (2016). Polarized localization of voltage-gated Na^+ channels is regulated by concerted FGF13 and FGF14 action. *Proc. Natl. Acad. Sci. U S A* 113, E2665–E2674. doi: 10.1073/pnas.1521194113

Palmer, L. M., and Stuart, G. J. (2006). Site of action potential initiation in layer 5 pyramidal neurons. *J. Neurosci.* 26, 1854–1863. doi: 10.1523/JNEUROSCI.4812-05.2006

Park, N., Juo, S. H., Cheng, R., Liu, J., Loth, J. E., Lilliston, B., et al. (2004). Linkage analysis of psychosis in bipolar pedigrees suggests novel putative loci for bipolar disorder and shared susceptibility with schizophrenia. *Mol. Psychiatry* 9, 1091–1099. doi: 10.1038/sj.mp.4001541

Reif, A., Schmitt, A., Fritzen, S., and Lesch, K. P. (2007). Neurogenesis and schizophrenia: dividing neurons in a divided mind? *Eur. Arch. Psychiatry Clin. Neurosci.* 257, 290–299. doi: 10.1007/s00406-007-0733-3

Rush, A. M., Wittmack, E. K., Tyrrell, L., Black, J. A., Dib-Hajj, S. D., and Waxman, S. G. (2006). Differential modulation of sodium channel $Na_V1.6$ by two members of the fibroblast growth factor homologous factor 2 subfamily. *Eur. J. Neurosci.* 23, 2551–2562. doi: 10.1111/j.1460-9568.2006.04789.x

Shakkottai, V. G., Xiao, M., Xu, L., Wong, M., Nerbonne, J. M., Ornitz, D. M., et al. (2009). FGF14 regulates the intrinsic excitability of cerebellar Purkinje neurons. *Neurobiol. Dis.* 33, 81–88. doi: 10.1016/j.nbd.2008.09.019

Shavkunov, A., Panova, N., Prasai, A., Veselenak, R., Bourne, N., Stoilova-McPhie, S., et al. (2012). Bioluminescence methodology for the detection of protein-protein interactions within the voltage-gated sodium channel macromolecular complex. *Assay Drug Dev. Technol.* 10, 148–160. doi: 10.1089/adt.2011.413

Shavkunov, A. S., Wildburger, N. C., Nenov, M. N., James, T. F., Buzhdygan, T. P., Panova-Elektronova, N. I., et al. (2013). The fibroblast growth factor 14·Voltage-gated sodium channel complex is a new target of glycogen synthase kinase 3 (GSK3). *J. Biol. Chem.* 288, 19370–19385. doi: 10.1074/jbc.M112.445924

Singh, H. N., and Rajeswari, M. R. (2015). Role of long purine stretches in controlling the expression of genes associated with neurological disorders. *Gene* 572, 175–183. doi: 10.1016/j.gene.2015.07.007

Smallwood, P. M., Munoz-Sanjuan, I., Tong, P., Macke, J. P., Hendry, S. H., Gilbert, D. J., et al. (1996). Fibroblast growth factor (FGF) homologous factors: new members of the FGF family implicated in nervous system development. *Proc. Natl. Acad. Sci. U S A* 93, 9850–9857. doi: 10.1073/pnas.93.18.9850

Sun, J., Sun, J., Ming, G.-L., and Song, H. (2011). Epigenetic regulation of neurogenesis in the adult mammalian brain. *Eur. J. Neurosci.* 33, 1087–1093. doi: 10.1111/j.1460-9568.2011.07607.x

Taupin, P. (2005). Adult neurogenesis in the mammalian central nervous system: functionality and potential clinical interest. *Med. Sci. Monit.* 11, RA247–RA252.

Taupin, P. (2008). Adult neurogenesis pharmacology in neurological diseases and disorders. *Expert Rev. Neurother.* 8, 311–320. doi: 10.1586/14737175.8.2.311

Tempia, F., Hoxha, E., Negro, G., Alshammari, M. A., Alshammari, T. K., Panova-Elektronova, N., et al. (2015). Parallel fiber to Purkinje cell synaptic impairment in a mouse model of spinocerebellar ataxia type 27. *Front. Cell. Neurosci.* 9:205. doi: 10.3389/fncel.2015.00205

van Swieten, J. C., Brusse, E., de Graaf, B. M., Krieger, E., van de Graaf, R., de Koning, I., et al. (2003). A mutation in the *fibroblast growth factor 14* gene is associated with autosomal dominant cerebellar ataxia [corrected]. *Am. J. Hum. Genet.* 72, 191–199. doi: 10.1086/345488

Verbeek, E. C., Bakker, I. M., Bevova, M. R., Bochdanovits, Z., Rizzu, P., Sondervan, D., et al. (2012). A fine-mapping study of 7 top scoring genes from a GWAS for major depressive disorder. *PLoS One* 7:e37384. doi: 10.1371/journal.pone.0037384

Walton, N. M., Zhou, Y., Kogan, J. H., Shin, R., Webster, M., Gross, A. K., et al. (2012). Detection of an immature dentate gyrus feature in human schizophrenia/bipolar patients. *Transl. Psychiatry* 2:e135. doi: 10.1038/tp.2012.56

Wang, Q., Bardgett, M. E., Wong, M., Wozniak, D. F., Lou, J., McNeil, B. D., et al. (2002). Ataxia and paroxysmal dyskinesia in mice lacking axonally transported FGF14. *Neuron* 35, 25–38. doi: 10.1016/s0896-6273(02)00744-4

Wang, C., Chung, B. C., Yan, H., Lee, S. Y., and Pitt, G. S. (2012). Crystal structure of the ternary complex of a NaV C-terminal domain, a fibroblast growth factor homologous factor, and calmodulin. *Structure* 20, 1167–1176. doi: 10.1016/j.str.2012.05.001

Wang, C., Wang, C., Hoch, E. G., and Pitt, G. S. (2011). Identification of novel interaction sites that determine specificity between fibroblast growth factor homologous factors, and voltage-gated sodium channels. *J. Biol. Chem.* 286, 24253–24563. doi: 10.1074/jbc.M111.245803

Wildburger, N. C., Ali, S. R., Hsu, W. C., Shavkunov, A. S., Nenov, M. N., Lichti, C. F., et al. (2015). Quantitative proteomics reveals protein-protein interactions with fibroblast growth factor 12 as a component of the voltage-gated sodium channel 1.2 (navl.2) macromolecular complex in Mammalian brain. *Mol. Cell. Proteomics* 14, 1288–1300. doi: 10.1074/mcp.M114.040055

Wittmack, E. K., Rush, A. M., Craner, M. J., Goldfarb, M., Waxman, S. G., and Dib-Hajj, S. D. (2004). Fibroblast growth factor homologous factor 2B: association with Nav1.6 and selective colocalization at nodes of Ranvier of dorsal root axons. *J. Neurosci.* 24, 6765–6775. doi: 10.1523/JNEUROSCI.1628-04.2004

Wozniak, D. F., Xiao, M., Xu, L., Yamada, K. A., and Ornitz, D. M. (2007). Impaired spatial learning and defective theta burst induced LTP in mice lacking fibroblast growth factor 14. *Neurobiol. Dis.* 26, 14–26. doi: 10.1016/j.nbd.2006.11.014

Xiao, M., Xu, L., Laezza, F., Yamada, K., Feng, S., and Ornitz, D. M. (2007). Impaired hippocampal synaptic transmission and plasticity in mice lacking fibroblast growth factor 14. *Mol. Cell. Neurosci.* 34, 366–377. doi: 10.1016/j.mcn.2006.11.020

Yan, H., Pablo, J. L., and Pitt, G. S. (2013). FGF14 regulates presynaptic Ca^{2+} channels and synaptic transmission. *Cell Rep.* 4, 66–75. doi: 10.1016/j.celrep.2013.06.012

Yang, T., Wang, J., Sun, Q., Hibar, D. P., Jahanshad, N., Liu, L., et al. (2015). Detecting genetic risk factors for alzheimer's disease in whole genome sequence data via lasso screening. *Proc. IEEE Int. Symp. Biomed. Imaging* 2015, 985–989. doi: 10.1109/ISBI.2015.7164036

7

Lactate Shuttles in Neuroenergetics—Homeostasis, Allostasis and Beyond

Shayne Mason *

Centre for Human Metabolomics, North-West University, Potchefstroom, South Africa

Edited by:
Andrew Harkin, Trinity College, Dublin, Ireland

Reviewed by:
Claude Messier, University of Ottawa, Canada
Fahmeed Hyder, Yale University, USA

***Correspondence:**
Shayne Mason
nmr.nwu@gmail.com

Understanding brain energy metabolism—neuroenergetics—is becoming increasingly important as it can be identified repeatedly as the source of neurological perturbations. Within the scientific community we are seeing a shift in paradigms from the traditional neurocentric view to that of a more dynamic, integrated one where astrocytes are no longer considered as being just supportive, and activated microglia have a profound influence. Lactate is emerging as the "good guy," contrasting its classical "bad guy" position in the now superseded medical literature. This review begins with the evolution of the concept of "lactate shuttles"; goes on to the recent shift in ideas regarding normal neuroenergetics (homeostasis)—specifically, the astrocyte–neuron lactate shuttle; and progresses to covering the metabolic implications whereby homeostasis is lost—a state of allostasis, and the function of microglia. The role of lactate, as a substrate and shuttle, is reviewed in light of allostatic stress, and beyond—in an acute state of allostatic stress in terms of physical brain trauma, and reflected upon with respect to persistent stress as allostatic overload—neurodegenerative diseases. Finally, the recently proposed astrocyte–microglia lactate shuttle is discussed in terms of chronic neuroinflammatory infectious diseases, using tuberculous meningitis as an example. The novelty extended by this review is that the directionality of lactate, as shuttles in the brain, in neuropathophysiological states is emerging as crucial in neuroenergetics.

Keywords: neuroenergetics, lactate, astrocyte-neuron lactate shuttle (ANLS), astrocyte-microglia lactate shuttle (AMLS), neuropathology, traumatic brain injury (TBI), neurodegenerative disease, infectious neuroinflammatory disease

INTRODUCTION

The human brain represents approximately 2% of total body weight and receives up to 15% of total blood flow, consuming up to 20% of oxygen and 25% of circulating glucose under normal conditions (Pellerin, 2010). The metabolism of this high energy consuming organ involves complex intercellular trafficking of metabolites and compartmentalization of numerous processes. Tight coupling exists between the supply and demand of energy in brain metabolism with changes in cerebral blood flow and glucose utilization in response to neuronal activity (i.e., neurovascular and neurometabolic coupling) (Bélanger et al., 2011) under normal homeostatic conditions. Mechanisms involved in brain energy metabolism adapt during periods of perturbation and trauma. The important role of lactate, and its shuttles, has been overlooked and merits acknowledgement.

The interconversion of lactate and pyruvate occurs via lactate dehydrogenase, with increased lactate typically being associated with anaerobic respiration. Thus, one could postulate that elevated levels of lactate present in the cerebrospinal fluid (CSF) due to neuroinflammation could be from hypoxia caused by ischemia—increased anaerobic respiration (Rossi et al., 2007), or by raised glucose levels and hence elevated flow through the glycolysis pathway. However, in most neuroinflammatory cases there are typically periods of low levels of glucose in the CSF. Furthermore, several studies have shown no correlation between CSF lactate levels and cerebral blood flow (i.e., they are unrelated to ischemia) (Brodersen and Jorgensen, 1974; DeSalles et al., 1986; De Salles et al., 1987). Thus, an alternative postulate is that the elevated levels of lactate in the CSF of neuroinflammatory cases is unlikely to be due to anaerobic respiration but instead is possibly a product of temporarily increased flux in the glycolysis pathway—using glycogen as a supplementary source of glucose.

The notion that lactate is not simply just a by-product of glycolysis but also a shuttle system was pioneered by Brooks (1985). In June the following year, Brooks provided more evidence for a "shuttling" system for lactate (Brooks, 1986a); by December Brooks (1986b) formally coined the term "lactate shuttle" in skeletal muscle during rest and exercise under fully aerobic conditions. Brooks further defined lactate shuttles as being either intracellular (cytosolic to mitochondrial) or cell-to-cell (extracellular) (Brooks, 2000, 2002). Later, Brooks (2009) provided evidence that glycolytic and oxidative pathways should be viewed as linked, as opposed to alternative processes, because lactate, the product of one pathway, is the substrate for the other (Brooks, 2009). The concept of intracellular lactate shuttles was challenged (Sahlin et al., 2002), and continues to be so (Laureys et al., 2014). A study by Cruz et al. (2012) discussed these challenges but ultimately reiterated Brooks' sentiment regarding interaction between energy systems—the product of one is the substrate of another. Soon after Brooks first introduced the concept of lactate shuttles in 1986, several studies by Schurr et al. (1988, 1997a,b,c, 1999a,b) provided experimental evidence that astrocytic lactate is even used preferentially over glucose by neurons after episodes of cerebral ischemia.

Thus, lactate plays an important role as a shuttle, even beyond the brain—in numerous systems, for example, in pregnancy (Zuo et al., 2015), in reproduction (Kuchiiwa et al., 2011), and, notably, within the human heart (Cruz et al., 2012; Rakus et al., 2016). This paper provides an overview of brain neuroenergetics and the crucial roles of lactate shuttles. These roles will be discussed: (1) with regard to the normal physiological function and relationship between astrocytes and neurons (homeostasis)—the astrocyte-neuron lactate shuttle (ANLS) model; (2) the dynamic role of microglia and their preferential utilization of lactate under perturbed conditions (allostasis); (3) the activity of lactate and its shuttles in neuropathological states (in particular in traumatic brain injury and neurodegenerative diseases); and (4) the brain in crisis—in response to a neuroinflammatory infectious disease—according to the astrocyte-microglia lactate shuttle (AMLS) model, using tuberculous meningitis (TBM) as an example.

HOMEOSTATIC NEUROENERGETICS

Shifting Neuroenergetics Paradigms

The classical view of neuroenergetics is that the blood supplies oxygen and glucose to the brain (Sokoloff, 1989). Glucose is the primary source of energy utilized by both neurons and astrocytes. It undergoes complete oxidation via glycolysis, the Krebs cycle and oxidative phosphorylation, which ultimately produces adenosine triphosphate (ATP) for energy-dependent reactions. Thus, glucose is used in the same way by all cell types. Since neurons consume the greatest quantity of energy of all brain elements, metabolic intermediates (e.g., in the Krebs cycle) are diverted toward neurons. Some of the pyruvate produced by glycolysis is converted to lactate and released into the extracellular space. In this classical view, lactate is considered a by-product with deleterious effects when in excess (Norenberg et al., 1987; Siesjö, 1988; Bender et al., 1997). Astrocytes have long been thought to play a passive role in supporting neuronal function, with the neuron being the star of the show. However, the dynamic involvement of astrocytes (Ranjbar and Amiri, 2015) in the forefront of neuroenergetics is now being recognized, shifting paradigms (Haydon and Carmignoto, 2006; Giaume et al., 2010). The neurocentric view of neuroenergetics is evolving into a more integrated one of complementary and co-operative metabolic interactions between astrocytes and neurons.

Astrocytes–More than a Supporting Role?

At the cellular level the human brain consists of the all-important neurons and up to 10 times more glial cells than neurons (Kimelberg and Norenberg, 1989). There are four types of glial cells: ependymal cells, oligodendrocytes, astrocytes, and microglia (resident macrophages in the brain). Astrocytes constitute about 50% of the total human brain volume and are classically divided into three types based on morphology and spatial organization. These three types are: (1) radial—orientated perpendicular to ventricular surfaces with long, unbranched processes (end-feet); (2) protoplasmic—displaying bushy morphology with numerous, highly branched, short processes; and (3) fibrous—manifesting stellate shapes with smooth, long processes that are less branched. The cytoarchitectural organization of astrocytes is such that, according to Pellerin (2010) particular sections cover 99% of the surface area of cerebral blood vessels; although, due to tissue shrinkage with chemical fixation (Korogod et al., 2015), this 99% value is likely an inflated estimate. These astrocytes are, however, the preferential site for glucose uptake from the blood, as well as having projections in peri-synaptic areas of neurons, providing close interaction with neuronal elements and acting as a cellular barrier between blood and neurons. The unique morphological and phenotypic characteristics of astrocytes ideally position them to sense and respond dynamically to changes in neuronal activity (Pellerin, 2010; Bélanger et al., 2011), lending them to conduct numerous critical functions (Chen and Swanson, 2003; Steele and Robinson, 2012), such as glutamate homeostasis (in the glutamate-glutamine cycle), maintaining brain ionic equilibrium (K^+ and H^+ buffering), the maintenance of reactive oxygen species (ROS) (in glutathione recycling) and osmotic regulation. Astrocytes therefore support neuronal activity via structural, trophic and metabolic means, suggesting a critical role in regulating neuroenergetics and homeostatic functions (Pellerin, 2010). Notably, neurons rely on astrocytes to supply precursors of the Krebs cycle intermediates, or their derivatives, as the enzyme pyruvate carboxylase is present in only astrocytes but not in neurons (Hertz et al., 1999).

Astrocytes exhibit a higher capacity for glucose utilization, as well as greater metabolic plasticity, than neurons; these characteristics are important for homeostatic and neuroprotective functions. The calculated energy needs of astrocytes only represent about 10–15% of the total brain energy needs (Attwell and Laughlin, 2001; Gjedde et al., 2002; Rothman et al., 2003; Shulman et al., 2004). Hence, approximately 85% of the glucose in the brain is used in the expenditure of energy in neurons via the glycolytic pathway and the Krebs cycle leading to the synthesis of ATP (Jueptner and Weiller, 1995; Attwell and Laughlin, 2001). The high glycolytic rate of astrocytes suggests a preference for the production and release of lactate. The neuroprotective role of lactate has been experimentally demonstrated by studies (Cater et al., 2001, 2003). Neuroprotection here is defined as an intervention that prevents the death of vulnerable neurons and slows disease progression. Hence, evidence that has emerged over the past two decades has begun to highlight lactate as a supplementary substrate for neurons, resulting in the (re)emergence of a dynamic nursing role for astrocytes (Bouzier-Sore et al., 2002).

Astrocyte–Neuron Lactate Shuttle (ANLS) Hypothesis

Magistretti and Pellerin (1996) presented the framework of a hypothesis that they have since developed and refined to become one of the prevailing contemporary viewpoints of neuroenergetics—the ANLS hypothesis. The hypothesis states that astrocytes respond to intensified neuron activity by increasing their rate of glucose uptake, glycolysis and the release of lactate into the extracellular space, as shown schematically in **Figure 1**. At the metabolic level, it begins with glutamatergic activity, a process whereby increased neuronal activity results in the release of glutamate, the main excitatory neurotransmitter in the brain, into the extracellular space along the glutamate transporter EAAT3, which is exclusively located in neurons. Astrocytes sense increased activity at the glutamatergic synapses, followed by glutamate uptake via the glia-specific glutamate transporters EAAT1 and EAAT2. The transport of glutamate is driven by a sodium gradient (i.e., by a Na^+-dependent mechanism), with a stoichiometry of three Na^+ ions co-transported with one glutamate, resulting in a significant increase in intracellular Na^+ concentrations in astrocytes (Magistretti and Pellerin, 1999; Pellerin and Magistretti, 2004; Bélanger et al., 2011). Glutamate taken up by astrocytes is converted to glutamine through an ATP-dependent reaction catalyzed by astrocyte-specific glutamine synthetase. Glutamine is released back into the extracellular space and taken up by neurons, where it is converted to glutamate by glutaminase (Magistretti and Pellerin, 1999; Bélanger et al., 2011). This reaction thereby replenishes the neurotransmitter pool of glutamate and completes the glutamate–glutamine cycle. Glutamate uptake by astrocytes stimulates glucose uptake with a stoichiometric relationship of 1:1 between uptake of glutamate and glucose. Increased concentrations of Na^+ in astrocytes activate the enzyme Na^+-K^+-ATPase, particularly the α_2 subunit. The result is the triggering of glycolysis, leading to the production and release of lactate into the extracellular space; the lactate is then taken up as an energy substrate by neurons for oxidative-derived ATP production (Debernardi et al., 1999; Magistretti and Pellerin, 1999; Pellerin, 2003; Pellerin and Magistretti, 2004; Pellerin et al., 2007; Bélanger et al., 2011). This demonstrates the presence of open astroglial metabolic networks—an intercellular route, allowing the trafficking of energy substrates through astrocytes from their source, which is blood vessels, to the site of high energy demand and use, the neurons (Giaume et al., 2010).

Fox et al. (1988) were the first to show that focal, physiological increase in neuronal activity induced by visual stimulation in humans was associated with increased glucose uptake and blood flow in the human visual cortex. This suggested that increased neuronal functional activity stimulates glycolysis. Prichard et al. (1991) and Sappey-Marinier et al. (1992) further developed this postulate by demonstrating increased levels of lactate in the human visual cortex using nuclear magnetic resonance (NMR) technology, following visual stimulation. Thus, a tight coupling was demonstrated between neuronal activation and glucose utilization in astrocytes (Magistretti, 2006), an intrinsic feature of astrocytes not specifically linked to culture conditions or cell origin (Pellerin et al., 2007). It is interesting to note that glucose uptake by astrocytes is disproportionately high compared to their energy requirements. This suggests that sustained astrocytic glycolysis occurs in order to maintain the extracellular lactate pool to meet the energy requirements of neurons. Most recently, data from Angamo et al. (2016) suggest that astrocytic neuronal lactate shuttles contribute to the regulation of ion homeostasis and synaptic signaling in the presence of ample glucose.

In addition to blood-borne glucose, the brain also makes use of an important energy reserve in the form of glycogen stores located almost exclusively in astrocytes. Mobilization of glycogen occurs without ATP requirement during extended periods of limited energy supply (e.g., in hypoglycemia) and leads to enhanced lactate production and release, thereby maintaining energetic homeostasis and preserving neuronal function and viability (Wender et al., 2000; Pellerin, 2003; Pellerin and Magistretti, 2004). Glycogen mobilization can thus be viewed as an extension of the ANLS concept instead of a competing hypothesis (Pellerin et al., 2007). But, as stated by Dienel and Cruz (2015), glycogen is very difficult to study in the human brain. Roles for glycogen in brain function continue to emerge, revealing increasing complexity of the signaling and regulatory mechanisms that integrate glycogen mobilization with physiological activities.

It is important to note that the ANLS hypothesis does not preclude glucose as a source of energy for the brain. Glucose remains an important energy substrate with concentration gradients facilitating the transport of glucose across the blood–brain barrier into the brain via glucose transporters (GLUTs).

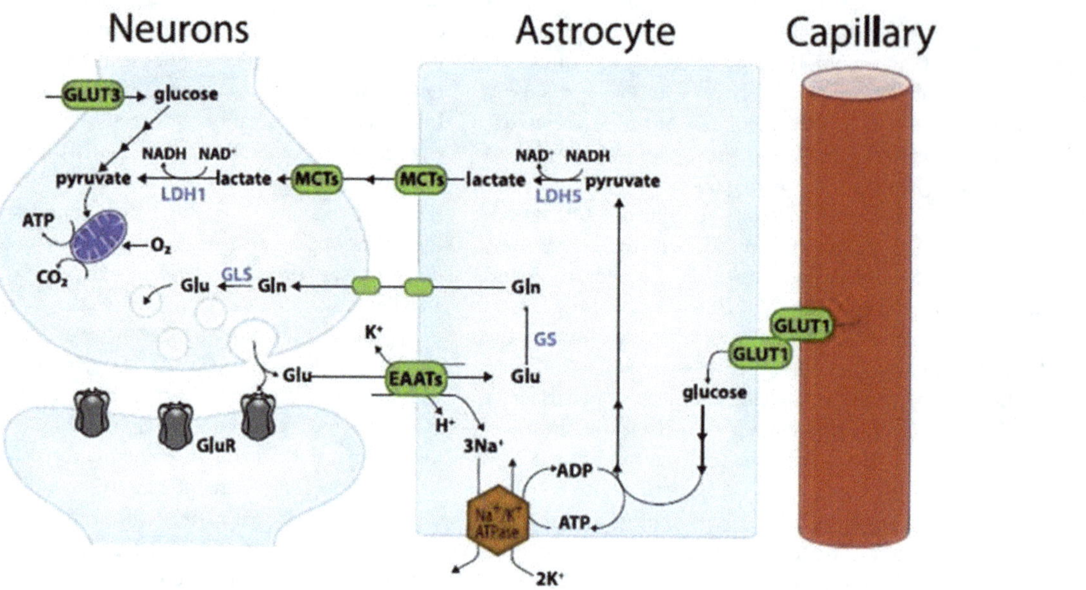

FIGURE 1 | Schematic representation of the astrocyte-neuron lactate shuttle model (with permission from Bélanger et al., 2011). Glu, glutamate; Gln, glutamine; GluR, glutamatergic receptor; EAATs, excitatory amino acid transporters; GLUT, glucose transporter; MCTs, monocarboxylate transporters; LDH, lactate dehydrogenase; GS, glutaminase; GLS, glutamine synthetase.

This gradient exists since concentrations of glucose in plasma and CSF are approximately 5 mM (Psychogios et al., 2011) and 3 mM (Wishart et al., 2008) respectively, with a CSF:plasma glucose ratio typically being approximately 0.4–0.8 (Leen et al., 2012). GLUT1 is specific to astrocytes and cerebral blood vessels, GLUT3 is exclusively localized at neurons, and GLUT5, primarily a fructose transporter, is found in microglia (Vannucci et al., 1997).

Other important regulating proteins in neuroenergetics are: pyruvate dehydrogenase, the rate-limiting enzyme that catalyzes lactate oxidation in astrocytes, with the inactive form being greater in astrocytes than in neurons (Itoh et al., 2003); lactate dehydrogenase (LDH), of which isoenzymes are found to be specific to astrocytes (LDH-5: associated with glycolysis) and neurons (LDH-1: associated with oxidative metabolism) (Bittar et al., 1996; Laughton et al., 2000); and monocarboxylate transporters (MCTs), proton-linked transporters of lactate with localization of subtypes MCT2 to neurons (with high affinity for lactate) and MCT1 and MCT4 to blood vessels and astrocytes, respectively (with lower affinity for lactate) (Bergersen, 2007). The kinetics of these regulating proteins supports the concept of a flux of lactate from astrocyte to neuron. Most recently in literature there has been renewed vigor in the research in the role of MCTs (Bourgeois et al., 2016; Chaumeil et al., 2016; Karagiannis et al., 2016; Kolko et al., 2016; Lee and Kang, 2016; Pérez-Escuredo et al., 2016; Rosafio et al., 2016). Hence, we are entering an era in science whereby we are recognizing that understanding not only shuttles, but the means by which shuttles operate—transporters (e.g., MCTs), are integral toward unraveling new information of the complex dynamic processes found in neuroenergetics.

Astrocytes are therefore viewed as "lactate sources" supplying the extracellular lactate pool, and neurons as "lactate sinks" consuming lactate oxidatively in response to energy demands. The transfer of lactate from astrocyte to neuron can be viewed as a spatially and temporally independent process (Pellerin and Magistretti, 2004). Thus, the metabolic plasticity of astrocytes is likely to be associated with synaptic plasticity (Magistretti, 2006). Magistretti (2000, 2009) sums up the ANLS model in terms of neurometabolic coupling in which sodium-coupled uptake of glutamate by astrocytes activates Na^+-K^+-ATPase, which triggers glucose uptake and its glycolytic processing. This results in the production and release of lactate that is used by neurons for activity-dependent energy demands. It has become generally accepted that lactate is a pivotal component in neuronal brain energy homeostasis (Schurr et al., 1999a; Pellerin, 2003, 2010; Gladden, 2004; Schurr, 2006; van Hall et al., 2009).

Controversy Surrounding the ANLS Hypothesis–Is this the New Paradigm?

Since its introduction, the ANLS has received much attention, some of which criticizes and refutes the concept; however, substantial evidence has accumulated from independent sources that supports the model. Based on *in vitro* and *in vivo* studies (Kuhr and Korf, 1988; Pellerin et al., 2002, 2007; Itoh et al., 2003; Smith et al., 2003; Pellerin and Magistretti, 2004; Hashimoto et al., 2008; Sampol et al., 2013), there exists experimental evidence that neurons use lactate derived from astroglial metabolism efficiently as energy substrates to preserve normal neuronal function. The lactate shuttle concept at the core of the ANLS was further supported by studies on the critical role of glutamate transporters (Pierre et al., 2000; Voutsinos-Porche et al., 2003) and distribution of MCTs in the brain (Pierre et al., 2000; Chiry et al., 2008; Erlichman et al., 2008; Robinet and Pellerin, 2011), particularly for long-term memory formation (Suzuki et al., 2011).

Molecular mechanisms provide further *in vitro* evidence that supports the ANLS hypothesis (Bliss et al., 2004; Porras et al., 2004), showing that upregulation of glycolysis in neurons decreased oxidation of glucose through the pentose phosphate pathway, resulting in impaired regeneration of reduced glutathione, and subsequently oxidative stress and apoptotic death. Thus, neurons downregulate glycolysis in order to use available glucose to maintain antioxidant status (a neuroprotective mechanism) at the expense of its use for bioenergetics purposes. Neuroenergetic demands can be met by other sources, such as lactate (Tabernero et al., 1996; Herrero-Mendez et al., 2009).

Rouach et al. (2008) demonstrated *in vitro* the change in character of astrocyte metabolic networks in response to local energy demand and trafficking of energetic metabolites from blood vessels, through astrocytes, to distal neurons. Using ^{13}C-NMR, this metabolic flux of lactate from astrocyte to neuron can be measured noninvasively in the human brain (Bouzier-Sore et al., 2003; Gallagher et al., 2009; Boumezbeur et al., 2010). Plasma lactate supports up to 10% of brain energy metabolism under physiological conditions, and up to 60% under supra-physiological conditions. Mathematical modeling studies have also described these dynamics, in particular brain lactate kinetics (Aubert et al., 2005) and compartmentalization of brain energy metabolism (Aubert and Costalat, 2005). However, as stated by Pellerin et al. (2007): "[mathematical modeling] ... can give a coherent, quantitative framework for the discussion, suggest possible mechanisms or, conversely, emphasize the contradictions or implausibility or some hypotheses." An example of the argument about the possible ambiguity of mathematical modeling is given by Genc et al. (2011). This sentiment is further expressed by Jolivet et al. (2010): "mathematical models are very powerful tools but they are ultimately only partial replicas of the system they model, not the system itself." Thus, mathematical models are useful guides but one should be mindful to draw definitive conclusions based on modeling studies alone. Jolivet et al. (2010) commented on two mathematical studies of hypotheses of opposing lactate flux in neuroenergetics—they compared the mathematical model of ANLS by Aubert et al. (2007) and the neuron-to-astrocyte lactate shuttle (NALS) by Mangia et al. (2009). Jolivet et al. (2010) concluded that the Aubert (ANLS) model currently remains the best biophysical representation of neuron–astrocyte metabolic interactions. Further multi-timescale mathematical modeling by Jolivet et al. (2015) has since provided further support for the ANLS hypothesis.

While less vocal, there remains strong opposition to the ANLS hypothesis, with various studies expressing divergent views. Dienel and Hertz (2001) emphasized the paradox of intense production of lactate by the brain and the slow rate of its uptake, thus disagreeing that lactate is used as a major neuronal fuel. Dienel and Cruz (2003, 2004) further argued that cerebral metabolic rates of oxygen consumption do not equal that of glucose plus glycogen and that this disproportionate consumption is strong evidence against stoichiometric transfer of lactate from astrocytes to neighboring neurons for oxidation. Gjedde et al. (2002) averred that, based on their experimental evidence, changes in metabolism in afferent phase (activity involving presynaptic terminals and astrocytes) and efferent phase (activity involving neurons) are additive. This view opposed the idea that changes in metabolism are characterized by significant transfer of lactate from astrocyte to neurons. Gjedde et al. (2002) conclude that there is no suggestion that astrocytic glycolysis supports oxidative metabolism of neurons in the baseline condition. Instead, neurons increase their oxidative metabolism in parallel with a rise in pyruvate generated by neuronal rather than astrocytic glycolysis (Gjedde and Marrett, 2001). Mangia et al. (2003a) discussed various ambiguities from other studies and conclude that astrocyte activation supports only the glutamate–glutamine cycle and that neurons primarily metabolize directly absorbed glucose to support neuronal activity. This behavior is demonstrated by an initial dip in lactate concentrations following visual stimulation (Mangia et al., 2003b). As mentioned above, Mangia et al. (2009) also proposed a model of opposite flux to the ANLS, namely the NALS hypothesis which utilized the mathematical model introduced by Simpson et al. (2007), suggesting that depending on the thermodynamic and kinetic status of the cytosolic and mitochondrial redox states, lactate transfers from neurons to astrocytes. The directionality of the ANLS hypothesis (i.e., lactate from astrocytes to neurons), has been covered in many reviews. However, the other perspective of shuttling direction (i.e., from neurons to astrocytes) is an intriguing one, albeit without substantiated experimental proof of the NALS, beyond modeling. Other divergent views come from studies by, for example, Bak et al. (2006), who suggested that synaptic activity does not induce corresponding upregulation of lactate metabolism in neurons; DiNuzzo et al. (2010a), who suggested that carbon recruitment by neurons relies upon glucose uptake rather than that of a lactate shuttle, and that glycogenolysis in astrocytes preserves glucose availability for neurons (DiNuzzo et al., 2010b).

Others have critically reviewed the ANLS hypothesis in defense of the traditional role of neuroenergetics (Chih et al., 2001; Chih and Roberts, 2003). Pellerin and Magistretti (2011) not only addressed all these divergent views by reviewing experimental evidence supporting the main tenets of the ANLS model, but also were able to confute several unfounded criticisms. With overwhelming support for the ANLS hypothesis, it was becoming clear that lactate is a crucial element in neuronal brain energy homeostasis (Schurr et al., 1999b; Pellerin, 2003, 2010; Gladden, 2004; Schurr, 2006; van Hall et al., 2009). However, as is the case in science, refuting evidence continues to challenge the foundations of the ANLS hypothesis, leading to it being redefined and strengthened over time. The tenets of this hypothesis continue to hold, begging the question—is this the new paradigm for homeostatic neuroenergetics?

NEUROPATHOLOGY AND THE HUMAN RESPONSE

Beyond Homeostasis

Biological processes maintain stability, by detecting environmental (external) and physiological (internal) changes, and activating specialized adaptive responses. The dynamic metabolic characteristics of astrocytes lend them to being particularly adept at such a task within the neuronal framework of homeostasis. Beyond homeostasis lies the comparatively new concept of allostasis. Allostasis is an extension of the concept of homeostasis and refers to the maintenance of stability by means of robust, energy-demanding adaptive mechanisms in response to severe physical, psychosocial or environmental challenges. Homeostasis involves maintaining a *stable* internal environment of an organism (i.e., by means of a *feedback* mechanism), whereas allostasis is more *dynamic* in that it involves the continuous response to physiological needs, resulting in biochemical *adaptive* mechanisms. These two concepts seem similar and are not intended to operate independently; instead, allostasis supports homeostasis, placing emphasis on flexible adaptation with the ultimate goal of maintaining a stable internal environment (McEwen, 2006, 2008; Logan and Barksdale, 2008; McEwen and Gianaros, 2011; Danese and McEwen, 2012). Frequent or chronic challenges (e.g., neuroinflammation) produce dysregulation of several major physiological systems by triggering chemical mediators of adaption that operate in a nonlinear network. The cumulative "wear and tear" associated with the inability to disengage these physiological systems is referred to as allostatic load. In vulnerable biological systems an allostatic overload prevails that results in the development of disease.

Since the term was first coined, by Sterling and Eyer (1988), the concept of allostasis has primarily been used in the literature to describe mild perturbations that are stress related, psychosomatic and/or psychopathological (Tannenbaum et al., 2002; Stewart, 2006; Shannon et al., 2007; Logan and Barksdale, 2008; Blair et al., 2011; Danese and McEwen, 2012; Tomiyama et al., 2012). As a concept allostasis is still being developed and so is gradually being applied to more diverse fields, such as metabolic diseases and lipidomics (Oresic et al., 2008) and metabolomics (Ramautar et al., 2013). Allostasis has also been used to explain extreme glucose fluctuations as reflecting the body's inability to cope with allostatic load in the case of chronic illness, predisposing the individual to serious harm as manifested by heightened mortality (Stumvoll et al., 2003, 2004; Rake et al., 2010).

Herein this review the typology, as given by Peters and McEwen (2015) to describe cardiovascular disease, has been adapted to define terms in neuroenergetics. Stress occurs in a state of increased cerebral energy demand to safeguard an individual's physical, mental and social well-being. A reversible stress response distinguishes allostasis from homeostasis and can be indicated by a relief result (restored homeostasis) in which the individual returns toward physiological normality. An allostatic load is indicated by an acute stress challenge—an irreversible or nearly irreversible state of allostatic stress from homeostasis—as seen in severely elevated CSF lactate in acute, physical damage to the brain (Gallagher et al., 2009). Chronic cases of persistently highly elevated CSF lactate and lactate:pyruvate ratios would be parameters to define the transition of allostatic load toward allostatic overload (disease).

Thus, allostasis encompasses typical dynamic adaptations to transient stress mediators; allostatic load pertains to an acute state of persistent perturbation and, ultimately, circumstances of allostatic overload are associated with disease and the body's inability to cope. These terms are henceforth discussed in terms of neuropathological conditions, with the focus on lactate and its shuttles.

Microglia–Addressing Neuronal Allostasis

Under pathological conditions, such as caused by infection, the brain enters a state of allostasis and microglia become activated. Microglia are immunocompetent cells that act as the intrinsic macrophages of the brain, bearing multiple similarities to those of macrophages in peripheral tissues. Some of the shared functions include phagocytosis, antigen presentation, effector inflammatory response and production of various cytotoxins and cytokines. Thus, microglia are an important component of both the innate and adaptive immune response to central nervous system (CNS) pathogens (Olson and Miller, 2004). They populate the entire brain parenchyma with a homogeneous distributed network with territorial organization and act as the first and only line of defense in the brain.

Under physiological conditions microglia exist in a resting ("ramified") state characterized by a small soma and numerous thin, branched processes (Giaume et al., 2007). Microglia remain quiescent until activated upon by brain insult (i.e., injury, disease or infection), characterized by proliferation and immunophenotypical (expression of various surface markers and ion channels) and morphological (transformation to amoeboid morphology) changes (Eder, 1998). The response of microglia to brain insult is first to detect the site of assault by constant dynamic monitoring of the surrounding micro-environment, and then to send out process extensions toward the lesion site where process tips reorganize to confine, control and eliminate the source of the disturbance.

Neuroinflammation, the reaction of surrounding brain tissue to brain insult, is characterized by synthesis of various inflammatory mediators and reactive gliosis, associated with phenotypic changes and proliferation of glia (both astrocytes and microglia), in response to a dynamically changing environment (Giaume et al., 2007). The modified phenotype of astrocytes, from basal to reactive state, results in them abandoning their neuroprotective role, allowing excessive oxidative stress and production of ROS, and subsequently ROS-induced neuronal damage (Pellerin, 2003). Chronic neuroinflammation, the response to sustained and widespread stimuli, typically occurs due to either disease (e.g., Alzheimer's and multiple sclerosis) or persistent infection by viruses (Olson et al., 2001; Ovanesov et al., 2008) or bacteria (e.g., chronic meningitis as in TBM). The role of microglia in CNS infections was extensively reviewed by Rock et al. (2004). Hence, metabolic coupling of microglia is essential during neuronal allostasis, especially in response to pathogens.

THE BRAIN IN CRISIS

Allostatic Load–Physical Brain Trauma

The topic of traumatic brain injury (TBI)—acute, physical damage to the brain—gained notoriety in 2009 when Jeanne Marie Laskas wrote an article titled "Game brain" in GQ magazine (Laskas, 2009), exposing the hidden, negative medical implications within some popular, professional contact sports. In 2015 this was expanded into a book (Laskas, 2015) and a film called "Concussion," about forensic pathologist Bennet Omalu and his attempts to publicize his scientific findings regarding physical contact sports (such as in the National Football League, the apex of American football). Omalu postulated that persistent mild TBI leads to chronic traumatic encephalopathy. Consequently, there has been renewed research into concussion and TBI (Sone et al., 2016; Sussman et al., 2016), making it another hot topic in neuroscience.

It is well recognized that there is an elevation of brain extracellular lactate and the lactate:pyruvate ratio in TBI cases (Gallagher et al., 2009). The group of Gallagher et al. (2009) and Carpenter et al. (2014) presented direct evidence of brain utilization of lactate in TBI cases by administration of ^{13}C-labeled lactate via a microdialysis catheter and using ^{13}C-NMR analysis. Based on these studies, Carpenter et al. (2015) suggested that where neurons are too damaged to use the lactate produced from glucose by astrocytes (i.e., by uncoupling of neuronal and glial metabolism), high extracellular levels of lactate would accumulate—explaining the association between high lactate and poor outcome. Thus, therapeutic intervention before metabolic uncoupling is imperative. Glucose administration after TBI has been shown to be beneficial but there is a correlation between hyperglycemia and increased infection or mortality; hence, alternative sources of energy, such as lactate, may improve outcome (Moro et al., 2013). However, as with the ANLS model, there are opposing opinions of the notion that lactate is a preferential fuel in TBI cases (Dienel, 2014).

Acute administration of exogenous fuels, such as lactate, after experimentally induced TBI in rats has been shown to attenuate histopathology and improve outcome (Chen et al., 2000). In two companion reports by Glenn et al. (2015a,b), evidence was provided that central venous tracer infusion of both glucose and lactate showed massive mobilization of mainly lactate—systematic lactate was preferentially being directly consumed and used by TBI cases. Thus, there is a high production and clearance rate of lactate in TBI cases. The role of this lactate in cerebral metabolism following TBI and the advantages of treatment by exogenous lactate infusions was reviewed by Brooks and Martin (2015). In recent clinical trials of TBI, and other neurocritical care cases, the beneficial properties of hypertonic lactate have been observed with respect to cerebral blood flow and intracranial pressure (Bouzat and Oddo, 2014; Patet et al., 2016). Thus, accumulating evidence points to lactate being an important component used during allostatic load caused by acute, physical damage to the brain—a therapeutic target.

Allostatic Overload–Neurodegenerative Diseases

A common trait among neurodegenerative diseases is perturbed brain energy metabolism (Magistretti and Pellerin, 1996; Beal, 2000; Bélanger et al., 2011; Albanese et al., 2016). Huntington's disease and multiple sclerosis have been linked to mitochondrial dysfunction, and so are susceptible to oxidative stress and energy deficits (Dutta et al., 2006; Regenold et al., 2008; Sack, 2010; Gouarné et al., 2013); with implications of perturbed lactate levels. In contradiction, two ^{1}H-NMR studies found conflicting results regarding lactate in Huntington's disease. An ^{1}H-NMR investigation by Gårseth et al. (2000) reported decreased levels of lactate, which they attributed to neuronal loss, but based upon only a small sample ($n = 7$). Another ^{1}H-NMR study, by Verwaest et al. (2011), found lactate to be significantly increased, but this result was also based on a small sample ($n = 10$). In a more comprehensive study, Gouarné et al. (2013) used cultured neuronal subpopulations from transgenic mice and provided evidence that neurons use lactate, along with pyruvate, as an energy source to support respiration. The importance of lactate was corroborated by a study (Covarrubias-Pinto et al., 2015) on Huntington's disease (HD) using ascorbic acid to inhibit use of neuronal glucose—showing the favoring of lactate uptake to sustain brain activity. Hence, experimental evidence is emerging that lactate is important and used preferentially as an energy source in HD cases.

Two reviews on neurodegenerative diseases support the ANLS hypothesis and its role in neuropathology—namely, lactate is neuroprotective and a therapeutic agent. A review by Newington et al. (2013) refers to their previous scientific work, which showed that increased lactate production proved to be protective against Aβ-induced neuronal toxicity that is inherently associated with Alzheimer's disease. A review by Finsterwald et al. (2015) summarizes numerous studies involving astrocytic lactate in treatments for multiple neurodegenerative diseases [Alzheimer's, Parkinson's disease and amyotrophic lateral sclerosis (ALS)]. Finsterwald et al. (2015) concluded that astrocytic function elicits intrinsic neuroprotective properties through, amongst others, the ANLS mechanism. One could go one step further and speculate that a "specialized" type of ANLS mechanism is necessary.

In multiple sclerosis (MS) there have been reports of the importance of CSF lactate. A negative correlation between the presence of lactate and the presence of inflammatory plaques and MS severity has been experimentally shown (Lutz et al., 2007; Albanese et al., 2016)—increased lactate in MS cases without plaques and vice versa, suggesting close metabolic coupling between plaque activity and lactate production. A gene expression study by Zeis et al. (2015) revealed alterations (downregulation) in the ANLS mechanism in MS, such that alternative lactate shuttle systems may be at play. Indeed, other studies have proposed such shuttle systems to supply demyelinated axons with lactate as an important energy source—namely, the astrocyte-axon lactate shuttle (Cambron et al., 2012; Nijland et al., 2015) and the oligodendrocyte-axon lactate shuttle (Campbell et al., 2014).

A common thread seen in these studies of neurodegenerative diseases is the perturbation of lactate. Evidence in neuropathophysiological cases indicates that lactate acts as an important, sometimes preferential, source of energy, and also has neuroprotective properties. The role of lactate shuttle systems is also emerging as being vital—imperative as supply and demand needs fluctuate to extremes in situations of allostatic overload. This is when normal physiological systems can no longer provide the required resources and/or effects. It is, however, important to note that neuropathologically activated astrocytes, as well as other glial cells, such as microglia, may support mechanisms, such as neuroinflammation, aggravating neuronal degeneration (Li et al., 2011). The dynamics behind addressing neuroinflammation caused by an invading pathogen involves the use of microglia.

In the remainder of this review an adaptation of the ANLS model—the AMLS model (Mason et al., 2015)—is discussed in terms of TBM; a chronic, infectious neuroinflammatory disease.

Pathogen-Induced Chronic Neuroinflammation

In the case of a chronic infection in the brain by a persistent pathogen, such as *Mycobacterium tuberculosis* (Mtb), the bacillus responsible for TBM, there is sustained allostatic overload. Here, the microglia strive to eradicate the scourge but unwittingly become the habitat of the persisting pathogen. Similar to the ANLS hypothesis, the AMLS model proposes that when the brain is in crisis due to infection, energy flow in brain metabolism is shifted away from the neurons, and shunted toward the microglia (see **Figure 2**). The initial mechanics of the AMLS remain the same as the ANLS, the only difference being the directionality of the lactate upon exiting the astrocyte. The AMLS hypothesis postulates that in neuroinflammatory infectious diseases, such as TBM, lactate produced through glycolysis in astrocytes participates in the activated immune response and, in association with ketones and gluconeogenic amino acids, is collectively directed from the neurons preferentially into microglia. Within the microglia, lactate is expected to enter the mitochondrial Krebs cycle, contributing to oxidative phosphorylation and hence producing high levels of ATP and forms of ROS, such as hydrogen peroxide, required for degradation of the invading pathogen. Thus, the AMLS hypothesis uses the same line of logic of the ANLS model, but instead the microglia are the prime focus under conditions of neuroinflammatory infectious diseases; increased astrocytic lactate is directed toward the microglia.

Using the same CSF samples from the study by Mason et al. (2015), it was shown in a targeted analysis (Mason et al., 2016a) that the highly elevated amounts of lactate observed in the CSF of confirmed TBM cases was only in the L-form (L-lactate is produced by the host, whereas D-lactate is of bacterial origin). Thus, elevated lactate found in the CSF of TBM cases is solely a response by the host to the infection. These results from this follow-up study by Mason et al. (2016a) provide experimental evidence to support the proposed AMLS model and highlight the fact that lactate plays an important role in neuroinflammatory diseases, such as TBM. Activation of microglia, as required in the AMLS hypothesis, does not, however, present a uniform process and involves intricate interactions and feedback loops between the microglia, astrocytes and neurons that hamper attempts to construct basic and linear cascades of cause and effect; TBM involves a complex integration of the responses from the various cell types present within the CNS, with microglia and the astrocytes as main players.

During the course of a neuroinflammatory infectious disease, such as TBM, the ANLS is not only inadequate but, indeed, a liability as activated neurons will only become vulnerable to neurodestructive components. The bypassing of metabolic energy intermediates from the neurons effectively inactivates them to protect them from neurodestructive agents in response to chronic neuroinflammation. This neuron inactivation is evident from a clinical viewpoint as the progression of TBM is reflected by reduced scoring in the Glasgow Coma Score—specifically, decreased consciousness and awareness. The AMLS hypothesis can thus be viewed as invoking a persistent allostatic overload state that becomes activated when allostatic mechanisms fail and the body enters into a diseased state. The regulation of dynamic systems that function within the brain, in terms of homeostasis, allostasis and disease states, is delicate. Chronic activation of microglia can lead to neuropathological sequelae (Streit et al., 2004), and is also linked to neuropathic pain (Raghavendra et al., 2003). The persistent activation of microglia can be viewed as the proverbial double-edged sword—simultaneously exhibiting neuroprotective and neurodestructive properties in an attempt to save the whole at the expense of the part (Hall et al., 1998; Giaume et al., 2007).

Using TBM as an example of an infectious neuroinflammatory disease—an extreme scenario of allostatic overload—it can be speculated that the Mtb-induced host and microbe markers can reflect: (1) the disease state on admission to hospital, and (2) differentiation in the restoration toward a new condition of homeostasis following treatment. Upon admission to hospital, most TBM patients present with moderate to severe symptoms of ketosis. Metabolomics analysis of the urine (Mason et al., 2016b) substantiates this clinical picture through a ketosis urinary biosignature—cases admitted to hospital with very high ketosis biomarkers tended to have a poor prognosis, leading to severe neurological complications irrespective of treatment. A similar profile was also reflected in the CSF biochemistry (Mason et al., 2016a); as the TBM disease progressed into its later stages there was a deterioration in patient prognosis. Hence, in more advanced TBM stages there is less CSF lactate and therefore fewer energy substrates available for microglia activity, and decreased protection of neurons. During this period, irreversible neurological damage can begin to occur—illustrating the importance of lactate levels during periods of chronic neuroinflammation.

The concept of lactate shuttle systems extends to other types of neuronal cells, such as the oligodendrocyte–axon lactate shuttle (Baltan, 2015) and the Bergmann glia (BG) Purkinje cell (PC) lactate shuttle (Sawada et al., 2016). Lactate shuttles extend beyond the brain—they are of particular interest in cancer research (Pizzuto et al., 2012). Several cancer studies have suggested a tumor-to-stroma coupling via a lactate shuttle in

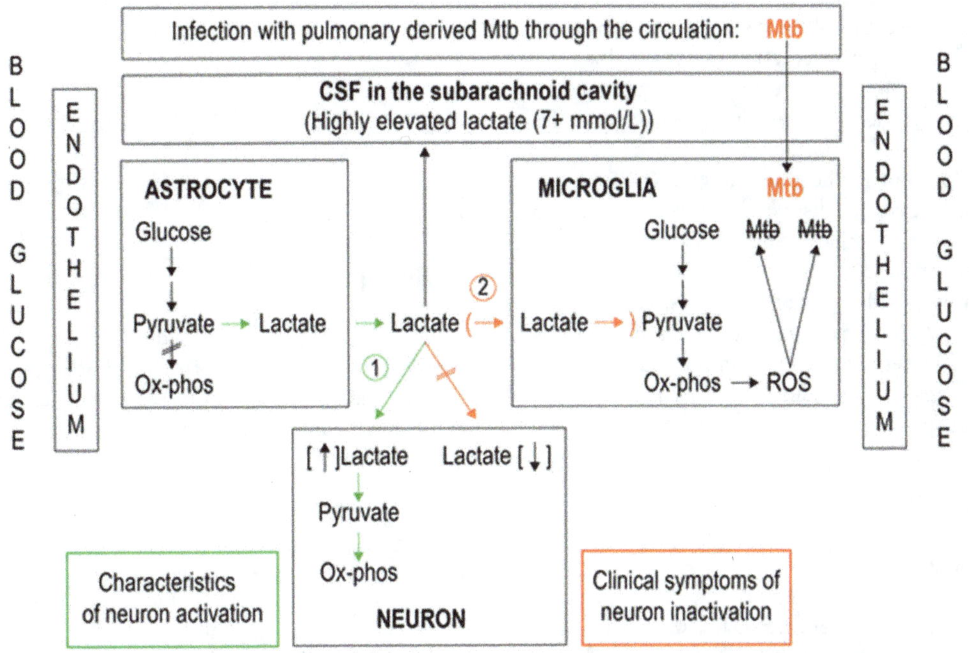

FIGURE 2 | Representation of metabolic pathways of two lactate shuttles within the central nervous system. (1) The astrocyte–neuron lactate shuttle (ANLS; green pathway) operates under normal physiological conditions with astrocytes responding to glutamatergic activation by increasing their rate of glucose utilization and release of lactate in the extracellular space, making the lactate available for neurons to sustain their energy demands. (2) The astrocyte–microglia lactate shuttle (AMLS; red pathway) proposed for tuberculous meningitis (TBM). Astrocytes respond to signaling from *Mycobacterium tuberculosis* (Mtb)-infected microglia by increasing glucose mobilization, leading to increased extracellular lactate, reflected in increased cerebrospinal fluid (CSF) lactate levels. Lactate used by microglia as an additional energy source for reactive oxygen species (ROS) production aimed at destroying the invading Mtb.

cancer cells (Pértega-Gomes et al., 2014; Sanità et al., 2014). These studies indicate that over-propagation of cells is strongly dependent upon the anaplerotic role of increased lactate uptake (Whitaker-Menezes et al., 2011; Fiaschi et al., 2012). This concept is supported by a large-scale *in silico* metabolic model (Capuani et al., 2015). Interestingly, Somashekar et al. (2011) stated that their most relevant metabolic observations in studying tuberculosis are similar to metabolic changes seen in cancer during tumor development—corroborated by Zhou et al. (2015). Conceptually, the "Reverse Warburg Effect" (Pavlides et al., 2009), proposed as operating in tumor cells, has been interpreted to be analogous to the astrocyte–neuron metabolic coupling (Pavlides et al., 2010), where the astrocytes resemble cancer-associated fibroblasts and the neuron the epithelial tumor cells, resulting in their higher proliferative capacity.

The regulation of lactate shuttles has been discussed as being a potential therapeutic target in cancer research (Draoui and Feron, 2011; Sanità et al., 2014). While disruption of transport of lactate into cancerous cells (i.e., reducing lactate shuttling into cancerous cells) is considered beneficial, upregulation in neuropathological cases shows merit for research. Several studies have demonstrated that intracerebroventricular or intravenous injection of lactate yields a neuroprotective effect during experimentally induced hypoglycemia or cerebral ischemia (Berthet et al., 2009, 2012; Wyss et al., 2011). In addition, other experimental work (Yamanishi et al., 2006; Gordon et al., 2008) has shown that lactate increases cerebral blood flow (vasodilation)—increasing the supply of metabolic (e.g., energy) substrates during allostasis. Thus, lactate has a potentially beneficial role in the clinical management of several neurological disorders (Taher et al., 2016). This review, like the others cited here, therefore shows that further research into the role of lactate and its shuttling mechanism(s) are certainly warranted to address neuroenergetics and neuropathology.

CONCLUDING REMARKS

In summary, we are seeing the prevailing school of thought moving away from the neurocentric paradigm, albeit with divergent views, toward that of one that is more integrated. Within this emerging new paradigm, an unraveling of the intricacies of the complex and diverse dynamic interactions of the human brain at the metabolic and cellular levels is occurring. Our current knowledge has led us to the realization that lactate shuttle systems, both intracellular and extracellular, play a far more pivotal role than originally considered. Indeed, there exist numerous other shuttles in neuroenergetics—for example: the lactate-alanine shuttle (Zwingman et al., 2000); the astrocyte–neuron ketone body shuttle (Guzmán and Blázquez, 2001); the glycerol phosphate shuttle (McKenna et al., 2006); and the malate-aspartate shuttle (McKenna et al., 2006; Moffett et al., 2013). Each in its own right is essential in terms of both homeostasis and allostasis. It is evident that transitions between different states of homeostasis and allostasis, and disease, are dynamic—they are often difficult to distinguish and/or control. However, the role of neuroenergetics is undeniable in the brain's constant objective of protecting itself and trying to maintain an optimum state. Here, we have discussed, in terms of neuroenergetics, the role of lactate in a shuttle system during homeostasis (ANLS) and in the infected state (AMLS). Other studies on neurodegenerative diseases have described complex pathophysiological changes that highlighted the importance of lactate (Newington et al., 2013; Finsterwald et al., 2015). There is thus overwhelming evidence that astrocytes, lactate and the associated shuttle systems so far recognized in combination are of crucial importance in neuroenergetics—in both the healthy and diseased state. Perhaps not surprisingly, the latest technology has revealed that neuro(patho)physiological metabolism is far more complex than originally thought and that further knowledge of the lactate shuttle systems apparently operating, as outlined in this article, is key to our understanding of the mechanisms involved.

AUTHOR CONTRIBUTIONS

The author confirms being the sole contributor of this work and approved it for publication.

FUNDING

Research funding was provided by the Technological Innovation Agency (TIA) of the Department of Science and Technology of South Africa. Opinions expressed and conclusions arrived at, are those of the author and are not necessarily to be attributed to the funding body TIA.

REFERENCES

Albanese, M., Zagaglia, S., Landi, D., Boffa, L., Nicoletti, C. G., Marciani, M. G., et al. (2016). Cerebrospinal fluid lactate is associated with multiple sclerosis disease progression. *J. Neuroinflamm.* 13:36. doi: 10.1186/s12974-016-0502-1

Angamo, E. A., Röesner, J., Liotta, A., Kovács, R., and Heinemann, U. (2016). A neuronal lactate uptake inhibitor slows recovery of extracellular ion concentration changes in the hippocampal CA3 region by affecting energy metabolism. *J. Neurophysiol.* 116, 2420–2430. doi: 10.1152/jn.003 27.2016

Attwell, D., and Laughlin, S. B. (2001). An energy budget for signaling in the grey matter of the brain. *J. Cereb. Blood Flow Metab.* 21, 1133–1145. doi: 10.1097/00004647-200110000-00001

Aubert, A., Costalat, R., Magistretti, P. J., and Pellerin, L. (2005). Brain lactate kinetics: modeling evidence for neuronal lactate uptake upon activation. *Proc. Natl. Acad. Sci. U.S.A.* 102, 16448–16453. doi: 10.1073/pnas.0505427102

Aubert, A., and Costalat, R. (2005). Interaction between astrocytes and neurons studied using a mathematical model of compartmentalized energy metabolism. *J. Cereb. Blood Flow Metab.* 25, 1476–1490. doi: 10.1038/sj.jcbfm. 9600144

Aubert, A., Pellerin, L., Magistretti, P. J., and Costalat, R. (2007). A coherent neurobiological framework for functional neuroimaging provided by a model integrating compartmentalized energy metabolism. *Proc. Natl. Acad. Sci. U.S.A.* 104, 4188–4193. doi: 10.1073/pnas.0605864104

Bak, L. K., Schousboe, A., Sonnewald, U., and Waagepetersen, H. S. (2006). Glucose is necessary to maintain neurotransmitter homeostasis during synaptic activity in cultured glutamatergic neurons. *J. Cereb. Blood Flow Metab.* 26, 1285–1297. doi: 10.1038/sj.jcbfm.9600281

Baltan, S. (2015). Can lactate serve as an energy substrate for axons in good times and in bad, in sickness and in health? *Metab. Brain Dis.* 30, 25–30. doi: 10.1007/s11011-014-9595-3

Beal, M. F. (2000). Energetics in the pathogenesis of neurodegenerative diseases. *Trends Neurosci.* 23, 298–304. doi: 10.1016/S0166-2236(00)01584-8

Bélanger, M., Allaman, I., and Magistretti, P. J. (2011). Brain energy metabolism: focus on astrocyte-neuron metabolic cooperation. *Cell Metab.* 14, 724–738. doi: 10.1016/j.cmet.2011.08.016

Bender, A. S., Young, L. P., and Norenberg, M. D. (1997). Effect of lactic acid on L-glutamate uptake in cultured astrocytes: mechanistic considerations. *Brain Res.* 750, 59–66. doi: 10.1016/S0006-8993(96)01331-5

Bergersen, L. H. (2007). Is lactate food for neurons? Comparison of monocarboxylate transporter subtypes in brain and muscle. *Neuroscience* 145, 11–19. doi: 10.1016/j.neuroscience.2006.11.062

Berthet, C., Lei, H., Thevenet, J., Gruetter, R., Magistretti, P. J., and Hirt, L. (2009). Neuroprotective role of lactate after cerebral ischemia. *J. Cereb. Blood Flow Metab.* 29, 1780–1789. doi: 10.1038/jcbfm.2009.97

Berthet, C., Castillo, X., Magistretti, P. J., and Hirt, L. (2012). New evidence of neuroprotection by lactate after transient focal cerebral ischaemia: extended benefit after intracerebroventricular injection and efficacy of intravenous administration. *Cerebrovasc. Dis.* 34, 329–335. doi: 10.1159/0003 43657

Bittar, P. G., Charnay, Y., Pellerin, L., Bouras, C., and Magistretti, P. J. (1996). Selective distribution of lactate dehydrogenase isoenzymes in neurons and astrocytes of human brain. *J. Cereb. Blood Flow Metab.* 16, 1079–1089. doi: 10.1097/00004647-199611000-00001

Blair, C., Raver, C. C., Granger, D., Mills-Koonce, R., and Hibel, L., (2011). Allostasis and allostatic load in the context of poverty in early childhood. *Dev. Psychopathol.* 23, 845–857. doi: 10.1017/S0954579411000344

Bliss, T. M., Ip, M., Cheng, E., Minami, M., Pellerin, L., Magistretti, P., et al. (2004). Dual-gene, dual-cell type therapy against an excitotoxic insult by bolstering neuroenergetics. *J. Neurosci.* 4, 6202–6208. doi: 10.1523/JNEUROSCI.0805-04.2004

Boumezbeur, F., Petersen, K. F., Cline, G. W., Mason, G. F., Behar, K. L., Shulman, G. I., et al. (2010). The contribution of blood lactate to brain energy metabolism in humans measured by dynamic 13C nuclear magnetic resonance spectroscopy. *J. Neurosci.* 30, 13983–13991. doi: 10.1523/JNEUROSCI.2040-10.2010

Bourgeois, N. M., Van Herck, S. L., Vancamp, P., Delbaere, J., Zevenbergen, C., Kersseboom, S., et al. (2016). Characterization of chicken thyroid hormone transporters. *Endocrinology* 157, 2560–2574. doi: 10.1210/en.2015-2025

Bouzat, P., and Oddo, M. (2014). Lactate and the injured brain: friend or foe? *Curr. Opin. Crit. Care* 20, 133–140. doi: 10.1097/MCC.0000000000000072

Bouzier-Sore, A. K., Merle, M., Magistretti, P. J., and Pellerin, L. (2002). Feeding active neurons: (re) emergence of a nursing role for astrocytes. *J. Physiol. Paris* 96, 273–282. doi: 10.1016/S0928-4257(02)00016-5

Bouzier-Sore, A. K., Serres, S., Canioni, P., and Merle, M. (2003). Lactate involvement in neuron–glia metabolic interaction: 13C-NMR spectroscopy contribution. *Biochimie* 85, 841–848. doi: 10.1016/j.biochi.2003.08.003

Brodersen, P., and Jorgensen, E. O. (1974). Cerebral blood flow and oxygen uptake, and cerebrospinal fluid biochemistry in severe coma. *J. Neurol. Neurosurg. Psychiatr.* 37, 384–391. doi: 10.1136/jnnp.37.4.384

Brooks, G. A. (1985). "Lactate: glycolytic end product and oxidative substrate during sustained exercise in mammals – the 'lactate shuttle'," in *Circulation, Respiration and Metabolism: Current Comparative Approaches*, ed R. Gilles (Berlin: Springer–Verlag), 208–218.

Brooks, G. A. (1986a). The lactate shuttle during exercise and recovery. *Med. Sci. Sports Exerc.* 18, 360–368.

Brooks, G. A. (1986b). Lactate production under fully aerobic conditions: the lactate shuttle during rest and exercise. *Fed. Proc.* 45, 2924–2929.

Brooks, G. A. (2000). Intra-and extra-cellular lactate shuttles. *Med. Sci. Sports Exerc.* 32, 790–799. doi: 10.1097/00005768-200004000-00011

Brooks, G. A. (2002). Lactate shuttles in nature. *Biochem. Soc. Trans.* 30, 258–264. doi: 10.1042/bst0300258

Brooks, G. A. (2009). Cell–cell and intracellular lactate shuttles. *J. Physiol.* 587, 5591–5600. doi: 10.1113/jphysiol.2009.178350

Brooks, G. A., and Martin, N. A. (2015). Cerebral metabolism following traumatic brain injury: new discoveries with implications for treatment. *Front. Neurosci.* 8:408. doi: 10.3389/fnins.2014.0040

Cambron, M., D'haeseleer, M., Laureys, G., Clinckers, R., Debruyne, J., and De Keyser, J. (2012). White-matter astrocytes, axonal energy metabolism, and axonal degeneration in multiple sclerosis. *J. Cereb. Blood Flow Metab.* 32, 413–424. doi: 10.1038/jcbfm.2011.193

Campbell, G. R., Worrall, J. T., and Mahad, D. J. (2014). The central role of mitochondria in axonal degeneration in multiple sclerosis. *Mult. Scler. J.* 20, 1806–1813. doi: 10.1177/1352458514544537

Capuani, F., De Martino, D., Marinari, E., and De Martino, A. (2015). Quantitative constraint-based computational model of tumor-to-stroma coupling via lactate shuttle. *Sci. Rep.* 5:11880. doi: 10.1038/srep11880

Carpenter, K. L., Jalloh, I., Gallagher, C. N., Grice, P., Howe, D. J., Mason, A., et al. (2014). 13C-labelled microdialysis studies of cerebral metabolism in TBI patients. *Eur. J. Pharm. Sci.* 57, 87–97. doi: 10.1016/j.ejps.2013.12.012

Carpenter, K. L., Jalloh, I., and Hutchinson, P. J. (2015). Glycolysis and the significance of lactate in traumatic brain injury. *Front. Neurosci.* 9:112. doi: 10.3389/fnins.2015.00112

Cater, H. L., Benham, C. D., and Sundstrom, L. E. (2001). Neuroprotective role of monocarboxylate transport during glucose deprivation in slice cultures of rat hippocampus. *J. Physiol.* 531, 459–466. doi: 10.1111/j.1469-7793.2001.0459i.x

Cater, H. L., Chandratheva, A., Benham, C. D., Morrison, B. III., and Sundstrom, L. E. (2003). Lactate and glucose as energy substrates during, and after, oxygen deprivation in rat hippocampal acute and cultured slices. *J. Neurochem.* 87, 1381–1390. doi: 10.1046/j.1471-4159.2003.02100.x

Chaumeil, M. M., Radoul, M., Najac, C., Eriksson, P., Viswanath, P., Blough, M. D., et al. (2016). Hyperpolarized 13C MR imaging detects no lactate production in mutant IDH1 gliomas: implications for diagnosis and response monitoring. *Neuroimage Clin.* 12, 180–189. doi: 10.1016/j.nicl.2016.06.018

Chen, T., Qian, Y. Z., Di, X., Rice, A., Zhu, J. P., and Bullock, R. (2000). Lactate/glucose dynamics after rat fluid percussion brain injury. *J. Neurotrauma* 17, 135–142. doi: 10.1089/neu.2000.17.135

Chen, Y., and Swanson, R. A. (2003). Astrocytes and brain injury. *J. Cereb. Blood Flow Metab.* 23, 137–149. doi: 10.1097/00004647-200302000-00001

Chih, C. P., Lipton, P., and Roberts, E. L. Jr. (2001). Do active cerebral neurons really use lactate rather than glucose? *Trends Neurosci.* 24, 573–578. doi: 10.1016/S0166-2236(00)01920-2

Chih, C. P., and Roberts, E. L. Jr. (2003). Energy substrates for neurons during neural activity: a critical review of the astrocyte-neuron lactate shuttle hypothesis. *J. Cereb. Blood Flow Metab.* 23, 1263–1281. doi: 10.1097/01.WCB.0000081369.51727.6F

Chiry, O., Fishbein, W. N., Merezhinskaya, N., Clarke, S., Galuske, R., Magistretti, P. J., et al. (2008). Distribution of the monocarboxylate transporter MCT2 in human cerebral cortex: an immunohistochemical study. *Brain Res.* 1226, 61–69. doi: 10.1016/j.brainres.2008.06.025

Covarrubias-Pinto, A., Moll, P., Solís-Maldonado, M., Acuña, A. I., Riveros, A., Miró, M. P., et al. (2015). Beyond the redox imbalance: oxidative stress contributes to an impaired GLUT3 modulation in Huntington's disease. *Free Radic. Biol. Med.* 89, 1085–1096. doi: 10.1016/j.freeradbiomed.2015.09.024

Cruz, R. S., de Aguiar, R. A., Turnes, T., Penteado Dos Santos, R., Fernandes Mendes de Oliveira, M., and Caputo, F. (2012). Intracellular shuttle: the lactate aerobic metabolism. *Scientific World J.* 2012:420984. doi: 10.1100/2012/420984

Danese, A., and McEwen, B. S. (2012). Adverse childhood experiences, allostasis, allostatic load, and age-related disease. *Physiol. Behav.* 106, 29–39. doi: 10.1016/j.physbeh.2011.08.019

Debernardi, R., Magistretti, P. J., and Pellerin, L. (1999). Trans-inhibition of glutamate transport prevents excitatory amino acid-induced glycolysis in astrocytes. *Brain Res.* 850, 39–46. doi: 10.1016/S0006-8993(99)02022-3

DeSalles, A. A., Kontos, H. A., Becker, D. P., Yang, M. S., Ward, J. D., Moulton, R., et al. (1986). Prognostic significance of ventricular CSF lactic acidosis in severe head injury. *J. Neurosurg.* 65, 615–624. doi: 10.3171/jns.1986.65.5.0615

De Salles, A. A., Muizelaar, J. P., and Young, H. F. (1987). Hyperglycemia, cerebrospinal fluid lactic acidosis, and cerebral blood flow in severely head-injured patients. *Neurosurgery* 21, 45–50. doi: 10.1227/00006123-198707000-00009

Dienel, G. A., and Hertz, L. (2001). Glucose and lactate metabolism during brain activation. *J. Neurosci. Res.* 66, 824–838. doi: 10.1002/jnr.10079

Dienel, G. A., and Cruz, N. F. (2003). Neighborly interactions of metabolically-activated astrocytes *in vivo*. *Neurochem. Int.* 43, 339–354. doi: 10.1016/S0197-0186(03)00021-4

Dienel, G. A., and Cruz, N. F. (2004). Nutrition during brain activation: does cell-to-cell lactate shuttling contribute significantly to sweet and sour food for thought? *Neurochem. Int.* 45, 321–351. doi: 10.1016/j.neuint.2003.10.011

Dienel, G. A. (2014). Lactate shuttling and lactate use as fuel after traumatic brain injury: metabolic considerations. *J. Cereb. Blood Flow Metab.* 34, 1736–1748. doi: 10.1038/jcbfm.2014.153

Dienel, G. A., and Cruz, N. F. (2015). Contributions of glycogen to astrocytic energetics during brain activation. *Metab. Brain Dis.* 30, 281–298. doi: 10.1007/s11011-014-9493-8

DiNuzzo, M., Mangia, S., Maraviglia, B., and Giove, F. (2010a). Changes in glucose uptake rather than lactate shuttle take center stage in subserving neuroenergetics: evidence from mathematical modeling. *J. Cereb. Blood Flow Metab.* 30, 586–602. doi: 10.1038/jcbfm.2009.232

DiNuzzo, M., Mangia, S., Maraviglia, B., and Giove, F. (2010b). Glycogenolysis in astrocytes supports blood-borne glucose channeling not glycogen-derived lactate shuttling to neurons: evidence from mathematical modeling. *J. Cereb. Blood Flow Metab.* 30, 1895–1904. doi: 10.1038/jcbfm.2010.151

Draoui, N., and Feron, O. (2011). Lactate shuttles at a glance: from physiological paradigms to anti-cancer treatments. *Dis. Model. Mech.* 4, 727–732. doi: 10.1242/dmm.007724

Dutta, R., McDonough, J., Yin, X., Peterson, J., Chang, A., Torres, T., et al. (2006). Mitochondrial dysfunction as a cause of axonal degeneration in multiple sclerosis patients. *Ann. Neurol.* 59, 478–489. doi: 10.1002/ana.20736

Eder, C. (1998). Ion channels in microglia (brain macrophages). *Am. J. Physiol. Cell Physiol.* 275, C327–C342.

Erlichman, J. S., Hewitt, A., Damon, T. L., Hart, M., Kurascz, J., Li, A., et al. (2008). Inhibition of monocarboxylate transporter 2 in the retrotrapezoid nucleus in rats: a test of the astrocyte–neuron lactate-shuttle hypothesis. *J. Neurosci.* 28, 4888–4896. doi: 10.1523/JNEUROSCI.5430-07.2008

Fiaschi, T., Marini, A., Giannoni, E., Taddei, M. L., Gandellini, P., De Donatis, A., et al. (2012). Reciprocal metabolic reprogramming through lactate shuttle coordinately influences tumor-stroma interplay. *Cancer Res.* 72, 5130–5140. doi: 10.1158/0008-5472.CAN-12-1949

Finsterwald, C., Magistretti, P. J., and Lengacher, S. (2015). Astrocytes: new targets for the treatment of neurodegenerative diseases. *Curr. Pharm. Des.* 21, 3570–3581. doi: 10.2174/1381612821666150710144502

Fox, P. T., Raichle, M. E., Mintun, M. A., and Dence, C. (1988). Nonoxidative glucose consumption during focal physiologic neural activity. *Science* 241, 462–464. doi: 10.1126/science.3260686

Gallagher, C. N., Carpenter, K. L., Grice, P., Howe, D. J., Mason, A., Timofeev, I., et al. (2009). The human brain utilizes lactate via the tricarboxylic acid cycle: a 13C-labelled microdialysis and high-resolution nuclear magnetic resonance study. *Brain* 132, 2839–2849. doi: 10.1093/brain/awp202

Gårseth, M., Sonnewald, U., White, L. R., Rød, M., Zwart, J. A., Nygaard, Ø., et al. (2000). Proton magnetic resonance spectroscopy of cerebrospinal fluid in neurodegenerative disease: indication of glial energy impairment in Huntington chorea, but not Parkinson disease. *J. Neurosci. Res.* 60, 779–782. doi: 10.1002/1097-4547(20000615)60:6<779::AID-JNR10>3.0.CO;2-M

Genc, S., Kurnaz, I. A., and Ozilgen, M. (2011). Astrocyte-neuron lactate shuttle may boost more ATP supply to the neuron under hypoxic conditions-*in silico* study supported by *in vitro* expression data. *BMC Syst. Biol.* 5:162. doi: 10.1186/1752-0509-5-162

Giaume, C., Kirchhoff, F., Matute, C., Reichenbach, A., and Verkhratsky, A. (2007). Glia: the fulcrum of brain diseases. *Cell Death Differ.* 14, 1324–1335. doi: 10.1038/sj.cdd.4402144

Giaume, C., Koulakoff, A., Roux, L., Holcman, D., and Rouach, N. (2010). Astroglial networks: a step further in neuroglial and gliovascular interactions. *Nature Rev. Neurosci.* 11, 87–99. doi: 10.1038/nrn2757

Gjedde, A., Marrett, S., and Vafaee, M. (2002). Oxidative and nonoxidative metabolism of excited neurons and astrocytes. *J. Cereb. Blood Flow Metab.* 22, 1–14. doi: 10.1097/00004647-200201000-00001

Gjedde, A., and Marrett, S. (2001). Glycolysis in neurons, not astrocytes, delays oxidative metabolism of human visual cortex during sustained checkerboard stimulation *in vivo*. *J. Cereb. Blood Flow Metab.* 21, 1384–1392. doi: 10.1097/00004647-200112000-00002

Gladden, L. B. (2004). Lactate metabolism: a new paradigm for the third millennium. *J. Physiol.* 558, 5–30. doi: 10.1113/jphysiol.2003.058701

Glenn, T. C., Martin, N. A., Horning, M. A., McArthur, D. L., Hovda, D. A., Vespa, P., et al. (2015a). Lactate: brain fuel in human traumatic brain injury: a comparison with normal healthy control subjects. *J. Neurotrauma* 32, 820–832. doi: 10.1089/neu.2014.3483

Glenn, T. C., Martin, N. A., McArthur, D. L., Hovda, D. A., Vespa, P., Johnson, M. L., et al. (2015b). Endogenous nutritive support after traumatic brain injury: peripheral lactate production for glucose supply via gluconeogenesis. *J. Neurotrauma* 32, 811–819. doi: 10.1089/neu.2014.3482

Gordon, G. R., Choi, H. B., Rungta, R. L., Ellis-Davies, G. C., and MacVicar, B. A. (2008). Brain metabolism dictates the polarity of astrocyte control over arterioles. *Nature* 456, 745–749. doi: 10.1038/nature07525

Gouarné, C., Tardif, G., Tracz, J., Latyszenok, V., Michaud, M., Clemens, L. E., et al. (2013). Early deficits in glycolysis are specific to striatal neurons from a rat model of huntington disease. *PLoS ONE* 8:e81528. doi: 10.1371/journal.pone.0081528

Guzmán, M., and Blázquez, C. (2001). Is there an astrocyte–neuron ketone body shuttle? *Trends Endocrinol. Metab.* 12, 169–173. doi: 10.1016/S1043-2760(00)00370-2

Hall, E. D., Oostveen, J. A., and Gurney, M. E. (1998). Relationship of microglial and astrocytic activation to disease onset and progression in a transgenic model of familial ALS. *Glia* 23, 249–256. doi: 10.1002/(SICI)1098-1136(199807)23:3<249::AID-GLIA7>3.0.CO;2-#

Hashimoto, T., Hussien, R., Cho, H. S., Kaufer, D., and Brooks, G. A. (2008). Evidence for the mitochondrial lactate oxidation complex in rat neurons: demonstration of an essential component of brain lactate shuttles. *PLoS ONE* 3:e2915. doi: 10.1371/journal.pone.0002915

Haydon, P. G., and Carmignoto, G. (2006). Astrocyte control of synaptic transmission and neurovascular coupling. *Physiol. Rev.* 86, 1009–1031. doi: 10.1152/physrev.00049.2005

Hertz, L., Dringen, R., Schousboe, A., and Robinson, S. R. (1999). Astrocytes: glutamate producers for neurons. *J. Neurosci. Res.* 57, 417–428. doi: 10.1002/(SICI)1097-4547(19990815)57:4<417::AID-JNR1>3.0.CO;2-N

Herrero-Mendez, A., Almeida, A., Fernández, E., Maestre, C., Moncada, S., and Bolaños, J. P. (2009). The bioenergetic and antioxidant status of neurons is controlled by continuous degradation of a key glycolytic enzyme by APC/C–Cdh1. *Nat. Cell Biol.* 11, 747–752. doi: 10.1038/ncb1881

Itoh, Y., Esaki, T., Shimoji, K., Cook, M., Law, M. J., Kaufman, E., et al. (2003). Dichloroacetate effects on glucose and lactate oxidation by neurons and astroglia *in vitro* and on glucose utilization by brain *in vivo*. *Proc. Natl. Acad. Sci. U.S.A.* 100, 4879–4884. doi: 10.1073/pnas.0831078100

Jolivet, R., Allaman, I., Pellerin, L., Magistretti, P. J., and Weber, B. (2010). Comment on recent modeling studies of astrocyte–neuron metabolic interactions. *J. Cereb. Blood Flow Metab.* 30, 1982–1986. doi: 10.1038/jcbfm.2010.132

Jolivet, R., Coggan, J. S., Allaman, I., and Magistretti, P. J. (2015). Multi-timescale modeling of activity-dependent metabolic coupling in the neuron-glia-vasculature ensemble. *PLoS Comput. Biol.* 11:e1004036. doi: 10.1371/journal.pcbi.1004036

Jueptner, M., and Weiller, C. (1995). Review: does measurement of regional cerebral blood flow reflect synaptic activity?—Implications for PET and fMRI. *Neuroimage* 2, 148–156. doi: 10.1006/nimg.1995.1017

Karagiannis, A., Sylantyev, S., Hadjihambi, A., Hosford, P. S., Kasparov, S., and Gourine, A. V. (2016). Hemichannel-mediated release of lactate. *J. Cereb. Blood Flow Metab.* 36, 1202–1211. doi: 10.1177/0271678X15611912

Kimelberg, H. K., and Norenberg, M. D. (1989). Astrocytes. *Sci. Am.* 260, 66–72. doi: 10.1038/scientificamerican0489-66

Kolko, M., Vosborg, F., Henriksen, U. L., Hasan-Olive, M. M., Diget, E. H., Vohra, R., et al. (2016). Lactate transport and receptor actions in retina: potential roles in retinal function and disease. *Neurochem. Res.* 41, 1229–1236. doi: 10.1007/s11064-015-1792-x

Korogod, N., Petersen, C. C., and Knott, G. W. (2015). Ultrastructural analysis of adult mouse neocortex comparing aldehyde perfusion with cryo fixation. *Elife* 4:e05793. doi: 10.7554/eLife.05793

Kuchiiwa, T., Nio-Kobayashi, J., Takahashi-Iwanaga, H., Yajima, T., and Iwanaga, T. (2011). Cellular expression of monocarboxylate transporters in the female reproductive organ of mice: implications for the genital lactate shuttle. *Histochem. Cell Biol.* 135, 351–360. doi: 10.1007/s00418-011-0794-2

Kuhr, W. G., and Korf, J. (1988). Extracellular lactic acid as an indicator of brain metabolism: continuous on-line measurement in conscious, freely moving rats with intrastriatal dialysis. *J. Cereb. Blood Flow Metab.* 8, 130–137. doi: 10.1038/jcbfm.1988.17

Laskas, J. M. (2009). *Game Brain*. Gentlemen's Quarterly. New York, NY: Condé Nast.

Laskas, J. M. (2015). *Concussion*. New York, NY: Random House.

Laughton, J. D., Charnay, Y., Belloir, B., Pellerin, L., Magistretti, P. J., and Bouras, C. (2000). Differential messenger RNA distribution of lactate dehydrogenase LDH-1 and LDH-5 isoforms in the rat brain. *Neuroscience* 96, 619–625. doi: 10.1016/S0306-4522(99)00580-1

Laureys, G., Valentino, M., Demol, F., Zammit, C., Muscat, R., Cambron, M., et al. (2014). β 2-Adrenergic receptors protect axons during energetic stress but do not influence basal glio-axonal lactate shuttling in mouse white matter. *Neuroscience* 277, 367–374. doi: 10.1016/j.neuroscience.2014.07.022

Lee, N. Y., and Kang, Y. S. (2016). *In vivo* and *in vitro* evidence for brain uptake of 4-phenylbutyrate by the monocarboxylate transporter 1 (MCT1). *Pharm. Res.* 33, 1711–1722. doi: 10.1007/s11095-016-1912-6

Leen, W. G., Willemsen, M. A., Wevers, R. A., and Verbeek, M. M. (2012). Cerebrospinal fluid glucose and lactate: age-specific reference values and implications for clinical practice. *PLoS ONE* 7:e42745. doi: 10.1371/journal.pone.004274

Li, C., Zhao, R., Gao, K., Wei, Z., Yin, Y. M., Lau, T. L., et al. (2011). Astrocytes: implications for neuroinflammatory pathogenesis of Alzheimer's disease. *Curr. Alzheimer Res.* 8, 67–80. doi: 10.2174/156720511794604543

Logan, J. G., and Barksdale, D. J. (2008). Allostasis and allostatic load: expanding the discourse on stress and cardiovascular disease. *J. Clin. Nurs.* 17, 201–208. doi: 10.1111/j.1365-2702.2008.02347.x

Lutz, N. W., Viola, A., Malikova, I., Confort-Gouny, S., Audoin, B., Ranjeva, J. P., et al. (2007). Inflammatory multiple-sclerosis plaques generate characteristic metabolic profiles in cerebrospinal fluid. *PLoS ONE* 2:e595. doi: 10.1371/journal.pone.0000595

Magistretti, P. J., and Pellerin, L. (1996). Cellular bases of brain energy metabolism and their relevance to functional brain imaging: evidence for a prominent role of astrocytes. *Cereb. Cortex* 6, 50–61. doi: 10.1093/cercor/6.1.50

Magistretti, P. J., and Pellerin, L. (1999). Astrocytes couple synaptic activity to glucose utilization in the brain. *Physiology* 14, 177–182.

Magistretti, P. J. (2000). Cellular bases of functional brain imaging: insights from neuron-glia metabolic coupling. *Brain Res.* 886, 108–112. doi: 10.1016/S0006-8993(00)02945-0

Magistretti, P. J. (2006). Neuron–glia metabolic coupling and plasticity. *J. Exp. Biol.* 209, 2304–2311. doi: 10.1242/jeb.02208

Magistretti, P. J. (2009). Role of glutamate in neuron-glia metabolic coupling. *Am. J. Clin. Nutr.* 90, 875S–880S. doi: 10.3945/ajcn.2009.27462CC

Mangia, S., Giove, F., Bianciardi, M., Di Salle, F., Garreffa, G., and Maraviglia, B. (2003a). Issues concerning the construction of a metabolic model for neuronal activation. *J. Neurosci. Res.* 71, 463–467. doi: 10.1002/jnr.10531

Mangia, S., Garreffa, G., Bianciardi, M., Giove, F., Di Salle, F., and Maraviglia, B. (2003b). The aerobic brain: lactate decrease at the onset of neural activity. *Neuroscience* 118, 7–10. doi: 10.1016/S0306-4522(02)00792-3

Mangia, S., Simpson, I. A., Vannucci, S. J., and Carruthers, A. (2009). The *in vivo* neuron-to-astrocyte lactate shuttle in human brain: evidence from modeling of measured lactate levels during visual stimulation. *J. Neurochem.* 109, 55–62. doi: 10.1111/j.1471-4159.2009.06003.x

Mason, S., van Furth, A. M., Mienie, L. J., Engelke, U. F., Wevers, R. A., Solomons, R., et al. (2015). A hypothetical astrocyte–microglia lactate shuttle derived from a 1H NMR metabolomics analysis of cerebrospinal fluid from a cohort of South African children with tuberculous meningitis. *Metabolomics* 11, 822–837. doi: 10.1007/s11306-014-0741-z

Mason, S., Reinecke, C. J., Kulik, W., van Cruchten, A., Solomons, R., and van Furth, A. M. (2016a). Cerebrospinal fluid in tuberculous meningitis exhibits only the L-enantiomer of lactic acid. *BMC Infect. Dis.* 16:251. doi: 10.1186/s12879-016-1597-9

Mason, S., van Furth, A. M. T., Solomons, R., Wevers, R. A., van Reenen, M., and Reinecke, C. J. (2016b). A putative urinary biosignature for diagnosis and follow-up of tuberculous meningitis in children: outcome of a metabolomics study disclosing host–pathogen responses. *Metabolomics* 12, 1–16. doi: 10.1007/s11306-016-1053-2

McEwen, B. S. (2006). Sleep deprivation as a neurobiologic and physiologic stressor: allostasis and allostatic load. *Metab. Clin. Exp.* 55, S20–S23. doi: 10.1016/j.metabol.2006.07.008

McEwen, B. S. (2008). Central effects of stress hormones in health and disease: understanding the protective and damaging effects of stress and stress mediators. *Eur. J. Pharmacol.* 583, 174–185. doi: 10.1016/j.ejphar.2007.11.071

McEwen, B. S., and Gianaros, P. J. (2011). Stress- and allostasis-induced brain plasticity. *Annu. Rev. Med.* 62, 431–445. doi: 10.1146/annurev-med-052209-100430

McKenna, M. C., Waagepetersen, H. S., Schousboe, A., and Sonnewald, U. (2006). Neuronal and astrocytic shuttle mechanisms for cytosolic-mitochondrial transfer of reducing equivalents: current evidence and pharmacological tools. *Biochem. Pharmacol.* 71, 399–407. doi: 10.1016/j.bcp.2005.10.011

Moffett, J. R., Arun, P., Ariyannur, P. S., and Namboodiri, A. M. (2013). N-Acetylaspartate reductions in brain injury: impact on post-injury neuroenergetics, lipid synthesis, and protein acetylation. *Front. Neuroenergetics* 5:11. doi: 10.3389/fnene.2013.00011

Moro, N., Ghavim, S., Harris, N. G., Hovda, D. A., and Sutton, R. L. (2013). Glucose administration after traumatic brain injury improves cerebral metabolism and reduces secondary neuronal injury. *Brain Res.* 1535, 124–136. doi: 10.1016/j.brainres.2013.08.044

Newington, J. T., Harris, R. A., and Cumming, R. C. (2013). Reevaluating metabolism in Alzheimer's disease from the perspective of the astrocyte-neuron lactate shuttle model. *J. Neurodegen. Dis.* 2013:234572. doi: 10.1155/2013/234572

Nijland, P. G., Molenaar, R. J., van der Pol, S. M., van der Valk, P., van Noorden, C. J., de Vries, H. E., et al. (2015). Differential expression of glucose-metabolizing enzymes in multiple sclerosis lesions. *Acta Neuropathol. Commun.* 3:79. doi: 10.1186/s40478-015-0261-8

Norenberg, M. D., Mozes, L. W., Gregorios, J. B., and Norenberg, L. O. (1987). Effects of lactic acid on astrocytes in primary culture. *J. Neuropathol. Exp. Neurol.* 46, 154–166. doi: 10.1097/00005072-198703000-00004

Olson, J. K., Girvin, A. M., and Miller, S. D. (2001). Direct activation of innate and antigen-presenting functions of microglia following infection with Theiler's virus. *J. Virol.* 75, 9780–9789. doi: 10.1128/JVI.75.20.9780-9789.2001

Olson, J. K., and Miller, S. D. (2004). Microglia initiate central nervous system innate and adaptive immune responses through multiple TLRs. *J. Immunol.* 173, 3916–3924. doi: 10.4049/jimmunol.173.6.3916

Oresic, M., Hänninen, V. A., and Vidal-Puig, A. (2008). Lipidomics: a new window to biomedical frontiers. *Trends Biotechnol.* 26, 647–652. doi: 10.1016/j.tibtech.2008.09.001

Ovanesov, M. V., Ayhan, Y., Wolbert, C., Moldovan, K., Sauder, C., and Pletnikov, M. V. (2008). Astrocytes play a key role in activation of microglia by persistent Borna disease virus infection. *J. Neuroinflamm.* 5:50. doi: 10.1186/1742-2094-5-50

Patet, C., Suys, T., Carteron, L., and Oddo, M. (2016). Cerebral lactate metabolism after traumatic brain injury. *Curr. Neurol. Neurosci. Rep.* 16, 1–7. doi: 10.1007/s11910-016-0638-5

Pavlides, S., Whitaker-Menezes, D., Castello-Cros, R., Flomenberg, N., Witkiewicz, A. K., Frank, P. G., et al. (2009). The reverse Warburg effect—aerobic glycolysis in cancer associated fibroblasts and the tumor stroma. *Cell Cycle* 8, 3984–4001. doi: 10.4161/cc.8.23.10238

Pavlides, S., Tsirigos, A., Vera, I., Flomenberg, N., Frank, P. G., Casimiro, M. C., et al. (2010). Transcriptional evidence for the "Reverse Warburg Effect" in human breast cancer tumor stroma and metastasis: similarities with oxidative stress, inflammation, Alzheimer's disease, and "Neuron-Glia Metabolic Coupling". *Aging* 2, 185–199. doi: 10.18632/aging.100134

Pellerin, L., Bonvento, G., Voutsinos-Porche, B., Tanaka, K., Chatton, J. Y., Brunet, J. F., et al. (2002). Role of astrocytes in coupling synaptic activity to glucose utilization. *Int. Congr. Ser.* 1235, 189–196. doi: 10.1016/S0531-5131(02)00186-3

Pellerin, L. (2003). Lactate as a pivotal element in neuron–glia metabolic cooperation. *Neurochem. Int.* 43, 331–338. doi: 10.1016/S0197-0186(03)00020-2

Pellerin, L., and Magistretti, P. J. (2004). Neuroenergetics: calling upon astrocytes to satisfy hungry neurons. *Neuroscientist* 10, 53–62. doi: 10.1177/1073858403260159

Pellerin, L., Bouzier-Sore, A. K., Aubert, A., Serres, S., Merle, M., Costalat, R., et al. (2007). Activity-dependent regulation of energy metabolism by astrocytes: an update. *Glia* 55, 1251–1262. doi: 10.1002/glia.20528

Pellerin, L. (2010). Food for thought: the importance of glucose and other energy substrates for sustaining brain function under varying levels of activity. *Diabetes Metab.* 36, S59–S63. doi: 10.1016/S1262-3636(10)70469-9

Pellerin, L., and Magistretti, P. J. (2011). Sweet sixteen for ANLS. *J. Cereb. Blood Flow Metab.* 32, 1152–1166. doi: 10.1038/jcbfm.2011.149

Pérez-Escuredo, J., Van Hée, V. F., Sboarina, M., Falces, J., Payen, V. L., Pellerin, L., et al. (2016). Monocarboxylate transporters in the brain and in cancer. *Biochim. Biophys. Acta* 1863, 2481–2497. doi: 10.1016/j.bbamcr.2016.03.013

Pértega-Gomes, N., Vizcaíno, J. R., Attig, J., Jurmeister, S., Lopes, C., and Baltazar, F. (2014). A lactate shuttle system between tumour and stromal cells is associated with poor prognosis in prostate cancer. *BMC Cancer* 14:352. doi: 10.1186/1471-2407-14-352

Peters, A., and McEwen, B. S. (2015). Stress habituation, body shape and cardiovascular mortality. *Neurosci. Biobehav. Rev.* 56, 139–150. doi: 10.1016/j.neubiorev.2015.07.001

Pierre, K., Pellerin, L., Debernardi, R., Riederer, B. M., and Magistretti, P. J. (2000). Cell-specific localization of monocarboxylate transporters, MCT1 and MCT2, in the adult mouse brain revealed by double immunohistochemical labeling and confocal microscopy. *Neuroscience* 100, 617–627. doi: 10.1016/S0306-4522(00)00294-3

Pizzuto, R., Paventi, G., Porcile, C., Sarnataro, D., Daniele, A., and Passarella, S. (2012). L-Lactate metabolism in HEP G2 cell mitochondria due to the L-lactate dehydrogenase determines the occurrence of the lactate/pyruvate shuttle and the appearance of oxaloacetate, malate and citrate outside mitochondria. *Biochim. Biophys. Acta* 1817, 1679–1690. doi: 10.1016/j.bbabio.2012.05.010

Porras, O. H., Loaiza, A., and Barros, L. F. (2004). Glutamate mediates acute glucose transport inhibition in hippocampal neurons. *J. Neurosci.* 24, 9669–9673. doi: 10.1523/JNEUROSCI.1882-04.2004

Prichard, J., Rothman, D., Novotny, E., Petroff, O., Kuwabara, T., Avison, M., et al. (1991). Lactate rise detected by 1H NMR in human visual cortex during physiologic stimulation. *Proc. Natl. Acad. Sci. U.S.A.* 88, 5829–5831. doi: 10.1073/pnas.88.13.5829

Psychogios, N., Hau, D. D., Peng, J., Guo, A. C., Mandal, R., Bouatra, S., et al. (2011). The human serum metabolome. *PLoS ONE* 6:e16957. doi: 10.1371/journal.pone.0016957

Raghavendra, V., Tanga, F., and DeLeo, J. A. (2003). Inhibition of microglial activation attenuates the development but not existing hypersensitivity in a rat model of neuropathy. *J. Pharm. Exp. Ther.* 306, 624–630. doi: 10.1124/jpet.103.052407

Rake, A. J., Srinivasan, V., Nadkarni, V., Kaptan, R., and Newth, C. J. L. (2010). Glucose variability and survival in critically ill children: allostasis or harm? *Pediatr. Crit. Care Med.* 11, 707–712. doi: 10.1097/PCC.0b013e3181e88b1f

Rakus, D., Gizak, A., and Wiśniewski, J. R. (2016). Proteomics unveils fibroblast-cardiomyocyte lactate shuttle and hexokinase paradox in mouse muscles. *J. Proteome Res.* 15, 2479–2490. doi: 10.1021/acs.jproteome.5b01149

Ramautar, R., Berger, R., van der Greef, J., and Hankemeier, T. (2013). Human metabolomics: strategies to understand biology. *Curr. Opin. Chem. Biol.* 17, 841–846. doi: 10.1016/j.cbpa.2013.06.015

Ranjbar, M., and Amiri, M. (2015). On the role of astrocyte analog circuit in neural frequency adaptation. *Neural Comput. Appl.* 26, 1–13. doi: 10.1007/s00521-015-2112-8

Regenold, W. T., Phatak, P., Makley, M. J., Stone, R. D., and Kling, M. A. (2008). Cerebrospinal fluid evidence of increased extra-mitochondrial glucose metabolism implicates mitochondrial dysfunction in multiple sclerosis disease progression. *J. Neurol. Sci.* 275, 106–112. doi: 10.1016/j.jns.2008.07.032

Robinet, C., and Pellerin, L. (2011). Brain-derived neurotrophic factor enhances the hippocampal expression of key postsynaptic proteins *in vivo* including the monocarboxylate transporter MCT2. *Neuroscience* 192, 155–163. doi: 10.1016/j.neuroscience.2011.06.059

Rock, R. B., Gekker, G., Hu, S., Sheng, W. S., Cheeran, M., Lokensgard, J. R., et al. (2004). Role of microglia in central nervous system infections. *Clin. Microbiol. Rev.* 17, 942–964. doi: 10.1128/CMR.17.4.942-964.2004

Rosafio, K., Castillo, X., Hirt, L., and Pellerin, L. (2016). Cell-specific modulation of monocarboxylate transporter expression contributes to the metabolic reprograming taking place following cerebral ischemia. *Neuroscience* 317, 108–120. doi: 10.1016/j.neuroscience.2015.12.052

Rossi, D. J., Brady, J. D., and Mohr, C. (2007). Astrocyte metabolism and signaling during brain ischemia. *Nat. Neurosci.* 10, 1377–1386. doi: 10.1038/nn2004

Rothman, D. L., Behar, K. L., Hyder, F., and Shulman, R. G. (2003). *In vivo* NMR studies of the glutamate neurotransmitter flux and neuroenergetics: implications for brain function. *Annu. Rev. Physiol.* 65, 401–427. doi: 10.1146/annurev.physiol.65.092101.142131

Rouach, N., Koulakoff, A., Abudara, V., Willecke, K., and Giaume, C. (2008). Astroglial metabolic networks sustain hippocampal synaptic transmission. *Science* 322, 1551–1555. doi: 10.1126/science.1164022

Sack, G. H. Jr. (2010). Mitochondrial matters in Huntington disease. *J. Bioenerg. Biomembr.* 42, 189–191. doi: 10.1007/s10863-010-9291-x

Sahlin, K., Fernström, M., Svensson, M., and Tonkonogi, M. (2002). No evidence of an intracellular lactate shuttle in rat skeletal muscle. *J. Physiol.* 541, 569–574. doi: 10.1113/jphysiol.2002.016683

Sampol, D., Ostrofet, E., Jobin, M. L., Raffard, G., Sanchez, S., Bouchaud, V., et al. (2013). Glucose and lactate metabolism in the awake and stimulated rat: a 13C-NMR study. *Front. Neuroenergetics* 5:5. doi: 10.3389/fnene.2013.00005

Sanità, P., Capulli, M., Teti, A., Galatioto, G. P., Vicentini, C., Chiarugi, P., et al. (2014). Tumor-stroma metabolic relationship based on lactate shuttle can sustain prostate cancer progression. *BMC Cancer* 14:154. doi: 10.1186/1471-2407-14-154

Sappey-Marinier, D., Calabrese, G., Fein, G., Hugg, J. W., Biggins, C., and Weiner, M. W. (1992). Effect of photic stimulation on human visual cortex lactate and phosphates using 1H and 31P magnetic resonance spectroscopy. *J. Cereb. Blood Flow Metab.* 12, 584–592. doi: 10.1038/jcbfm.1992.82

Sawada, Y., Konno, A., Nagaoka, J., and Hirai, H. (2016). Inflammation-induced reversible switch of the neuron-specific enolase promoter from Purkinje neurons to Bergmann glia. *Sci. Rep.* 6:27758. doi: 10.1038/srep27758

Schurr, A., West, C. A., and Rigor, B. M. (1988). Lactate-supported synaptic function in the rat hippocampal slice preparation. *Science* 240, 1326–1328. doi: 10.1126/science.3375817

Schurr, A., Payne, R. S., Miller, J. J., and Rigor, B. M. (1997a). Glia are the main source of lactate utilized by neurons for recovery of function posthypoxia. *Brain Res.* 774, 221–224.

Schurr, A., Payne, R. S., Miller, J. J., and Rigor, B. M. (1997b). Brain lactate is an obligatory aerobic energy substrate for functional recovery after hypoxia: further *in vitro* validation. *J. Neurochem.* 69, 423–426.

Schurr, A., Payne, R. S., Miller, J. J., and Rigor, B. M. (1997c). Brain lactate, not glucose, fuels the recovery of synaptic function from hypoxia upon reoxygenation: an *in vitro* study. *Brain Res.* 744, 105–111.

Schurr, A., Payne, R. S., Tseng, M. T., Miller, J. J., and Rigor, B. M. (1999a). The glucose paradox in cerebral ischemia: new insights. *Ann. N.Y. Acad. Sci.* 893, 386–390.

Schurr, A., Miller, J. J., Payne, R. S., and Rigor, B. M. (1999b). An increase in lactate output by brain tissue serves to meet the energy needs of glutamate-activated neurons. *J. Neurosci.* 19, 34–39.

Schurr, A. (2006). Lactate: the ultimate cerebral oxidative energy substrate? *J. Cereb. Blood Flow Metab.* 26, 142–152. doi: 10.1038/sj.jcbfm.9600174

Shannon, M., King, T. L., and Kennedy, H. P. (2007). Allostasis: a theoretical framework for understanding and evaluating perinatal health outcomes. *J. Obstet. Gynecol. Neonatal Nurs.* 36, 125–134. doi: 10.1111/j.1552-6909.2007.00126.x

Shulman, R. G., Rothman, D. L., Behar, K. L., and Hyder, F. (2004). Energetic basis of brain activity: implications for neuroimaging. *Trends Neurosci.* 27, 489–495. doi: 10.1016/j.tins.2004.06.005

Siesjö, B. K. (1988). Acidosis and ischemic brain damage. *Neurochem. Pathol.* 9, 31–88.

Simpson, I. A., Carruthers, A., and Vannucci, S. J. (2007). Supply and demand in cerebral energy metabolism: the role of nutrient transporters. *J. Cereb. Blood Flow Metab.* 27, 1766–1791. doi: 10.1038/sj.jcbfm.9600521

Smith, D., Pernet, A., Hallett, W. A., Bingham, E., Marsden, P. K., and Amiel, S. A. (2003). Lactate: a preferred fuel for human brain metabolism *in vivo*. *J. Cereb. Blood Flow Metab.* 23, 658–664. doi: 10.1097/01.WCB.0000063991.19746.11

Sokoloff, L. (1989). Circulation and energy metabolism of the brain. *Basic Neurochemistry* 2, 338–413.

Somashekar, B. S., Amin, A. G., Rithner, C. D., Troudt, J., Basaraba, R., Izzo, A., et al. (2011). Metabolic profiling of lung granuloma in Mycobacterium tuberculosis infected guinea pigs: *ex vivo* 1H magic angle spinning NMR studies. *J. Proteome Res.* 10, 4186–4195. doi: 10.1021/pr2003352

Sone, J. Y., Kondziolka, D., Huang, J. H., and Samadani, U. (2016). Helmet efficacy against concussion and traumatic brain injury: a review. *J. Neurosurg.* 124, 1–14. doi: 10.3171/2016.2.jns151972

Steele, M. L., and Robinson, S. R. (2012). Reactive astrocytes give neurons less support: implications for Alzheimer's disease. *Neurobiol. Aging* 33, 423–e1. doi: 10.1016/j.neurobiolaging.2010.09.018

Sterling, P., and Eyer, J. (1988). "Allostasis: a new paradigm to explain arousal pathology," in *Handbook of Life Stress, Cognition and Health*, eds S. Fisher and J. Reason (Oxford: John Wiley & Sons), 629–649.

Stewart, J. A. (2006). The detrimental effects of allostasis: allostatic load as a measure of cumulative stress. *J. Physiol. Anthropol.* 25, 133–145. doi: 10.2114/jpa2.25.133

Streit, W. J., Mrak, R. E., and Griffin, W. S. (2004). Microglia and neuroinflammation: a pathological perspective. *J. Neuroinflamm.* 1:14. doi: 10.1186/1742-2094-1-14

Stumvoll, M., Tataranni, P. A., Stefan, N., Vozarova, B., and Bogardus, C. (2003). Perspective in diabetes: glucose allostasis. *Diabetes* 52, 903–909. doi: 10.2337/diabetes.52.4.903

Stumvoll, M., Tataranni, P. A., and Bogardus, C. (2004). The role of glucose allostasis in type 2 diabetes. *Rev. Endocr. Metab. Disord.* 5, 99–103. doi: 10.1023/B:REMD.0000021430.56457.2c

Sussman, E. S., Ho, A. L., Pendharkar, A. V., and Ghajar, J. (2016). Clinical evaluation of concussion: the evolving role of oculomotor assessments. *Neurosurg. Focus* 40, E7. doi: 10.3171/2016.1.FOCUS15610

Suzuki, A., Stern, S. A., Bozdagi, O., Huntley, G. W., Walker, R. H., Magistretti, P. J., et al. (2011). Astrocyte-neuron lactate transport is required for long-term memory formation. *Cell* 144, 810–823. doi: 10.1016/j.cell.2011.02.018

Tabernero, A., Vicario, C., and Medina, J. M. (1996). Lactate spares glucose as a metabolic fuel in neurons and astrocytes from primary culture. *Neurosci. Res.* 26, 369–376. doi: 10.1016/S0168-0102(96)01121-2

Taher, M., Leen, W. G., Wevers, R. A., and Willemsen, M. A. (2016). Lactate and its many faces. *Eur. J. Paediatr. Neurol.* 20, 3–10. doi: 10.1016/j.ejpn.2015.09.008

Tannenbaum, B., Tannenbaum, G. S., and Anisman, S. H. (2002). Neurochemical and behavioural alterations elicited by a chronic intermittent stressor regimen: implications for allostatic load. *Brain Res.* 963, 82–92. doi: 10.1016/S0006-8993(02)03273-0

Tomiyama, A. J., O'Donovan, A., Lin, J., Puterman, E., Lazaro, A., Chan, J., et al. (2012). Does cellular aging relate to patterns of allostasis? An examination of basal and stress reactive HPA axis activity and telomere length. *Physiol. Behav.* 106, 40–45. doi: 10.1016/j.physbeh.2011.11.016

van Hall, G., Strømstad, M., Rasmussen, P., Jans, O., Zaar, M., Gam, C., et al. (2009). Blood lactate is an important energy source for the human brain. *J. Cereb. Blood Flow Metab.* 29, 1121–1129. doi: 10.1038/jcbfm.2009.35

Vannucci, S. J., Maher, F., and Simpson, I. A. (1997). Glucose transporter proteins in brain: delivery of glucose to neurons and glia. *Glia* 21, 2–21. doi: 10.1002/(SICI)1098-1136(199709)21:1<2::AID-GLIA2>3.0.CO;2-C

Verwaest, K. A., Vu, T. N., Laukens, K., Clemens, L. E., Nguyen, H. P., Van Gasse, B., et al. (2011). 1H NMR based metabolomics of CSF and blood serum: a metabolic profile for a transgenic rat model of Huntington disease. *Biochim. Biophys. Acta* 1812, 1371–1379.

Voutsinos-Porche, B., Bonvento, G., Tanaka, K., Steiner, P., Welker, E., Chatton, J. Y., et al. (2003). Glial glutamate transporters mediate a functional metabolic crosstalk between neurons and astrocytes in the mouse developing cortex. *Neuron* 37, 275–286. doi: 10.1016/S0896-6273(02)01170-4

Wender, R., Brown, A. M., Fern, R., Swanson, R. A., Farrell, K., and Ransom, B. R. (2000). Astrocytic glycogen influences axon function and survival during glucose deprivation in central white matter. *J. Neurosci.* 20, 6804–6810.

Whitaker-Menezes, D., Martinez-Outschoorn, U. E., Lin, Z., Ertel, A., Flomenberg, N., Witkiewicz, A. K., et al. (2011). Evidence for a stromal-epithelial "lactate shuttle" in human tumors: MCT4 is a marker of oxidative stress in cancer-associated fibroblasts. *Cell Cycle* 10, 1772–1783. doi: 10.4161/cc.10.11.15659

Wishart, D. S., Lewis, M. J., Morrissey, J. A., Flegel, M. D., Jeroncic, K., Xiong, Y., et al. (2008). The human cerebrospinal fluid metabolome. *J. Chromatogr. B Analyt. Technol. Biomed. Life Sci.* 871, 164–173. doi: 10.1016/j.jchromb.2008.05.001

Wyss, M. T., Jolivet, R., Buck, A., Magistretti, P. J., and Weber, B. (2011). *In vivo* evidence for lactate as a neuronal energy source. *J. Neurosci.* 31, 7477–7485. doi: 10.1523/JNEUROSCI.0415-11.2011

Yamanishi, S., Katsumura, K., Kobayashi, T., and Puro, D. G. (2006). Extracellular lactate as a dynamic vasoactive signal in the rat retinal microvasculature. *Am. J. Physiol. Heart Circ. Physiol.* 290, H925–H934. doi: 10.1152/ajpheart.01012.2005

Zeis, T., Allaman, I., Gentner, M., Schroder, K., Tschopp, J., Magistretti, P. J., et al. (2015). Metabolic gene expression changes in astrocytes in Multiple Sclerosis cerebral cortex are indicative of immune-mediated signaling. *Brain Behav. Immun.* 48, 313–325. doi: 10.1016/j.bbi.2015.04.013

Zhou, A., Ni, J., Xu, Z., Wang, Y., Zhang, W., Wu, W., et al. (2015). Metabolomics specificity of tuberculosis plasma revealed by 1H NMR spectroscopy. *Tuberculosis* 95, 294–302. doi: 10.1016/j.tube.2015.02.038

Zuo, R. J., Gu, X. W., Qi, Q. R., Wang, T. S., Zhao, X. Y., Liu, J. L., et al. (2015). Warburg-like glycolysis and lactate shuttle in mouse decidua during early pregnancy. *J. Biol. Chem.* 290, 21280–21291. doi: 10.1074/jbc.M115.656629

Zwingman, C., Richter-Landsberg, C., Brand, A., and Leibfritz, D. (2000). NMR spectroscopic study on the metabolic fate of [3-(13)C] alanine in astrocytes, neurons, and cocultures: implications for glia-neuron interactions in neurotransmitter metabolism. *Glia* 32, 286–303. doi: 10.1002/1098-1136(200012)32:3<286::AID-GLIA80>3.0.CO;2-P

8

New Insights into the Crosstalk between NMDARs and Iron: Implications for Understanding Pathology of Neurological Diseases

Huamin Xu [1,2]*, *Hong Jiang* [1,2] *and Junxia Xie* [1,2]*

[1] *Collaborative Innovation Center for Brain Science, Department of Physiology, Shandong Provincial Key Laboratory of Pathogenesis and Prevention of Neurological Disorders and State Key Disciplines: Physiology, Medical College of Qingdao University, Qingdao, China,* [2] *Shandong Provincial Collaborative Innovation Center for Neurodegenerative Disorders, Qingdao University, Qingdao, China*

Edited by:
Andrew Harkin,
Trinity College, Dublin, Ireland

Reviewed by:
Christian Gonzalez-Billault,
University of Chile, Chile
Daniela Tropea,
Trinity College, Dublin, Ireland
Fabrizio Gardoni,
University of Milan, Italy

***Correspondence:**
Huamin Xu
huamin102@163.com
Junxia Xie
jxiaxie@public.qd.sd.cn

Both iron dyshomeostasis and N-methyl-D-aspartate receptors (NMDARs)-mediated neurotoxicity have been shown to have an important role in neurological diseases such as Parkinson's disease (PD) and Alzheimer's disease (AD). Evidence proved that activation of NMDARs could promote iron overload and iron-induced neurotoxicity by enhancing iron importer divalent metal transporter 1 (DMT1)-mediated iron uptake and iron releasing from lysosome. Also, iron overload could regulate NMDARs-mediated synaptic transmission. This indicates that there might be a possible relationship between iron and activation of NMDARs in neurological diseases. Understanding this interaction between iron and activation of NMDARs may provide new therapeutic avenues for a more targeted neurotherapeutic strategy for these diseases. Therefore, in this review article, we will describe the dysfunction of iron metabolism and NMDARs in neurological diseases including PD and AD, and summarize the new insight into the mechanisms underlying the interaction between iron and activation of NMDARs.

Keywords: Parkinson's disease, Alzheimer's disease, iron, NMDA receptor, divalent metal transporter 1

INTRODUCTION

Iron is an important cofactor in many proteins such as heme-containing proteins and iron-containing enzymes. It is required for many physiological processes for life (Zucca et al., 2015). In the central nervous system (CNS), iron also participates in myelin synthesis, development of dendritic spines in the hippocampus and synthesis of neurotransmitters including monoamine transmitters and gamma-aminobutyric acid (GABA; Li, 1998; Jorgenson et al., 2003; Todorich et al., 2009; Zucca et al., 2015; Bastian et al., 2016). However, excess iron is toxic due to its ability to produce cytotoxic hydroxyl radicals, which could cause damages to proteins, nucleic acids and cell membranes (Whitnall and Richardson, 2006). Therefore, intracellular iron metabolism is tightly regulated. There are two pathways for iron uptake: the classical transferrin (Tf)-mediated iron uptake pathway and the non-Tf bound iron (NTBI) uptake pathway (Qian and Shen, 2001). Traditionally, the Tf-transferrin receptor 1 (Tf-TfR1) pathway is considered as major pathway for cellular iron uptake in the brain. Divalent metal transporter 1 (DMT1) is identified as the main NTBI pathway, responsible for ferrous iron uptake. There are four DMT1 mRNA isoforms: N-terminus (1A, 1B) generated from alternative promoters with subsequent, exclusive splicing of the respective first exon to exon 2 and C-terminus splice variants (+iron-responsive element (IRE), −IRE) due to alternative splice mechanisms (Hubert and Hentze, 2002). DMT1 + IRE contains an IRE in the 3′-untranslated region (UTR) and DMT1 − IRE has no IRE. Additionally, 1A/DMT1 is predominantly expressed in kidney and duodenum and 1B/DMT1 is ubiquitously expressed in the peripheral organs and brain (Hubert and Hentze, 2002). Ferroportin 1 (FPN1), also known as metal transport protein1 (Abboud and Haile, 2000) or iron-regulated transporter 1 (IREG1) is the only known iron transporter responsible for cellular iron export (Ganz, 2005). Disturbance in iron metabolism plays a key role in the pathogenesis of neurodegenerative disorders such as Parkinson's disease (PD) and Alzheimer's disease (AD) (LaVaute et al., 2001; Lieu et al., 2001; Perez et al., 2008; Zhu et al., 2009). Elevated iron levels were found in the substantia nigra (SN) in PD patients (Sofic et al., 1988). Studies also showed that iron accumulation was observed in the hippocampus and cerebral cortex in AD patients (Piñero et al., 2000, 2001; Altamura and Muckenthaler, 2009). Increased import, decreased export or redistribution of intracellular iron might be responsible for iron metabolism disturbance in these diseases, which may increase the vulnerability of neurons to iron.

Glutamate is the major excitatory neurotransmitter in the CNS, exerting its functions by binding to different receptors. Among them, N-methyl-D-aspartate receptors (NMDARs) are cation channels that mediate entry of Na^{+} and Ca^{2+} ions and are activated by the co-agonists glutamate (or NMDA) and glycine or D-serine. There are several subunits of NMDARs: NR1, NR2A, NR2B, NR2C and NR2D and NR3. Among them, NR1 is a fundamental subunit of the receptor. Appropriate activation of NMDARs plays a critical role in physiological functions such as excitatory neurotransmission, synaptic plasticity (Carvajal et al., 2016). However, excitotoxicity induced by excessive activation of NMDARs contributes to pathological changes in the CNS (Ambrosi et al., 2014; Gonzalez et al., 2015). Influx of Ca^{2+} through NMDARs might lead to neuronal loss in several neurodegenerative diseases such as PD and AD (Hynd et al., 2004). NMDARs have both synaptic and extrasynaptic locations. One hypothesis posits that synaptic NMDARs were neuroprotective and extrasynaptic NMDARs were neurotoxic (Hardingham and Bading, 2010). The death signaling induced by extrasynaptic NMDARs or relocalization of NMDARs to extrasynaptic sites has been shown to contribute to pathology of neurodegenerative diseases (Bading, 2017). Fine-tuning might provide a promising operation to optimize the activity of the glutamatergic system in order to maintain normal function of neurons (Köles et al., 2016). Activation of NMDARs as well as iron deposits in neurological diseases including PD and AD suggest that there might be a correlation between iron deposition and activation of NMDARs. Therefore, in this article, we reviewed the studies about the involvement of iron dyshomeostasis and NMDARs-mediated neurotoxicity in PD and AD. We then described the advanced knowledge on interaction of iron and NMDARs activation. This will provide implications for understanding pathology of these neurological diseases.

DYSFUNCTION OF IRON METABOLISM AND NMDARs IN PD

PD is a common neurodegenerative disorder characterized by loss of dopamine (DA) neurons in the SN pars compacta (SNpc), resulting in depletion of DA in the striatum (Parkinson, 2002; Hornykiewicz, 2008). Although the etiology of PD has not been clarified until now, iron accumulation and excitatory neurotoxicity are considered as contributing factors to the etiology of PD. It has become increasingly evident that elevated iron levels in the SNpc play a key role in the degeneration of DA neurons in PD (Jiang et al., 2016; Muñoz et al., 2016). Nigral iron levels increased with age, and PD patients showed an even greater increase, which correlates with clinical PD status (Wu et al., 2014; Du G. et al., 2016). Experimental evidence also showed that iron was involved in the degeneration of SNpc dopaminergic neurons in 1-methyl-4-phenyl-1,2,3,6-tetrahydropyridine (MPTP) and 6-hydroxydopamine (6-OHDA)-induced animal models of PD (Salazar et al., 2008; Jiang et al., 2010). Mechanisms underlying iron-induced neurodegeneration of DA neurons have been reported: First, iron participates in Fenton reaction to generate ·OH, which could damage proteins, nucleic acids and cell membranes (Mohanakumar et al., 1994). Second, iron-induced α-synuclein oligomers can form ion-permeable pores in lipid bilayers and give rise to α-synuclein-dependent toxicity in neuronal cells (Kostka et al., 2008). Our previous studies also showed iron could promote α-synuclein aggregation (He et al., 2013). Third, iron overload induced mitochondrial fragmentation via increasing intracellular calcium (Ca^{2+}) and activated calcineurin via Ca^{2+}/calmodulin and Ca^{2+}/calpain pathways. This mitochondrial fragmentation and neuronal cell death could be rescued by chelation of intracellular Ca^{2+} (Lee et al., 2016). Recently, it was reported that ferroptosis, an iron-dependent regulated cell death process, is an important cell death pathway for DA neurons in PD (Do Van et al., 2016).

A recent research showed that increase in DMT1 expression, rather than TfR1 and Fpn1 expression might be partly responsible for age-dependent increase in brain iron (Lu et al., 2016). This indicated the importance of DMT1 in age-induced iron overload. Our previous studies showed that increased expression of DMT1 + IRE and decreased expression of FPN1 were responsible for nigral-specific iron accumulation in PD models (Wang et al., 2007; Jiang et al., 2010; Song et al., 2010). DMT1 was found in the SNpc and associated predominantly with neuromelanin-containing DA neurons. It was consistently less intense in DA neurons of the ventral tegmental area (VTA) than in those of the SNpc in the same tissue sections of human brain older than 60 years (Salazar et al., 2008). In addition, postmortem studies have shown an increase of DMT1 in the SN of PD patients (Salazar et al., 2008). And a mutation in DMT1 that impaired iron transport protected rodents against parkinsonism-inducing neurotoxins MPTP and 6-OHDA (Salazar et al., 2008). Recent study demonstrated that DMT1 polymorphisms might be a risk factor for PD (Saadat et al., 2015). This indicated that higher DMT1 expression and consequently higher iron levels in nigral DA neurons might contribute to increased vulnerability of nigral

DA neurons to PD-related neurotoxins (Huang E. et al., 2004). The mechanisms underlying the expression of iron transporters DMT1 + IRE and FPN1 are IRE/iron regulatory proteins (IRPs)-dependent in 6-OHDA-induced PD models and IRE/IRPs-independent in MPP^+-treated dopaminegic cells (Zhang et al., 2009; Jiang et al., 2010). In addition, ceruloplasmin (CP) is the strongest ferroxidase to stabilize iron exporter FPN1. It was reported that the activity of CP in PD brains was reduced in SN (Ayton et al., 2013). In CP-knockout mice, iron overload was found in several tissues, including the brain (Kaneko et al., 2008). In our previous report, we also showed that decreased expression of CP in the SN was involved in the nigral iron accumulation of 6-OHDA-induced PD rats (Wang et al., 2015). These results suggested that CP might also play an important role in iron deposit in PD.

In addition, NMDARs-mediated excitotoxicity also contributed to the progressive degeneration of nigral DA neurons in PD (Ambrosi et al., 2014). Research has showed that ligand-gated ion channel NMDARs were vital in the glutamate-induced excitotoxicity in primary dopaminergic cell culture (Oster et al., 2014). Furthermore, glutamate exposure induced Parkin accumulation at mitochondria in a calcium- and NMDARs-dependent manner (Van Laar et al., 2015). It has been confirmed that SNpc DA neurons express functional triheteromeric NMDARs composed of NR1, NR2B and NR2D subunits (Jones and Gibb, 2005). A selective decrease of NR1 pan mRNA levels in layer IV of frontal cortex was found in PD patients (Meoni et al., 1999). However, NR1 expression increased in surviving SN DA neurons from PD brains compared with neurons from controls (Schiemann et al., 2012). Meanwhile, intracellular Ca^{2+} overload triggered by activation of NMDARs is believed to be responsible for inducing of nitric oxide synthases (NOS) activity, affecting mitochondrial integrity and functions (Yamauchi et al., 1998; Sattler and Tymianski, 2000). It has been reported that NMDARs antagonists were considered as potential therapies for patients with PD (Little and Brown, 2014). Among the NMDARs antagonists, memantine has been reported to preferentially blocks extrasynaptic NMDARs of SNpc DA neurons in slices of rat midbrain using whole-cell patch-clamp recordings (Wu and Johnson, 2015). This selective effect on NMDARs might be protective due to the neurotoxic effect of extrasynaptic NMDARs.

DYSFUNCTION OF IRON METABOLISM AND NMDARs IN AD

AD is a progressive neurodegenerative disorder, clinically characterized by a progressive loss of cognitive abilities and dementia, which is closely related to a degree of neuronal and synaptic loss (Selkoe, 1996; Hardy, 1997; Mattson, 1997). The key features of the disease are the accumulation of extracellular amyloid-β (Aβ) plaques and neurofibrillary tangles inside neurons. Although genetic and non-genetic factors are involved in the etiology of AD, the exact reason is still unknown. Increasing evidence suggests that iron might play an important role in the development or progression of AD (Mandel et al., 2007; Ward et al., 2014; Belaidi and Bush, 2016; Van Bergen et al., 2016). The first evidence is that iron accumulates in the same brain regions which are characterized by Aβ deposition such as hippocampus, parietal cortex and motor cortex in AD patients (Dedman et al., 1992; Good et al., 1992). High levels of iron have also been reported in the amyloid plaques in PS/amyloid precursor protein (APP) and APP [V717I] transgenic mice (Falangola et al., 2005), resembling those seen in the brains of AD patients. In addition, higher cortical iron was associated with increased Aβ-plaque-load in mild cognitive impairment (MCI; Van Bergen et al., 2016). Another important link between iron and AD is based on the observation that APP expression is iron-regulated. APP is a single transmembrane metalloprotein that is cleaved to generate the 40–42-amino-acid Aβs by β- and γ-secretases. The existence of a functional IRE in the 5′- UTR of APP mRNA makes it possible to be controlled at the level of mRNA translation by the action of IRE/IRP's response to iron (Rogers et al., 2002). This implied that high intracellular iron levels could cause increased APP translation and Aβ formation via this mechanism. In addition, iron could induce Aβ precipitation (Mantyh et al., 1993; Huang X. et al., 2004) and significantly enhance the toxicity of Aβ in cultured neuronal cells, whereas iron chelators protect the neurons from Aβ toxicity (Schubert and Chevion, 1995). This provided a direct link between excessive iron and loss of neuronal function seen in AD patients.

However, the underlying mechanisms involved in disturbance of iron homeostasis in AD brain remain unclear. It is reported that Aβ is a metalloprotein that binds transition metal ions through three histidine residues (His6, His13 and His14) located in the N-terminal domain (Nakamura et al., 2007; Altamura and Muckenthaler, 2009). And other protein that accumulates in AD such as tau protein also possesses metal-binding sites (Perry et al., 2003). These might account for the iron accumulation in the affected brain regions in AD. Furthermore, it is reported that DMT1 was colocalized with Aβ in the plaques of postmortem AD brain and the levels of DMT1 was significantly increased in the cortex and hippocampus in APP/PS1 transgenic mouse model compared with wild type-control (Zheng et al., 2009). And the mean serum p97 concentration was elevated 3- to 4-fold in patients with AD as compared to non-AD dementia and normal controls (Kim et al., 2001). In addition, HO-1 is increased in neurofibrillary tangles, senile plaque neurites, granulovacuolar degeneration and neuropil threads in human AD brains (Smith et al., 1994; Perry et al., 2003), suggesting the redistribution of iron due to release from heme proteins in affected areas of the AD brain.

NMDARs–mediated excitotoxicity also contributed to the pathology of AD. Evidence proved that impaired glutamate uptake in astrocytes and neurons in AD can lead to increased concentrations of glutamate at the synapse, which can subsequently trigger NMDARs–mediated excitotoxicity via increase of intracellular Ca^{2+} concentrations (Greenamyre et al., 1988; Tong et al., 2017). It has been shown that extrasynaptic NMDARs were largely associated with NMDARs-mediated excitotoxicity in AD (Hardingham and Bading, 2010). Prolonged activation of extrasynaptic NMDARs increases APP processing, leads to neuronal Aβ release, and ultimately results in AD pathology (Bordji et al., 2010). It has been reported that an open channel blocker memantine could preferentially antagonize excessively activated NMDARs (Lipton, 2004). *In vitro* and *in vivo* studies have demonstrated the neuroprotective effect of memantine in AD models. Memantine could prevent oligomeric Aβ-induced oxidative stress in mature hippocampal neurons (De Felice et al., 2007). More interestingly, memantine decreased the levels of secreted APP and Aβ peptide in human neuroblastoma cells (Ray et al., 2010) and lowered cortical levels of Aβ1–42 in APP/PS1 transgenic mice (Alley et al., 2010). This indicated the important role of excessively activated NMDARs in AD.

INTERACTION OF IRON AND NMDARs ACTIVATION

NMDARs Activation Promoted Iron Accumulation

Results revealed that activation of NMDARs significantly promoted Fe^{2+} entry into cells (Cheah et al., 2006). It was reported that NMDARs activation might promote iron accumulation by accelerating DMT1-mediated iron influx (Cheah et al., 2006), enhancing iron releasing from lysosome and regulation the expression of DMT1 (White et al., 2016). Elevated intracellular iron then aggravated iron-induced cell damage.

NMDARs Activation Increased NTBI Influx

It has been demonstrated that ferrous iron could block the influx of Ca^{2+} across NMDARs channels in cultured neurons (Nakamichi et al., 2004). This indicated that Fe^{2+} competed with Ca^{2+} for NMDARs to enter primary neurons. This iron entry can be harmful for neurons during aging due to increased NTBI levels. An investigation with interest to the involvement of NMDARs in NTBI influx pathways showed that activation of NMDARs significantly promoted Fe^{2+} entry into cells using fluorescence-based single cell analysis in rat hippocampal primary cultures (Pelizzoni et al., 2011). This elevation of iron was accompanied by a corresponding increase in reactive oxygen species (ROS) production and higher susceptibility of neurons to death.

Another investigation demonstrated a novel signaling cascade for glutamate in regulating iron uptake in the brain (Cheah et al., 2006). It is increasingly appreciated that glutamate via NMDARs triggers calcium influx, then activates neuronal NOS (nNOS) to produce NO, which causes excitability toxicity (Guix et al., 2005; Cheah et al., 2006; Chen et al., 2013; Courtney et al., 2014). Research has identified a signaling cascade whereby NMDARs regulated iron homeostasis (Cheah et al., 2006). Their results showed that the activation of NMDARs could increase intracellular iron levels in PC12 cells via NO-Dexras1-peripheral benzodiazepine receptor-associated protein 7 (PAP7)-DMT1 signaling cascade to enhance iron uptake (Cheah et al., 2006). Additionally, chelation of intracellular iron blocked formation of free radicals in brain cultures and also markedly attenuated NMDA neurotoxicity (Cheah et al., 2006). Furthermore, subsequent investigation showed that Dexras1 was required for NMDA-elicited neuronal toxicity via NO and iron influx (Chen et al., 2013). This implies that NMDA-NO activation-induced iron uptake might play an important role in neurotoxicity and misregulation of this pathway might participate in iron accumulation in PD. It has been shown that nNOS binding to CAPON leading to NO delivery to Dexras1 and S-nitrosylation of Dexras1. Then S-nitrosylation of Dexras1 could enhance iron uptake by regulating the function of iron importer DMT1. It was also reported that Dexras1 could be phosphorylated by protein kinase A (PKA) on serine 253. This PKA activation reduced Dexras1 S-nitrosylation, leading to an inhibition of iron influx (Chen et al., 2015). This indicated the important role of Dexras1 S-nitrosylation in iron uptake. In addition, PAP7 might presumably serve as a scaffold delivering Dexras1 into proximity to DMT1 (Cheah et al., 2006). However, another research showed that PAP7 played a role in cellular iron metabolism. They found that PAP7 was internalized in parallel with the internalization of DMT1 following iron feeding. And downregulated PAP7 expression in K562 cells with small interfering RNA led to downregulation of DMT1 (IRE) protein but not DMT1 (−IRE) mRNA. However, they did not measure iron uptake after downregulation of PAP7 expression. The levels of TfR1 and ferritin were not affected following transfection with siPAP7, indicating that the intracellular iron level might not change (Okazaki et al., 2012). Moreover, they also reported that overexpression of PAP7 had no effect on DMT1 (IRE) expression which is consist with the results of Cheah et al. (2006). Further research should be conducted to figure out the mechanisms underlying the effect of PAP7 on DMT1 and DMT1-induced iron uptake.

Rhes (Dexras2), a homolog of Dexras1, is a highly conserved small GTP binding protein belonging to the Ras superfamily. Rhes shares 67% identity with Dexras1. Although the physiological role of Rhes is not fully understood, results showed that Rhes physiologically interacted with PAP7 and participated in DMT1-induced iron uptake via pathway similar to Dexras1 (Choi et al., 2013). However, the mechanisms underlying the effect of Rhes on DMT1-induced iron uptake are different from Dexras1. They showed that Rhes was not S-nitrosylated after NO-treatment, however was phosphorylated by PKA at serine-239 (Choi et al., 2013). Rhes is selectively localized to the corpus striatum (Errico et al., 2008), so might involved in NMDARs-induced iron entry into the striatal neurons and maintain striatal iron homeostasis via PKA-Rhes-DMT1 pathway. In addition, striatum received nigral dopaminergic synapses projection and is responsible for movement balance. Imbalance of iron metabolism in striatum might contribute to the degeneration of striatal neurons and dysregulation of dopaminergic function in the striatum due to iron-induced oxidative stress, then affecting motor function.

NMDARs Activation Enhanced Iron Releasing from Lysosome

In fact, Dexras1 also could regulate TfR-mediated iron uptake as well as NTBI uptake (DMT1-mediated iron uptake) (Cheah et al., 2006). However, the exact mechanisms underlying this effect are not elucidated. Subcellular localization experiments showed that DMT1 + IRE had higher surface expression and was internalized from the plasma membrane with slower kinetics than DMT1 − IRE. And it was not efficiently recycled and was targeted to lysosomes. While DMT1 − IRE is efficiently sorted to recycling endosomes upon internalization (Lam-Yuk-Tseung and Gros, 2006). This implicated that different isoforms of DMT1 might have different functions on regulation of the subcellular localization of Fe^{2+} transport. As lysosomal iron serves as a main source for intracellular iron and DMT1 plays a role in iron recycling from lysosome to cytoplasm, DMT1-mediated iron release from lysosome might be responsible for increased intracellular iron levels. Findings from patch-clamping of individual lysosomes showed that they could transmit iron through their membrane (Dong et al., 2008). Recently, an investigation confirmed that the Dexras1/ACBD3(PAP7)/DMT1 complex was located on the lysosomes (White et al., 2016). Collapsing the proton gradient or blocking DMT1 channel both could reduce cytosolic iron pool (White et al., 2016), indicating that Dexras1/ACBD3/DMT1 complex played roles in iron release from lysosome. Therefore, NMDA activation not only led to Dexras1/DMT1 mediated increase in iron uptake, but also enhanced Dexras1-dependent iron release from lysosome.

NMDARs Activation Increased DMT1 Expression

Activation of NMDARs not only could affect the iron uptake function of DMT1, but also could regulate its expression. It has been reported that mRNA expression of DMT1-1B and DMT1 + IRE increased after 5 min exposure of 50 μM NMDA to primary hippocampal cultures, but not mRNA expression of DMT1 − IRE (Haeger et al., 2010). NMDA also enhanced DMT1 protein expression, which was abolished by the transcription inhibitor actinomycin D and NMDARs antagonist MK-801 (Haeger et al., 2010). This stimulation on iron entry pathway via DMT1 could ensure an adequate iron supply. This is of potential importance because iron deficiency hinders learning processes and impairs cognitive performance (Carlson et al., 2009; Muñoz et al., 2011; Estrada et al., 2014). This implicated that NMDARs-activation stimulated expression of the iron transporter DMT1-1B + IRE, which presumably played a significant role in hippocampal spatial memory formation. Interestingly, both excessive activation of NMDARs and upregulation of DMT1 were contributing factors in degeneration of DA neurons in PD, indicating the link between activation of NMDARs and upregulation of DMT1 in PD. Further studied should be conducted to elucidate this possibility and the underlying mechanisms.

NMDARs-Induced Co-Activation of ATP-Sensitive Potassium (K_{ATP}) Channels Might Promote Iron Influx via DMT1

K_{ATP} channel was first discovered by Akinori Noma in cardiac myocytes and was demonstrated to be important for regulation of cellular energy metabolism in the control of membrane excitability (Noma, 1983). Liss et al. (2005) provided evidence that selective activation of K_{ATP} channels of DA midbrain neurons in the SN was a potential mechanism for the selective degeneration of DA neurons in PD. Increased activity of K_{ATP} channels due to metabolic stress leads to membrane potential hyperpolarization and reduced SN DA activity (Liss et al., 2005). Although in adult mice K_{ATP} channels in DA neurons of both SN and VTA are formed by the same subunits (four Kir6.2 subunits and four regulatory SUR1 subunits), the activation of nigral K_{ATP} channels of DA neurons was responsible for the selective degeneration of DA neurons in PD (Liss et al., 2005). Moreover, genetic inactivation of the pore-forming subunit Kir6.2 of K_{ATP} channels induced a selective rescue of SN DA (but not VTA DA) neurons in MPTP-induced PD models (Liss et al., 2005). This indicated that activation of nigral K_{ATP} channels contributed to the selective degeneration of DA neurons in the SN.

It is reported that the activation of K_{ATP} channels induced hyperpolarization of the membrane potential of DA neurons in the SN following MPP^+ treatment (Liss et al., 2005). Furthermore, it was reported DMT1-mediated iron transport was driven at higher rates of hyperpolarized potentials (Gunshin et al., 1997). This makes the possibility that the hyperpolarization of cell membrane induced by activation of K_{ATP} channels might increase DMT1-mediated iron transport, and enhance iron influx into the DA neurons. Results in our experiments demonstrated that activation of the K_{ATP} channels in the DA cells caused hyperpolarization of the cell membrane and subsequently enhanced ferrous iron uptake function (Du X. et al., 2016). Results showed that activation of K_{ATP} channels resulted in increased free iron levels in the SK-N-SH cells and this was partially blocked by DMT1 knockdown. Further studies showed that activation of K_{ATP} channels by diazoxide prolonged Fe^{2+}-evoked currents in DMT1-transfected HEK293 cells using whole cell patch clamp recordings (Du X. et al., 2016). And inhibition of the K_{ATP} channels protected the DA neurons from the ferrous iron insult (Du X. et al., 2016). These results suggest that the activation of K_{ATP} channels could enhance DMT1-mediated iron uptake, resulting in an increased intracellular iron contents and oxidative stress, and ultimately cell damage.

It has been proved that there is a relationship between NMDARs and K_{ATP} channels. Elevated mRNA expressions of K_{ATP} channels and NMDARs subunits were found in human SN DA neurons from PD patients (Schiemann et al., 2012). NMDARs stimulation *in vitro* induced the co-activation of K_{ATP} channels in subthalamic neurons (Shen and Johnson, 2010). Activity of K_{ATP} channels in medial DA neurons of the SN enabled NMDA-mediated bursting *in vitro* and *in vivo* in anesthetized mice (Schiemann et al., 2012). Furthermore, activation of K_{ATP} channels in already metabolically challenged SN DA neurons could promote excitotoxicity and increase NMDARs-mediated calcium loading (Schiemann et al., 2012). Calcium-triggered ROS production from mitochondria in turn activated K_{ATP} channels in highly vulnerable SN DA neurons (Liss et al., 2005). In addition, NMDARs-mediated NO production might activate K_{ATP} channels in large DRG neurons via direct S-nitrosylation of SUR1 subunit (Kawano et al., 2009). The link of K_{ATP} channels and DMT1 indicated that co-activation of NMDARs and K_{ATP}

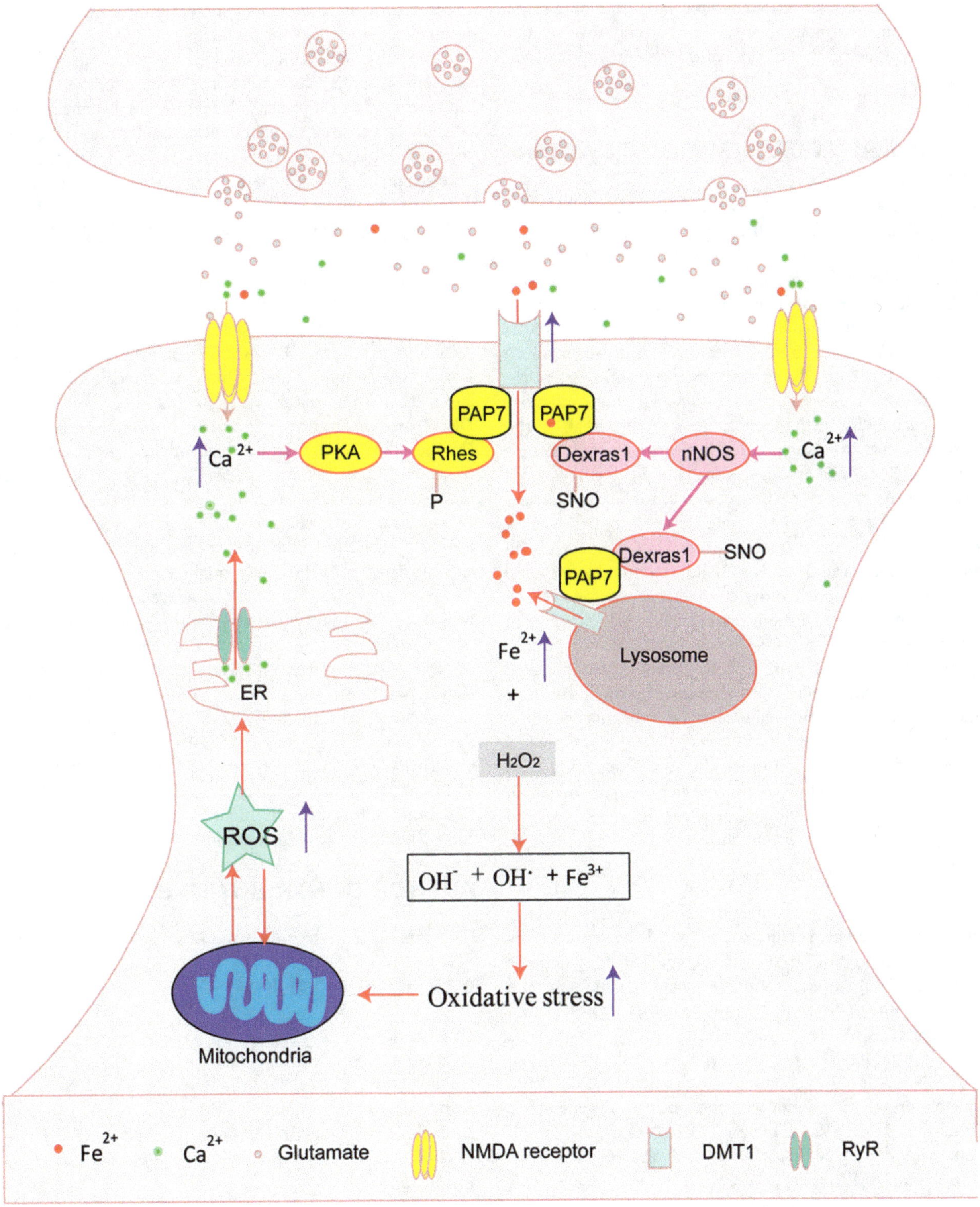

FIGURE 1 | Possible interaction between N-methyl-D-aspartate receptors (NMDARs) activation and iron overload. NMDARs activation might promote divalent metal transporter 1 (DMT1)-mediated iron influx via protein kinase A (PKA)-Rhes-DMT1, NO-Dexras1-peripheral benzodiazepine receptor-associated protein 7 (PAP7)-DMT1 signaling cascade pathway and enhance iron releasing from lysosome, then aggravated iron-induced cell damage. In addition, iron overload might stimulate calcium release from endoplasmic reticulum (ER). This indicated that glutamate-induced neurotoxicity and iron participated to a vicious cycle of neuronal death.

channels could affect iron uptake function of DMT1, which might contribute to iron accumulation and the degeneration of neurons in neurological diseases. Further investigation should be conducted in the future to reveal the underlying mechanisms.

Iron Affected NMDARs-Mediated Synaptic Transmission

It was reported that iron has an effect on NMDARs-mediated synaptic plasticity. Investigation demonstrated that glutamatergic neurotransmission pathways were regulated by dietary iron (Han and Kim, 2015). They showed that NMDARs were significantly elevated in the prefrontal cortex and hippocampus of iron-loaded rats. These findings indicate the important role of iron in learning and memory via regulation NMDARs-mediated neurotransmission. In addition, study showed that intracellular iron signaling could modulate neuronal excitability in the hippocampus (White et al., 2016). They showed that iron was released in neurons from lysosome can regulate NMDARs mediated glutamatergic excitability via PKC/Src/NR2A pathway (White et al., 2016). This indicates that iron can act in a feedback manner to modulate NMDA function and thus maintain the excitability of neurons in normal condition. In addition, NMDARs activation induce rapid opening of Ca^{2+} channel across cell membranes, followed by an increase in free Ca^{2+} ions in the cytoplasm and subsequent signaling cascade in the CNS (Paul and Connor, 2010). Hippocampal neurons require iron to generate RyR-mediated calcium signals after NMDARs stimulation, which in turn promotes ERK1/2 activation, an essential step of sustained LTP (Muñoz et al., 2011). It was reported that iron stimulated RyR-mediated Ca^{2+} release from endoplasmic reticulum (ER) in PC12 cells (Múñoz et al., 2006). Further study showed that iron-induced ROS generation is required for RyR-mediated Ca^{2+} release for long-term potentiation in primary hippocampal neurons (Muñoz et al., 2011).

However, evidence has also proved that iron was involved in glutamate excitotoxicity (Yu et al., 2009). As is known that glutamate excitotoxicity could be induced by threohydroxyaspartate (THA), which could inhibit glutamate uptake and lead to accumulation of synaptic glutamate and over stimulation of the postsynaptic receptors. It was found that increased iron level was involved in THA-induced glutamate excitotoxicity in rat spinal cord tissue (Yu et al., 2009). And iron chelator deferoxamine (DFO) could completely prevent THA-induced motor neuron degeneration. Importantly, NMDARs inhibitor MK-801 could inhibit glutamate and hypoxia/reperfusion-mediated damage, but not the kainate/AMPA antagonist CNQX (Yu et al., 2009). This supports the idea that iron contributed to glutamate-induced excitotoxicity via NMDARs and regulation of iron level might be an effective strategy for protection against glutamate-induced excitotoxicity. Therefore, iron is required for NMDARs-mediated synaptic plasticity in physiologic conditions. However, iron overload might promote NMDARs-mediated excitotoxicity possibly by enhancing RyR-mediated Ca^{2+} release and calcium-induced cell damage. Further studies should be conducted to investigate this possibility and the underlying mechanisms.

CONCLUSION AND PERSPECTIVES

In this review article, we describe the possible relationship between NMDARs activation and iron deposit, which both contributed to the pathogenesis of neurological diseases including PD and AD. NMDARs activation might promote iron accumulation by enhancing DMT1-mediated iron influx, stimulating iron releasing from lysosome, and regulating DMT1 expression, thus aggravating iron-induced cell damage. On the other hand, iron overload might aggravate NMDARs-mediated glutamate excitotoxicity. This suggests that glutamate-induced neurotoxicity and iron participate to a vicious cycle of neuronal death (**Figure 1**). Therefore, regulation of iron levels might be effective for protection against glutamate-induced excitotoxicity and NMDARs might be a potential target for the treatment of iron-induced neurodegenerative processes. The drug discovery strategy is being oriented toward the development of new molecules targeting both iron overload and activation of NMDARs. However, NMDARs-mediated excitotoxicity and iron deposit were also reported in other neurological diseases such as stroke, Huntington' disease (Carvajal et al., 2016; Li and Reichmann, 2016; Petrova et al., 2016). The exact mechanisms underlying interaction between NMDARs activation and iron accumulation in these diseases should be conducted in the future. The future of this research might have significant impact on the clinical treatment of these neurological diseases.

AUTHOR CONTRIBUTIONS

HX wrote the manuscript. HJ and JX revised the manuscript.

ACKNOWLEDGMENTS

This work was supported by grants from the National Foundation of Natural Science of China (31371081, 81430024 and 31471114), the Department of Science and Technology of Shandong Province (ZR2015JL011) and the Bureau of Science and Technology of Qingdao (15-9-1-20-jch), Taishan Scholarship and Program for New Century Excellent Talents in University.

REFERENCES

Abboud, S., and Haile, D. J. (2000). A novel mammalian iron-regulated protein involved in intracellular iron metabolism. *J. Biol. Chem.* 275, 19906–19912. doi: 10.1074/jbc.m000713200

Alley, G. M., Bailey, J. A., Chen, D., Ray, B., Puli, L. K., Tanila, H., et al. (2010). Memantine lowers amyloid-β peptide levels in neuronal cultures and in APP/PS1 transgenic mice. *J. Neurosci. Res.* 88, 143–154. doi: 10.1002/jnr.22172

Altamura, S., and Muckenthaler, M. U. (2009). Iron toxicity in diseases of aging: Alzheimer's disease, Parkinson's disease and atherosclerosis. *J. Alzheimers Dis.* 16, 879–895. doi: 10.3233/JAD-2009-1010

Ambrosi, G., Cerri, S., and Blandini, F. (2014). A further update on the role of excitotoxicity in the pathogenesis of Parkinson's disease. *J. Neural Transm. (Vienna)* 121, 849–859. doi: 10.1007/s00702-013-1149-z

Ayton, S., Lei, P., Duce, J. A., Wong, B. X., Sedjahtera, A., Adlard, P. A., et al. (2013). Ceruloplasmin dysfunction and therapeutic potential for Parkinson disease. *Ann. Neurol.* 73, 554–559. doi: 10.1002/ana.23817

Bading, H. (2017). Therapeutic targeting of the pathological triad of extrasynaptic NMDA receptor signaling in neurodegenerations. *J. Exp. Med.* doi: 10.1084/jem.20161673 [Epub ahead of print].

Bastian, T. W., von Hohenberg, W. C., Mickelson, D. J., Lanier, L. M., and Georgieff, M. K. (2016). Iron deficiency impairs developing hippocampal neuron gene expression, energy metabolism, and dendrite complexity. *Dev. Neurosci.* 38, 264–276. doi: 10.1159/000448514

Belaidi, A. A., and Bush, A. I. (2016). Iron neurochemistry in Alzheimer's disease and Parkinson's disease: targets for therapeutics. *J. Neurochem.* 139, 179–197. doi: 10.1111/jnc.13425

Bordji, K., Becerril-Ortega, J., Nicole, O., and Buisson, A. (2010). Activation of extrasynaptic, but not synaptic, NMDA receptors modifies amyloid precursor protein expression pattern and increases amyloid-β production. *J. Neurosci.* 30, 15927–15942. doi: 10.1523/JNEUROSCI.3021-10.2010

Carlson, E. S., Tkac, I., Magid, R., O'Connor, M. B., Andrews, N. C., Schallert, T., et al. (2009). Iron is essential for neuron development and memory function in mouse hippocampus. *J. Nutr.* 139, 672–679. doi: 10.3945/jn.108.096354

Carvajal, F. J., Mattison, H. A., and Cerpa, W. (2016). Role of NMDA receptor-mediated glutamatergic signaling in chronic and acute neuropathologies. *Neural Plast.* 2016:2701526. doi: 10.1155/2016/2701526

Cheah, J. H., Kim, S. F., Hester, L. D., Clancy, K. W., Patterson, S. E. III., Papadopoulos, V., et al. (2006). NMDA receptor-nitric oxide transmission mediates neuronal iron homeostasis via the GTPase Dexras1. *Neuron* 51, 431–440. doi: 10.1016/j.neuron.2006.07.011

Chen, Y., Khan, R. S., Cwanger, A., Song, Y., Steenstra, C., Bang, S., et al. (2013). Dexras1, a small GTPase, is required for glutamate-NMDA neurotoxicity. *J. Neurosci.* 33, 3582–3587. doi: 10.1523/JNEUROSCI.1497-12.2013

Chen, Y., Mathias, L., Falero-Perez, J. M., and Kim, S. F. (2015). PKA-mediated phosphorylation of Dexras1 suppresses iron trafficking by inhibiting S-nitrosylation. *FEBS Lett.* 589, 3212–3219. doi: 10.1016/j.febslet.2015.08.041

Choi, B.-R., Bang, S., Chen, Y., Cheah, J. H., and Kim, S. F. (2013). PKA modulates iron trafficking in the striatum via small GTPase, Rhes. *Neuroscience* 253, 214–220. doi: 10.1016/j.neuroscience.2013.08.043

Courtney, M. J., Li, L.-L., and Lai, Y. Y. (2014). Mechanisms of NOS1AP action on NMDA receptor-nNOS signaling. *Front. Cell. Neurosci.* 8:252. doi: 10.3389/fncel.2014.00252

Dedman, D. J., Treffry, A., Candy, J. M., Taylor, G. A., Morris, C. M., Bloxham, C. A., et al. (1992). Iron and aluminium in relation to brain ferritin in normal individuals and Alzheimer's-disease and chronic renal-dialysis patients. *Biochem. J.* 287, 509–514. doi: 10.1042/bj2870509

De Felice, F. G., Velasco, P. T., Lambert, M. P., Viola, K., Fernandez, S. J., Ferreira, S. T., et al. (2007). Aβ oligomers induce neuronal oxidative stress through an N-methyl-D-aspartate receptor-dependent mechanism that is blocked by the Alzheimer drug memantine. *J. Biol. Chem.* 282, 11590–11601. doi: 10.1074/jbc.m607483200

Dong, X.-P., Cheng, X., Mills, E., Delling, M., Wang, F., Kurz, T., et al. (2008). The type IV mucolipidosis-associated protein TRPML1 is an endolysosomal iron release channel. *Nature* 455, 992–996. doi: 10.1038/nature07311

Do Van, B., Gouel, F., Jonneaux, A., Timmerman, K., Gelé, P., Pétrault, M., et al. (2016). Ferroptosis, a newly characterized form of cell death in Parkinson's disease that is regulated by PKC. *Neurobiol. Dis.* 94, 169–178. doi: 10.1016/j.nbd.2016.05.011

Du, G., Liu, T., Lewis, M. M., Kong, L., Wang, Y., Connor, J., et al. (2016). Quantitative susceptibility mapping of the midbrain in Parkinson's disease. *Mov. Disord.* 31, 317–324. doi: 10.1002/mds.26417

Du, X., Xu, H., Shi, L., Jiang, Z., Song, N., Jiang, H., et al. (2016). Activation of ATP-sensitive potassium channels enhances DMT1-mediated iron uptake in SK-N-SH cells *in vitro*. *Sci. Rep.* 6:33674. doi: 10.1038/srep33674

Errico, F., Santini, E., Migliarini, S., Borgkvist, A., Centonze, D., Nasti, V., et al. (2008). The GTP-binding protein Rhes modulates dopamine signalling in striatal medium spiny neurons. *Mol. Cell. Neurosci.* 37, 335–345. doi: 10.1016/j.mcn.2007.10.007

Estrada, J. A., Contreras, I., Pliego-Rivero, F. B., and Otero, G. A. (2014). Molecular mechanisms of cognitive impairment in iron deficiency: alterations in brain-derived neurotrophic factor and insulin-like growth factor expression and function in the central nervous system. *Nutr. Neurosci.* 17, 193–206. doi: 10.1179/1476830513y.0000000084

Falangola, M. F., Lee, S.-P., Nixon, R. A., Duff, K., and Helpern, J. A. (2005). Histological co-localization of iron in Aβ plaques of PS/APP transgenic mice. *Neurochem. Res.* 30, 201–205. doi: 10.1007/s11064-004-2442-x

Ganz, T. (2005). Cellular iron: ferroportin is the only way out. *Cell Metab.* 1, 155–157. doi: 10.1016/j.cmet.2005.02.005

Gonzalez, J., Jurado-Coronel, J. C., Ávila, M. F., Sabogal, A., Capani, F., and Barreto, G. E. (2015). NMDARs in neurological diseases: a potential therapeutic target. *Int. J. Neurosci.* 125, 315–327. doi: 10.3109/00207454.2014.940941

Good, P. F., Perl, D. P., Bierer, L. M., and Schmeidler, J. (1992). Selective accumulation of aluminum and iron in the neurofibrillary tangles of Alzheimer's disease: a laser microprobe (LAMMA) study. *Ann. Neurol.* 31, 286–292. doi: 10.1002/ana.410310310

Greenamyre, J. T., Maragos, W. F., Albin, R. L., Penney, J. B., and Young, A. B. (1988). Glutamate transmission and toxicity in Alzheimer's disease. *Prog. Neuropsychopharmacol. Biol. Psychiatry* 12, 421–430. doi: 10.1016/0278-5846(88)90102-9

Guix, F. X., Uribesalgo, I., Coma, M., and Muñoz, F. J. (2005). The physiology and pathophysiology of nitric oxide in the brain. *Prog. Neurobiol.* 76, 126–152. doi: 10.1016/j.pneurobio.2005.06.001

Gunshin, H., Mackenzie, B., Berger, U. V., Gunshin, Y., Romero, M. F., Boron, W. F., et al. (1997). Cloning and characterization of a mammalian proton-coupled metal-ion transporter. *Nature* 388, 482–488. doi: 10.1038/41343

Haeger, P., Alvarez, A., Leal, N., Adasme, T., Núñez, M. T., and Hidalgo, C. (2010). Increased hippocampal expression of the divalent metal transporter 1 (DMT1) mRNA variants 1B and +IRE and DMT1 protein after NMDA-receptor stimulation or spatial memory training. *Neurotox. Res.* 17, 238–247. doi: 10.1007/s12640-009-9096-z

Han, M., and Kim, J. (2015). Effect of dietary iron loading on recognition memory in growing rats. *PLoS One* 10:e0120609. doi: 10.1371/journal.pone.0120609

Hardingham, G. E., and Bading, H. (2010). Synaptic versus extrasynaptic NMDA receptor signalling: implications for neurodegenerative disorders. *Nat. Rev. Neurosci.* 11, 682–696. doi: 10.1038/nrn2911

Hardy, J. (1997). Amyloid, the presenilins and Alzheimer's disease. *Trends Neurosci.* 20, 154–159. doi: 10.1016/s0166-2236(96)01030-2

He, Q., Song, N., Jia, F., Xu, H., Yu, X., Xie, J., et al. (2013). Role of α-synuclein aggregation and the nuclear factor E2-related factor 2/heme oxygenase-1 pathway in iron-induced neurotoxicity. *Int. J. Biochem. Cell Biol.* 45, 1019–1030. doi: 10.1016/j.biocel.2013.02.012

Hornykiewicz, O. (2008). Basic research on dopamine in Parkinson's disease and the discovery of the nigrostriatal dopamine pathway: the view of an eyewitness. *Neurodegener. Dis.* 5, 114–117. doi: 10.1159/000113678

Huang, X., Moir, R. D., Tanzi, R. E., Bush, A. I., and Rogers, J. T. (2004). Redox-active metals, oxidative stress, and Alzheimer's disease pathology. *Ann. N Y Acad. Sci.* 1012, 153–163. doi: 10.1196/annals.1306.012

Huang, E., Ong, W. Y., and Connor, J. R. (2004). Distribution of divalent metal transporter-1 in the monkey basal ganglia. *Neuroscience* 128, 487–496. doi: 10.1016/j.neuroscience.2004.06.055

Hubert, N., and Hentze, M. W. (2002). Previously uncharacterized isoforms of divalent metal transporter (DMT)-1: implications for regulation and cellular function. *Proc. Natl. Acad. Sci. U S A* 99, 12345–12350. doi: 10.1073/pnas.192423399

Hynd, M. R., Scott, H. L., and Dodd, P. R. (2004). Glutamate-mediated excitotoxicity and neurodegeneration in Alzheimer's disease. *Neurochem. Int.* 45, 583–595. doi: 10.1016/j.neuint.2004.03.007

Jiang, H., Song, N., Xu, H., Zhang, S., Wang, J., and Xie, J. (2010). Up-regulation of divalent metal transporter 1 in 6-hydroxydopamine intoxication is IRE/IRP dependent. *Cell Res.* 20, 345–356. doi: 10.1038/cr.2010.20

Jiang, H., Wang, J., Rogers, J., and Xie, J. (2016). Brain iron metabolism dysfunction in Parkinson's disease. *Mol. Neurobiol.* doi: 10.1007/s12035-016-9879-1 [Epub ahead of print]

Jones, S., and Gibb, A. J. (2005). Functional NR2B- and NR2D-containing NMDA receptor channels in rat substantia nigra dopaminergic neurones. *J. Physiol.* 569, 209–221. doi: 10.1113/jphysiol.2005.095554

Jorgenson, L. A., Wobken, J. D., and Georgieff, M. K. (2003). Perinatal iron deficiency alters apical dendritic growth in hippocampal CA1 pyramidal neurons. *Dev. Neurosci.* 25, 412–420. doi: 10.1159/000075667

Kaneko, K., Hineno, A., Yoshida, K., and Ikeda, S. (2008). Increased vulnerability to rotenone-induced neurotoxicity in ceruloplasmin-deficient mice. *Neurosci. Lett.* 446, 56–58. doi: 10.1016/j.neulet.2008.08.089

Kawano, T., Zoga, V., Kimura, M., Liang, M. Y., Wu, H. E., Gemes, G., et al. (2009). Nitric oxide activates ATP-sensitive potassium channels in mammalian sensory neurons: action by direct S-nitrosylation. *Mol. Pain* 5:12. doi: 10.1186/1744-8069-5-12

Kim, D. K., Seo, M. Y., Lim, S. W., Kim, S., Kim, J. W., Carroll, B. J., et al. (2001). Serum melanotransferrin, p97 as a biochemical marker of Alzheimer's disease. *Neuropsychopharmacology* 25, 84–90. doi: 10.1016/s0893-133x(00)00230-x

Köles, L., Kató, E., Hanuska, A., Zádori, Z. S., Al-Khrasani, M., Zelles, T., et al. (2016). Modulation of excitatory neurotransmission by neuronal/glial signalling molecules: interplay between purinergic and glutamatergic systems. *Purinergic Signal.* 12, 1–24. doi: 10.1007/s11302-015-9480-5

Kostka, M., Högen, T., Danzer, K. M., Levin, J., Habeck, M., Wirth, A., et al. (2008). Single particle characterization of iron-induced pore-forming α-synuclein oligomers. *J. Biol. Chem.* 283, 10992–11003. doi: 10.1074/jbc.M709634200

Lam-Yuk-Tseung, S., and Gros, P. (2006). Distinct targeting and recycling properties of two isoforms of the iron transporter DMT1 (NRAMP2, Slc11A2). *Biochemistry* 45, 2294–2301. doi: 10.1021/bi052307m

LaVaute, T., Smith, S., Cooperman, S., Iwai, K., Land, W., Meyron-Holtz, E., et al. (2001). Targeted deletion of the gene encoding iron regulatory protein-2 causes misregulation of iron metabolism and neurodegenerative disease in mice. *Nat. Genet.* 27, 209–214. doi: 10.1038/84859

Lee, D. G., Park, J., Lee, H. S., Lee, S. R., and Lee, D. S. (2016). Iron overload-induced calcium signals modulate mitochondrial fragmentation in HT-22 hippocampal neuron cells. *Toxicology* 365, 17–24. doi: 10.1016/j.tox.2016.07.022

Li, D. (1998). Effects of iron deficiency on iron distribution and γ-aminobutyric acid (GABA) metabolism in young rat brain tissues. *Hokkaido Igaku Zasshi* 73, 215–225.

Li, K., and Reichmann, H. (2016). Role of iron in neurodegenerative diseases. *J. Neural Transm. (Vienna)* 123, 389–399. doi: 10.1007/s00702-016-1508-7

Lieu, P. T., Heiskala, M., Peterson, P. A., and Yang, Y. (2001). The roles of iron in health and disease. *Mol. Aspects Med.* 22, 1–87. doi: 10.1016/s0098-2997(00)00006-6

Lipton, S. A. (2004). Paradigm shift in NMDA receptor antagonist drug development: molecular mechanism of uncompetitive inhibition by memantine in the treatment of Alzheimer's disease and other neurologic disorders. *J. Alzheimers Dis.* 6, S61–S74.

Liss, B., Haeckel, O., Wildmann, J., Miki, T., Seino, S., and Roeper, J. (2005). K-ATP channels promote the differential degeneration of dopaminergic midbrain neurons. *Nat. Neurosci.* 8, 1742–1751. doi: 10.1038/nn1570

Little, S., and Brown, P. (2014). Focusing brain therapeutic interventions in space and time for Parkinson's disease. *Curr. Biol.* 24, R898–R909. doi: 10.1016/j.cub.2014.08.002

Lu, L. N., Qian, Z. M., Wu, K. C., Yung, W. H., and Ke, Y. (2016). Expression of iron transporters and pathological hallmarks of Parkinson's and Alzheimer's diseases in the brain of young, adult and aged rats. *Mol. Neurobiol.* doi: 10.1007/s12035-016-0067-0 [Epub ahead of print].

Mandel, S., Amit, T., Bar-Am, O., and Youdim, M. B. (2007). Iron dysregulation in Alzheimer's disease: multimodal brain permeable iron chelating drugs, possessing neuroprotective-neurorescue and amyloid precursor protein-processing regulatory activities as therapeutic agents. *Prog. Neurobiol.* 82, 348–360. doi: 10.1016/j.pneurobio.2007.06.001

Mantyh, P. W., Ghilardi, J. R., Rogers, S., Demaster, E., Allen, C. J., Stimson, E. R., et al. (1993). Aluminum, iron and zinc ions promote aggregation of physiological concentrations of β-amyloid peptide. *J. Neurochem.* 61, 1171–1174. doi: 10.1111/j.1471-4159.1993.tb03639.x

Mattson, M. P. (1997). Cellular actions of β-amyloid precursor protein and its soluble and fibrillogenic derivatives. *Physiol. Rev.* 77, 1081–1132.

Meoni, P., Bunnemann, B. H., Kingsbury, A. E., Trist, D. G., and Bowery, N. G. (1999). NMDA NR1 subunit mRNA and glutamate NMDA-sensitive binding are differentially affected in the striatum and pre-frontal cortex of Parkinson's disease patients. *Neuropharmacology* 38, 625–633. doi: 10.1016/s0028-3908(98)00219-6

Mohanakumar, K. P., de Bartolomeis, A., Wu, R. M., Yeh, K. J., Sternberger, L. M., Peng, S. Y., et al. (1994). Ferrous-citrate complex and nigral degeneration: evidence for free-radical formation and lipid peroxidation. *Ann. N Y Acad. Sci.* 738, 392–399. doi: 10.1111/j.1749-6632.1994.tb21828.x

Muñoz, Y., Carrasco, C. M., Campos, J. D., Aguirre, P., and Núñez, M. T. (2016). Parkinson's disease: the mitochondria-iron link. *Parkinsons Dis.* 2016:7049108. doi: 10.1155/2016/7049108

Muñoz, P., Humeres, A., Elgueta, C., Kirkwood, A., Hidalgo, C., and Núñez, M. T. (2011). Iron mediates N-methyl-D-aspartate receptor-dependent stimulation of calcium-induced pathways and hippocampal synaptic plasticity. *J. Biol. Chem.* 286, 13382–13392. doi: 10.1074/jbc.M110.213785

Múñoz, P., Zavala, G., Castillo, K., Aguirre, P., Hidalgo, C., and Nunez, M. T. (2006). Effect of iron on the activation of the MAPK/ERK pathway in PC12 neuroblastoma cells. *Biol. Res.* 39, 189–190. doi: 10.4067/s0716-97602006000100021

Nakamichi, N., Oikawa, H., Kambe, Y., and Yoneda, Y. (2004). Relevant modulation by ferrous ions of N-methyl-D-aspartate receptors in ischemic brain injuries. *Curr. Neurovasc. Res.* 1, 429–440. doi: 10.2174/1567202043361910

Nakamura, M., Shishido, N., Nunomura, A., Smith, M. A., Perry, G., Hayashi, Y., et al. (2007). Three histidine residues of amyloid-β peptide control the redox activity of copper and iron. *Biochemistry* 46, 12737–12743. doi: 10.1021/bi701079z

Noma, A. (1983). ATP-regulated K^+ channels in cardiac muscle. *Nature* 305, 147–148. doi: 10.1038/305147a0

Okazaki, Y., Ma, Y., Yeh, M., Yin, H., Li, Z., Yeh, K. Y., et al. (2012). DMT1 (IRE) expression in intestinal and erythroid cells is regulated by peripheral benzodiazepine receptor-associated protein 7. *Am. J. Physiol. Gastrointest. Liver Physiol.* 302, G1180–G1190. doi: 10.1152/ajpgi.00545.2010

Oster, S., Radad, K., Scheller, D., Hesse, M., Balanzew, W., Reichmann, H., et al. (2014). Rotigotine protects against glutamate toxicity in primary dopaminergic cell culture. *Eur. J. Pharmacol.* 724, 31–42. doi: 10.1016/j.ejphar.2013.12.014

Parkinson, J. (2002). An essay on the shaking palsy. 1817. *J. Neuropsychiatry Clin. Neurosci.* 14, 223–236; discussion 222. doi: 10.1176/appi.neuropsych.14.2.223

Paul, S., and Connor, J. A. (2010). NR2B-NMDA receptor-mediated increases in intracellular Ca^{2+} concentration regulate the tyrosine phosphatase, STEP and ERK MAP kinase signaling. *J. Neurochem.* 114, 1107–1118. doi: 10.1111/j.1471-4159.2010.06835.x

Pelizzoni, I., Macco, R., Morini, M. F., Zacchetti, D., Grohovaz, F., and Codazzi, F. (2011). Iron handling in hippocampal neurons: activity-dependent iron entry and mitochondria-mediated neurotoxicity. *Aging Cell* 10, 172–183. doi: 10.1111/j.1474-9726.2010.00652.x

Perez, C. A., Tong, Y., and Guo, M. (2008). Iron chelators as potential therapeutic agents for Parkinson's disease. *Curr. Bioact. Compd.* 4, 150–158. doi: 10.2174/157340708786305952

Perry, G., Taddeo, M. A., Petersen, R. B., Castellani, R. J., Harris, P. L., Siedlak, S. L., et al. (2003). Adventiously-bound redox active iron and copper are at the center of oxidative damage in Alzheimer disease. *Biometals* 16, 77–81. doi: 10.1023/A:1020731021276

Petrova, J., Manolov, V., Vasilev, V., Tzatchev, K., and Marinov, B. (2016). Ischemic stroke, inflammation, iron overload—connection to a hepcidin. *Int. J. Stroke* 11, 16–17. doi: 10.1177/1747493015607509

Piñero, D. J., Hu, J., and Connor, J. R. (2000). Alterations in the interaction between iron regulatory proteins and their iron responsive element in normal and Alzheimer's diseased brains. *Cell. Mol. Biol. (Noisy-le-grand)* 46, 761–776.

Piñero, D. J., Li, N., Hu, J., Beard, J. L., and Connor, J. R. (2001). The intracellular location of iron regulatory proteins is altered as a function of iron status in cell cultures and rat brain. *J. Nutr.* 131, 2831–2836.

Qian, Z. M., and Shen, X. (2001). Brain iron transport and neurodegeneration. *Trends Mol. Med.* 7, 103–108. doi: 10.1016/s1471-4914(00)01910-9

Ray, B., Banerjee, P. K., Greig, N. H., and Lahiri, D. K. (2010). Memantine treatment decreases levels of secreted Alzheimer's amyloid precursor protein (APP) and amyloid beta (Aβ) peptide in the human neuroblastoma cells. *Neurosci. Lett.* 470, 1–5. doi: 10.1016/j.neulet.2009.11.016

Rogers, J. T., Randall, J. D., Cahill, C. M., Eder, P. S., Huang, X., Gunshin, H., et al. (2002). An iron-responsive element type II in the 5'-untranslated region of the Alzheimer's amyloid precursor protein transcript. *J. Biol. Chem.* 277, 45518–45528. doi: 10.1074/jbc.M207435200

Saadat, S. M., Değirmenci, I., Özkan, S., Saydam, F., Özdemir Köroğlu, Z., Çolak, E., et al. (2015). Is the 1254T > C polymorphism in the DMT1 gene associated with Parkinson's disease? *Neurosci. Lett.* 594, 51–54. doi: 10.1016/j.neulet.2015.03.054

Salazar, J., Mena, N., Hunot, S., Prigent, A., Alvarez-Fischer, D., Arredondo, M., et al. (2008). Divalent metal transporter 1 (DMT1) contributes to neurodegeneration in animal models of Parkinson's disease. *Proc. Natl. Acad. Sci. U S A* 105, 18578–18583. doi: 10.1073/pnas.0804373105

Sattler, R., and Tymianski, M. (2000). Molecular mechanisms of calcium-dependent excitotoxicity. *J. Mol. Med.* 78, 3–13. doi: 10.1007/s001090000077

Schiemann, J., Schlaudraff, F., Klose, V., Bingmer, M., Seino, S., Magill, P. J., et al. (2012). K-ATP channels in dopamine substantia nigra neurons control bursting and novelty-induced exploration. *Nat. Neurosci.* 15, 1272–1280. doi: 10.1038/nn.3185

Schubert, D., and Chevion, M. (1995). The role of iron in beta amyloid toxicity. *Biochem. Biophys. Res. Commun.* 216, 702–707. doi: 10.1006/bbrc.1995.2678

Selkoe, D. J. (1996). Amyloid β-protein and the genetics of Alzheimer's disease. *J. Biol. Chem.* 271, 18295–18298. doi: 10.1074/jbc.271.31.18295

Shen, K. Z., and Johnson, S. W. (2010). Ca^{2+} influx through NMDA-gated channels activates ATP-sensitive K^+ currents through a nitric oxide-cGMP pathway in subthalamic neurons. *J. Neurosci.* 30, 1882–1893. doi: 10.1523/JNEUROSCI.3200-09.2010

Smith, M. A., Kutty, R. K., Richey, P. L., Yan, S. D., Stern, D., Chader, G. J., et al. (1994). Heme oxygenase-1 is associated with the neurofibrillary pathology of Alzheimer's disease. *Am. J. Pathol.* 145, 42–47.

Sofic, E., Riederer, P., Heinsen, H., Beckmann, H., Reynolds, G. P., Hebenstreit, G., et al. (1988). Increased iron (III) and total iron content in post mortem substantia nigra of parkinsonian brain. *J. Neural Transm.* 74, 199–205. doi: 10.1007/bf01244786

Song, N., Wang, J., Jiang, H., and Xie, J. (2010). Ferroportin 1 but not hephaestin contributes to iron accumulation in a cell model of Parkinson's disease. *Free Radic. Biol. Med.* 48, 332–341. doi: 10.1016/j.freeradbiomed.2009.11.004

Todorich, B., Pasquini, J. M., Garcia, C. I., Paez, P. M., and Connor, J. R. (2009). Oligodendrocytes and myelination: the role of iron. *Glia* 57, 467–478. doi: 10.1002/glia.20784

Tong, H., Zhang, X., Meng, X., Xu, P., Zou, X., and Qu, S. (2017). Amyloid-beta peptide decreases expression and function of glutamate transporters in nervous system cells. *Int. J. Biochem. Cell Biol.* 85, 75–84. doi: 10.1016/j.biocel.2017.01.017

Van Bergen, J. M., Li, X., Hua, J., Schreiner, S. J., Steininger, S. C., Quevenco, F. C., et al. (2016). Colocalization of cerebral iron with amyloid beta in mild cognitive impairment. *Sci. Rep.* 6:35514. doi: 10.1038/srep35514

Van Laar, V. S., Roy, N., Liu, A., Rajprohat, S., Arnold, B., Dukes, A. A., et al. (2015). Glutamate excitotoxicity in neurons triggers mitochondrial and endoplasmic reticulum accumulation of Parkin and, in the presence of N-acetyl cysteine, mitophagy. *Neurobiol. Dis.* 74, 180–193. doi: 10.1016/j.nbd.2014.11.015

Wang, J., Bi, M., and Xie, J. (2015). Ceruloplasmin is involved in the nigral iron accumulation of 6-OHDA-lesioned rats. *Cell. Mol. Neurobiol.* 35, 661–668. doi: 10.1007/s10571-015-0161-2

Wang, J., Jiang, H., and Xie, J. X. (2007). Ferroportin1 and hephaestin are involved in the nigral iron accumulation of 6-OHDA-lesioned rats. *Eur. J. Neurosci.* 25, 2766–2772. doi: 10.1111/j.1460-9568.2007.05515.x

Ward, R. J., Zucca, F. A., Duyn, J. H., Crichton, R. R., and Zecca, L. (2014). The role of iron in brain ageing and neurodegenerative disorders. *Lancet Neurol.* 13, 1045–1060. doi: 10.1016/s1474-4422(14)70117-6

White, R. S., Bhattacharya, A. K., Chen, Y., Byrd, M., McMullen, M. F., Siegel, S. J., et al. (2016). Lysosomal iron modulates NMDA receptor-mediated excitation via small GTPase, Dexras1. *Mol. Brain* 9:38. doi: 10.1186/s13041-016-0220-8

Whitnall, M., and Richardson, D. R. (2006). Iron: a new target for pharmacological intervention in neurodegenerative diseases. *Semin. Pediatr. Neurol.* 13, 186–197. doi: 10.1016/j.spen.2006.08.008

Wu, Y. N., and Johnson, S. W. (2015). Memantine selectively blocks extrasynaptic NMDA receptors in rat substantia nigra dopamine neurons. *Brain Res.* 1603, 1–7. doi: 10.1016/j.brainres.2015.01.041

Wu, S. F., Zhu, Z. F., Kong, Y., Zhang, H. P., Zhou, G. Q., Jiang, Q. T., et al. (2014). Assessment of cerebral iron content in patients with Parkinson's disease by the susceptibility-weighted MRI. *Eur. Rev. Med. Pharmacol. Sci.* 18, 2605–2608.

Yamauchi, M., Omote, K., and Ninomiya, T. (1998). Direct evidence for the role of nitric oxide on the glutamate-induced neuronal death in cultured cortical neurons. *Brain Res.* 780, 253–259. doi: 10.1016/s0006-8993(97)01201-8

Yu, J., Guo, Y., Sun, M., Li, B., Zhang, Y., and Li, C. (2009). Iron is a potential key mediator of glutamate excitotoxicity in spinal cord motor neurons. *Brain Res.* 1257, 102–107. doi: 10.1016/j.brainres.2008.12.030

Zhang, S., Wang, J., Song, N., Xie, J., and Jiang, H. (2009). Up-regulation of divalent metal transporter 1 is involved in 1-methyl-4-phenylpyridinium (MPP^+)-induced apoptosis in MES23.5 cells. *Neurobiol. Aging* 30, 1466–1476. doi: 10.1016/j.neurobiolaging.2007.11.025

Zheng, W., Xin, N., Chi, Z. H., Zhao, B. L., Zhang, J., Li, J. Y., et al. (2009). Divalent metal transporter 1 is involved in amyloid precursor protein processing and Aβ generation. *FASEB J.* 23, 4207–4217. doi: 10.1096/fj.09-135749

Zhu, W. Z., Zhong, W. D., Wang, W., Zhan, C. J., Wang, C. Y., Qi, J. P., et al. (2009). Quantitative MR phase-corrected imaging to investigate increased brain iron deposition of patients with Alzheimer disease. *Radiology* 253, 497–504. doi: 10.1148/radiol.2532082324

Zucca, F. A., Segura-Aguilar, J., Ferrari, E., Muñoz, P., Paris, I., Sulzer, D., et al. (2015). Interactions of iron, dopamine and neuromelanin pathways in brain aging and Parkinson's disease. *Prog. Neurobiol.* doi: 10.1016/j.pneurobio.2015.09.012 [Epub ahead of print].

9

Insulin-Like Growth Factor 1: At the Crossroads of Brain Development and Aging

Sarah Wrigley[1], *Donia Arafa*[1] *and Daniela Tropea*[2,3]*

[1]*School of Medicine, Trinity College Dublin, Dublin, Ireland,* [2]*Neuropsychiatric Genetics, Trinity Translational Medicine Institute St. James Hospital, Dublin, Ireland,* [3]*Institute of Neuroscience, Trinity College Dublin, Dublin, Ireland*

Edited by:
Hansen Wang,
University of Toronto, Canada

Reviewed by:
Enrique Cadenas,
University of Southern California, USA
Carlos Vicario-Abejón,
Spanish National Research Council, Spain
Derek LeRoith,
Icahn School of Medicine at Mount Sinai, USA

***Correspondence:**
Daniela Tropea
tropead@tcd.ie

Insulin-like growth factor 1 (IGF1) is a polypeptide hormone structurally similar to insulin. It is central to the somatotropic axis, acting downstream of growth hormone (GH). It activates both the mitogen-activated protein (MAP) kinase and PI3K signaling pathways, acting in almost every tissue in the body to promote tissue growth and maturation through upregulation of anabolic processes. Overall GH and IGF1 signaling falls with age, suggesting that it is this reduced IGF1 activity that leads to age-related changes in organisms. However, mutations that reduce IGF1-signaling activity can dramatically extend the lifespan of organisms. Therefore, the role of IGF1 in the overall aging process is unclear. This review article will focus on the role of IGF1 in brain development and aging. The evidence points towards a role for IGF1 in neurodevelopment both prenatally and in the early post-natal period, and in plasticity and remodeling throughout life. This review article will then discuss the hallmarks of aging and cognitive decline associated with falls in IGF1 levels towards the end of life. Finally, the role of IGF1 will be discussed within the context of both neuropsychiatric disorders caused by impaired development of the nervous system, and neurodegenerative disorders associated with aging. IGF1 and its derivatives are shown to improve the symptoms of certain neuropsychiatric disorders caused by deranged neurodevelopment and these effects have been correlated with changes in the underlying biology in both *in vitro* and *in vivo* studies. On the other hand, studies looking at IGF1 in neurodegenerative diseases have been conflicting, supporting both a role for increased and decreased IGF1 signaling in the underlying pathogenesis of these diseases.

Keywords: insulin-like growth factor 1, aging, neurodevelopment, growth factors

Insulin-like growth factor 1 (IGF1) signaling is an essential factor for early brain development, but its role in the aging brain remains unclear. In fact, while reduced IGF1 signaling with age has been historically observed as a causative factor in the aging process, correlation does not imply causation, and falling IGF1 signaling with age may in fact attenuate the effects of aging. Further work must be done in order to truly discern the role and effects of IGF1 signaling in the aging brain.

INSULIN-LIKE GROWTH FACTOR-1: DOWNSTREAM SIGNALING CASCADES AND CELLULAR EFFECTS

IGF-1 is synthesized primarily in the liver, where its synthesis is regulated by pituitary secretion of growth hormone (GH). It is central to the somatrotropic axis, acting downstream of GH to promote anabolic processes and tissue growth throughout life. IGF1 is also synthesized locally in many organs, including the brain. Both in circulation and in tissues, IGF1 is bound to high affinity IGF1-binding proteins (IGFBPs), which modulate interactions between IGF1 and its receptor.

The biological actions of IGF1 are mediated through IGF1R, a membrane-bound receptor tyrosine kinase (RTK). Binding of IGF1 to its receptor causes autophosphorylation of the intracellular component, leading to enzymatic activation and subsequent phopshorylation of the insulin receptor substrate-1 (IRS1) protein on multiple tyrosine sites. These phosphotyrosine sites then serve as docking sites for numerous intracellular signaling proteins. By bringing these interacting proteins together, complex signaling pathways are begun, including the canonical PI3-kinase and mitogen-activated protein (MAP) kinase pathways.

IGF-1R activation triggers the PI3kinase-Akt signaling pathway, which promotes cell growth and maturation. IRS1 binds PI3kinase which phosphorylates PIP2 to PIP3. PIP3 binds two protein kinases; Akt and PDK1, leading to activation of Akt, which acts on numerous proteins throughout the cell to promote cell growth and survival. Downstream substrates of Akt include mammalian target of rapamycin (mTOR), which stimulates ribosome production and protein synthesis, and Bad, a pro-apoptopic protein that is inhibited by Akt phosphorylation. Another effect of IGF1R activation through PI3kinase-Akt signaling is inhibitory phosphorylation of pro-apoptopic glycogen synthase 3β (GSK3β), which is associated with increased glycogen storage in projection neurons in the post-natal brain, as well as reduced tau hyperphosphorylation which causes neuronal death (Bondy and Cheng, 2004). IGF1-induced PI3K-Akt signaling is also linked to production of GLUT4 glucose transporters and translocation to neuronal cell membranes, promoting glucose uptake into neurons (Bondy and Cheng, 2004). This corresponds to studies demonstrating increased glucose utilization in areas of higher IGF1 and IGF1R expression in the developing brain, and reduced glucose utilization in IGF1 null brains (Cheng et al., 2000). This pathway also leads to inactivation of FOXO1, preventing FOXO-driven transcription of pro-apoptopic genes (Yin et al., 2013). Hence, PI3K signaling directly inhibits the pro-apoptopic machinery via multiple pathways.

IGF1R also phosphorylates the Sch protein, which recruits the GDP2/SOS complex, leading to activation of Ras, thereby triggering the MAP kinase pathway central to growth-related gene transcription and mitogenesis (**Figure 1**).

IGF1-SIGNALING, AGING AND LIFESPAN IN MODEL ORGANISMS

IGF1 signaling is central to pathways that promote cell growth and survival, maturation and proliferation, allowing for tissue growth and renewal. Furthermore, the activity of the GH-IGF1 somatotrophic axis decreases with age, and is almost undetectable in people over 60 years (Junnila et al., 2013). This has led to many theories that upregulation of the GH/IGF1 pathway may delay aging. However, studies of IGF1 signaling on nematodes and many other species have suggested that, on the contrary, downregulation of IGF1 signaling delays aging and increases lifespan.

The IGF1 signaling pathway is an evolutionarily ancient pathway, conserved from *C. elegans* through to modern humans. The *C. elegans* IR-IGF1 receptor homolog is Daf-2. Mutations that lower the level of Daf-2 double the lifespan of the *C. elegans* model (Kenyon et al., 1993). Exactly how Daf-2 mutations increase *C. elegans* lifespan in unclear. Some daf-2 mutants adopt a quiescent state of reduced movement and fertility known as the dauer state, whereas other mutants are shown to have a lower metabolic rate, and other mutants again demonstrate a metabolic shift to fat production. However, these findings are not consistent among all daf-2 mutants, and can therefore not be coupled to lifespan extension (Kenyon, 2010). Another theory is that daf-2 mutants are better able to withstand oxidative stress (Holzenberger et al., 2003). Reduced Daf-2 activity downregulates Akt-mediated inhibition of Daf-16 (FOXO homolog), allowing Daf-16 translocation to the nucleus for target gene activation. The transcriptional targets of Daf-16/FOXO may be at least in part responsible for the stress resistance and longevity associated with Daf-2 mutants (Lin et al., 1997; Gami and Wolkow, 2006).

The impact of altered Daf-2 activity on lifespan varies between different cell lineages. While present in ectodermal, mesodermal and endodermal lineages, it is reduction in ectodermal (neuronal, skin tissue) daf-2 activity that induces a dauer state (Guarente and Kenyon, 2000). Restoration of insulin-like signaling alone in Daf-2 mutants reverts these mutants back to a wild-type lifespan, whereas restoration of insulin-like signaling in muscle or adipose tissue had no effect on lifespan (Wolkow et al., 2000). This study provides persuasive evidence that insulin/IGF1 signaling in neurons regulates lifespan. Interestingly, reduction in sensory input to the olfactory system by mutations in sensory cilia or olfactory support cell ablation can increase lifespan by up to 50% without affecting development or reproduction. This suggests that sensory neurons influence lifespan and this is at least partly mediated through Daf-2 signaling (Apfeld and Kenyon, 1999). Downstream of Daf-2 (IGF1R), mutations in age-1 (PI3K homolog) also increase lifespan, suggesting that reduction in factors downstream of IGF1 signaling are sufficient to extend lifespan (Morris et al., 1996).

The effect on lifespan by inhibition of insulin/IGF1 signaling observed in the *C. elegans* model is conserved in other species,

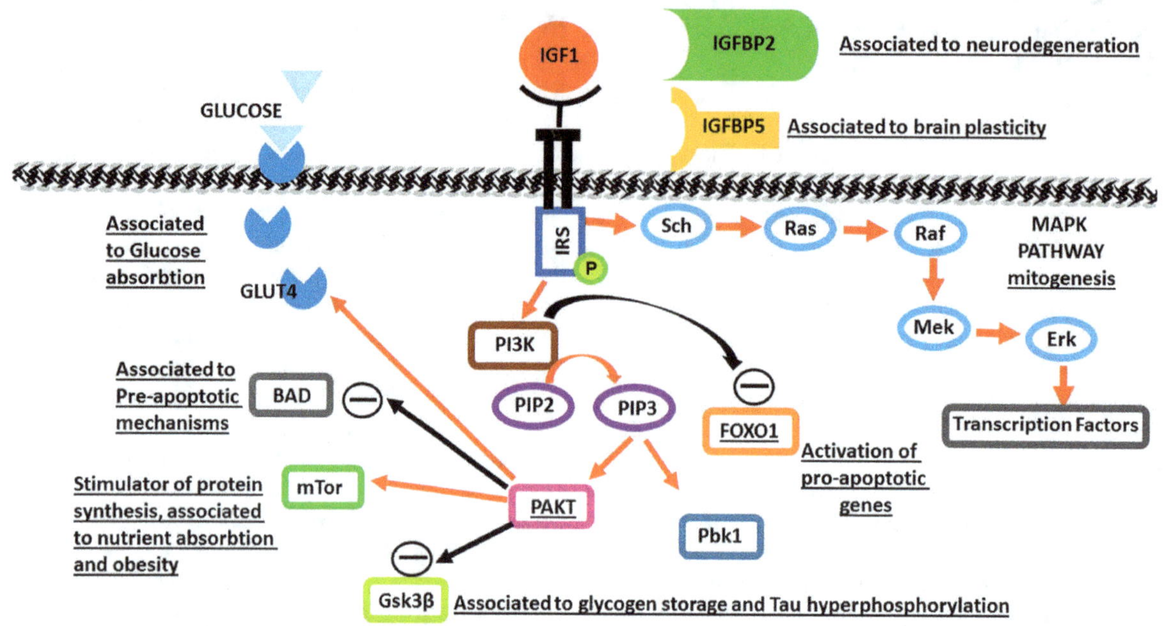

FIGURE 1 | A schematic of Insulin-like growth factor 1 (IGF1) molecular pathways activated in brain maturation and aging. Black rows indicate inhibition, red rows indicate activation. The underlined proteins have been identified to be genetically associated to aging.

including the *Drosophila* fly, whereby inhibiting IGF1 signaling or increasing the activity of FOXO (the Daf-16 homolog) in adipose tissue increases lifespan (Kenyon, 2010). Heterozygous mutation of the insulin receptor (IR) in *Drosophila* extends lifespan by up to 85% (Tatar et al., 2001). Furthermore, mutation of CHICO, the IRS homolog, extends lifespan by 48% in homozygotes and 36% in heterozygotes (Clancy et al., 2001). A striking inverse correlation between IGF1 levels and lifespan is also observed in mice (Kenyon, 2010). While IGF1R null mice die shortly after birth (Liu et al., 1993), heterozygous knockout (KO) of IGF1R extends lifespan by 26% compared to wild-type littermates (Holzenberger et al., 2003). This mouse model of reduced IGF1 signaling were normal in size, and displayed normal energy metabolism, but showed greater resistance to oxidative stress (Holzenberger et al., 2003).

Interestingly, this is in contrast to mice with IR or IRS KO, which show severe insulin resistance and die earlier due to hyperglycemia. From invertebrates to mammals, IGF1 signaling and insulin signaling became distinct cellular pathways with different downstream effects. Therefore, IGF1 signaling in mammals can be manipulated without interfering with systemic glucose metabolism.

In humans, lowered IGF signaling is also shown to improve longevity. Mutations known to impair IGFR function are observed in Ashkenazi Jewish centenarians (Suh et al., 2008). Additionally, Akt, FOXO3A and FOXO1A mutations are linked to longevity in numerous patient cohorts (Willcox et al., 2008; Flachsbart et al., 2009; Kenyon, 2010).

The findings that reductions in Daf-2/IGF1R signaling can radically increase lifespan would suggest that IGF1 signaling is directly linked to the aging of organisms, which is in contradiction to the theory that a fall in the activity of GH-IGF1 somatotropic axis underlies the mechanism of aging.

Although in the whole organism a general decrease of IGF signaling delays aging, this review will focus on the role of IGF1 signaling in the developing and aging brain, where IGF1 signaling in the brain promotes development and, in some cases, appears to attenuate age-related changes. Numerous studies outlined below demonstrate the neurotrophic effects of IGF1 signaling, giving evidence for promotion of neurogenesis, development and maturation, myelination, prolonged survival and resistance to injury.

IGF1 AND THE DEVELOPING BRAIN: EXPRESSION PATTERNS OF IGF1 AND IGF1R IN THE DEVELOPING BRAIN

IGF1 is produced by all major cell types in the CNS. IGF1 expression peaks perinatally and falls throughout life, though it persists in discrete brain regions associated with continual renewal and remodeling. This is in contrast to the IGF1 receptor, which is shown to be widely expressed throughout the brain, and concentrated in neuron-rich areas including the granule cell layers of olfactory bulb, dentate gyrus and cerebellar cortex, with little hybridization in white matter regions (Bondy et al., 1992a). IGF1R is expressed in all neuroepithelial cell types, and shows a relatively stable pattern of expression from early development to maturity (Bondy et al., 1992b). There is, however, a period of increased IGF1R expression coinciding with increased IGF1 expression in specific sensory and cerebellar projecting neurons during late post-natal development (Bondy et al., 1992b). Early post-natal IGF1 expression was identified in brain regions where neurogenesis persisted after birth, including the cerebellum, olfactory bulb and hippocampus, and was shown to fall after this period of neuronal proliferation (Bach et al., 1991; Bartlett et al., 1991).

IGF1 expression persists in these areas in adult brains, but at levels much lower than that of early neonatal animals (García-Segura et al., 1991). These expression patterns highlight the association between regions of increased neurogenesis and local IGF1 and IGF1R expression during early development.

While local IGF1 expression falls shortly after birth, there exists throughout life an active transport mechanism that allows peripheral circulating IGF1 to cross the blood brain barrier (Fernandez and Torres-Alemán, 2012). This finding, combined with the fact that IGF1 receptor expression in the brain persists throughout life, suggests a role for peripherally produced IGF1 in adult brain function. Therefore, while locally produced IGF1 appears to play a role in brain function during prenatal and early post-natal development, peripherally produced IGF1 may have a continued role in the adult brain.

IGF1 AND THE DEVELOPING BRAIN: EVIDENCE FROM *IN VITRO* AND *IN VIVO* STUDIES ON THE EFFECT OF IGF1 ON BRAIN SIZE, NEURONAL CELL NUMBER, AXONAL GROWTH AND MYELINATION DURING EARLY DEVELOPMENT

IGF1 has been shown to have pleiotropic actions in all neural cells, including neurons, oligodendrocytes and astrocytes, by increasing cell number and promoting maturation and myelination. This has been proven through *in vitro* culture studies, and through both overexpression and under-expression studies in transgenic mice.

IGF1 and the Developing Brain: Effects of IGF1 on Neural Stem Cells

In vitro studies examining the effect of IGF1 in neural stem cells report increased neural progenitor cell proliferation and maintenance in cell culture following treatment with IGF1 (Drago et al., 1990; Supeno et al., 2013). IGF1 was found to be more potent than insulin in stimulating mitosis of sympathetic neuroblasts (DiCicco-Bloom and Black, 1988). Furthermore, numbers of neurons produced from neural stem cell clones was increased following administration of IGF1 or heparin or withdrawal of FGF2 from cell culture, the effects of which were negated by administration of IGF1 and IGF1BP antibodies (Brooker et al., 2000). Examination of adult rat hippocampal progenitor cells showed uniform IGF1R expression, and the combined addition of IGF1 and FGF2 to these cells in culture increased DNA synthesis and cell division, without significant changes in the rate of cell death (Åberg et al., 2003).

IGF1 and the Developing Brain: Evidence from Prenatal Overexpression and Underexpression Studies

Popken et al. (2004) demonstrated through nestin-driven overexpression of IGF1 early in the embryonic development of transgenic mice a 6% increase in brain weight by embryonic day 16, associated with a cortical plate volume 42% greater and a total cell number 54% greater in the transgenic mice compared to controls. This increase in total cell number was attributed to a 15% increase in proliferating cells in the ventricular and subventricular zones of the embryonic cerebral cortex, which give rise to the neuronal and glial cell types respectively. At post-natal day 12, a 27% increase in overall brain weight was observed, with significant increases in volume and total cell number in certain brain regions including the cerebral cortex, subcortical white matter, caudate-putamen, hippocampus, dentate gyrus and habernacular complex (Popken et al., 2004). This enhancement in neuroepithelial cell proliferation by IGF1 during embryonic neurogenesis has been shown to result from acceleration through the cell cycle (Hodge et al., 2004). Further studies in the same mouse model reported that, in ddition to enhanced proliferation of neural progenitors, there are reduced numbers of apoptopic cells throughout the cerebral cortex both prenatally and post-natally in the mice showing IGF1 overexpression, correlating with overall increased brain weight 9 months post-natally (Hodge et al., 2007).

Conversely, examination of homozygous IGF$^{-/-}$ KO mice at 2 months demonstrates a grossly structurally normal brain, but a 38% reduction in brain weight. A reduction in parvalbumin-containing neurons in the hippocampus and striatum was shown, as well as a significant reduction in the thickness of the dentate gyrus granule cell layer (Beck et al., 1995). IGF1$^{-/-}$ mice also show reduced dendritic length and complexity, and a 16% reduction in synaptotagmin levels, suggesting a reduction in the number of synapses, in the frontoparietal cortex (Cheng et al., 2003). A study by Liu et al. (2009) showed that brain-specific IGF1R heterozygous KO mice had brain weights 56% lower than controls at birth and 60% lower at post-natal day 90. The hippocampus was particularly affected, where the rate of growth post-natally was much lower in IGF1R heterozygous KOs compared to wild-type controls, with a greater fall in the numbers of neurons in the CA1–3 region and a smaller rise in the neuronal cell number in the dentate gyrus post-natally. This was attributed to a higher rate of cell death in IGF1R heterozygous KO mice. In all experiments performed, the phenotype was more severe in the two IGF1R homozygous KO mice that survived to adulthood, suggesting that degree of brain growth retardation was related to the level of IGF1R expression (Liu et al., 2009).

IGF1 and the Developing Brain: Evidence from Post-Natal Overexpression and Underexpression Studies

While the above studies examined the downstream effect of prenatal IGF1 over-and under-expression on subsequent brain development, other studies had focused on the role of IGF1 in the post-natal period, given that IGF1 mRNA expression in the developing rodent brain peaks in the first two post-natal weeks of life. Using a line of transgenic mice that begin to express the transgene at birth, causing brain-restricted overexpression of IGF1, studies have shown that IGF1 overexpression causes increases in brain weight after day 10, with enlargement of the brainstem, cerebellum, cerebral cortex and hippocampus (Ye et al., 1996; Dentremont et al., 1999; O'Kusky et al., 2000). Cerebellar weight was increased by 90%, with concomitant increases in granule and Purkinje cell numbers by 82% and 20% respectively (Ye et al., 1996).

Specifically, given the persistence of IGF1 expression in the hippocampal subventricular zone and dentate gyrus post-natally, the *in vivo* actions of IGF1 on growth and development of the hippocampal dentate gyrus up to 130 post-natal days have been investigated. Transgenic IGF1 overexpression was shown to increase granule cell layer and molecular cell layer by 27%–69%, total number of neurons by 29%–61%, and total number of synapses in the molecular layer by 42%–105% compared to control littermates (O'Kusky et al., 2000). Increased neuronal numbers in the dentate gyrus in the post-natal period is thought to be due not only to increased neurogenesis but also reduced neuronal death.

Numerous studies have reported that IGF1 promotes cell survival in the post-natal brain. Transgenic mice overexpressing IGF1 have significantly fewer apoptopic cerebellar neurons at post-natal day 7 compared to wild-type controls, with increased expression of anti-apoptopic proteins and reduced expression of pro-apoptopic proteins (Chrysis et al., 2001). Similarly, in the dentate gyrus of post-natal brains, IGF1 null mice had higher rates of granule cell proliferation but lower numbers of mature granule cells, suggesting the IGF1 promotes survival of granule cells in the post-natal period (Cheng et al., 2001). For a focused review on the function of IGF1 in brain development and plasticity see Dyer et al. (2016). The role of IGF1 in improving neuronal survival and reorganization following injury in both the developing and aging brain are outlined further on in this article.

IGF1 and the Developing Brain: Oligodendrocyte Development and Myelination

In addition to the effect of IGF1 on neuronal proliferation and survival in the developing brain, the effect on glial cells, especially oligodendrocytes, has been investigated through *in vitro* and *in vivo* studies.

In vitro studies show that administration of IGF1 to oligodendrocyte cells in culture promotes oligodendrocyte proliferation, differentiation, myelin production and survival (McMorris and Dubois-Dalcq, 1988; Mozell and McMorris, 1991; Barres et al., 1992; Ye and D'Ercole, 1999).

In vivo studies comparing transgenic mice with increased IGF-1 expression to those with IGFBP-1 expression (an inhibitor of IGF1) have shown that the mice with increased IGF-1 expression demonstrate higher numbers of oligodendrocytes, increased percentage of myelinated axons and increased thickness of myelin sheath compared to the transgenic mice with increased IGFBP-1 expression (Ye et al., 1995). In another study, prenatal overexpression of IGF1 in transgenic mice produced a mouse brain 55% larger, owing to an overall increase in total cell number, and a total myelin brain content 130% higher than that found in their non-transgenic littermates, which was not associated with a higher percentage increase in oligodendrocyte number, suggesting that increased meylin content was due to increased myelin production per oligodendrocyte (Carson et al., 1993).

Conversely, examination of IGF1 KO mice reported reduced cerebral and spinal cord white matter volume due to fewer myelinated axons and oligodendrocytes at post-natal day 55 (Beck et al., 1995). Further detailed study of IGF-1 KO mice showed consistently reduced overall brain weight 1 week post-natally compared to wild-type littermates, affecting all brain regions, as well as reduced myelination in all brain regions during the first 3 weeks of life, though this normalized and became similar to that of wild-type mice thereafter. Ths coincided with reduced levels of myelin-binding protein (MPB) and proteolipid protein (PLP) in IGF-1 KO mice during the first 3 weeks, which also normalized and became similar to controls by 10 weeks, while percentage oligodendrocyte number was persistently reduced in IGF-1 KO mice at weeks 1, 3 and 10. Additionally, reduced levels of the median subunit of neurofilament (a neuron-specific intermediate filament which acts a s a marker of axon growth) was reduced in IGF-1 KO mice and did not recover as the brain matured (Ye et al., 2002).

These studies suggest the importance of prenatal IGF1 expression in the developing brain for axon growth and CNS myelination in the early post-natal brain.

IGF1 AND THE DEVELOPING BRAIN: EVIDENCE FROM STUDIES OF EXTERNAL STIMULI KNOWN TO PROMOTE PAST-NATAL CORTICAL MATURATION

Certain external stimuli have been shown to promote neurodevelopment, and in many cases these studies show that the effect is mediated by IGF1 signaling. In particular, the visual cortex is studied in the context of how brain development is affected by external sensory input. For instance, environmental enrichment (EE), defined as "a complex of inanimate and social stimulation," is known to promote hippocampal neurogenesis and increase dendritic branching and synaptogenesis. It accelerates development of the visual cortex, causing enhanced visual acuity and increased expression of BDNF, which is known to act through the GABAergic system to promote neuroplasticity (Cancedda et al., 2004). A further study showed that this effect of EE on post-natal visual cortical development is inhibited by treatment of enriched pups with IGF1 antagonists and mimicked by treatment of non-EE pups with IGF1 infusion (Ciucci et al., 2007). Similarly, maturation of the visual system in preterm infants was accelerated by massage therapy, as evidenced both through electrophysoiogical studies and through visual acuity testing performed 3 months later. This correlated with higher serum levels of IGF1 and IGFBP3 in massaged infants. This was similarly shown in rat pups undergoing tactile stimulation, who showed faster maturation of electrophysiological tracings and higher levels of IGF1 in the brain compared to controls (Guzzetta et al., 2009).

While the above studies use the EE model to investigate the role of IGF1 in post-natal cortical maturation, other studies have used the model of monocular deprivation (MD) to assess the role of IGF1 in neuroplasticity and reorganization, whereby blocking visual input from one eye leads to structural organization of the visual cortex, allowing for ocular dominance of the intact eye. Expression of regulatory IGFBP5 gene is highly upregulated after MD, and the effects of MD on ocular dominance plasticity are negated by exogenous application of IGF1 (Tropea et al., 2006). Given that the capacity of ocular dominance plasticity in response to short deprivation is a marker of circuit immaturity, this study further supports the theory that IGF1 signaling promotes brain maturation in juvenile animals.

IGF1 AND THE ADULT BRAIN: ADULT NEUROGENESIS

As well as the role of IGF1 in early brain development, much research has been done into the role of IGF1 in ongoing neurogenesis and CNS plasticity in the adult brain. In most regions of the brain, neurogenesis ceases after birth. IGF1 mRNA expression correlates both temporally and spatially with these periods of rapid neurogenesis in the perinatal brain. Similarly, there are certain brain regions, namely the dentate gyrus and subventricular zone of the hippocampus, where neurogenesis persists into adulthood, and this correlates with the finding that IGF1 expression in the brain is diffuse during antenatal development, but persists only in the subventricular zone and dentate gyrus of the hippocampus after birth (Anderson et al., 2002). IGF1 expression levels decrease again later in life, again at a time that corresponds with a decrease in hippocampal neurogenesis. Therefore, much research has been done to investigate how manipulation of IGF1 signaling affects adult hippocampal neurogenesis.

It has already been noted in *in vitro* studies that adult hippocampal neural progenitor cells express IGF1R, and that administration of IGF1 with FGF2 increased progenitor cell proliferation (Åberg et al., 2003). This group further suggested that low-dose IGF1 treatment triggered a small increase in the differentiation of neuronal progenitors into neurons. A further *in vivo* study used hypophysectomied rats, as this model would have low levels of circulating IGF1. Six days of peripheral subcutaneous IGF1 administration increased proliferation of neuronal progenitors in the hippocampal dentate gyrus, as evidenced by BrdU uptake. After 20 days of subcutaneous IGF1 administration, these new cells expressed neuronal-specific proteins, suggesting stimulation of neurogenesis (Aberg et al., 2000). This suggests that, while local IGF1 mRNA expression levels fall after birth, peripheral IGF1 plays a role in adult hippocampal neurogenesis.

Another study looked at the effect of local IGF1 administration on neuronal cell numbers in the dentate gyrus. Mice aged 5, 18 and 28 months were examined. The dentate gyrus was divided for analysis into the proliferative subgranular zone (PZ), the granular cell layer (GCL) and the hilus, and the numbers of new cells were quantified using BrdU labeling. This study showed that the number of BrdU labeled cells decreases with age, with 80% fewer BrdU labeled cells in the PZ of the 18 month old rats than the 5 month old rats, with a much smaller but significant decrease in BrdU labeled cells in the hilus, though no age-related changes were observed in the GCL. Intracerebroventricular infusion of IGF-I maintained an approximately three-fold increase in the number of BrdU-labeled cells in the PZ, GCL and hilus in old rats examined 31 days after BrdU injection. IGF-I did not, however, selectively induce a neuronal fate since the percentage of BrdU-labeled cells in IGF-I-treated animals that colocalized NeuN was identical to that observed in age-matched controls (Lichtenwalder et al., 2001). Transgenic overexpression of IGF1 was similarly shown to increase the proliferation of neural stem cells in the subgranular and subventricular zones of adult mice brains (Yuan et al., 2015). In this study, however, IGF1 overexpression also led to an increase in the differentiation of neuronal stem cells into neurons, in contrast to the previous study (Yuan et al., 2015).

A recent study has looked in detail at the effects of both global and brain-specific KO of IGF1 in adult hippocampal neurogenesis. Global IGF1 KO mice had both low brain IGF1 expression and low serum IGF1 levels, and showed a 2.4-fold reduction in hippocampal volume compared to controls. Using extensive immunohistochemisty studies, this group demonstrated higher staining for markers of immature differentiation from neural progenitor cells to neurons in $IGF^{-/-}$ mice compared to controls, reduced staining for markers of the later stages of differentiation, and disorganized staining for markers of differentiated granule cells in the GCL of the dentate gyrus compared to controls (Nieto-Estévez et al., 2016b). $IGF1^{-/-}$ cells in the GCL showed greater proliferative capacity but more immature morphology compared to controls (Nieto-Estévez et al., 2016b). The group then studied the effects of brain-specific IGF1 KO on adult hippocampal neurogenesis. These mice had normal body size and total brain volume compared to controls, but reduced volume of the GCL of the dentate gyrus. As with the global IGF1 KO mice, these mice demonstrated greater immunostaining for immature differentiation markers and more disorganized distribution of mature differentiation markers in the GCL of the dentate gyrus (Nieto-Estévez et al., 2016b). In all, this study of two $IGF1^{-/-}$ mouse models demonstrates that a lack of IGF1 in the brain is associated with accumulation of neuronal progenitor cells, impaired transition from neural progenitor to mature granule cell neurons, a reduction in mature morphology of granule cells and disorganization of the GCL (Nieto-Estévez et al., 2016b), all of which supports the idea that IGF1 signaling is key in promoting organized adult hippocampal neurogenesis. Thus, IGF1 not only promotes adult neurogenesis through increased stem cell proliferation, but also through organized cell migration. This is similarly demonstrated in the study of IGF1 KO mice who showed reduced neuroblast migration from the subventricular zone to the olfactory bulb and poor organization of immature neurons in the olfactory bulb compared to normal mice (Hurtado-Chong et al., 2009).

Multiple processes are thought to stimulate adult neurogenesis, the best studied of which is exercise, and recent studies show that this effect is mediated through IGF1 signaling. This was shown through administration of an antibody that blocked systemic IGF1 uptake into the brain parenchyma, which reversed the exercise-induced effects on hippocampal neurogenesis (Trejo et al., 2001). Blocking IGF1R reverses exercise-induced increases in BDNF, suggesting that the downstream effects of IGF1 signaling are at least in part medicated though upregulation of brain-derived neurotrophic factor (Ding et al., 2006).

Exercise promotes functional recovery of spatial memory acquisition in rats who have undergone hippocampal injury, and attenuated the loss of motor coordination in rats following brainstem injury or Purkinje cell degeneration (Carro et al., 2001). The neuroprotective effects of exercise demonstrated in this study were reduced in rats who received subcutaneous IGF1 antibody treatment (Carro et al., 2001). Memory deficits are frequently reported in depression, and imaging studies have shown decreased hippocampal volume in patients with depression. Antidepressant therapy, including SSRIs and ECT, is known to cause upregulation of BDNF, and this has recently been shown to be IGF1-dependent (Chen and Russo-Neustadt, 2007). For a focused review on IGF1 and neurogenesis please see Nieto-Estévez et al. (2016a).

IGF1 AND THE ADULT BRAIN: PROLONGED SURVIVAL, REDUCED CELL DEATH, RESISTANCE TO INJURY, REPARATION AND NEUROPLASTICITY IN RESPONSE TO ENVIRONMENTAL CUES

In addition to its role in neurogenesis in the adult brain, IGF1 has been studied for its effect on CNS reparation and plasticity using injury and sensory deprivation models. These studies may indicate that falling levels of IGF1 in the aging brain may indirectly lead to aging through reduced reparation, remodeling and resistance to stress.

One model of injury is the cerebellar deafferentiation model, whereby the olivocerebellar pathway is transected. The remaining olivocerebellar fibers reinnervate the hemicerebellum, but only in the early post-natal period (days 7–10). However, injection of IGF1 into the cerebellum of rats aged 11–30 days allowed for reinnervation of this pathway, indicating that this period of neuroplasticity is extended with use of IGF1 (Sherrard and Bower, 2003). IGF1-mediated reinnervation of the olivocerebellar pathway caused full motor recovery in rats rendered ataxic after 3-acetylpyridine-induced cerebellar injury (Fernandez et al., 1998).

More evidence for its role in reparative neuroplasticity is shown through the use of excitotoxicity models. Chronic intracerebral administration of IGF1 following an excitotoxic lesion in the dentate gyrus caused increased dendritic formation in young neurons in the dentate gyrus compared to untreated controls, and recovery of contextual fear memory, which is a dentate gyrus-dependent function (Liquitaya-Montiel et al., 2012). Another model of dentate gyrus injury is injection of trimethyltin, which is shown to cause elevated IGF1 mRNA levels in the hippocampus. Mice deficient in IGF1 had a significant level of CA1 hippocampal cell death, implying a role for IGF1 in CA1 hippocampal cell survival (Wine et al., 2009).

IGF1 is also thought to be protective in hypoxic-ischemic injury. Intracerebroventricular infusion of IGF1 during perinatal asphyxia in near-term foetal sheep was linked to reduced loss of striatal cholinergic and GABAergic neurons compared to controls on post-mortem examination (Guan et al., 2000). A single dose of intracerebroventricular IGF1 2 h hypoxic-ischemic injury reduced somatosensory deficits for up to 20 days after the initial insult (Guan et al., 2001). The effects of malnourishment in the post-natal period are also attenuated by IGF1 administration. Malnourished mice treated with IGF1 comparable brain weights and cell numbers compared to nourished controls, and higher numbers of oligodendrocytes and expression of myelin markers MPB and PLP, suggesting that this protective effect is through increased myelination (Ye et al., 2000).

The effects of IGF1 signaling following traumatic brain injury (TBI) have also been studied. Overexpression of IGF1 was shown to increase the density of hippocampal immature neurons following TBI. This was shown to be the result of post-traumatic proliferation and differentiation of neural stem cells into immature neurons, rather than through protection against initial insult. IGF1 overexpression also enhanced dendritic arborization of immature neurons compared to normal controls (Carlson et al., 2014). Thus, through enhanced neurogenesis and maturation, IGF1 overexpression accelerated recovery.

The role of IGF1 in activity-dependent neuroplasticity is also demonstrated through the use of sensory deprivation models. MD is a model of reduced activity-dependent activity, whereby one eye is deprived of visual stimuli, which leads to neuronal network reorganization with subsequent ocular dominance of the normal eye. IGFBP-5 is highly upregulated after MD, and administration of IGF1 promotes recovery of normal visual function in these models (Tropea et al., 2006) through upregulation of BDNF (Landi et al., 2009). Based on these findings, studies were performed to investigate whether administration of IGF1 in adult brains restores neuroplasticity. Adult rats underwent MD by eyelid suturing, and were then treated with IGF1. This was shown to trigger ocular dominance plasticity compared to MD rats untreated with IGF1 (Maya-Vetencourt et al., 2012). Furthermore, in rats rendered amblyopic by long-term sensory deprivation, those treated with IGF1 prior to restoration of sensory input showed full recovery of visual acuity compared to rats untreated with IGF1 (Maya-Vetencourt et al., 2012).

Downregulation of intracortical inhibitory GABA activity, increased utilization of glucose, and interaction with 5-HT were offered as potential mechanisms through which IGF1 mediates this restoration of plasticity. An alternative sensory deprivation model is that of hindlimb unloading (HU). In adult rats, 14 days of HU decreases IGF1 levels in the somatosensory cortex (Mysoet et al., 2014) and shrinks the somatotopic representation of the hindpaw. Administration of IGF1 prevents this change in somatotopic representation (Papadakis et al., 1996; Mysoet et al., 2015). These interventional studies have demonstrated that IGF1 administration alters neuronal plasticity in response to sensory deprivation in adult animals.

The above studies outline the role of IGF1 in adult neurogenesis, reparation and reorganization in response to stressors. It is therefore possible that loss of these IGF1-driven mechanisms with age leads to age-related cognitive changes. However, numerous studies outlined later in this article report the contrary theory that it is a reduction IGF1 signaling that is neuroprotective following CNS insult.

IGF1 AND THE AGING BRAIN: EVIDENCE FROM MOLECULAR BIOLOGY

The GH-IGF1 signaling pathway is the best characterized hormonal pathway in the process of aging. Pulsatile pituitary secretion of GH in response to stimuli such as induced hypoglycemia or arginine administration declines with age (Laron et al., 1969). This is associated with concomitant declines of circulating IGF1 levels (Johanson and Blizzard, 1981). Numerous age-related changes in the brain have been identified that suggest changes in IGF1 signaling. The density of GH receptors decreases with age, while reports are conflicting regarding age-related changes in IGF1 receptor density, with one group reporting increased density of IGF1R expression in the CA3 region of the hippocampus (Chung et al., 2002) and others reporting reduced decreased hippocampal and cortical IGF1R density in aging rats (D'Costa et al., 1993; Sonntag et al., 1999). Expression of IGF1 mRNA was reported to be reduced in the cerebellum of aging rats (Pañeda et al., 2003). These findings would suggest that IGF1 signaling is reduced in the aging brain. How this is linked to functional changes in the aging brain is unclear.

IGF1 AND THE AGING BRAIN: EVIDENCE FROM COGNITIVE TESTING

Therefore, studies have been done to examine whether reduced IGF1 signaling is linked to cognitive dysfunction. Studies in humans found a significant correlation between better perceptual motor performance, information processing speed and fluid intelligence and higher circulating IGF1 levels (Aleman et al., 1999, 2001). Others have found a correlation between higher IGF1 levels and higher MMSE scores (Paolisso et al., 1997; Rollero et al., 1998). The MMSE is a well-validated test in terms of repeat-test reliability and tracking of cognitive function over time. In a 2 year prospective study, higher levels of circulating IGF1 levels were associated with reduced cognitive decline over the study period. However, these findings are inconsistent, with many studies also reporting no correlation between IGF1 and attention, fluid intelligence, memory or cognitive decline (Papadakis et al., 1995; Aleman et al., 1999, 2001).

IGF1 AND THE AGING BRAIN: EVIDENCE FROM INTERVENTIONAL STUDIES

In any case, correlation does not imply causation. Therefore interventional studies in human were performed to assess if GH or IGF1 levels improved cognitive function, but the results were conflicting and ultimately inconclusive (Papadakis et al., 1996; Friedlander et al., 2001). In mice, intracerebroventricular infusion of IGF1 attenuated age-related deficits in working and reference memory as assessed by Morris water maze and object recognition tasks (Markowska et al., 1998).

Further work has been done in mice studies to assess the downstream molecular effects of IGF1 administration in an aging brain. Intracerebroventricular infusion of IGF1 has been shown to increase microvascular density in aged animals (Sonntag et al., 2000b). Furthermore, it increases hippocampal NMDAR2A/B subunit expression (Sonntag et al., 2000a), which is relevant because NMDAR2B subunit ablation has been shown to impair spatial learning (Clayton et al., 2002). Local IGF1 increases local glucose utilization in the anterior cingulate cortex of aged rats (Lynch et al., 2001). Finally administration of IGF1 attenuates the age-related decline in neurogenesis in aged rats (Lichtenwalder et al., 2001).

IGF1 AND DISEASE: EVIDENCE FROM DISORDERS OF NEURODEVELOPMENT AND NEURODEGENERATION

IGF1 and Disorders of Impaired Neurodevelopment

In order to better understand the physiological roles of IGF1 in normal neurodevelopment and aging, one can look at IGF1 activity in the context of known disorders of neurodevelopment and neurodegeneration. For instance, Rett Syndrome is an X-linked neurological disorder characterized by seemingly normal post-natal development initially, followed by a sudden deterioration in function, with loss of acquired functional and motor skills at 12–18 months of age. Rather than being a neurodegenerative process, the underlying pathology is thought to be a stagnation in neuronal maturation. It is caused by a mutation in the MECP2 gene, which codes a transcriptional modulator. It is abundant in neuronal tissue and its expression correlates with that of synaptic maturation. A downstream factor of MECP2 is BDNF, which activates the same PI3K and MAPK pathways that are activated by IGF1 signaling. Therefore, subcutaneous injections if IGF1 have been administered to both mouse models and human subjects to assess if this intervention can reverse the Rett Syndrome phenotype. IGF1 has been shown to increase brain weight, dendritic spine density and levels of PSD-95, a post-synaptic scaffold protein that promotes synaptic maturation, in MECP2 null mice, as well as partially reverse the reduction in amplitude of excitatory post-synaptic current in MECP2 mice (Tropea et al., 2009). Interestingly, persistence of ocular dominance plasticity following MD, a marker of neuronal immaturity, is a feature of MECP2 mouse models of Rett syndrome. It is prevented by pre-treatment with IGF1, giving further evidence for the role of IGF1 in neuronal circuit maturation and reduction in neuroplasticity (Tropea et al., 2009; Castro et al., 2014). These studies indicate the role of IGF1 signaling in neuronal circuit maturation. Similarly, work in SHANK3 deficient models of autism have showed that treatment with IGF1 promotes maturation of excitatory synapses (Shcheglovitov et al., 2013), and reverses deficits in LTP, AMPA signaling and motor function (Bozdagi et al., 2013). Therefore, through the study of IGF1 in the context of disorders caused by poor brain development, it appears that IGF1 promotes neuronal development and brain maturation. For a review focused on IGF1 function in neurodevelopmental disorders, see Vahdatpour et al. (2016).

IGF1 and Disorders Associated with Brain Aging

Findings through the study of IGF1 in age-related neurodegenerative disorders, however, have been contradictory, with some studies reporting that reduced IGF1 signaling is neuroprotective, while others claim that reduced IGF1 signaling with age contributes to brain aging. For instance, Alzheimer's disease (AD) is a neurodegenerative disease associated with aging, and one group have shown that a reduction in IGF1 signaling rescues mice from AD-like pathology. An AD mouse model with reduced IGF1 signaling was created, and was reported as having reduced neuronal loss and behavioral deficits compared to the control AD mouse model with normal levels of IGF1 signaling (Cohen et al., 2009). This was attributed to tighter aggregation of Aβ plaques leading to reduced proteotoxicity. These mice also show greater resistance to oxidative stress than mice with intact IGF1 signaling (Holzenberger et al., 2003), suggesting that these findings may be due to an enhanced capacity to protect against the inflammatory effects of Aβ plaques. Similarly, another group demonstrated protection of the aging brain from amyloid pathology by knocking out neuronal IGF1R activity in the brains of adult rats (Gontier et al., 2015). In this study, IGF1R KO in adult neurons led to reduced Aβ pathology and neuroinflammation, along with preservation of spatial memory. Another study reported reduction in Aβ plaques and improved learning and memory following IRS2 KO compared to controls in APP transgenic mice (Killick et al., 2009).

This is in contrast to the prevailing theory that AD is a disorder of insulin and IGF1 resistance. AD has recently been termed "Type 3 Diabetes," given the observation that the spectrum of Mild Cognitive Impairment—AD is associated with global reductions in glucose uptake and utilization occurring early in the course of the disease (Steen et al., 2005; Mosconi et al., 2013). In particular, hippocampal hypometabolism has been observed to correlate with faster progression to dementia (Mosconi et al., 2013). AD could therefore represent a form of CNS insulin resistance. Expression patterns of IR, IGF1 receptor (IGF1R), the intracellular substrate proteins IRS1 and IRS2, and the regulatory IGFBP-2, have been studied in brains affected by AD. One study reported increased IGF1R and decreased IGFBP-2 expression in AD brains, with higher IGF1R expression levels concentrated around amyloid plaques and in neurons with neurofibrillary tangles. These AD neurons showed decreased intracellular levels of IRS1 and IRS2, in association with greater levels of the phosphorylated inactivated forms of these proteins. These findings would suggest that AD neurons show resistance to IGF1 signaling (Moloney et al., 2010). Similarly, another study showed that cerebral neurons in AD brains demonstrate reduced responses to insulin and IGF1 signaling, mainly through phosphorylation and subsequent inactivation of IRS1 (Talbot et al., 2012). Another group that found that mutant rats with lower circulating levels of IGF1 have higher levels of Aβ plaques in the brain, and that levels of Aβ can be reduced in aging rats to levels similar to that in young rats by increasing serum levels of IGF1 (Carro et al., 2002). This is thought to be due to increased clearance of Aβ by albumin and transthyretin carrier proteins due to increased choroid plexus permeability to these proteins (Carro et al., 2002). Furthermore, IGF1R blockade in the choroid plexus worsens AD like pathology, causing amyloidosis, tau hyperphosphorylation and cognitive disturbance (Carro et al., 2006). These studies would therefore suggest that decreased insulin-IGF1 signaling in the brain at least correlates with the development of AD.

The effect of IGF1 signaling in the pathogenesis of Huntington's disease (HD) has also been investigated. This is a triple repeat disorder caused by mutation of the HTT protein, whereby elongation of the CAG triple repeat leads to a resultant HTT protein with a prolonged polyglutamine tract. This prolongated protein is cut into toxic fragments that aggregate, causing neurotoxicity and degeneration. Reduced IGF1 signaling is linked to pathological and symptomalogical improvements in mouse models of HD. The R6/2 mouse model of HD showed more rapid neurodegeneration following increased expression of IRS2, while decreasing IRS2 expression is associated with a longer lifespan in this model (Sadagurski et al., 2011). This is attributed to fewer polyQ-HTT aggregates in the brain. Conversely, another study showed that treatment of neurons transfected with the HTT mutation with IGF1 reduced polyQ-htt aggregation through Akt-mediated huntingtin phosphorylation (Humbert et al., 2002).

IGF1 AND METABOLISM: TARGETING IGF1

IGF1 signaling has many effects on metabolism, at the tissue and cellular levels. This signaling is not limited to glucose and lipid homeostasis but also influences protein turnover (Sharples et al., 2015).

Manipulating IGF1 depends on our understanding of the metabolic trade-offs, especially in the brain, adipose tissue and skeletal muscle, that are associated with it. IGF and its related molecules are important in protein metabolism and the regulation of skeletal muscle mass. KO of IGFI, IGFII or the IGFI receptor causes neonatal lethality and decreases in skeletal muscle mass in rodents (Sharples et al., 2015). The role of IGF1 and its related molecules in the maintenance of skeletal muscle mass in humans is especially important for elderly individuals whose IGF1 levels decrease with age and are at risk of frailty (Maggio et al., 2013) and sarcopenia (Sharples et al., 2015). Manipulating metabolism by using dietary restriction offers a similar mechanism to reduced IGF1 signaling in that it results in the inhibition of mTOR and it has also been linked to reduced IGF1 levels. It has the potential to be used in combination with an increase in protein or amino acid intake to counteract the losses in skeletal muscle that accompany a reduction in IGF1 (Sharples et al., 2015).

Choosing which pathway to target poses an obstacle to the modification of IGF1 signaling. mTOR, which functions through complexes mTORC1 and mTORC2, might be a promising target. mTORC1 is responsive to nutrients, energy and growth factors and its inhibition has been shown to decrease aging rate and age-related weight gain in mice (Hu and Liu, 2014). KO of RAPTOR, an mTORC1-specific accessory protein, in adipose tissue preserves the lifespan extension seen in other models reducing Insulin/IGF1 signaling while also improving metabolic markers such as glucose tolerance and insulin sensitivity (Hu and Liu, 2014). This, taken with the detrimental effects of KO on tissues such as skeletal muscle and the importance of IGF1 in metabolism in the developing brain, suggests that tissue-specific reductions in signaling may be one way of overcoming this obstacle. In addition to approaches which take into account specific pathways and tissues, it may also be beneficial to investigate the differences in the effects of IGF1 reductions at different time points. Human population studies point to a positive impact of IGF1 reductions at a young age and elevations at an old age (Sharples et al., 2015).

It has been questioned whether the extended longevity afforded by reduced IGF-1 signaling and its effects on metabolism are mediated in the same way. In fact, it has recently been suggested that extended lifespan in the Ames and Snell dwarf mice is not due to IGF1 levels but rather the decrease in GH (Brown-Borg and Bartke, 2012). Furthermore, it is thought that distinct sets of neurons mediate the functions of insulin/IGF1 in the brain. KO of IRS2 in the entire brain in mice does result in lifespan extension but at 22 months these mice are also overweight, hyperinsulinemic and glucose-intolerant, demonstrating the centrality of this pathway in metabolic homeostasis. Nutrient-sensing which is central to the regulation of glucose and lipid homeostasis is carried out by the leptin-sensitive neurons of the arcuate nucleus which contain IRS2 and the IR. While it is in these neurons that insulin/IGF1 exert profound effects on metabolism, IRS2 is not required for leptin action. So then, IRS2 in these neurons mediates the functions of insulin/IGF1 ad not those of leptin, once again highlighting the importance of insulin-like signaling in metabolism. Interestingly, the decrease of IRS2 on leptin receptor-expressing neurons did not result in the increase in lifespan seen with overall IRS2 decrease. These results indicate that the neurons which act as the metabolic mediators of insulin/IGF1 signaling in the CNS are distinct from those which underlie mammalian lifespan extension due to a reduction in insulin/IGF1 signaling (Sadagurski and White, 2013; White, 2014). This provides a powerful starting point for the potential development of strategies to manipulate IGF1 function without causing metabolic dysfunction.

There is a paradox presented by the Insulin/IGF1 signaling pathway in metabolism which warrants further research. In the CNS, this paradox could well be due to the existence of neuronal subsets which mediate the effects of IGF1/Insulin and in the periphery could be owed to the differing actions of IGF1 on various tissues. The importance of IGF1 and its related molecules on metabolism is undeniable and if manipulated correctly could prove to be viable therapeutically.

THE DEBATE CONTINUES

In conclusion, the above studies largely support a role for IGF1 signaling in brain development, and adult neuroplasticity and neurogenesis. However, while numerous studies report that IGF1 signaling serves to delay brain aging, and that the known fall in IGF1 signaling with age acts as a causative factor in age-related brain changes, there remain as many studies that stand in contradiction, and suggest that a reduction in IGF1 signaling delays age-related changes and diseases.

IGF1 levels are higher in the developing brain, and this is shown, through the studies outlined above, to promote neuronal development. It activates the PI3K pathway, which promotes survival by directly inactivating pro-apoptopic machinery (van der Heide et al., 2006), and increases glucose uptake by neurons (Bondy and Cheng, 2004). Post-natally, IGF1 promotes neuronal maturation, and has been shown to partially correct the phenotype of certain neurodevelopmental disorders. IGF1 is associated, in the adult brain, with regions of continued neurogenesis. These findings would suggest that IGF1 signaling exerts an overall neuroprotective effect, and that falling IGF1 levels with age contribute to the effects of aging in the brain.

However, there also exists a body of evidence suggesting that reduced IGF1 signaling attenuates the effects of aging, both in the brain and in the whole organism. A reduction in IGF1 signaling increases the life span of *C. elegans*, as DAF-2 mutants with a lower level of DAF-2 signaling have a lifespan double that of normal controls (Kenyon et al., 1993). With regards to brain function, age-related decline in axonal regeneration in *C.elegans* was shown to be regulated by DAF-2 signaling. While the rate of axonal regeneration following injury was 65% in day1 *C.elegans* worms and 28% in day 5 worms, the same experiment in DAF2$^{-/-}$ worms had no reduction in axonal degeneration. Reduced DAF-2 signaling allowed for increased DAF-16 activity, stimulating neuronal regeneration in response to injury (Byrne et al., 2014). However, in the *C. elegans*, the insulin and IGF1 pathways are not diverged, and therefore the effects of IGF1 on aging cannot be studied in isolation. Studies of IGF1 signaling and lifespan in mammals have also been done, and an IGF1R$^{+/-}$ transgenic mouse model with a reduced level of IGF1 signaling activity has been created that has a longer lifespan than control mice, and demonstrated greater resistance to oxidative stress (Holzenberger et al., 2003). These findings would therefore suggest that the fall in IGF1 signaling with age is not in fact the cause of aging, but is perhaps a protective mechanism that occurs as to attenuate the effects of aging.

These contradictions may arise partly because of the differential activity of IGF1 signaling in the brain compared to the whole body in different experimental models. One particular study characterizes the distinction in Ames mice, which have a primary deficiency in GH, leading to low levels of circulating IGF1. These mice demonstrate a longer lifespan, which has been attributed to absence of GH-IGF1 signaling, thereby affording evidence that IGF1 signaling contributes to aging. However, Sun et al. (2005) demonstrated that while these Ames mice show lower levels of GH and IGF1 peripherally, they have elevated levels of IGF1 in the hippocampus compared to normal mice. Furthermore, this correlated with higher levels of neurogenesis in the dentate gyrus, compared to the controls (Sun et al., 2005). This elevated level of neurogenesis in the Ames mice may underlie the observation that these mice showed less age-related cognitive deficits. Therefore, while globally reduced IGF1 signaling appears to extend the lifespan of these organisms, one should not assume that brain-specific IGF1 signaling is also reduced, or that the effect of IGF1 activity in the brain compared to the rest of the organism on the process of aging is necessarily the same.

Contradictions again arise when studying the neuroprotective effect of IGF1 signaling in hypoxic-ischemic injury. While above studies describe reduced neuronal loss following intracerebroventricular infusion of IGF1 (see above), other studies report that following Cre-LoxP-mediated inactivation of IGF1R in forebrain neurons, there was reduced neuronal damage, inflammation and edema in response to hypoxic-ischemic insult (De Maghalaes Filho et al., 2016).

These contradictions between different studies may be due to the different approaches taken: decreasing IGF1 or the receptor, or the IRS receptor, or the targeting of the modulators IGFBPs. In fact, the systems are highly regulated and the changes in each factor may have a different effect. For example, a moderate decrease in IGF1R increases life span, contrary to what happens to decreases in IGF1. Another factor to take into account is the integration insulin-IGF1 in the brain. In neurons, IRSBPs proteins and IGF1R form a complex which also binds insulin and may activate different intracellular signals. This interaction should be taken into account in therapies which use IGF1 to improve brain function, because the variability of the results may be due to different levels of insulin in the body. This theory is in line with the homeostatic function of IGF1 as a connector between body and brain. In addition, as demonstrated by Sun et al. (2005), inconsistencies also arise when the differential activity and effect of IGF1 in different organ systems is not taken into account, for it may be the case that peripheral and brain IGF1 signaling have opposing effects, with the former leading to overall acceleration of aging in the body while the latter continues to promote renewal and reparation. Furthermore, it is possible that while IGF1 signaling continues to promote neuronal development and plasticity throughout life, through its effects on cellular apoptotic machinery, glucose utilization and other neurotrophic factors, such anabolic process may simultaneously contribute to aging through accumulation of reactive oxygen species and resultant prolonged oxidative stress over time.

In all, there remains much to be done in elucidating the role of IGF1 signaling in the brain as it develops, matures and ages. IGF1 appears to act in concert with BDNF and other neurotrophic factors to promote neurogenesis and remodeling in the brain. However, its overall effects on energy metabolism and cellular oxidation may contribute to aging in all organs. What is obvious is that it is not simply a matter of high IGF1 signaling early in life promoting development and falling levels thereafter underlying the process of aging. An evolutionarily ancient pathway, IGF1 signaling has likely taken on numerous differential roles in different body tissues in health and disease (Forbes, 2016), and its complex effects on cellular maturation, tissue development and energy metabolism may contribute to organismal development and aging simultaneously.

AUTHOR CONTRIBUTIONS

SW wrote a consistent part of the manuscript. DA wrote part of the manuscript and contributed to the figures. DT designed the structure of the review, wrote part of the manuscript and contributed to the figures.

REFERENCES

Aberg, M., Aberg, N., Hedbäcker, H., Oscarsson, J., and Eriksson, P. (2000). Peripheral infusion of IGF-I selectively induces neurogenesis in the adult rat hippocampus. *J. Neurosci.* 20, 2896–2903.

Åberg, M. A. I., Åberg, N. D., Palmer, T. D., Allborn, A.-M., Carlsson-Skwirut, C., Bang, P., et al. (2003). IGF-1 has a direct proliferative effect in adult hippocampal progenitor cells. *Mol. Cell. Neurosci.* 24, 23–40. doi: 10.1016/s1044-7431(03)00082-4

Aleman, A., de Vries, W., Koppeschaar, H., Osman-Dualeh, A., Verhaar, H., Samson, M., et al. (2001). Relationship between circulating levels of sex hormones and insulin-like growth factor-1 and fluid intelligence in older men. *Exp. Aging Res.* 27, 283–291. doi: 10.1080/036107301300208718

Aleman, A., Verhaar, H., De Haan, E., De Vries, W., Samson, M., Drent, M., et al. (1999). Insulin-like growth factor-1 and cognitive function in healthy older men. *J. Clin. Endocrinol. Metab.* 84, 471–475. doi: 10.1210/jc.84.2.471

Anderson, M., Åberg, M., Nilson, M., and Erikkson, P. (2002). Insulin-like growth factor-1 and neurogenesis in the adult mammalian brain. *Brain Res.* 134, 115–122. doi: 10.1016/s0165-3806(02)00277-8

Apfeld, J., and Kenyon, C. (1999). Regulation of lifespan by sensory perception in *Caenorhabditis elegans. Nature* 402, 804–809. doi: 10.1038/45544

Bach, M., Shen-Orr, Z., Lowe, W., Roberts, C., and Leroith, D. (1991). Insulin-like growth factor 1 mRNA levels are developmentally regulated in specific regions of the rat brain. *Mol. Brain Res.* 10, 43–48. doi: 10.1016/0169-328x(91)90054-2

Barres, B., Hart, I., Coles, H., Burne, J., Voyvodic, J., Richardson, W., et al. (1992). Cell death and control of cell survival in the oligodendrocyte lineage. *Cell* 70, 31–46. doi: 10.1016/0092-8674(92)90531-g

Bartlett, W. P., Li, X.-S., Williams, M., and Benkovic, S. (1991). Localisation of insulin-like growth factor-1 mRNA in murine central nervous system during post-natal development. *Dev. Biol.* 147, 239–250. doi: 10.1016/s0012-1606(05)80021-1

Beck, K. D., Powel-Braxton, L., Widmer, H., Valverde, J., and Hefti, F. (1995). IGF1 disruption results in reduced brain size, CNS hypomelination, and loss of hippocampal granule and striatal parvalbumin-containing neurons. *Neuron* 14, 717–730. doi: 10.1016/0896-6273(95)90216-3

Bondy, C., Bach, M., and Lee, W.-H. (1992a). Mapping of brain insulin and insulin-like growth factor receptor gene expression by *in situ* hybridization. *Neuroprotocols* 1, 240–259. doi: 10.1016/1058-6741(92)90034-u

Bondy, C., Werner, H., Roberts, C. T., and LeRoith, D. (1992b). Cellular pattern of type-I insulin-like growth factor receptor gene expression during maturation of the rat brain: comparison with insulin-like growth factors I and II. *Neuroscience* 46, 909–923. doi: 10.1016/0306-4522(92)90193-6

Bondy, C. A., and Cheng, C. M. (2004). Signalling by insulin-like growth factor 1 in brain. *Eur. J. Pharmacol.* 490, 25–31. doi: 10.1016/j.ejphar.2004.02.042

Bozdagi, O., Tavassoli, T., and Buxbaum, J. (2013). Insulin-like growth factor-1 rescues synaptic and motor deficits in a mouse model of autism and developmental delay. *Mol. Autism* 4:9. doi: 10.1186/2040-2392-4-9

Brooker, G. J. F., Kalloniatis, M., Russo, V. C., Murphy, M., Werther, G. A., and Bartlett, P. F. (2000). Endogenous IGF-1 regulates the neuronal differentiation of adult stem cells. *J. Neurosci. Res.* 59, 332–341. doi: 10.1002/(sici)1097-4547(20000201)59:3<332::aid-jnr6>3.0.co;2-2

Brown-Borg, H., and Bartke, A. (2012). GH and IGF1: roles in energy metabolism of long-living GH mutant mice.*J. Gerontol. A Biol. Sci. Med. Sci.* 67A, 652–660. doi: 10.1093/gerona/gls086

Byrne, A. B., Walradt, T., Gardner, K. E., Hubbert, A., Reinke, V., and Hammarlund, M. (2014). Insulin/IGF1 signaling inhibits age-dependent axon regeneration. *Neuron* 81, 561–573. doi: 10.1016/j.neuron.2013.11.019

Cancedda, L., Putignano, E., Sale, A., Viegi, A., Berardi, N., and Maffei, L. (2004). Acceleration of visual system development by environmental enrichment. *J. Neurosci.* 24, 4840–4848. doi: 10.1523/JNEUROSCI.0845-04.2004

Carlson, S. W., Madathil, S. K., Sama, D. M., Gao, X., Chen, J., and Saatman, K. E. (2014). Conditional overexpression of insulin-like growth factor-1 enhances hippocampal neurogenesis and restores immature neuron dendritic processes after traumatic brain injury. *J. Neuropathol. Exp. Neurol.* 73, 734–746. doi: 10.1097/NEN.0000000000000092

Carro, E., Trejo, J., Busiguina, S., and Torres-Aleman, I. (2001). Circulating insulin-like growth factor I mediates the protective effects of physical exercise against brain insults of different aetiology and anatomy. *J. Neurosci.* 21, 5678–5684.

Carro, E., Trejo, J. L., Gomez-Isla, T., LeRoith, D., and Torres-Aleman, I. (2002). Serum insulin-like growth factor I regulates brain amyloid-β levels. *Nat. Med.* 8, 1390–1397. doi: 10.1038/nm793

Carro, E., Trejo, J. L., Spuch, C., Bohl, D., Heard, J. M., and Torres-Aleman, I. (2006). Blockade of the insulin-like growth factor I receptor in the choroid plexus originates Alzheimer's-like neuropathology in rodents: new cues into the human disease? *Neurobiol. Aging* 27, 1618–1631. doi: 10.1016/j.neurobiolaging.2005.09.039

Carson, M. J., Behringer, R. R., Brinster, R. L., and McMorris, F. (1993). Insulin-like growth factor-1 increases brain growth and central nervous system myelination in tTransgenic mice. *Neuron* 10, 729–740. doi: 10.1016/0896-6273(93)90173-o

Castro, J., Garcia, R. I., Kwok, S., Banerjee, A., Petravicz, J., Woodson, J., et al. (2014). Functional recovery with recombinant human IGF1 treatment in a mouse model of Rett syndrome. *Proc. Natl. Acad. Sci. U S A* 111, 9941–9946. doi: 10.1073/pnas.1311685111

Chen, M. J., and Russo-Neustadt, A. A. (2007). Running exercise- and antidepressant-induced increases in growth and survival-associated signaling molecules are IGF-dependent. *Growth Factors* 25, 118–131. doi: 10.1080/08977190701602329

Cheng, C., Cohen, M., Tseng, V., and Bondy, C. (2001). Endogeneous IGF1 enhances cell survival in the post-natal dentate gyrus. *J. Neurosci. Res.* 64, 341–347. doi: 10.1002/jnr.1084

Cheng, C. M., Mervis, R. F., Niu, S. L., Salem, N., Witters, L. A., Tseng, V., et al. (2003). Insulin-like growth factor 1 is essential for normal dendritic growth. *J. Neurosci. Res.* 73, 1–9. doi: 10.1002/jnr.10634

Cheng, C. M., Reinhardt, R. R., Lee, W.-H., Joncas, G., Patel, S. C., and Bondy, C. A. (2000). Insulin-like growth factor 1 regulates developing brain glucose metabolism. *Proc. Natl. Acad. Sci. U S A* 97, 10236–10241. doi: 10.1073/pnas.170008497

Chrysis, D., Calikoglu, A., Ye, P., and D'Ercole, A. (2001). Insulin-like growth factor 1 overexpression attenuates cerebellar apoptosis by altering expression of Bcl family proteins in a developmentally specific manner. *J. Neurosci.* 21, 1481–1489.

Chung, Y. H., Shin, C. M., Joo, K. M., Kim, M., and Cha, C. I. (2002). Region-specific alterations in insulin-like growth factor receptor type 1 in the cerebral cortex and hippocampus of aged rats. *Brain Res.* 946, 307–313. doi: 10.1016/s0006-8993(02)03041-x

Ciucci, F., Putignano, E., Baroncelli, L., Landi, S., Berardi, N., and Maffei, L. (2007). Insulin-like growth factor-1 (IGF-1) mediates the effects of enriched environment (EE) on visual cortical development. *PLoS One* 2:e475. doi: 10.1371/journal.pone.0000475

Clancy, D. J., Gems, D., Harshman, L. G., Oldham, S., Stocker, H., Hafen, E., et al. (2001). Extension of life-span by loss of CHICO, a Drosophila insulin receptor substrate protein. *Science* 292, 104–106. doi: 10.1126/science.1057991

Clayton, D., Mesches, M., Alvarez, E., Bickford, P., and Browning, M. (2002). A hippocampal NR2B deficit can mimic age-related changes in long-term potentiation and spatial learning in the Fsicher 344 rat. *J. Neurosci.* 22, 3628–3637.

Cohen, E., Paulsson, J. F., Blinder, P., Burstyn-Cohen, T., Du, D., Estepa, G., et al. (2009). Reduced IGF-1 signaling delays age-associated proteotoxicity in mice. *Cell* 139, 1157–1169. doi: 10.1016/j.cell.2009.11.014

D'Costa, A. P., Lenham, J. E., Ingram, R. L., and Sonntag, W. E. (1993). Moderate calorie restriction increases type 1 IGF receptors and protein synthesis in aging rats. *Mech. Aging Dev.* 71, 59–71. doi: 10.1016/0047-6374(93)90035-p

Dentremont, K. D., Ye, P., D'Ercole, A. J., and O'Kusky, J. R. (1999). Increased insulin-like growth factor-I (IGF-I) expression during early postnatal development differentially increases neuron number and growth in medullary nuclei of the mouse. *Dev. Brain Res.* 114, 135–141. doi: 10.1016/s0165-3806(99)00024-3

DiCicco-Bloom, E., and Black, I. B. (1988). Insulin growth factors regulate the mititic cycle in cultured rat sympathetic neuroblasts. *Proc. Natl. Acad. Sci. U S A* 85, 4066–4070. doi: 10.1073/pnas.85.11.4066

Ding, Q., Vaynman, S., Akhavan, M., Ying, Z., and Gomez-Pinilla, F. (2006). Insulin-like growth factor I interfaces with brain-derived neurotrophic factor-mediated synaptic plasticity to modulate aspects of exercise-induced cognitive function. *Neuroscience* 140, 823–833. doi: 10.1016/j.neuroscience.2006.02.084

Drago, J., Murohy, M., Carrol, S. M., Harvey, R. P., and Bartlett, P. F. (1990). Fibroblast growth factor-mediated proliferation of central nervous system precursors depends on endogenous production of insulin-like growth factor-1. *Proc. Natl. Acad. Sci. U S A* 88, 2199–2203. doi: 10.1073/pnas.88.6.2199

Dyer, A. H., Vahdatpour, C., Sanfeliu, A., and Tropea, D. (2016). The role of insulin-like growth factor 1 (IGF1-1) in brain development, maturation and plasticity. *Neuroscience* 325, 89–99. doi: 10.1016/j.neuroscience.2016.03.056

Fernandez, A. M., de la Vega, A. G., and Torres-Aleman, I. (1998). Insulin-like growth factor I restores motor coordination in a rat model of of cerebellar ataxia. *Proc. Natl. Acad. Sci. U S A* 95, 1253–1258. doi: 10.1073/pnas.95.3.1253

Fernandez, A. M., and Torres-Alemán, I. (2012). The many faces of insulin-like peptide signalling in the brain. *Nat. Rev. Neurosci.* 13, 225–239. doi: 10.1038/nrn3209

Flachsbart, F., Caliebe, A., Kleindorp, R., Blanché, H., von Eller-Eberstein, H., Nikolaus, S., et al. (2009). Association of FOXO3A variation with human longevity confirmed in German centenarians. *Proc. Natl. Acad. Sci. U S A* 106, 2700–2705. doi: 10.1073/pnas.0809594106

Forbes, B. E. (2016). Two years in IGF1 research. *Growth Horm. IGF Res.* 30–31, 70–74. doi: 10.1016/j.ghir.2016.09.006

Friedlander, A., Butterfield, G., Moynihan, S., Grillo, J., Pollack, M., Holloway, L., et al. (2001). One year of insulin-like growth factor 1 treatment does not affect bone density, body composition, or psychological measures in postmenopausal women. *J. Clin. Endocrinol. Metab.* 85, 1496–1503. doi: 10.1210/jc.86.4.1496

Gami, M. S., and Wolkow, C. A. (2006). Studies of *Caenorhabditis elegans* DAF-2/insulin signaling reveal targets for pharmacological manipulation of lifespan. *Aging Cell* 5, 31–37. doi: 10.1111/j.1474-9726.2006.00188.x

García-Segura, L. M., Pérez, J., Pons, S., Rejas, M., and Torres-Alemán, I. (1991). Localization of insulin-like growth factor I (IGF-I)-like immunoreactivity in the developing and adult rat brain. *Brain Res.* 560, 167–174. doi: 10.1016/0006-8993(91)91228-s

Gontier, G., George, C., Chaker, Z., Holzenberger, M., and Aïd, S. (2015). Blocking IGF signaling in adult neurons alleviates Alzheimer's disease pathology through amyloid-β clearance. *J. Neurosci.* 35, 11500–11513. doi: 10.1523/JNEUROSCI.0343-15.2015

Guan, J., Bennett, T. L., George, S., Waldvogel, H. J., Faull, R. L., Gluckman, P., et al. (2000). Selective neuroprotective effects with insulin-like growth factor 1 in phenotypic striatal neurons following ischemic brain injury in fetal sheep. *Neuroscience* 95, 831–839. doi: 10.1016/s0306-4522(99)00456-x

Guan, J., Miller, O. T., Waugh, K. M., McCarthy, D. C., and Gluckman, P. D. (2001). Insulin-like growth factor-1 improves somatosensory function and reduces the extent of cortical infarction and ongoing neuronal loss after hypoxia-ischaemia in rats. *Neuroscience* 105, 299–306. doi: 10.1016/s0306-4522(01)00145-2

Guarente, L., and Kenyon, C. (2000). Genetic pathways that regulate aging in model organisms. *Nature* 408, 255–262. doi: 10.1038/35041700

Guzzetta, A., Baldini, S., Bancale, A., Baroncelli, L., Ciucci, F., Ghirri, P., et al. (2009). Massage accelerates brain development and the maturation of visual function. *J. Neurosci.* 29, 6042–6051. doi: 10.1523/JNEUROSCI.5548-08.2009

van der Heide, L., Ramakers, G., and Smidt, M. (2006). Insulin signalling in the central nervous system: learning to survive. *Prog. Neurobiol.* 79, 205–221. doi: 10.1016/j.pneurobio.2006.06.003

Hodge, R. D., D'Ercole, A. J., and O'Kusky, J. R. (2004). Insulin-like growth factor-I accelerates the cell cycle by decreasing G1 phase length and increases cell cycle reentry in the embryonic cerebral cortex. *J. Neurosci.* 24, 10201–10210. doi: 10.1523/JNEUROSCI.3246-04.2004

Hodge, R. D., D'Ercole, A. J., and O'Kusky, J. R. (2007). Insulin-like growth factor-I (IGF-I) inhibits neuronal apoptosis in the developing cerebral cortex *in vivo*. *Int. J. Dev. Neurosci.* 25, 233–241. doi: 10.1016/j.ijdevneu.2007.03.004

Holzenberger, M., Dupont, J., Ducos, B., Leneuve, P., Géloën, A., Even, P. C., et al. (2003). IGF-1 receptor regulates lifespan and resistance to oxidative stress in mice. *Nature* 421, 182–187. doi: 10.1038/nature01298

Hu, F., and Liu, F. (2014). Targeting tissue-specific metabolic signalling pathways in aging: the promise and limitations. *Protein Cell* 5, 21–35. doi: 10.1007/s13238-013-0002-3

Humbert, S., Bryson, E. A., Cordelières, F. P., Connors, N. C., Datta, S. R., Finkbeiner, S., et al. (2002). The IGF-1/Akt pathway is neuroprotective in Huntington's disease and involves Huntingtin phosphorylation by Akt. *Dev. Cell* 2, 831–837. doi: 10.1016/s1534-5807(02)00188-0

Hurtado-Chong, A., Yusta-Boyo, M. J., Vergaño-Vera, E., Bulfone, A., de Pablo, F., and Vicario-Abejón, C. (2009). IGF-I promotes neuronal migration and positioning in the olfactory bulb and the exit of neuroblasts from the subventricular zone. *Eur. J. Neurosci.* 30, 742–755. doi: 10.1111/j.1460-9568.2009.06870.x

Johanson, A. J., and Blizzard, R. M. (1981). Low somatomedin-C levels in older men rise in response to growth hormone administration. *John Hopkins Med. J.* 149, 115–117.

Junnila, R. K., List, E. O., Berryman, D. E., Murrey, J. W., and Kopchick, J. J. (2013). The GH/IGF-1 axis in ageing and longevity. *Nat. Rev. Endocrinol.* 9, 366–376. doi: 10.1038/nrendo.2013.67

Kenyon, C. J. (2010). The genetics of ageing. *Nature* 464, 504–512. doi: 10.1038/nature08980

Kenyon, C., Chang, J., Gensch, E., Rudner, A., and Tabtiang, R. (1993). A C. elegans mutant that lives twice as long as wild type. *Nature* 366, 461–464. doi: 10.1038/366461a0

Killick, R., Scales, G., Leroy, K., Causevic, M., Hooper, C., Irvine, E. E., et al. (2009). Deletion of *Irs2* reduces amyloid deposition and rescues behavioural deficits in APP transgenic mice. *Biochem. Biophys. Res. Commun.* 386, 257–262. doi: 10.1016/j.bbrc.2009.06.032

Landi, S., Ciucci, F., Maffei, L., Berardi, N., and Cenni, M. (2009). Setting the pace for retinal development: environmental enrichment acts thorugh insulin-like growth factor-1 and brain-derived neurotrophic factor. *J. Neurosci.* 29, 10809–10819. doi: 10.1523/JNEUROSCI.1857-09.2009

Laron, Z., Doron, M., and Amikan, B. (1969). Plasma growth hormone in men and women over 70 years of age. *Med. Sports Phys.* 4, 126–131. doi: 10.1159/000387283

Lichtenwalder, R. J., Forbes, M. E., Lynch, C. D., Sonntag, W. E., and Riddle, D. R. (2001). Intracerebroventricular infusion of insulin-like growth factor-1 ameliorates age-related decline in hippocampal neurogenesis. *Neuroscience* 107, 603–613. doi: 10.1016/s0306-4522(01)00378-5

Lin, K., Dorman, J. B., Rodan, A., and Kenyon, C. (1997). daf-16: an HNF-3/forkhead family member that can function to double the life-span of *Caenorhabditis elegans*. *Science* 278, 1319–1322. doi: 10.1126/science.278.5341.1319

Liquitaya-Montiel, A., Aguilar-Arredondo, A., Arias, C., and Zepeda, A. (2012). Insulin growth factor-I promotes functional recovery after a focal lesion in the dentate gyrus. *CNS Neurol. Disord. Drug Targets* 11, 818–828. doi: 10.2174/1871527311201070818

Liu, J.-P., Baker, J., Perkins, J. A., Robertson, E. J., and Efstratiadis, A. (1993). Mice carrying null mutations of the genes encoding insulin-like growth factor, I (lgf-1) and type 1 IGF receptor (lgflr). *Cell* 75, 59–72. doi: 10.1016/s0092-8674(05)80084-4

Liu, W., Ye, P., O'Kusky, J., and D'Ercole, A. (2009). Type 1 insulin-like growth factor receptor signalling is essential for the development of the hippocampal formation and dentate gyrus. *J. Neurosci. Res.* 87, 2821–2832. doi: 10.1002/jnr.22129

Lynch, C., Lyons, D., Khan, A., Bennett, S., and Sonntag, W. E. (2001). Insulin-like growth factor-1 increases glucose utilisation in brains of aged animals. *Endocrinology* 142, 506–509. doi: 10.1210/en.142.1.506

Maggio, M., De Vita, F., Lauretani, F., Buttò, V., Bondi, G., Cattabiani, C., et al. (2013). IGF1, the cross road of the nutritional, inflammatory and hormonal pathways to frailty. *Nutrients* 5, 4184–4205. doi: 10.3390/nu5104184

De Maghalaes Filho, C. D., Kappeler, L., Dupont, J., Solinc, J., Villapol, S., Denis, C., et al. (2016). Deleting IGF-1 receptor from forebrain neurons confers neuroprotection during stroke and upregulates endocrine somatotropin. *J. Cereb. Blood Flow Metab.* doi: 10.1177/0271678x15626718 [Epub ahead of print].

Markowska, A. L., Mooney, M., and Sonntag, W. E. (1998). Insulin-like growth factor-1 ameliorates age-related behavioral deficits. *Neuroscience* 87, 559–569. doi: 10.1016/s0306-4522(98)00143-2

Maya-Vetencourt, J. F., Baroncelli, L., Viegi, A., Tiraboschi, E., Castren, E., Cattaneo, A., et al. (2012). IGF-1 restores visual cortex plasticity in adult life by reducing local GABA levels. *Neural Plast.* 2012:250421. doi: 10.1155/2012/250421

McMorris, F., and Dubois-Dalcq, M. (1988). Insulin-like growth factor 1 promotes cell proliferation and oligodendroglial commitment in rat progenitor cells *in vitro*. *J. Neurosci. Res.* 21, 199–209. doi: 10.1002/jnr.490210212

Moloney, A. M., Griffin, R. J., Timmons, S., O'Connor, R., Ravid, R., and O'Neill, C. (2010). Defects in IGF-1 receptor, insulin receptor and IRS-1/2 in Alzheimer's disease indicate possible resistance to IGF-1 and insulin signalling. *Neurobiol. Aging* 31, 224–243. doi: 10.1016/j.neurobiolaging.2008.04.002

Morris, J. Z., Tissenbaum, H. A., and Ruvkun, G. (1996). A phosphatidylinositol-3-OH kinase family member regulating longevity and diapause in *Caenorhabditis elegans*. *Nature* 382, 536–539. doi: 10.1038/382536a0

Mosconi, L., Pupi, A., and De Leon, M. (2013). Brain glucose hypometabolism and oxidatice stress in preclinical Alzheimer's disease. *Ann. N Y Acad. Sci.* 1147, 180–195. doi: 10.1196/annals.1427.007

Mozell, R., and McMorris, F. (1991). Insulin like growth factor 1 stimulates oligodendrocyte development and myelination in rat brain aggregate cultures. *J. Neurosci. Res.* 30, 382–390. doi: 10.1002/jnr.490300214

Mysoet, J., Canu, M., Cieniewski-Bernard, C., Bastide, B., and Dupont, E. (2014). Hypoactivity affects IGF-1 level and PI3K/AKT signaling pathway in cerebral structures implied in motor control. *PLoS One* 9:e107631. doi: 10.1371/journal.pone.0107631

Mysoet, J., Dupont, E., Bastide, B., and Canu, M. (2015). Role of IGF-1 in cortical plasticity and functional deficit induced by sensorimotor restriction. *Behav. Brain Res.* 290, 117–123. doi: 10.1016/j.bbr.2015.04.055

Nieto-Estévez, V., Defterali, Ç., and Vicario-Abejón, C. (2016a). IGF-I: a key growth factor that regulates neurogenesis and synaptogenesis from embryonic to adult stages of the brain. *Front. Neurosci.*, 10:52. doi: 10.3389/fnins.2016.00052

Nieto-Estévez, V., Oueslati-Morales, C. O., Lingling, L., Pickel, J., Morales, A. V., and Vicario-Abejón, C. (2016b). Brain insulin-like growth factor-1 directs the transition from stem cells to mature neurons during postnatal/adult hippocampal neurogenesis. *Stem Cells* 34, 2194–2209. doi: 10.1002/stem.2397

O'Kusky, J. R., Ye, P., and D'Ercole, A. J. (2000). Insulin-like growth factor-I promotes neurogenesis and synaptogenesis in the hippocampal dentate gyrus during postnatal development. *J. Neurosci.* 20, 8435–8442.

Pañeda, C., Arroba, A. I., Frago, L. M., Holm, A. M., Rømer, J., Argente, J., et al. (2003). Growth hormone releasing peptide-6 inhibits cerebellar cell death in aged rats. *Neuroreport* 14, 1633–1635. doi: 10.1097/00001756-200308260-00018

Paolisso, G., Ammendola, S., Del Buono, A., Gambardella, A., Riondino, M., Tagliamonte, M., et al. (1997). Serum levels of insulin-like growth factor-1 (IGF1) and IGF-binding protein-3 in healthy centenarians: relationship with plasma leptin and lipid concentrations, insulin action, and cognitive function. *J. Clin. Endocrinol. Metab.* 82, 2204–2209. doi: 10.1210/jc.82.7.2204

Papadakis, M. A., Grady, D., Black, D., Tierney, M. J., Gooding, G. A., Schambelan, M., et al. (1996). Growth hormone replacement in healthy older men improves body composition but not functional ability. *Ann. Int. Med.* 124, 708–716. doi: 10.7326/0003-4819-124-8-199604150-00002

Papadakis, M. A., Grady, D., Tierney, M. J., Black, D., Wells, L., and Grunfeld, C. (1995). Insulin-like growth factor-1 and functional status in healthy older men. *J. Am. Geriatr. Soc.* 43, 1350–1355. doi: 10.1111/j.1532-5415.1995.tb06613.x

Popken, G. J., Hodge, R. D., Ye, P., Zhang, J., Ng, W., O'Kusky, J. R., et al. (2004). *In vivo* effects of insulin-like growth factor-I (IGF-I) on prenatal and early postnatal development of the central nervous system. *Eur. J. Neurosci.* 19, 2056–2068. doi: 10.1111/j.0953-816x.2004.03320.x

Rollero, A., Murialdo, G., Fonzi, S., Garrone, S., Gianelli, M. V., Gazzerro, E., et al. (1998). Relationship between cognitive function, growth hormone and insulin-like growth factor 1 plasma levels in aged subjects. *Neuropsychobiology* 38, 73–79. doi: 10.1159/000026520

Sadagurski, M., Cheng, Z., Rozzo, A., Palazzolo, I., Kelley, G. R., Dong, X., et al. (2011). IRS2 increases mitochondrial dysfunction and oxidative stress in a mouse model of Huntington disease. *J. Clin. Invest.* 121, 4070–4081. doi: 10.1172/JCI46305

Sadagurski, M., and White, M. F. (2013). Integrating metabolism and longevity through insulin and IGF-1 signalling. *Endocrinol. Metab. Clin. North Am.* 42, 127–148. doi: 10.1016/j.ecl.2012.11.008

Sharples, A. P., Hughes, D. C., Deane, C. S., Saini, A., Selman, C., and Stewart, C. E. (2015). Longevity and skeletal muscle mass: the role of the sirtuins, dietary restriction and protein intake. *Aging Cell* 14, 511–523. doi: 10.1111/acel.12342

Shcheglovitov, A., Shcheglovitova, O., Yazawa, M., Portmann, T., Shu, R., Sebastiano, V., et al. (2013). SHANK3 and IGF1 restore synaptic deficits in neurons from 22q13 deletion syndrome patients. *Nature* 503, 267–271. doi: 10.1038/nature12618

Sherrard, R. M., and Bower, A. J. (2003). IGF-1 induces neonatal climbing-fibre plasticity in the mature rat cerebellum. *Neuroreport* 14, 1713–1716. doi: 10.1097/01.wnr.0000087732.58565.f2

Sonntag, W. E., Bennett, S. A., Khan, A. S., Thornton, P. L., Xu, X., Ingram, R. L., et al. (2000a). Age and insulin-like growth factor-1modulate N-methyl-D-aspartate receptor subtype expression in rats. *Brain Res. Bull.* 51, 331–338. doi: 10.1016/s0361-9230(99)00259-2

Sonntag, W. E., Lynch, C., Thornton, P., Khan, A., Bennett, S., and Ingam, R. (2000b). The effects of growth hormone and IGF1 deficiency on cerebrovascular and brain ageing. *J. Anat.* 197, 575–585. doi: 10.1046/j.1469-7580.2000.19740575.x

Sonntag, W. E., Lynch, C. D., Bennett, S. A., Khan, A. S., Thornton, P. L., Cooney, P. T., et al. (1999). Alterations in insulin-like growth factor-1 gene and protein expression and type-1 insulin-like growth factor receptors in the brains of aging rats. *Neuroscience* 88, 269–279. doi: 10.1016/s0306-4522(98)00192-4

Steen, E., Terry, B. M., Rivera, E. J., Cannon, J. L., Neely, T. R., Tavares, R., et al. (2005). Impaired insulin resistance and insulin-like growth factor expression and sginalling mechanisms in Alzheimer's disease—is this type 3 diabetes? *J. Alzheimers Dis.* 7, 63–80.

Suh, Y., Atzmon, G., Cho, M. O., Hwang, D., Liu, B., Leahy, D. J., et al. (2008). Functionally significant insulin-like growth factor I receptor mutations in centenarians. *Proc. Natl. Acad. Sci. U S A* 105, 3438–3442. doi: 10.1073/pnas.0705467105

Sun, L. Y., Evans, M. S., Hsieh, J., Oanici, J., and Bartke, A. (2005). Increased neurogenesis in dentate gyrus of long-lived Ames dwarf mice. *Endocrinology* 146, 1138–1144. doi: 10.1210/en.2004-1115

Supeno, N., Pati, S., Hadi, R., Ghani, A., Mustafa, Z., Abdullah, J., et al. (2013). IGF-1 acts as a controlling switch for long-term proliferation and maintenance of EGF/FGF-responsive striatal neural stem cells. *Int. J. Med. Sci.* 10, 522–531. doi: 10.7150/ijms.5325

Talbot, K., Wang, H. Y., Kazi, H., Han, L. Y., Bakshi, K. P., Stucky, A., et al. (2012). Demonstrated brain insulin resistance in Alzheimer's disease patients is associated with IGF-1 resistance, IRS-1 dysregulation, and cognitive decline. *J. Clin. Invest.* 122, 1316–1338. doi: 10.1172/JCI59903

Tatar, M., Kopelman, A., Epstein, D., Tu, M.-P., Yin, C. M., and Garofalo, R. S. (2001). A mutant *Drosophila* insulin receptor homolog that extends life-span and impairs neuroendocrine function. *Science* 292, 107–110. doi: 10.1126/science.1057987

Trejo, J., Carro, E., and Torres-Aleman, I. (2001). Circulating insulin-like growth factor-1 mediates exercise-induced increases in the of new neurons in the adult hippocampus. *J. Neurosci.* 21, 1628–1634.

Tropea, D., Giacometti, E., Wilson, N. R., Beard, C., McCurry, C., Fu, D. D., et al. (2009). Patrial reversal of Rett syndrome-like symptoms in MECP2 mutant mice. *Proc. Natl. Acad. Sci. U S A* 106, 2029–2034. doi: 10.1073/pnas.0812394106

Tropea, D., Krerman, G., Lyckman, A., Mukherjee, S., Yu, H., Horng, S., et al. (2006). Gene expression changes and molecular pathways mediating activity-dependent plasticity in the visual cortex. *Nat. Neurosci.* 9, 660–668. doi: 10.1038/nn1689

Vahdatpour, C., Dyer, A. H., and Tropea, D. (2016). Insulin-like growth factor 1 and related compounds in the treatment of childhood-onset neurodevelopmental disorders. *Front. Neurosci.* 10:450. doi: 10.3389/fnins.2016.00450

White, M. (2014). IRS2 integrates insulin/IGF1 signalling with metabolism, neurodegeneration and longevity. *Diabetes Obes. Metab.* 16, 4–15. doi: 10.1111/dom.12347

Willcox, B. J., Donlon, T. A., He, Q., Chen, R., Grove, J. S., Yano, K., et al. (2008). FOXO3A genotype is strongly associated with human longevity. *Proc. Natl. Acad. Sci. U S A* 105, 13987–13992. doi: 10.1073/pnas.0801030105

Wine, R. N., McPherson, C. A., and Harry, G. J. (2009). IGF-1 and pAKT signaling promote hippocampal CA1 neuronal survival following injury to dentate granule cells. *Neurotox. Res.* 16, 280–292. doi: 10.1007/s12640-009-9060-y

Wolkow, C. A., Kimura, K. D., Lee, M.-S., and Ruvkun, G. (2000). Regulation of *C. elegans* life-span by insulin like signaling in the nervous system. *Science* 290, 147–150. doi: 10.1126/science.290.5489.147

Ye, P., Carson, J., and D'Ercole, A. (1995). *In vivo* actions of insulin-like growth factor-1 (IGF-1) on brain myelination: studies of IGF-1 and IGF-binding protein (IGFBP-1) transgenic mice. *J. Neuro.* 15, 7344–7356.

Ye, P., and D'Ercole, A. J. (1999). Insulin-like growth factor I protects oligodendrocytes from tumor necrosis factor-α-induced injury. *Endocrinology* 140, 3063–3072. doi: 10.1210/en.140.7.3063

Ye, P., Lee, K., and D'Ercole, A. (2000). Insulin-like growth factor-1 (IGF-1) protects myelination from under-nutritional insult: studies of transgenic mice overexpressing IGF1 in the brain. *J. Neurosci. Res.* 62, 700–708. doi: 10.1002/1097-4547(20001201)62:5<700::aid-jnr9>3.0.co;2-1

Ye, P., Li, L., Richards, R. G., DiAugustine, R. P., and D'Ercole, A. J. (2002). Myelination is altered in insulin-like growth factor null mice. *J. Neurosci.* 22, 6041–6051.

Ye, P., Xing, Y., Dai, Z., and D'Ercole, A. J. (1996). *In vivo* actions of insulin-like growth factor-I (IGF-I) on cerebellum development in transgenic mice: evidence that IGF-I increases proliferation of granule cell progenitors. *Dev. Brain Res.* 95, 44–54. doi: 10.1016/0165-3806(96)00492-0

Yin, F., Jiang, T., and Cadenas, E. (2013). Metabolic traid in brain aging: mitochondria, insulin/IGF1 signalling and JNK signalling. *Biochem. Soc. Trans.* 41, 101–105. doi: 10.1042/BST20120260

Yuan, H., Chen, R., Wu, L., Chen, Q., Hu, A., Zhang, T., et al. (2015). The regulatory mechanisms of neurogenesis by IGF1 in adult mice. *Mol. Neurobiol.* 51, 512–522. doi: 10.1007/s12035-014-8717-6

10

Inhibition of Histone Deacetylase 3 (HDAC3) Mediates Ischemic Preconditioning and Protects Cortical Neurons against Ischemia in Rats

*Xiaoyu Yang†, Qimei Wu†, Lei Zhang and Linyin Feng**

CAS Key Laboratory of Receptor Research, Shanghai Institute of Materia Medica, Chinese Academy of Sciences, Shanghai, China

Edited by:
Andrew Harkin,
Trinity College, Dublin, Ireland

Reviewed by:
Daniela Christiane Dieterich,
Leibniz Institute for Neurobiology, Germany
Natalia N. Nalivaeva,
University of Leeds, UK

***Correspondence:**
Linyin Feng
lyfeng@simm.ac.cn

† These authors have contributed equally to this work.

Brain ischemic preconditioning (PC) provides vital insights into the endogenous protection against stroke. Genomic and epigenetic responses to PC condition the brain into a state of ischemic tolerance. Notably, PC induces the elevation of histone acetylation, consistent with evidence that histone deacetylase (HDAC) inhibitors protect the brain from ischemic injury. However, less is known about the specific roles of HDACs in this process. HDAC3 has been implicated in several neurodegenerative conditions. Deletion of HDAC3 confers protection against neurotoxicity and neuronal injury. Here, we hypothesized that inhibition of HDAC3 may contribute to the neuronal survival elicited by PC. To address this notion, PC and transient middle cerebral artery occlusion (MCAO) were conducted in Sprague-Dawley rats. Additionally, primary cultured cortical neurons were used to identify the modulators and effectors of HDAC3 involved in PC. We found that nuclear localization of HDAC3 was significantly reduced following PC *in vivo* and *in vitro*. Treatment with the HDAC3-specific inhibitor, RGFP966, mimicked the neuroprotective effects of PC 24 h and 7 days after MCAO, causing a reduced infarct volume and less Fluoro-Jade C staining. Improved functional outcomes were observed in the neurological score and rotarod test. We further showed that attenuated recruitment of HDAC3 to promoter regions following PC potentiates transcriptional initiation of genes including *Hspa1a*, *Bcl2l1*, and *Prdx2*, which may underlie the mechanism of protection. In addition, PC-activated calpains were implicated in the cleavage of HDAC3. Pretreatment with calpeptin blockaded the attenuated nuclear distribution of HDAC3 and the protective effect of PC *in vivo*. Collectively, these results demonstrate that the inhibition of HDAC3 preconditions the brain against ischemic insults, indicating a new approach to evoke endogenous protection against stroke.

Keywords: preconditioning (PC), HDAC3, MCAO, RGFP966, calpain

---

Abbreviations: ChIP, chromatin immunoprecipetition; DIV, days *in vitro*; HAT, histone transacetylase; HDAC, histone deacetylase; MCAO, middle cerebral artery occlusion; MTT, 3-(4,5-dimethylthiazolyl)-2,5-diphenyltetrazolium bromide; OGD/R, oxygen-glucose deprivation and reoxygenation and restored energy supply; PC, preconditioning; TTC, 2,3,5-Triphenyltetrazolium chloride.

INTRODUCTION

Brain ischemia, induced by transient or permanent interruption of the blood supply, is a major cause of mortality and morbidity worldwide (Johnston et al., 2009; Feigin et al., 2014). The mechanisms of neuronal death in stroke are complex; involving cell membrane depolarization, free radical generation, excitotoxicity, and neuroinflammation (Dirnagl et al., 1999; Moskowitz et al., 2010). Despite extensive efforts, therapeutic strategies focusing on the pathological signaling cascades have not been successful (Moretti et al., 2015). Effective treatments for ischemic brain damage remain one of the major unfulfilled medical needs of clinical care (Fisher and Saver, 2015). Ischemic PC is an approach in which a sub-lethal ischemic exposure evokes endogenous protection against a subsequent, more severe ischemic insult. Not only can this therapy be applied in individuals, induced ischemic tolerance is also a strategy to obtain insights into neuroprotective mechanisms (Dirnagl et al., 2009; Stevens et al., 2014). PC stimuli may be identified by diverse sensors and transducers, and consequently initiate protection such as temporal gene profiles resistant to typically lethal ischemic insults by effectors.

Different genomic profiles and epigenetic reprogramming of the brain have been reported between ischemic PC and ischemic injury (Stenzel-Poore et al., 2003; Thompson et al., 2013). Thereby identification of epigenetic determinants of PC is the key for pharmacological manipulation to evoke conditioning. *In vivo* studies have shown that pan-HDAC inhibitors protected the brain from ischemic injury, by elevating the severe decrease of histone acetylation (Chuang et al., 2009; Langley et al., 2009). The treatment of myocardial ischemia with HDAC inhibitors triggers the PC effects against ischemia/reperfusion injury. Likewise, studies in retina and brain ischemia revealed an elevation of histone acetylation following PC, which may be associated with regulation of the deacetylase activity of HDAC or HAT recruitment (Yildirim et al., 2014; Fan et al., 2016). These studies have raised the hypotheses that HDACs might converge in the conditioning signaling pathways. However, considering the significant effects of HDAC inhibitors against ischemia, less is known about the specific role of HDACs in brain PC.

HDAC3, a homologue of Rpd3 from budding yeast, has been linked to neurotoxicity in several neuropathological conditions (Butler and Bates, 2006; Yang and Seto, 2008). In *Caenorhabditis elegans* knock-down of the homolog of HDAC3, HDA-3, suppressed Htn-Q150 toxicity in a model of Huntington's disease (Bates et al., 2006). In rat cerebellar granule neurons, mutant *Htt* disrupted the sequestration of HDAC3 and the liberation of HDAC3 resulted in neurotoxic activity (Bardai et al., 2013). Additionally, suppression by HDAC3 shRNA protected cerebellar granule neurons against a low-potassium insult, while overexpression of HDAC3 promoted the death of neurons (Bardai and D'Mello, 2011). Conditional knock-out of *Hdac3* in retinal ganglion cells displayed a significant amelioration of nuclear atrophy and reduction in cell death induced by optic nerve injury (Schmitt et al., 2014).

Given the properties of HDAC3 in neurodegeneration, we speculate whether inhibition of HDAC3 contributes to the neuronal survival elicited by PC. We first investigated histone acetylation and class I HDAC subcellular localization following PC. We found that PC-induced acetyl-histone 3 Lysine 9 (H3K9ac) elevation was accompanied by reduced HDAC3 nuclear localization in cortical neurons. Based on this, efficient and specific pharmacological inhibition of HDAC3 *in vivo* and knock-down of HDAC3 *in vitro* in models of ischemia were performed. The results showed that specific inhibition of HDAC3 could precondition the brain against ischemic injury 24 h and 7 days after MCAO *in vivo*, via the initiation of a gene-expressing program associated with neuroprotection. Furthermore, we identified that calpains were implicated in the cleavage of HDAC3, which blocked the nuclear distribution of HDAC3. Overall, the results demonstrate the importance of HDAC3 in the process of PC, providing a new pharmacological approach to evoke protection due to ischemic conditioning.

MATERIALS AND METHODS

Animals

Adult male Sprague-Dawley rats weighing 250–280 g were used in this study (Laboratory Animal Center, Chinese Academy of Sciences, Shanghai, China). All experimental procedures were performed in accordance with the Guide for the Care and Use of Laboratory Animals (National Institutes of Health) and approved by the Institutional Animal Care and Use Committee of Shanghai Institute of *Materia Medica*.

MCAO and Ischemic Preconditioning

All animals were acclimatized for 2 weeks before pharmacological treatment or surgery. The induction of transient focal cerebral ischemia was performed as previously described (Longa et al., 1989), with minor modifications. Briefly, the animals were anesthetized with chloral hydrate (400 mg/kg, i.p.). A 4-0 monofilament nylon surgical suture (Sunbio Biotech Co. Ltd., Beijing, China) with a rounded tip was introduced through the external carotid artery to the internal carotid artery and advanced up to 18–20 mm to block the middle cerebral artery. After a period of occlusion, 5 min for ischemic PC and 90 min for injurious ischemia, the suture was withdrawn to allow reperfusion. Regional cerebral blood flow was monitored throughout surgery using a laser Doppler (moorVMS-LDF2, Axminster, UK) to exclude rats that showed a cerebral blood flow (CBF) reduction of less than 80%. Rectal temperature was monitored and the core body temperature was maintained at 37 ± 0.5°C by a feed-back-controlled heat pad (Hugo Sachs Elektronik, March-Hugstetten, Germany). Rats were transferred back to their cages after recovery from anesthesia and rested in home cages before sacrifice. Sham operation were conducted using an identical procedure but without the insertion of a filament.

Experimental Design

Rats were randomly grouped ($n = 8$–14 per group) and subjected to different MCAO and pharmaceutical treatments as follows (Supplementary Figures S2A,B):

Sham group: Sham surgery was performed on day 1 and at the same time on day 2. Rats received vehicle injections at the same time as the RGFP966 group or the calpeptin group below.
MCAO group: Rats underwent sham operation on day 1 and 90 min of MCAO on day 2. Rats received vehicle injections at the same time as RGFP966 group or calpeptin group below.
PC group: Rats were subjected to 5 min of MCAO to induce ischemic PC on day 1, and 90 min of MCAO on day 2.
RGFP966 group: Rats were treated with RGFP966 (7.5 mg/kg, i.p) when subjected to a sham operation. The second RGFP966 was injected 6 h prior to the MCAO of 90 min on day 2.
Calpeptin group: Rats were treated with calpeptin (125 μg/kg, i.p) 6 h before surgery, and then underwent the same procedure as the PC group.
Rats were sacrificed 24 h or 7 days after injurious MCAO.

Pharmacological Treatment

Drugs were administrated at a volume of 5 ml/kg. RGFP966 (S7229, Selleckchem, Houston, TX, USA) was dissolved in DMSO, and diluted in a vehicle of 100 mM sodium acetate (PH 5.4) and 30% (wt/vol) hydroxypropyl-beta-cyclodextrin, with the final DMSO less than 10% (vol/vol). Calpeptin (C8999, Sigma–Aldrich, St Louis, MO, USA) was dissolved in DMSO and diluted in saline. Vehicles were obtained by identical procedures without drugs. The doses were determined based on pervious report to obtain proper concentrations in the brain (Malvaez et al., 2013; Samantaray et al., 2015).

Infarct Volume Quantification

The cerebral infract volumes were measured using TTC (T8877, Sigma–Aldrich) staining. Rat brains were harvested and sectioned into 2 mm thick coronal sections 24 h or 7 days after MCAO. Then sections were stained with 1% TTC at 37 °C for 5 min, and fixed in 4% paraformaldehyde (PFA) solution for 48 h. The images were captured and analyzed using Image-Pro Plus 7.0 (Media Cybernetics, Silver Spring, MD, USA). The infarct volume (%) for the brain was calculated with the following formula: (the volume of the contralateral hemisphere – the volume of the non-lesioned ipsilateral hemisphere)/(the volume of the contralateral hemisphere × 2). The ipsilateral hemisphere underwent occlusive treatment in the MCA, while the contralateral hemisphere did not. Investigators were kept blind to the treatment assignments.

Neurological Function Analysis

The neurological deficits score after surgery was evaluated according to validated scoring analyses with minor modifications (Longa et al., 1989): 0, no observable deficit; 1, unable to fully stretch the forelimb of the right side (the left MCA was occluded in this study); 2, decreased resistance to lateral push, circling to the right side but normal gesture at rest; 3, unilateral rolling to the right side; 4, occasionally leaning to the right side, declined locomotor activity; 5, unable to sustain normal gesture at rest, unresponsive. Investigators were kept blind to treatment assignments.

Rotarod Test

Rats were trained and tested on rotarod (IITC Life Science, Woodland Hills, CA, USA) which gradually accelerated from 4 to 40 rpm over 5 min (Hunter et al., 2000). The latency to fall was recorded as the time before rats fell off the rod or gripped and spun around for two successive revolutions. Rats underwent three training trails a day for 3 days. The base line control was recorded 1 day before the surgery. The mean latency was obtained from 3 trials with 30 min interval on the testing day. Investigators were kept blind to treatment assignments.

Primary Culture of Rat Cortical Neurons and Treatment

Primary cortical neurons were prepared from embryonic E17 Sprague-Dawley rats and cultured with Neurobasal medium and B27 supplement (Thermo Fisher Scientific, USA) as described previously (Xie et al., 2009). Neurons were cultured at 37°C in a humidified 5% CO_2 atmosphere and the medium was replaced by fresh every 3 days. Neurons at 7 DIV were used for experimentation. In the OGD treatment, the glucose-free Dulbecco's Modified Eagle Medium (DMEM) (Thermo Fisher Scientific) was bubbled with 95% N_2/5% CO_2. The chamber was pre-warmed, humidified, and flushed with 95% N_2/5% CO_2 at 3 liter/min for 5 min. The oxygen content was under 0.50% (v/v) throughout the experimental period detected with oxygen monitor (Jiande Analytical Instrument, Hangzhou, China). For PC treatment, the culture medium was replaced with and cells were placed glucose-free DMEM in an experimental hypoxia chamber for 45 min for neurons or 1.5 h for PC12. The cells were then removed from the chamber and cultured under normal conditions for the indicated periods (see figure legends). For the OGD/R model, neurons were cultured in glucose-free DMEM in a hypoxia chamber for 90 min and returned to normal culture conditions for 24 h. The control cells were cultured in a medium with glucose in a normal oxygen-condition incubator for the same time periods.

Tissue Preparation

After anesthetization, brains were immediately removed. Brain tissue were obtained by coronal sectioning and harvested along the core region of occlusion underlying the middle cerebral artery. The tissues were immediately frozen in liquid nitrogen, and stored at −80°C.

Western Blot

The brain tissue or cultured cells were lysed in a RIPA buffer with proteinase and phosphatase inhibitor cocktail (Sigma–Aldrich) for whole cell protein. The nuclear and cytoplasmic fractions were extracted with NE-PER Nuclear and Cytoplasmic Extraction Reagents Kit (Pierce, Rockford, IL, USA) following the manufacturer's instruction. The protein concentration was quantified using a BCA assay kit (Thermo Fisher Scientific). Samples were separated by sodium dodecyl sulfate-polyacrylamide gel electrophoresis (SDS-PAGE) and transferred to PVDF membranes (Merck-Millipore, Bedford, MA, USA). Blots were then probed with specific antibodies:

anti-H3K9ac (ab12179, Abcam, Cambridge, MA, USA), anti-HDAC1 (WH0003065M2, Sigma–Aldrich), anti-HDAC2 (ab16032, Abcam), anti-HDAC3 (ab47237, Abcam), anti-lamin A/C (2032, Cell Signaling Technology, Beverly, MA, USA), anti-β-actin (A8481, Sigma–Aldrich), anti-Bcl-xL (2764, Cell Signaling Technology), anti-Prdx2 (10545-2-AP, Proteintech Group, Chicago, IL, USA), anti-HSP70 (sc-32239, Santa Cruz, Dallas, TX). After incubation with HRP-conjugated secondary antibodies (Santa Cruz), chemiluminescence signals were detected with ECL reagents (GE Health, Little Chalfont, UK).

Histological and Immunohistochemical Assessment

After anesthesia with chloral hydrate, rats were injected transcardially with ice-cold 4% PFA in PBS. Brains were post-fixed in PFA for 24 h and dehydrated with 30% (wt/vol) sucrose for 48 h. Next, 25 μm coronal slices were obtained with a Leica freezing microtome. Primary antibodies used in immunofluorescence staining were: anti-H3K9ac (ab12179, Abcam), anti-HDAC3 (ab47237, Abcam) and anti-MAP2 (ab11267, Abcam). The sections were incubated with 300 nM 4,6-diamidino-2-phenylindole (DAPI, Sigma), Alexa Fluor 488 and Alexa Fluor 555 secondary antibodies (Thermo Fisher Scientific) for 45 min at 25°C. An Olympus FV1000 confocal laser scanning microscope was applied for acquisition of fluorescence images. 3,3′-diaminobenzidine immunostaining was performed with primary antibodies against: HSP70 (sc-32239, Santa Cruz), following with SignalStain Boost IHC Detection Reagent and visualized with SignalStain DAB Substrate Kit (Cell Signaling Technology). Images were acquired using a Leica microscope. Fluoro-Jade C (FJC) staining was performed according to the protocol provided by the manufacturer (Chemicon, Merck-Millipore). Images were obtained using an Olympus FV1000 confocal microscope. For histological quantification of H3K9ac intensity and FJC positive cells, images were obtained from two random 20× fields of the cortical area in three coronal sections (Interaural 10.60 mm/Bregma 1.60 mm, Interaural 9.20 mm/Bregma 0.20 mm, Interaural 7.12 mm/Bregma −1.88 mm) (Supplementary Figure S2C). Average intensities or cell counts were calculated from 5 rats per group with Image Pro Plus 7.0. Investigators were kept blind to treatment assignments.

Co-immunoprecipitation (Co-IP) Assay

Cell lysates were generated by incubating cells with an NP-40 lysis buffer with proteinase inhibitor cocktail on ice and then centrifuged at 10000 *g* for 10 min. Immunoprecipitation was carried out by incubating the lysate with the corresponding antibodies: anti-HDAC3 (ab47237, Abcam), anti-calpain1 (ab28258, Abcam), anti-calpain2 (ab39165, Abcam) and anti-HA (3724, Cell Signaling Technology) with slow agitation overnight at 4°C. Next, 20 μl PureProteome Protein A/G Mix Magnetic Beads (Merck-Millipore) was added and incubated with slow agitation for 4 h at 4°C. Immune complexes were washed extensively, boiled in SDS-sample buffer and analyzed using SDS-PAGE.

Quantitative Reverse Transcription Polymerase Chain Reaction (qRT-PCR)

Total RNA was extracted from cortical neurons after treatment using TRIzol reagent (Thermo Fisher Scientific). Next, 1 μg total RNA was converted to cDNA using a reverse transcription kit (Takara, Cat# RR047A). After the RT reaction, cDNA was used for subsequent real time PCR (SYBR Premix Ex TaqII Kit) following the manufacturer's protocol. The qPCR and data collection were carried out on ABI 7500 real-time PCR system (Applied Biosystems, Foster City, CA, USA). The results relative to the quantitation value for each target gene were expressed as $2^{-\Delta\Delta Ct}$. All PCR primers are shown in Supplementary Table S1.

Chromatin Immunoprecipetition and Real-Time PCR

Chromatin immunoprecipetition was carried out according to the protocol of the EZ-Magna ChIP kit (17-10086, Millipore). Briefly, the nuclear content of cortical neurons was extracted and the chromatin inside was sonicated into fragments. Fragmented chromatin was incubated and immunoprecipitated using anti-H3K9ac antibody (17-609, Millipore) and anti-HDAC3 antibody (17-10238, Millipore). After the de-crosslink, immunoprecipitated DNA and whole-cell extract DNA were then eluted and subjected to real-time PCR analysis using SYBR Premix Ex TaqII Kit (Takara, Shiga, Japan). All PCR primers are shown in Supplementary Table S2.

Plasmid Constructs and Transfection

Full-length human HDAC3 cDNA was synthesized by GENEWIZ (South Plainfield, NJ, USA) and ligated into the expression vector, HA-pcDNA3.0. C-terminus-truncated construct HDAC3 mutant (ΔC-HDAC3, 1-312) was amplified with primers: 5′GATATCGATGGCCAAGACCGTGGCGTATTTC3′ and 5′CTCGAGTTAAGATGTTTCATATGTCCAGCACCG3′ using full length HDAC3 cDNA as the template. Transient transfection was conducted using the FuGENE HD transfection reagent (Promega, Madison, WI, USA) according to the manufacturer's instructions. siRNA-HDAC3 (s136736, Dharmacon) was transfected into cortical neurons by the FuGENE HD transfection reagent. The silencing effect of protein expression was confirmed by western blot analysis.

Cell Viability

Neuron viability was assessed using the MTT assay as described previously. Briefly, MTT solution (0.5 mg/ml) was added to each well and incubated with cells for an additional 3 h at 37°C. The formazan was then dissolved with DMSO and the absorbance at 595 nm was read by a microplate reader (NOVOstar, BMG LABTECH, Offenburg, Germany).

Statistical Analysis

Quantifications and statistical analysis were carried out using GraphPad Prism 6 (Graphpad Software, San Diego, CA, USA). All values are presented as means ± SEM. Differences between groups were compared with a one-way ANOVA followed by group comparisons using a *post hoc* Bonferroni test or two-tailed Student's *t*-test. Neurological deficit scores were analyzed using the Kruskal-Wallis non-parametric test followed by Dunn's multiple comparisons test.

RESULTS

Acetylation of H3K9 Increased in Cortical Neurons in Preconditioning, Accompanied by Reduction of Nuclear Localization of HDAC3

Histone acetylation was shown to be differentially regulated depending on the duration of ischemia. While injurious ischemia led to a severe decline of histone acetylation in stroke models (Supplementary Figure S1A) (Ren et al., 2004; Faraco et al., 2006; Kim et al., 2007), PC for 5 min followed by 2 h reperfusion in rats induced increased levels of acetyl-H3K9 in the cortex, as assessed with both immunoblotting ($p < 0.05$, $n = 5$) and immunohistochemistry ($p < 0.001$, $n = 5$) (**Figure 1A**). We next measured levels of expression of the three class I HDAC subtypes with which the deacetylation of histone lysine residuals is largely associated. Western blot assay on nuclear lysates revealed that the levels of HDAC3, but not HDAC1 or HDAC2, were reduced in the nuclei following PC ($p < 0.05$, $n = 4$–6) (**Figure 1B**). To further determine the involvement of HDAC3 in PC, the subcellular localization of HDAC3 was assessed with immunofluorescence. The results showed that HDAC3 was distributed both in the nucleus and cytoplasm in cortical neurons before PC, while it was localized mainly in the cytoplasm following PC treatment (**Figure 1C**). Meanwhile, the modulation of histone acetylation (**Figure 1D**) and the nuclear reduction of HDAC3 following PC were verified with primary cortical neuron cultures (**Figure 1E**, Supplementary Figures S1C,D). These results indicated that a diminished recruitment of HDAC3 to the genomic arena might contribute to the modulation of the histone acetylation profile following PC.

Inhibition of HDAC3 Mimicked the Neuroprotective Effects of PC *In vivo*

Given the changes in redistribution of HDAC3 following PC, we wondered whether inhibition of HDAC3 mimics the neuroprotective effect of PC. Rats with different treatments were subjected to MCAO (Supplementary Figure S2A). RGFP966, a known HDAC3-specific inhibitor, was injected 24 and 6 h prior to MCAO. The RGFP966-treated group exhibited significantly reduced infarct volume compared with the vehicle-treated group 24 h (7.68 ± 2.90% versus 19.09 ± 2.91%, $p < 0.05$, $n = 7$–9) and 7 days (8.62 ± 2.00% versus 18.25 ± 3.75%, $p < 0.05$, $n = 8$–10) after reperfusion. Furthermore, the anterior-posterior analysis of infarct distribution revealed that the infarction mostly occupied the striatum and temporal cortex, which was decreased in slices 2, 3, 4 in the PC and RGFP966 group (**Figures 2A,B**). Brain coronal sections obtained 24 h and 7 days after MCAO were stained with FJC to label degenerating neurons (**Figures 2C,D**). Higher levels of FJC staining were observed in the MCAO group compared to with the Sham group, and significantly decreased labeling with FJC in the RGFP966-treated group compared with the MCAO group in both 24 h and 7 days assessments ($n = 5$). Furthermore, we analyzed the counterstain of FJC with GFAP or Iba with brain sections obtained 24 h after MCAO. The schematic brain section and outlined box showed the area where images were acquired in the ipsilateral hemisphere (Supplementary Figure S5A). Activated astrocytes and microglia were observed in MCAO group, while less activation in PC and RGFP966 group (Supplementary Figures S5B,C). Meanwhile, neurological function was evaluated using the neurological deficit score and rotarod test. Rats treated with RGFP966 displayed lower neurological deficit scores ($n = 8$–10) and improved rotarod performance ($n = 8$–10) throughout 7-day test compared with the Sham group (**Figures 2E,F**).

Attenuated Recruitment of HDAC3 to Promoter Regions Following PC Potentiated Transcriptional Initiation of Oxidation Relative Genes

Concomitant with the data *in vivo*, the reduction in cell viability elicited by OGD/R was blocked by both RGFP966 pretreatment and HDAC3 knock-down in primary cultured cortical neurons, as determined by the MTT assay (**Figure 3A**). To further elaborate the underlying role of HDAC3 in PC, data mining linking HDAC3 targeting genes (Feng et al., 2011) and ischemia was performed and determined a group of associated genes. ChIP analysis revealed that promoter occupancy of HDAC3 on *Hspa1a*, *Prdx2* and *Bcl2l1* were markedly reduced in response to PC, and concomitantly H3K9 acetylation levels were significantly elevated. Furthermore, RGFP966 pretreatment or HDAC3 knock-down also induced increases in H3K9 acetylation near the HDAC3 binding sites of indicated genes (**Figures 3B,C**). Consistently the expression of indicated genes increased significantly in PC, RGFP966 treatment or HDAC3 knock-down (**Figure 3D**). We next exposed primary neurons to injurious OGD/R with the same procedure in **Figure 3A**. Western blot analysis showed that OGD/R slightly induced HSP70 expression, but suppressed Bcl-xL and Prdx-2 expression, while RGFP966 treatment or HDAC3 knock-down, consistent with PC, enhanced expression of all indicated genes compared with OGD/R (**Figure 3E**, Supplementary Figure S6). Taken together, we have demonstrated that the diminished recruitment of HDAC3 observed in PC led to up-regulation of HDAC3 related genes associated with neuroprotection.

Inhibition of Calpain1/Calpain2 Blocked the Reduction of HDAC3 Nuclear Localization Following PC

Subcellular localization of HDAC3 was shown to be controlled by protein-protein interaction or proteolytic cleavage (Karagianni and Wong, 2007). The unique C-terminus of HDAC3 is essential for nuclear localization and assembly into co-repression complexes (Yang et al., 2002). Several cleavages of HDAC3 by different proteases, which are activated with temporal specificity

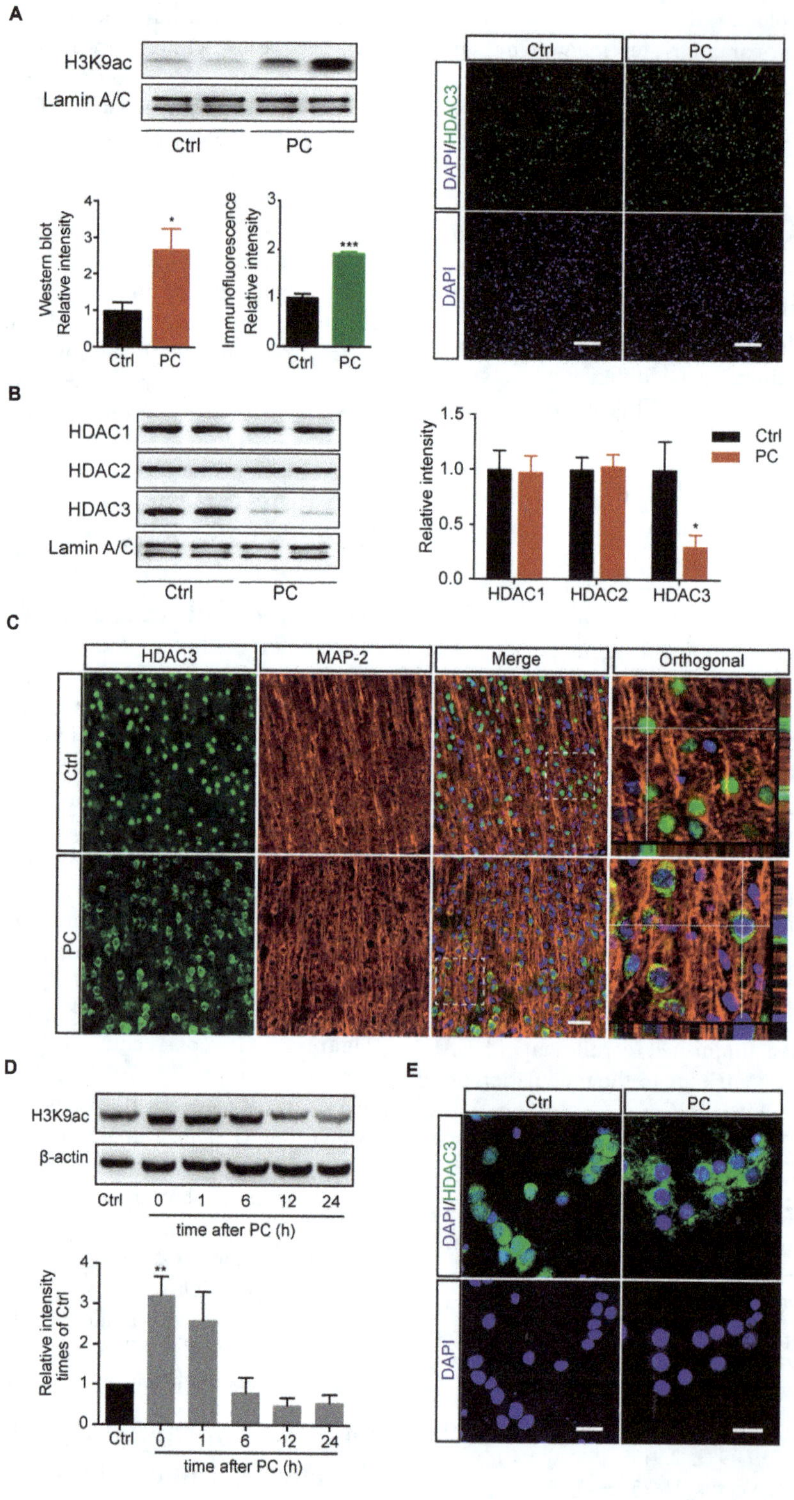

FIGURE 1 | Preconditioning induced the elevation of acetyl-H3K9 levels and reduced HDAC3 nuclear localization in rat cortical neurons *in vivo* and *in vitro*. Rats underwent 5 min PC treatment followed by 2 h reperfusion **(A–C)**. **(A)** Acetyl-H3K9 levels in the cortex by immunoblotting (Left, $n = 5$) and immunohistochemistry (Right, $n = 5$). $^{*}p < 0.05$, $^{***}p < 0.001$ Student's *t*-test. Scale bar: 100 μm. **(B)** Quantification of class I HDAC subtypes in nuclear lysates ($n = 4–6$). $^{*}p < 0.05$, Student's *t*-test. **(C)** Representative images of HDAC3 subcellular localization following sham or PC treatment *in vivo*. Scale bar: 50 μm. **(D)** Primary cultured cortical neurons underwent PC for 45 min followed by reoxygenation and restored energy supply for indicated period. Levels of H3K9 acetylation were assessed with whole cell lysates. Data are mean ± SEM. $^{**}p < 0.01$ versus control, ANOVA. **(E)** Representative images of HDAC3 subcellular localization in rat cortical neurons after PC. Scale bar: 25 μm.

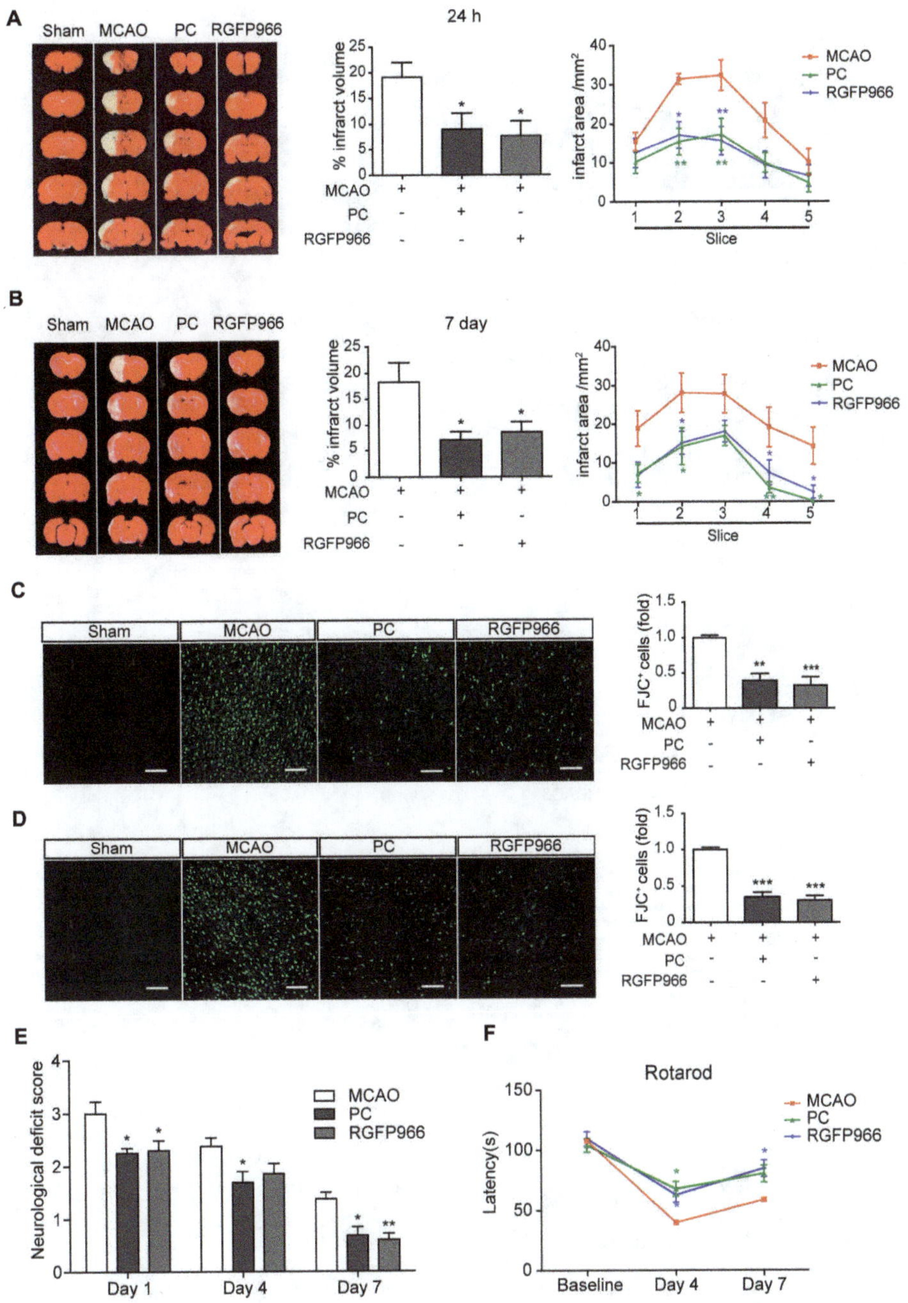

FIGURE 2 | RGFP966 protected the brain from ischemic injury *in vivo*. Infarct measurements were performed 24 h ($n = 7$–9) **(A)** and 7 days ($n = 8$–10) **(B)** after MCAO. Representative images of TTC staining (Left), infarct volume percentage (Middle) and infarct area for each slice (Right) from each group. $^{**}p < 0.01$, $^{*}p < 0.05$ versus MCAO group, ANOVA. Representative images of Fluoro-Jade C staining in each group. The histogram shows the numbers of degenerating neurons in the cortex 24 h **(C)** or 7 days **(D)** after MCAO (over 30 slices from five rats per group). $^{**}p < 0.01$, $^{***}p < 0.001$ versus MCAO group, ANOVA. Functional outcomes were assessed using the neurological deficits score (day 1, 4, and 7 after MCAO) **(E)** and rotarod test (day 4 and 7 after MCAO) **(F)** ($n = 8$–10). $^{*}p < 0.05$, $^{**}p < 0.01$ versus MCAO group, ANOVA.

in the process of cerebral ischemia, are involved in regulating the cellular distribution of HDAC3. We pretreated neurons with three major proteolytic pathway inhibitors including bortezomib (proteasome inhibitor), Z-VAD-FMK (pan-caspase inhibitor), and calpeptin (calpain inhibitor). PC was then conducted. Immunofluorescence results showed that calpeptin pretreatment, but not bortezomib or Z-VAD-FMK rescued the reduction of nuclear HDAC3 (**Figure 4A**). Western blot analysis with whole cell lysates showed a lower band of HDAC3 in PC treated neurons, suggesting a cleavage of HDAC3 induced by PC (**Figure 4B**). Furthermore, immunoprecipitation was performed with anti-HDAC3 or anti-calpain1/calpain2

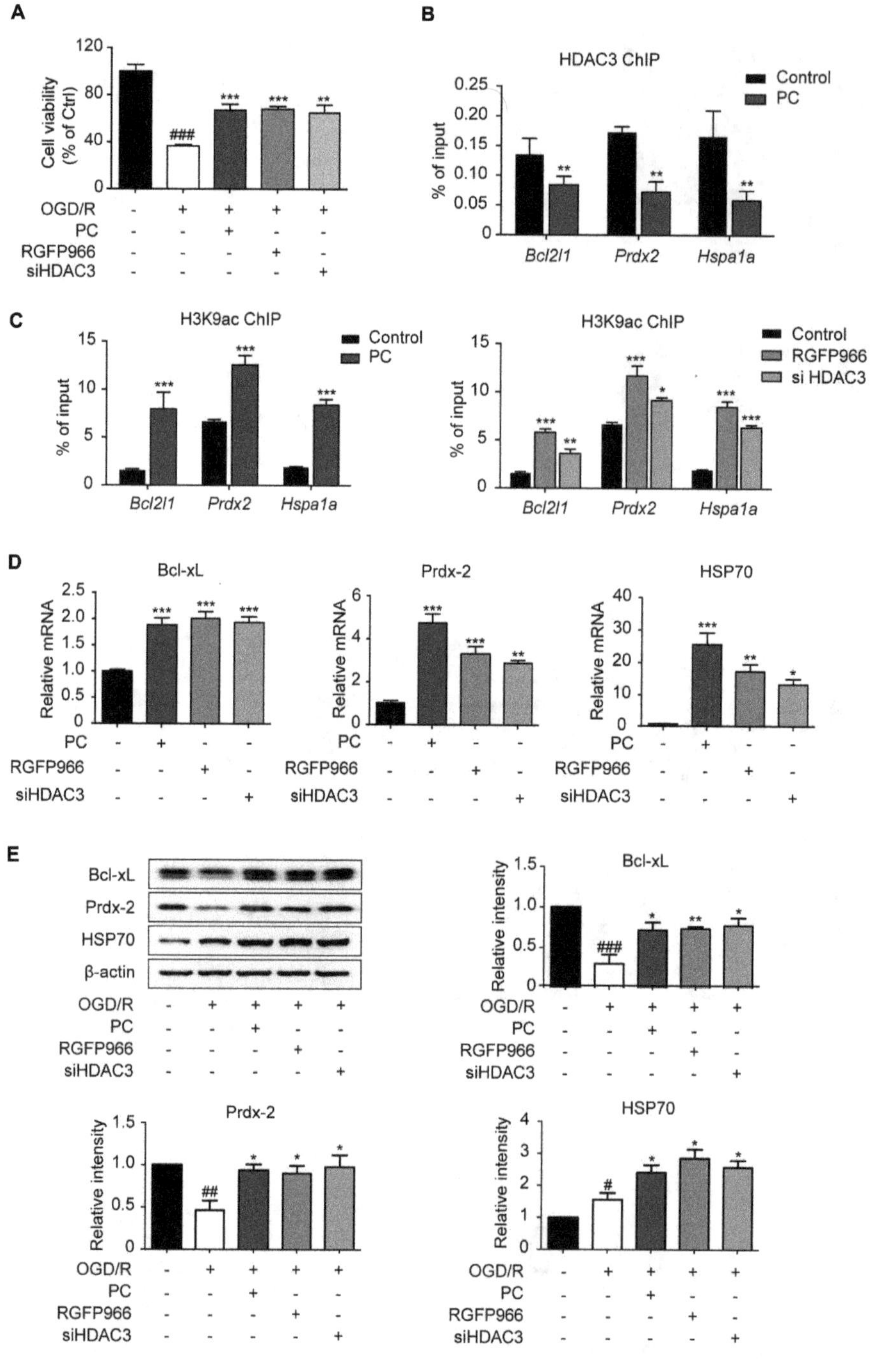

FIGURE 3 | Diminished recruitment of HDAC3 to the promoter region following PC potentiated the transcriptional initiation of oxidation relative genes. (A) For non-PC groups, cortical neurons at 7 DIV were pretreated with RGFP966 (2 μM) for 2 h, or transfected with siRNA targeting HDAC3 at 5.5 DIV 36 h in advance. For PC group, PC was induced at 6 DIV followed by reoxygenation. All groups underwent OGD/R at the same time at 7 DIV. At the end of the OGD/R period, cell viability was assessed using an MTT assay and calculated as the percentage of the non-treatment control. $^{###}p < 0.001$ versus control; $^{**}p < 0.01$, $^{***}p < 0.001$ versus OGD/R, ANOVA. Primary cultured neurons were subjected to PC or pretreated with RGFP966 for 2 h at 7 DIV, or transfected with siRNA targeting HDAC3 at 5.5 DIV 36 h in advance. Samples for ChIP were collected right after PC or RGFP966 and siHDAC3 treatment **(B,C)**. For mRNA test samples were collected 6 h after PC followed by reoxygenation **(D)**. **(B)** ChIP with HDAC3 antibodies was conducted followed by qPCR analysis using primers for HDAC3 binding sites near the promoter of the indicated genes. **(C)** Acetylation of H3K9 near the HDAC3-targeting gene promoters were analyzed by ChIP-qPCR. **(D)** RT-qPCR analysis for indicated genes. $^{*}p < 0.05$, $^{**}p < 0.01$, $^{***}p < 0.001$ versus control, Student's *t*-test and ANOVA. **(E)** Neurons were induced with PC, pretreated with RGFP966 or siHDAC3 and then exposed to OGD/R (the same procedure with **A**). The expression of oxidative relative genes was analyzed at the protein levels. Cell lysates were analyzed with specific antibodies. Data are presented as means ± SEM from three independent experiments. $^{#}p < 0.05$, $^{##}p < 0.01$, $^{###}p < 0.001$ versus control; $^{*}p < 0.05$, $^{**}p < 0.01$ versus OGD/R, ANOVA.

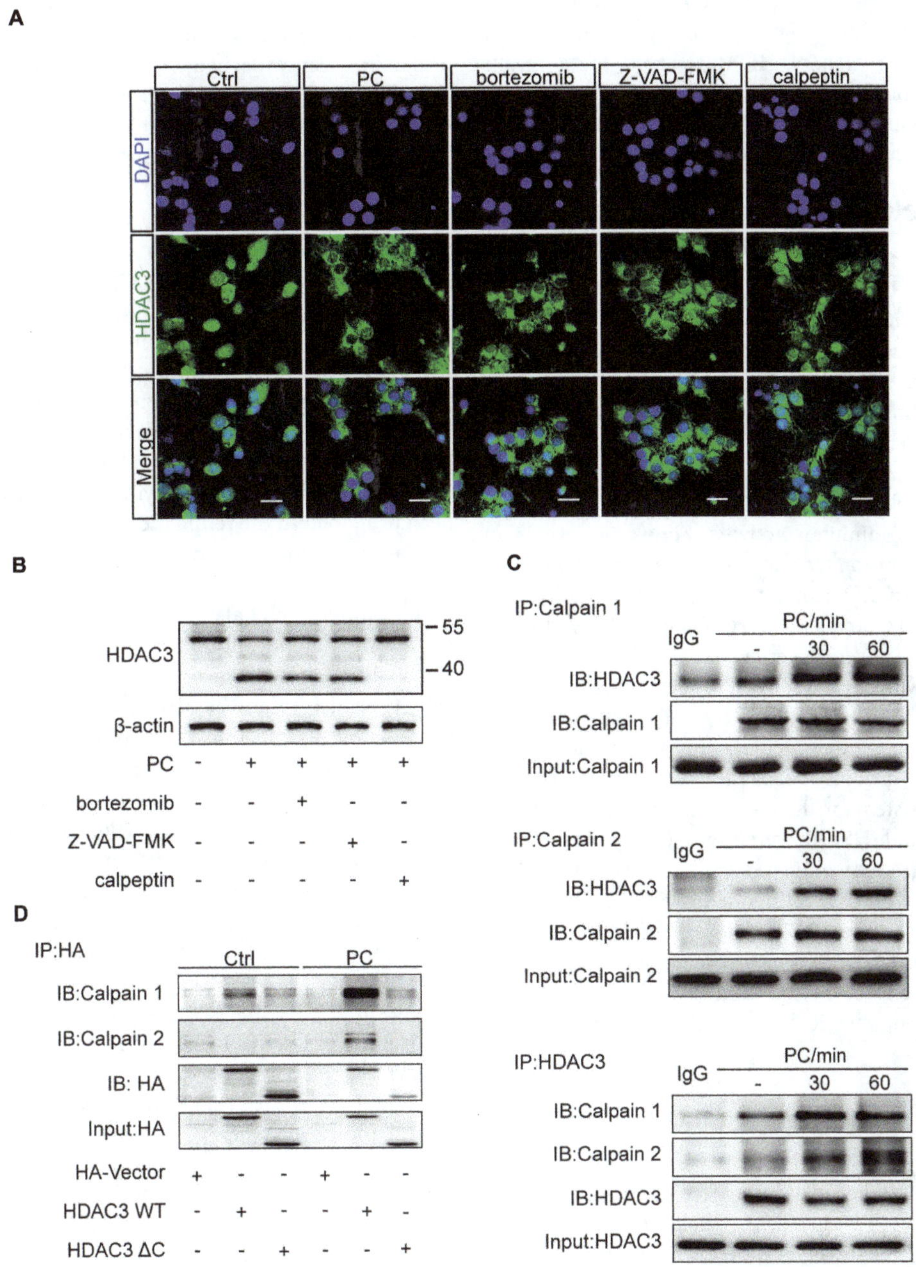

FIGURE 4 | Inhibition of calpains rescued the reduction of nuclear localization of HDAC3 following PC in neurons. (A) Primary cultured neurons were treated with bortezomib (4 nM), Z-VAD-FMK (50 nM) or calpeptin (5 μM) for 2 h prior to PC. Immunohistochemistry was conducted after PC. HDAC3 localization was visualized using immunofluorescence. Scale bars: 20 μm. **(B)** Cleavage products were analyzed by immunoblotting with an antibody against the N-terminus of HDAC3 (ab47237, Abcam) after PC. **(C)** Bands of HDAC3 were obtained by immunoprecipitating calpain1 or calpain2 and immunoblotting with the anti-HDAC3 antibody. Bands of calpain1 and calpain2 were obtained by immunoprecipitating HDAC3 and immunoblotting with the anti-calpain1 and anti-calpain2 antibodies respectively. **(D)** Plasmids encoding HA-tag, HA-HDAC3 WT, HA-HDAC3 ΔC were transfected into PC12 cells and PC was performed 36 h later. Whole cell lysates were immunoprecipitated with anti-HA antibody after PC and immunoblotted with anti-calpain1 or anti-calpain2 antibodies.

antibodies. We found that direct interactions between HDAC3 and calpain1/calpain2 were strengthened after PC (**Figure 4C**). To further identify the interaction domain between HDAC3 and calpain, we constructed HA-tagged WT HDAC3 and truncated HDAC3 (aa1-312, HDAC3 ΔC) plasmids. Consistent with previous reports (Yang et al., 2002), HA-HDAC3 WT displayed both cytoplasmic and nuclear distributions, while HA-HDAC3 ΔC specifically localized in the cytoplasm of neurons (Supplementary Figure S3). A PC12 cell line was transfected with HDAC3 constructs and underwent PC. As expected, PC significantly increased the interaction of HA-HDAC3 WT with calpains, while truncated mutation, HA-HDAC3 ΔC, reduced the interaction with calpains after PC compared with control group (**Figure 4D**), indicating that the interaction domain may lie in the C-terminal region of HDAC3. From these results we concluded that blockade of HDAC3 nuclear localization following PC treatment resulted from the C-terminal cleavage of HDAC3 mediated by calpain1/calpain2.

Calpeptin Blocked the Attenuated Nuclear Localization of HDAC3 and the Neuroprotective Effect of PC *In vivo*

Rats were treated with calpeptin 6 h prior to surgery. To determine the subcellular localization of HDAC3, brain sections were obtained 2 h after PC. Immunofluorescence results showed that calpeptin pretreatment blocked the reduction of nuclear HDAC3 induced by PC (**Figure 5A**). For pathological assessment, rats subjected to MCAO were sacrificed 24 h or 7 d later (Supplementary Figure S2B). TTC staining (**Figure 5B**) and FJC immunoreactivity (**Figure 5C**) revealed that calpeptin had significantly attenuated the protective effect of PC 24 h after MCAO, consistent with results observed 7 days after MCAO (Supplementary Figure S4). Activated astrocytes and microglia were observed in MCAO and calpeptin group compared with PC group (Supplementary Figures S5D,E). Furthermore, we compared the expression level of indicated genes in all experimental groups, including the RGFP966 treatment group. Specimens were obtained 24 h after MCAO. Consistent with results *in vitro*, the levels of Prdx-2, Bcl-xL and HSP70 were significantly elevated in PC and RGFP966 groups compared with the MCAO group, while pretreatment with calpeptin attenuated the expression enhancement of PC (**Figure 5D**). HSP70 regulation was further assessed by immunohistochemistry, which revealed that HSP70 expression was enhanced by PC and RGFP966 treatment, whereas its expression was blocked by calpeptin pretreatment (**Figure 5E**).

DISCUSSION

Ischemic PC has been studied in order to develop new therapeutic approaches to benefit patients with stroke (Dirnagl et al., 2003; Gidday, 2006; Stetler et al., 2014). The present study provides evidence that HDAC3 inhibition may have a role in PC the brain against ischemia. We found that the reduction of HDAC3 nuclear localization following PC resulted in elevated acetylation of H3K9. Acting as one of the leading causes of PC, release of the HDAC3 co-repressor complex facilitated the transcription of relevant genes including *Hspa1a*, *Bcl2l1*, and *Prdx2*, which contributed to the endogenous protection elicited by PC. Further, we showed that C-terminal cleavage of HDAC3 by calpain underlies the failure of HDAC3 nuclear localization, and inhibition of calpain attenuated the PC protection exerted by HDAC3 inhibition.

There has been increasing interest in targeting epigenetic process as potential treatment for stroke (Langley et al., 2009; Aune et al., 2015). Several HDAC inhibitors such as VPA (Kim et al., 2007; Wang et al., 2012b), TSA (Yildirim et al., 2008; Wang et al., 2012a) and SAHA (Faraco et al., 2006) have previously shown protective effects against cerebral ischemia. Meanwhile, epigenetic modification is believed to play a fundamental role in ischemic tolerance. Yet the precise roles of HDACs in PC remains less clearly understood. Notably, it has been reported that total histone-H3 acetylation was down-regulated in cerebral ischemic injury but up-regulated following PC both *in vitro* and *in vivo* (Yildirim et al., 2014). Another study revealed a significant increase in retinal acetyl histone-H3 labeling after PC but a pronounced decrease after ischemia (Fan et al., 2016). In our study we further illustrated the time course of histone modification in both PC and OGD/R *in vitro*. Acetyl-H3K9 was elevated within 2 h following PC and returned to normal levels 6 h later (**Figure 1C**), while it was decreased profoundly 12 h after OGD followed by reoxygenation (Supplementary Figures S1A,B). Different mechanisms underlying the opposite regulation have been proposed. In the retina the deacetylase activity of HDAC1/2 displayed an increase in ischemia but a decrease following PC, which was closely correlated with histone acetylation modification (Fan et al., 2016). Whereas in the brain, a decrease in histone H3 acetylation was observed for 6 h after MCAO, strikingly without concomitant change in HAT or HDAC activity, which might be associated with decreased acetyl-CoA contents after ischemia (Faraco et al., 2006). In the brain following PC, increased histone acetylation was reported to result from enhanced CBP recruitment at the promoter of the neuroprotective gene *gelsolin* (Yildirim et al., 2014). Here, we reported that additional regulation is involved in this process, whereby cleaved HDAC3 is distributed in the cytoplasm and reducing the recruitment to targeted genes following PC, which consequently elevated the level of acetyl-H3K9. All these finding present a new perspective in explaining the protective role of HDAC inhibitors that reinstatement of the decreased histone acetylation level may exert the PC protection following ischemic injury.

Numerous studies have identified the mechanisms of PC against injurious ischemia. Gene profile analysis demonstrated that PC induced an extensive down-regulation of genes responsible for metabolic pathways and ion-channel activity, indicating lowered cellular activity (Stenzel-Poore et al., 2003, 2007). Similar regulation is implicated in the response to resveratrol treatment, which functions via the activation of SIRT1 (NAD-dependent deacetylase sirtuin-1; Raval et al., 2006; Koronowski et al., 2015). HIF-1-alpha also plays a fundamental role in adapting the metabolism to hypoxic conditions via transcriptional regulation (Prass et al., 2003; Tang et al., 2006). Apart from the known effectors that suppress energy turnover, cumulative evidence has suggested that epigenetic modulators may be involved in PC paradigms. The volume of ischemic tissue was reduced by the inhibition of DNA methylation and histone acetylation, which elicited a reprogramming of ischemic tolerance (Thompson et al., 2013). In our study, ChIP assays have revealed that the induction of PC, HDAC3 knock-down and HDAC3 inhibition elevated the histone acetylation level of related gene including *Hspa1a*, *Bcl2l1*, and *Prdx2*, and were further permissive to

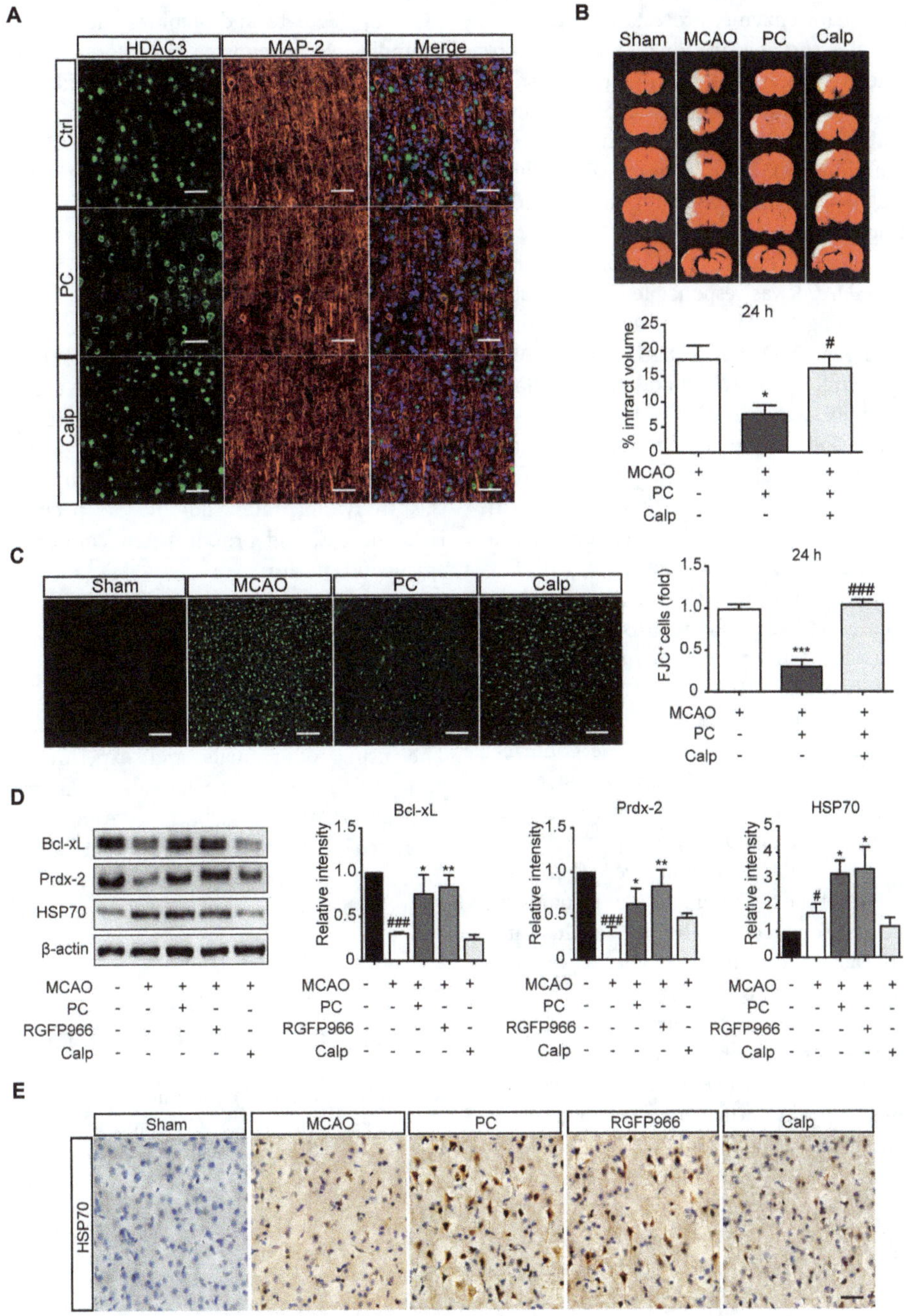

FIGURE 5 | Calpeptin pretreatment blocked the protective effect of PC *in vivo*. (A) Representative images of HDAC3 subcellular localization in cortex. Scale bar: 50 μm. **(B)** Representative images of TTC staining from each group are shown. Infarct volume percentage from each slice were determined ($n = 8$–10). $^{*}p < 0.05$ versus MCAO group, $^{\#}p < 0.05$ versus PC group, ANOVA. **(C)** Representative images of Fluoro-Jade C staining and the numbers of degenerating neurons (over 30 slices from six rats per group). $^{***}p < 0.001$ versus MCAO group, $^{\#\#\#}p < 0.001$ versus PC group, ANOVA. **(D)** Expression levels of Prdx-2, Bcl-xL and HSP70 in each group ($n = 3$–4) 24 h after MCAO. $^{\#}p < 0.05$, $^{\#\#\#}p < 0.001$ versus Sham group; $^{*}p < 0.05$, $^{**}p < 0.01$ versus MCAO group, ANOVA. **(E)** Representative images of Cerebral HSP70 immunohistochemistry. Scale bar: 50 μm. Calp, calpeptin.

transcriptional initiation. Notably, over 12-fold up-regulation of HSP70 transcription was observed 12 h in PC, siHDAC3 and RGFP966 treated cortical neurons 6 h after PC induction or mimicking. It has been reported that HSP70 was induced in the penumbra, but not core, of the ischemic region, as well as in neurons which survive PC (Masada et al., 2001). Delaying administration of HSP70 by 2.25 and 3 h after the onset of ischemia significantly decreased infarct volume by 68% (Zhan et al., 2010). Bcl-xL is required for neurite outgrowth and potentially inhibits programmed cell death through changing the topology of the mitochondrial membrane (Park et al., 2015). Peroxiredoxin, an antioxidant enzyme, protects cells from the insults due to free radical accumulation (Finkel and Holbrook, 2000). These observations suggest that like other methods of manipulating PC, HDAC3 inhibition triggers signaling cascades in neurons leading to increased levels of free radical species and superoxide clearance, inhibition of the endogenous cell apoptosis program, and improved overall protein integrity, which shield the brain from ischemic injury.

In our study we demonstrated that calpain-mediated C-terminus cleavage of HDAC3 was responsible for the absence of HDAC3 in nuclei following PC. HDAC3 is a member of the class I HDAC family (HDAC1, HDAC2, HDAC3, and HDAC8), which share homology with Rpd3 from budding yeast (Yang and Seto, 2008). The unique C-terminus of HDAC3 is essential for its deacetylase activity and nuclear localization (Yang et al., 2002). Several ways of HDAC3 cleavage have been reported to affect its distribution. Etoposide treatment resulted in the cleavage of HDAC3 by caspase-3 and its subsequent cytoplasmic accumulation (Choi et al., 2015). Following treatment with FasL or ultraviolet irradiation, HDAC3 was cleaved in an indirect caspase-dependent manner and subsequently distributed in the cytoplasm (Escaffit et al., 2007). In the present study, minimum amount of interaction between HDAC3 and calpains were observed under normal conditions. While following PC and pretreatment with different protease inhibitors, we confirmed HDAC3 was cleaved by calpains, but not caspase or proteasome. From our results we cannot determine the difference in cleavage participation between calpain1 and calpain2. Through truncation research, we confirmed that the non-conserved C-terminal region of HDAC3 is required for the interaction of calpain with HDAC3, but the specific sequence remains to be illustrated. Calpains are a family of calcium-dependent proteases, which are profoundly and causally linked to post-ischemic insults (Bevers and Neumar, 2008), and calpain inhibitors have been investigated as potential therapeutics for cerebral ischemia (Koumura et al., 2008). The sustained calcium overload in stroke led to pathological activation of calpains, which resulted in extensive degradation of structural proteins and enzymes and neuronal cell death. The spectrin cleavages generated by calpains, SBDP150 and SBDP145, appeared 60 min after ischemia, and followed by a second expansion between 24 and 48 h after reperfusion (Neumar et al., 2001; Lin et al., 2013). These two steps of calpain activation may indicate that the controlled activation of calpain was induced at the beginning of ischemia, whereas sustained calcium overload resulted in pathological hyper-activation of calpains, which played predominant pathologic protease activity in vulnerable neurons following ischemia (Zhang et al., 2002; Liu et al., 2008). Regulated activation of calpain in the brain are involved in synaptic function and memory formation, but the mechanism underlying the controlled activation of calpain in PC has not been illustrated. We propose that firstly, PC is not an injurious stimulus, whereby transient signaling cascades may not lead to loss of Ca^{2+} homeostasis and pronounced activation of proteases. Secondly, other signaling pathways involved in PC may regulate and stabilize the homeostasis of Ca^{2+}. For example, A1 adenosine receptors are reported to mediate the protection against infarction afforded by PC (Liu et al., 1991). And adenosine release from astrocytes down-regulated the synaptic activity level in transient hypoxia by negatively modulating the external or internal Ca^{2+} concentrations (Martín et al., 2007).

Here, we demonstrated that HDAC3 inhibition increased the resistance of the CNS to ischemic insult. Controlled activation of calpains in PC was involved in the cleavage of HDAC3, which reduced nuclear localization of HDAC3 and led to elevated acetylation of H3K9 and initiation of neuroprotective genes. Consistent with the role of HDAC inhibitors in neuroprotection, this study illustrates the role of specific HDAC subtypes in ischemic PC, and proposes new connections between PC and epigenetic effectors.

ETHICS STATEMENT

The using of animals and experimental procedures were performed following the rules of the Association for Assessment and Accreditation of Laboratory Animal Care International and approved by the Institutional Animal Care and Use Committee of the Shanghai Institute of Material Medica, Chinese Academy of Sciences. No endangered animals were applied in this research.

AUTHOR CONTRIBUTIONS

XY and LF designed experiments. XY and QW performed most of the experiments. XY, QW, and LZ contributed to the animal behavior studies. XY, QW, and LZ analyzed the data. XY and LF wrote the paper.

ACKNOWLEDGMENTS

This work was supported by grants from "Key New Drug Creation and Manufacturing Program" of the National Science and Technology Major Project (2014ZX09102-001-05), and the "Personalized Medicines—Molecular Signature-based Drug Discovery and Development," Strategic Priority Research Program of the Chinese Academy of Sciences (XDA12040304). All experiments were conducted in compliance with the ARRIVE guidelines.

REFERENCES

Aune, S. E., Herr, D. J., Kutz, C. J., and Menick, D. R. (2015). Histone deacetylases exert class-specific roles in conditioning the brain and heart against acute ischemic injury. *Front. Neurol.* 6:145. doi: 10.3389/fneur.2015.00145

Bardai, F. H., and D'Mello, S. R. (2011). Selective toxicity by HDAC3 in neurons: regulation by Akt and GSK3beta. *J. Neurosci.* 31, 1746–1751. doi: 10.1523/JNEUROSCI.5704-10.2011

Bardai, F. H., Verma, P., Smith, C., Rawat, V., Wang, L., and D'Mello, S. R. (2013). Disassociation of histone deacetylase-3 from normal huntingtin underlies mutant huntingtin neurotoxicity. *J. Neurosci.* 33, 11833–11838. doi: 10.1523/JNEUROSCI.5831-12.2013

Bates, E. A., Victor, M., Jones, A. K., Shi, Y., and Hart, A. C. (2006). Differential contributions of *Caenorhabditis elegans* histone deacetylases to huntingtin polyglutamine toxicity. *J. Neurosci.* 26, 2830–2838. doi: 10.1523/JNEUROSCI.3344-05.2006

Bevers, M. B., and Neumar, R. W. (2008). Mechanistic role of calpains in postischemic neurodegeneration. *J. Cereb. Blood Flow Metab.* 28, 655–673. doi: 10.1038/sj.jcbfm.9600595

Butler, R., and Bates, G. P. (2006). Histone deacetylase inhibitors as therapeutics for polyglutamine disorders. *Nat. Rev. Neurosci.* 7, 784–796. doi: 10.1038/nrn1989

Choi, H. K., Choi, Y., Park, E. S., Park, S. Y., Lee, S. H., Seo, J., et al. (2015). Programmed cell death 5 mediates HDAC3 decay to promote genotoxic stress response. *Nat. Commun.* 6:7390. doi: 10.1038/ncomms8390

Chuang, D. M., Leng, Y., Marinova, Z., Kim, H. J., and Chiu, C. T. (2009). Multiple roles of HDAC inhibition in neurodegenerative conditions. *Trends Neurosci.* 32, 591–601. doi: 10.1016/j.tins.2009.06.002

Dirnagl, U., Becker, K., and Meisel, A. (2009). Preconditioning and tolerance against cerebral ischaemia: from experimental strategies to clinical use. *Lancet Neurol.* 8, 398–412. doi: 10.1016/S1474-4422(09)70054-7

Dirnagl, U., Iadecola, C., and Moskowitz, M. A. (1999). Pathobiology of ischaemic stroke: an integrated view. *Trends Neurosci.* 22, 391–397. doi: 10.1016/S0166-2236(99)01401-0

Dirnagl, U., Simon, R. P., and Hallenbeck, J. M. (2003). Ischemic tolerance and endogenous neuroprotection. *Trends Neurosci.* 26, 248–254. doi: 10.1016/S0166-2236(03)00071-7

Escaffit, F., Vaute, O., Chevillard-Briet, M., Segui, B., Takami, Y., Nakayama, T., et al. (2007). Cleavage and cytoplasmic relocalization of histone deacetylase 3 are important for apoptosis progression. *Mol. Cell. Biol.* 27, 554–567. doi: 10.1128/MCB.00869-06

Fan, J., Alsarraf, O., Chou, C. J., Yates, P. W., Goodwin, N. C., Rice, D. S., et al. (2016). Ischemic preconditioning, retinal neuroprotection and histone deacetylase activities. *Exp. Eye Res.* 146, 269–275. doi: 10.1016/j.exer.2016.03.026

Faraco, G., Pancani, T., Formentini, L., Mascagni, P., Fossati, G., Leoni, F., et al. (2006). Pharmacological inhibition of histone deacetylases by suberoylanilide hydroxamic acid specifically alters gene expression and reduces ischemic injury in the mouse brain. *Mol. Pharmacol.* 70, 1876–1884. doi: 10.1124/mol.106.027912

Feigin, V. L., Forouzanfar, M. H., Krishnamurthi, R., Mensah, G. A., Connor, M., Bennett, D. A., et al. (2014). Global and regional burden of stroke during 1990–2010: findings from the Global Burden of Disease Study 2010. *Lancet* 383, 245–255. doi: 10.1016/S0140-6736(13)61953-4

Feng, D., Liu, T., Sun, Z., Bugge, A., Mullican, S. E., Alenghat, T., et al. (2011). A circadian rhythm orchestrated by histone deacetylase 3 controls hepatic lipid metabolism. *Science* 331, 1315–1319. doi: 10.1126/science.1198125

Finkel, T., and Holbrook, N. J. (2000). Oxidants, oxidative stress and the biology of ageing. *Nature* 408, 239–247. doi: 10.1038/35041687

Fisher, M., and Saver, J. L. (2015). Future directions of acute ischaemic stroke therapy. *Lancet Neurol.* 14, 758–767. doi: 10.1016/s1474-4422(15)00054-x

Gidday, J. M. (2006). Cerebral preconditioning and ischaemic tolerance. *Nat. Rev. Neurosci.* 7, 437–448. doi: 10.1038/nrn1927

Hunter, A., Hatcher, J., Virley, D., Nelson, P., Irving, E., Hadingham, S., et al. (2000). Functional assessments in mice and rats after focal stroke. *Neuropharmacology* 39, 806–816. doi: 10.1016/S0028-3908(99)00262-2

Johnston, S. C., Mendis, S., and Mathers, C. D. (2009). Global variation in stroke burden and mortality: estimates from monitoring, surveillance, and modelling. *Lancet Neurol.* 8, 345–354. doi: 10.1016/S1474-4422(09)70023-7

Karagianni, P., and Wong, J. (2007). HDAC3: taking the SMRT-N-CoRrect road to repression. *Oncogene* 26, 5439–5449. doi: 10.1038/sj.onc.1210612

Kim, H. J., Rowe, M., Ren, M., Hong, J. S., Chen, P. S., and Chuang, D. M. (2007). Histone deacetylase inhibitors exhibit anti-inflammatory and neuroprotective effects in a rat permanent ischemic model of stroke: multiple mechanisms of action. *J. Pharmacol. Exp. Ther.* 321, 892–901. doi: 10.1124/jpet.107.120188

Koronowski, K. B., Dave, K. R., Saul, I., Camarena, V., Thompson, J. W., Neumann, J. T., et al. (2015). Resveratrol preconditioning induces a novel extended window of ischemic tolerance in the mouse brain. *Stroke* 46, 2293–2298. doi: 10.1161/STROKEAHA.115.009876

Koumura, A., Nonaka, Y., Hyakkoku, K., Oka, T., Shimazawa, M., Hozumi, I., et al. (2008). A novel calpain inhibitor,((1S)-1 ((((1S)-1-benzyl-3-cyclopropylamino-2, 3-di-oxopropyl) amino) carbonyl)-3-methylbutyl) carbamic acid 5-methoxy-3-oxapentyl ester, protects neuronal cells from cerebral ischemia-induced damage in mice. *Neuroscience* 157, 309–318. doi: 10.1016/j.neuroscience.2008.09.007

Langley, B., Brochier, C., and Rivieccio, M. A. (2009). Targeting histone deacetylases as a multifaceted approach to treat the diverse outcomes of stroke. *Stroke* 40, 2899–2905. doi: 10.1161/STROKEAHA.108.540229

Lin, Y., Zhang, J.-C., Fu, J., Chen, F., Wang, J., Wu, Z.-L., et al. (2013). Hyperforin attenuates brain damage induced by transient middle cerebral artery occlusion (MCAO) in rats via inhibition of TRPC6 channels degradation. *J. Cereb. Blood Flow Metab.* 33, 253–262. doi: 10.1038/jcbfm.2012.164

Liu, G., Thornton, J., Van Winkle, D., Stanley, A., Olsson, R., and Downey, J. (1991). Protection against infarction afforded by preconditioning is mediated by A1 adenosine receptors in rabbit heart. *Circulation* 84, 350–356. doi: 10.1161/01.CIR.84.1.350

Liu, J., Liu, M. C., and Wang, K. (2008). Calpain in the CNS: from synaptic function to neurotoxicity. *Sci. Signal.* 1:re1. doi: 10.1126/stke.114re1

Longa, E. Z., Weinstein, P. R., Carlson, S., and Cummins, R. (1989). Reversible middle cerebral artery occlusion without craniectomy in rats. *Stroke* 20, 84–91. doi: 10.1161/01.STR.20.1.84

Malvaez, M., McQuown, S. C., Rogge, G. A., Astarabadi, M., Jacques, V., Carreiro, S., et al. (2013). HDAC3-selective inhibitor enhances extinction of cocaine-seeking behavior in a persistent manner. *Proc. Natl. Acad. Sci. U.S.A.* 110, 2647–2652. doi: 10.1073/pnas.1213364110

Martín, E. D., Fernández, M., Perea, G., Pascual, O., Haydon, P. G., Araque, A., et al. (2007). Adenosine released by astrocytes contributes to hypoxia-induced modulation of synaptic transmission. *Glia* 55, 36–45. doi: 10.1002/glia.20431

Masada, T., Hua, Y., Xi, G., Ennis, S. R., and Keep, R. F. (2001). Attenuation of ischemic brain edema and cerebrovascular injury after ischemic preconditioning in the rat. *J. Cereb. Blood Flow Metab.* 21, 22–33. doi: 10.1097/00004647-200101000-00004

Moretti, A., Ferrari, F., and Villa, R. F. (2015). Pharmacological therapy of acute ischaemic stroke: achievements and problems. *Pharmacol. Ther.* 153, 79–89. doi: 10.1016/j.pharmthera.2015.06.004

Moskowitz, M. A., Lo, E. H., and Iadecola, C. (2010). The science of stroke: mechanisms in search of treatments. *Neuron* 67, 181–198. doi: 10.1016/j.neuron.2010.07.002

Neumar, R. W., Meng, F. H., Mills, A. M., Xu, Y. A., Zhang, C., Welsh, F. A., et al. (2001). Calpain activity in the rat brain after transient forebrain ischemia. *Exp. Neurol.* 170, 27–35. doi: 10.1006/exnr.2001.7708

Park, H. A., Licznerski, P., Alavian, K. N., Shanabrough, M., and Jonas, E. A. (2015). Bcl-xL is necessary for neurite outgrowth in hippocampal neurons. *Antioxid. Redox. Signal.* 22, 93–108. doi: 10.1089/ars.2013.5570

Prass, K., Scharff, A., Ruscher, K., Lowl, D., Muselmann, C., Victorov, I., et al. (2003). Hypoxia-induced stroke tolerance in the mouse is mediated by erythropoietin. *Stroke* 34, 1981–1986. doi: 10.1161/01.STR.0000080381.76409.B2

Raval, A. P., Dave, K. R., and Perez-Pinzon, M. A. (2006). Resveratrol mimics ischemic preconditioning in the brain. *J. Cereb. Blood Flow Metab.* 26, 1141–1147. doi: 10.1038/sj.jcbfm.9600262

Ren, M., Leng, Y., Jeong, M., Leeds, P. R., and Chuang, D. M. (2004). Valproic acid reduces brain damage induced by transient focal cerebral ischemia in rats: potential roles of histone deacetylase inhibition and heat shock protein induction. *J. Neurochem.* 89, 1358–1367. doi: 10.1111/j.1471-4159.2004.02406.x

Samantaray, S., Knaryan, V. H., Shields, D. C., Cox, A. A., Haque, A., and Banik, N. L. (2015). Inhibition of calpain activation protects MPTP-Induced nigral and spinal cord neurodegeneration, reduces inflammation, and improves gait dynamics in mice. *Mol. Neurobiol.* 52, 1054–1066. doi: 10.1007/s12035-015-9255-6

Schmitt, H. M., Pelzel, H. R., Schlamp, C. L., and Nickells, R. W. (2014). Histone deacetylase 3 (HDAC3) plays an important role in retinal ganglion cell death after acute optic nerve injury. *Mol. Neurodegen* 9:1. doi: 10.1186/1750-1326-9-39

Stenzel-Poore, M. P., Stevens, S. L., King, J. S., and Simon, R. P. (2007). Preconditioning reprograms the response to ischemic injury and primes the emergence of unique endogenous neuroprotective phenotypes: a speculative synthesis. *Stroke* 38 2(Suppl.), 680–685. doi: 10.1161/01.STR.0000251444.56487.4c

Stenzel-Poore, M. P., Stevens, S. L., Xiong, Z., Lessov, N. S., Harrington, C. A., Mori, M., et al. (2003). Effect of ischaemic preconditioning on genomic response to cerebral ischaemia: similarity to neuroprotective strategies in hibernation and hypoxia-tolerant states. *Lancet* 362, 1028–1037. doi: 10.1016/S0140-6736(03)14412-1

Stetler, R. A., Leak, R. K., Gan, Y., Li, P., Zhang, F., Hu, X., et al. (2014). Preconditioning provides neuroprotection in models of CNS disease: paradigms and clinical significance. *Prog. Neurobiol.* 114, 58–83. doi: 10.1016/j.pneurobio.2013.11.005

Stevens, S. L., Vartanian, K. B., and Stenzel-Poore, M. P. (2014). Reprogramming the response to stroke by preconditioning. *Stroke* 45, 2527–2531. doi: 10.1161/STROKEAHA.114.002879

Tang, Y., Pacary, E., Freret, T., Divoux, D., Petit, E., Schumann-Bard, P., et al. (2006). Effect of hypoxic preconditioning on brain genomic response before and following ischemia in the adult mouse: identification of potential neuroprotective candidates for stroke. *Neurobiol. Dis.* 21, 18–28. doi: 10.1016/j.nbd.2005.06.002

Thompson, J. W., Dave, K. R., Young, J. I., and Perez-Pinzon, M. A. (2013). Ischemic preconditioning alters the epigenetic profile of the brain from ischemic intolerance to ischemic tolerance. *Neurotherapeutics* 10, 789–797. doi: 10.1007/s13311-013-0202-9

Wang, B., Zhu, X., Kim, Y., Li, J., Huang, S., Saleem, S., et al. (2012a). Histone deacetylase inhibition activates transcription factor Nrf2 and protects against cerebral ischemic damage. *Free Radic. Biol. Med.* 52, 928–936. doi: 10.1016/j.freeradbiomed.2011.12.006

Wang, Z., Tsai, L. K., Munasinghe, J., Leng, Y., Fessler, E. B., Chibane, F., et al. (2012b). Chronic valproate treatment enhances postischemic angiogenesis and promotes functional recovery in a rat model of ischemic stroke. *Stroke* 43, 2430–2436. doi: 10.1161/STROKEAHA.112.652545

Xie, K. Q., Zhang, L. M., Cao, Y., Zhu, J., and Feng, L. Y. (2009). Adenosine A(1) receptor-mediated transactivation of the EGF receptor produces a neuroprotective effect on cortical neurons in vitro. *Acta Pharmacol. Sin.* 30, 889–898. doi: 10.1038/aps.2009.80

Yang, W. M., Tsai, S. C., Wen, Y. D., Fejer, G., and Seto, E. (2002). Functional domains of histone deacetylase-3. *J. Biol. Chem.* 277, 9447–9454. doi: 10.1074/jbc.M105993200

Yang, X. J., and Seto, E. (2008). The Rpd3/Hda1 family of lysine deacetylases: from bacteria and yeast to mice and men. *Nat. Rev. Mol. Cell Biol.* 9, 206–218. doi: 10.1038/nrm2346

Yildirim, F., Gertz, K., Kronenberg, G., Harms, C., Fink, K. B., Meisel, A., et al. (2008). Inhibition of histone deacetylation protects wildtype but not gelsolin-deficient mice from ischemic brain injury. *Exp. Neurol.* 210, 531–542. doi: 10.1016/j.expneurol.2007.11.031

Yildirim, F., Ji, S., Kronenberg, G., Barco, A., Olivares, R., Benito, E., et al. (2014). Histone acetylation and CREB binding protein are required for neuronal resistance against ischemic injury. *PLoS ONE* 9:e95465. doi: 10.1371/journal.pone.0095465

Zhan, X., Ander, B. P., Liao, I. H., Hansen, J. E., Kim, C., Clements, D., et al. (2010). Recombinant Fv-Hsp70 protein mediates neuroprotection after focal cerebral ischemia in rats. *Stroke* 41, 538–543. doi: 10.1161/STROKEAHA.109.572537

Zhang, C., Siman, R., Xu, Y. A., Mills, A. M., Frederick, J. R., and Neumar, R. W. (2002). Comparison of calpain and caspase activities in the adult rat brain after transient forebrain ischemia. *Neurobiol. Dis.* 10, 289–305. doi: 10.1006/nbdi.2002.0526

11

Richness in Functional Connectivity Depends on the Neuronal Integrity within the Posterior Cingulate Cortex

Anton R. Lord[1,2,3*], *Meng Li*[2,4], *Liliana R. Demenescu*[1,2], *Johan van den Meer*[2,4,5], *Viola Borchardt*[2], *Anna Linda Krause*[2,6], *Hans-Jochen Heinze*[1,4,7], *Michael Breakspear*[3,8] *and Martin Walter*[1,2,6,7,9*]

[1] *Department of Behavioral Neurology, Leibniz Institute for Neurobiology, Magdeburg, Germany,* [2] *Clinical Affective Neuroimaging Laboratory, Otto-von-Guericke University, Magdeburg, Germany,* [3] *QIMR Berghofer Medical Research Institute, Brisbane, QLD, Australia,* [4] *Department of Neurology, Otto-von-Guericke University, Magdeburg, Germany,* [5] *Department of Cognition and Emotion, Netherlands Institute for Neuroscience, An Institute of the Royal Academy of Arts and Sciences, Amsterdam, Netherlands,* [6] *Department of Psychiatry and Psychotherapy, Otto-von-Guericke University, Magdeburg, Germany,* [7] *Center of Behavioral Brain Sciences, Otto-von-Guericke University, Magdeburg, Germany,* [8] *Metro North Mental Health Service, Royal Brisbane and Women's Hospital, Brisbane, QLD, Australia,* [9] *Department of Psychiatry, Eberhad Karls University Tuebingen, Tuebingen, Germany*

Edited by:
Andrew Harkin,
Trinity College, Dublin, Ireland

Reviewed by:
Andreas Hahn,
Medical University of Vienna, Austria
Vesa J. Kiviniemi,
University of Oulu, Finland

****Correspondence:***
Martin Walter
Martin.walter@uni-tuebingen.de
Anton R. Lord
Anton.Lord@qimrberghofer.edu.au

The brain's connectivity skeleton—a rich club of strongly interconnected members—was initially shown to exist in human structural networks, but recent evidence suggests a functional counterpart. This rich club typically includes key regions (or hubs) from multiple canonical networks, reducing the cost of inter-network communication. The posterior cingulate cortex (PCC), a hub node embedded within the default mode network, is known to facilitate communication between brain networks and is a key member of the "rich club." Here, we assessed how metabolic signatures of neuronal integrity and cortical thickness influence the global extent of a functional rich club as measured using the functional rich club coefficient (fRCC). Rich club estimation was performed on functional connectivity of resting state brain signals acquired at 3T in 48 healthy adult subjects. Magnetic resonance spectroscopy was measured in the same session using a point resolved spectroscopy sequence. We confirmed convergence of functional rich club with a previously established structural rich club. N-acetyl aspartate (NAA) in the PCC is significantly correlated with age ($p = 0.001$), while the rich club coefficient showed no effect of age ($p = 0.106$). In addition, we found a significant quadratic relationship between fRCC and NAA concentration in PCC ($p = 0.009$). Furthermore, cortical thinning in the PCC was correlated with a reduced rich club coefficient after accounting for age and NAA. In conclusion, we found that the fRCC is related to a marker of neuronal integrity in a key region of the cingulate cortex. Furthermore, cortical thinning in the same area was observed, suggesting that both cortical thinning and neuronal integrity in the hub regions influence functional integration of at a whole brain level.

Keywords: fMRI, MRS, graph metric, aged, cortical thickness

INTRODUCTION

Functionally, human brains are known to exhibit a highly organized structure (Meunier et al., 2010). Sub-networks within the brain have been identified which activate while performing various tasks related to visual stimuli (Calhoun et al., 2001), action (Karni et al., 1995), cognitive tasks (Buckner et al., 1996), or at rest (Damoiseaux et al., 2006). Brain regions involved in each of these tasks organize into distinct communities (Meunier et al., 2009). Underlying these segregated communities is a set of highly inter-connected regions facilitating functional connectivity between communities (Sporns et al., 2007). Typically highly influential regions are both structurally (van den Heuvel and Sporns, 2011) and functionally (van den Heuvel et al., 2009) interconnected, forming the so called rich club (Colizza et al., 2006). Despite advancements in imaging analysis techniques regarding graph theoretical analysis for functional MRI, there is currently little knowledge of the biochemical and biological neurotransmitter underpinnings of graph outcome metrics.

The rich club in human brains was first characterized structurally using diffusion tensor imaging (DTI) (van den Heuvel et al., 2013; Collin et al., 2014a), highlighting a consistent set of key regions. High resolution DTI studies have identified a myriad of rich club regions including frontal-temporal, anterior and posterior midline regions, and posterior cingulate cortex (van den Heuvel and Sporns, 2011). Functionally, there are few studies exploring the rich club in human brains at rest. One such study that found a significant enrichment of the fRCC in healthy adults when compared to adolescents (Grayson et al., 2014). While rich club like properties have been observed in both structural and functional modalities of brain imaging, fundamental underlying differences in imaging techniques and their subsequent analysis preclude meaningful direct comparison of the two. Most importantly, resting state functional connectivity is susceptible to the transitive property, particularly between highly correlated regions (Langford et al., 2001), an effect that structural imaging does not suffer from.

Recent studies have identified a number of regions which typically enter their active state during periods of rest with eyes closed (Zhang and Raichle, 2010), commonly known as the default mode network (DMN). Within the DMN the posterior cingulate cortex (PCC) plays an important role, being directly structurally connected to both the medial temporal lobe (MTL) and the medial prefrontal cortex (MPFC) (Greicius et al., 2009). Functionally, PCC is predominantly known as a core component of the default mode network (Greicius et al., 2003). However, it is also involved in other networks, such as the dorsal attention network and the executive control network (Leech and Sharp, 2014). Due to the extensive functional importance of the PCC across multiple networks, we hypothesize that it is a key hub node facilitating communication between multiple canonical networks. While the importance of the PCC in widespread communication between numerous brain networks is well documented, little is currently known about the impact of biochemical and structural alterations within the PCC on its functional connectivity with other key areas. Hence, we sought to elicit the impact of local biochemical and structural factors in the PCC on the fRCC in a healthy population.

Proton magnetic resonance spectroscopy (MRS) enables the identification of regionally specific metabolic signatures non-invasively (Duncan, 1996). Of particular importance to the present study, one particular metabolite, *N-acetyl Aspartate* (NAA), can be identified using this technique. NAA is thought to be present predominantly in neuronal cells, which has been shown to be a biomarker for neuronal and axonal integrity (Dautry et al., 2000; Demougeot et al., 2001). Another measure, which can be acquired using T1-weighted structural images allows for the quantification of neuronal and glial density (Li et al., 2014), known as cortical thickness (CTh).

Cortical thinning has been shown to occur due to aging in a healthy population (Salat et al., 2004). Furthermore, decreased cortical thickness within the pregenual cingulate cortex has been observed in patients suffering from late onset depression (Mayberg, 2003; Lim et al., 2012). One recent study identified a positive correlation between CTh and NAA in the dorsal anterior cingulate cortex (Li et al., 2014). However, the relationship between CTh, NAA, and the rich club coefficient are to our knowledge unexplored.

Due to the highly influential nature of the PCC at a functional level, we hypothesized that it exerts a substantial influence on the functional backbone of the network. Furthermore, we conjectured that both local metabolic and structural properties impact on the extent of its influence. Hence, we sought to elicit the impact of local metabolic and structural properties of the PCC on the overall importance of the rich club.

MATERIALS AND METHODS

Forty eight healthy volunteers (33.08 ± 8.68 years) were recruited in Magdeburg, Germany. The sample consisted of 35 males and 13 females. Participants were excluded based on major medical illness, pregnancy, history of seizures, current psychiatric disorder or general MRI contradictions. The study was approved by the institutional review board of the University of Magdeburg and all subjects gave written informed consent before inclusion.

Data Acquisition

The fMRI data were acquired on a 3 Tesla Siemens MAGNETOM Trio scanner (Siemens, Erlangen, Germany) with an eight-channel phased-array head coil. Subjects were requested to lie still with their eyes closed for the duration of the resting state scan. A total of 488 volumes were acquired with an echo-planar imaging sequence. The following acquisition parameters were used: echo time = 25 ms, field of view = 22 cm, acquisition matrix = 44 × 44, isometric voxel size = 5 × 5 × 5 mm^3. Whole brain coverage was achieved with 26 contiguous axial slices, using a repetition time of 1,250 ms and flip angle of 70°. The first 10 volumes were discarded to allow for magnetic field homogenization. High resolution T1-weighted structural MRI scans of the brain were acquired for structural reference using a 3D-MPRAGE sequence (TE = 4.77 ms, TR = 2,500 ms, T1 = 1,100 ms, flip angle = 7°, bandwidth = 140 Hz/pixel, acquisition matrix = 256 × 256 × 192, isometric voxel size = 1.0 mm^3).

Data Preprocessing

Functional data were corrected for differences in slice time acquisition, motion-corrected using a least squares approach and a six-parameter (rigid body) linear transformation and spatially normalized. The data were linearly detrended. All subjects had less than 1 mm head motion in any direction during the scanning session. An additional regression of nuisance covariates was applied during which the functional data was corrected for global mean signal as well as for white matter and cerebrospinal fluid signal and bandpass filtering between the frequencies of 0.01 and 0.1 Hz. Data were preprocessed using spm8 (Wellcome Trust Center for Neuroimaging, London, England) using the data processing assistant for resting-state fMRI (DPARSF version 2.3, Yan and Zang, 2010).

The resulting volumes were parcellated into 102 nodes using a modified version of the automatic anatomic labeling (AAL) atlas (Tzourio-Mazoyer et al., 2002) containing a fine grained parcellation for the cingulate and insular cortices (Horn et al., 2010; Lord et al., 2012). To compute the resting state functional connectivity (rsFC) of the ROIs, the mean time course of every voxel within each ROI was extracted and Pearsons correlation coefficients were calculated pair-wise for all pairs of ROI's, resulting in 102 by 102 symmetric matrices.

MRS Data Acquisition and Analysis

Proton MRS data were acquired from a single voxel ($10 \times 20 \times 20$ mm^3), located in the PCC for each subject at rest (**Figure 1**). MRS data were acquired using a point resolved spectroscopy (PRESS) sequence with an echo time of 80 ms, repetition time of 2,000 ms, 256 averages, 1,200 Hz bandwidth, 853 ms acquisition time and water suppression. Shimming was performed automatically, with manual fine tuning to improve field homogeneity. To correct for eddy currents, four pulses without water suppression (TR = 10 s) were averaged. Voxel acquisition time was 8 min and 40 s. Spectra were analyzed using LCModel version 6.3.0 (Provencher, 2001). Sixteen different metabolites (Creatine, Glutamate, myo-Inositole, Lactate, NAA, Phosphocholine, Taurine, Aspartate, GABA, Glutamine, Glucose, Alanine, NAAG, Phosphocreatine, Guanine, and Glycerophosphocholine) were fitted using a basis set including all these substances. The concentration of NAA was calculated as its ratio to creatine (Cr) as it is known to be an appropriate reference (Yildiz-Yesiloglu and Ankerst, 2006). Model fit error was estimated using the Cramer-Rao lower bounds (CRLB) (Cavassila et al., 2001) measure, with spectra deemed to be reliable if CRLB was less than 20%. Other minimum quality criteria included a full width half maximum value of smaller than 12 Hz and a signal to noise ratio of greater than eight.

Cortical Thickness

Cortical thickness (CTh) was measured across the whole brain using the CIVET pipeline (Zijdenbos et al., 2002). MR-images were linearly transformed (rigid body, 6 degrees of freedom) to standard Montreal Neurological Institute (MNI) space with intensity and non-uniformity also corrected (Sled et al., 1998). These images were then segmented into gray matter (GM), white matter (WM), cerebral spinal fluid using a neural net classifier. Next cortical surfaces were extracted for both the pial-cortical surface and GM-WM boundary for each hemisphere separately using a deformable mesh model implemented inside the Constrained Laplacian Anatomic Segmentation using Proximity algorithm (June et al., 2005). Both surfaces were non-linearly registered to a high resolution standard template to ensure the co-registration of all subjects to a common space (Lyttelton et al., 2007). To minimize morphological distortion, the inverse of the aforementioned transformation was applied for each subject and CTh was measured in native space. To calculate the GM percentage in the MRS voxel, the voxel was co-registered to the subjects T1 image using SPM8. MRS voxels for each subject were projected into template space using each subject's affine matrix calculated to transform each hemisphere to standard space earlier.

Rich Club Coefficient

These matrices were rendered sparse by recursively removing connections, starting with the lowest correlation until only 10% of connections remain. The sparsity of 10% was selected as networks with more edges tends to introduce weaker, noisy effects obscuring between-group effects (Rubinov et al., 2009; Lord et al., 2012; Borchardt et al., 2015). After thresholding

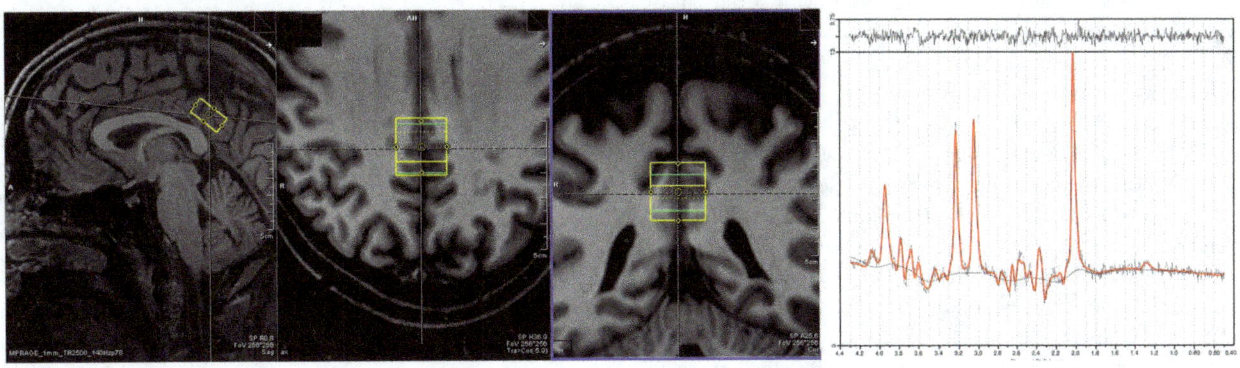

FIGURE 1 | Placement of MRS voxel in the PCC. An exemplar spectra for the MRS signal is on the right.

no negative edges remained. To ensure that the graph didn't disconnect, edges which would cause a disconnection if removed were retained even if their correlation was below the cutoff threshold. These sparse networks were then binarized, and the degree of each node is calculated.

The fRCC was then calculated across a range of degree thresholds. This was done by removing nodes with a degree of less than the chosen threshold and dividing the number of connections in the remaining subnetwork with the maximum possible number of connections. This ratio in and of itself is known not to be a good measure of interconnectedness (van den Heuvel and Sporns, 2011), thus we reference this information against what we would expect by random chance. To this end, we randomly move connections in the thresholded connectivity matrix, creating a randomized matrix with the same degree distribution (Maslov and Sneppen, 2002), preserving the degree distribution of the network while destroying the connection pattern. The rich club coefficient for each randomized graph was then calculated and the ratio of the raw RCC to the mean RCC of all randomized graphs at each degree threshold was computed. As such, a normalized RCC of 1 speaks to the connectivity pattern of the rich club being equal to a random graph, that is, high degree nodes are no more or less likely to connect to each other than by random chance. A value greater than 1 shows an affinity of rich nodes to cluster more tightly than expected together, while a value below 1 shows rich nodes predominantly connect with non-rich nodes. Since all analysis using the rich club refers to the normalized rich club and not the raw rich club, the normalized rich club will be henceforth described solely as the rich club. The regions included as rich club members were also extracted.

Rich club membership was defined on an individual level. That is, for each individual the degree threshold giving the highest RCC was identified, then the regions identified as members at this threshold were selected. At the group level, rich club members were identified as those regions appearing in at least 50% of subjects.

RESULTS

A positive rich club coefficient was observed for all subjects, with the largest fRCC across the group at a degree threshold of 9 (Figure S1). Twenty-one rich club members were consistent in at least half of the participants (**Figure 2**), with seven out of 21 regions from within the cingulate cortex, including the PCC (**Table 1**). No correlation between global signal and fRCC was observed (Figure S2).

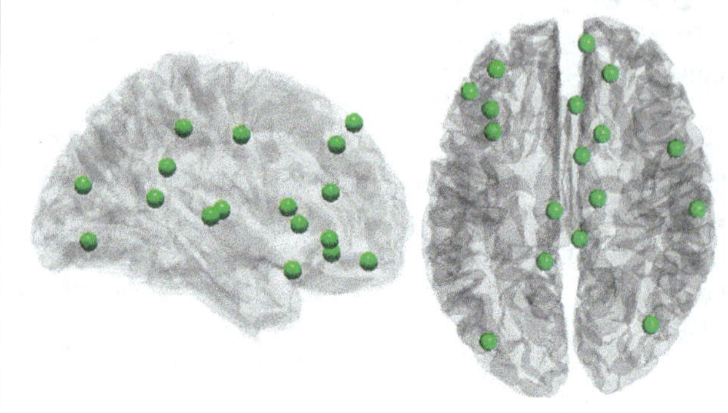

FIGURE 2 | Rich club members.

TABLE 1 | Rich club members.

Subjects	Region
45	Frontal Sup Orb R
44	Frontal Mid L
43	Rostral ACC R
43	Pregenual ACC R
42	Temporal Sup R
41	Rostal ACC L
40	Post Insula R
38	Temporal Sup L
37	Thalamus R
36	Temporal Pole Sup L
35	Frontal Inf Tri L
34	Posterior MCC R
33	Caudate R
33	23d L
32	dPCC R
31	Frontal Inf Orb L
31	vPCC L
30	Occipital Mid R
30	Occipital Inf L
28	Medial Prefront Upper R
26	Anterior Insula L

NAA in the PCC negatively correlated with age (**Figure 3A**, $r = -0.456$, $p = 0.001$, $t = -3.475$, $df = 46$), while no significant correlation exists between rich club coefficient and age ($r = 0.2356$, $p = 0.107$, $t = 1.644$, $df = 46$, **Figure 3B**). Furthermore, a significant quadratic relationship was identified between RCC and NAA/Cr in the PCC (Equation 1, **Figure 4**, $p = 0.009$). This relationship was not observed using a linear model ($r = -0.041$, $p = 0.093$, $t = -1.708$, $df = 46$). The model fit was formally tested using the bayesian information criterion (BIC), which revealed that a quadratic model fit the data better than a linear model (delta BIC $= -3.16$) or any higher order polynomial (Figure S3).

Linear correlates between low and high RCC values were assessed *post hoc*. The data were split into two groups, below the RCC value predicted to give the lowest concentration of NAA/Cr (2.44), and above this value. A negative linear correlation was observed in the low RCC values ($r = -0.365$, $p = 0.036$, $t = -2.185$, $df = 31$), while a trending positive linear correlation was observed in the high RCC values ($r = 0.473$, $p = 0.075$, $t = 1.935$, $df = 13$). Using a Fisher R-to-Z transformation, these two correlations were significantly different ($z = -2.62$, $p = 0.009$, Figure S4). In contrast this did not translate into dependency of global metrics (SWI and CC), which did not correlate with PCC-NAA.

Nonlinear relationship between NAA/Cr in the PCC and the RCC. $F = 5.206, p = 0.009254$.

$$y = 1.933 - 0.621x + 0.127x^2 \quad (1)$$

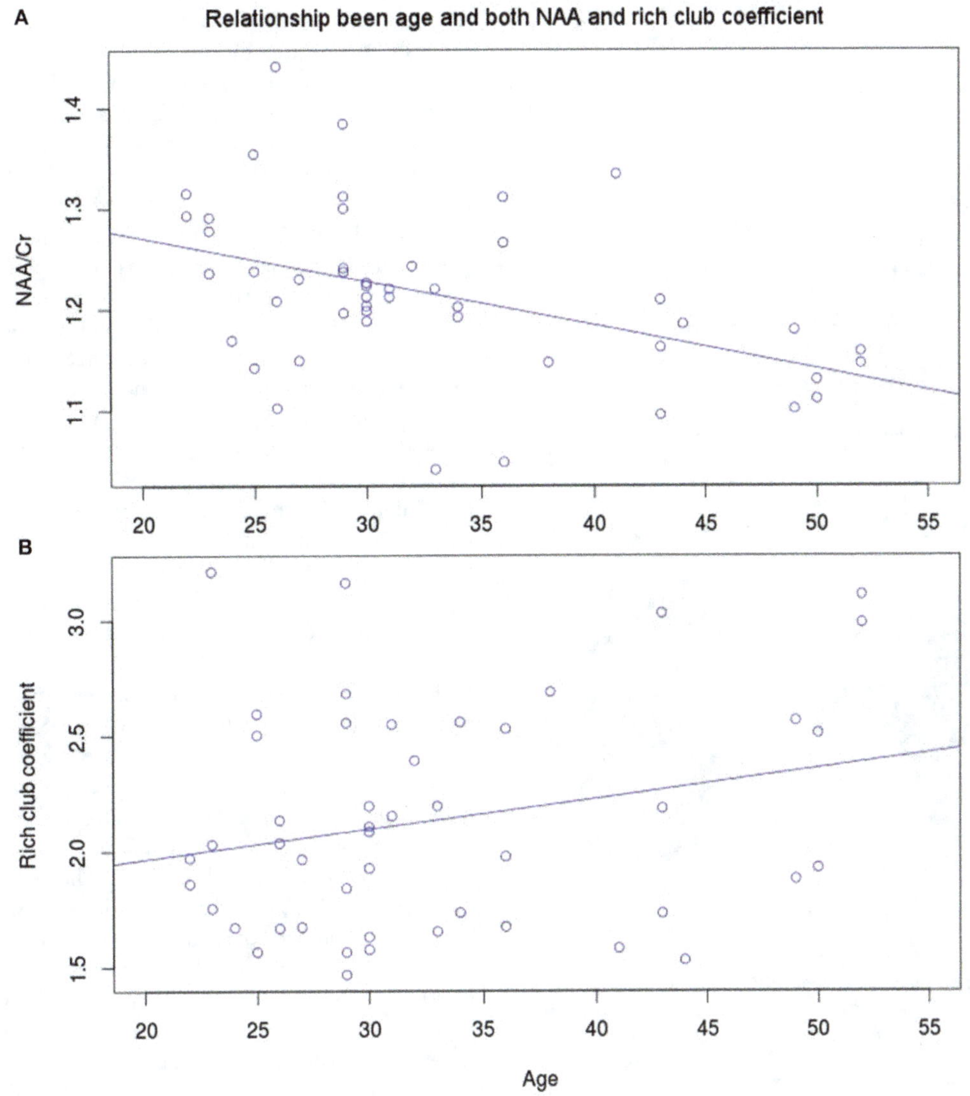

FIGURE 3 | Linear correlates of age with (A) NAA ($r = -0.456, p = 0.001, t = -3.475, df = 46$) and **(B)** rich club coefficient ($r = 0.2356, p = 0.107, t = 1.644, df = 46$).

Cortical thickness in the PCC positively correlated with the rich club coefficient after accounting for age and NAA/Cr as covariates (**Figure 5**, FDR corrected). Although extensive parts of the cortex showed reduced CT as a factor of age (Figure S5), this did not overlap with the previous finding. CT was also positively correlated with NAA/Cr, predominantly in the mid cingulate cortex, but did not overlap with the fRCC correlation with CT in the PCC (Figure S6). After accounting for age as a covariate, fRCC and mean CTh in the PCC was positively correlated ($r = 0.339$, $p = 0.015$, $t = 2.519$, **Figure 6**). When considering only age as a covariate, a cluster of vertices in the same location is observed at an uncorrected threshold only (Figure S7).

DISCUSSION

Although the rich club coefficient has become increasingly studied in both functional and structural networks in human brains (van den Heuvel et al., 2012; Collin et al., 2014b; Grayson et al., 2014), little is currently known about the impact of local metabolic and structural properties of key rich club regions on the integrity of the club as a whole. Hence, we sought to identify effects of neuronal integrity and cortical thinning in the PCC on the density of connections within this functional backbone of the human brain.

Regional distribution of rich club members in this study were in line with previous work (van den Heuvel and Sporns, 2011; van den Heuvel et al., 2013), showing most of the members of the rich

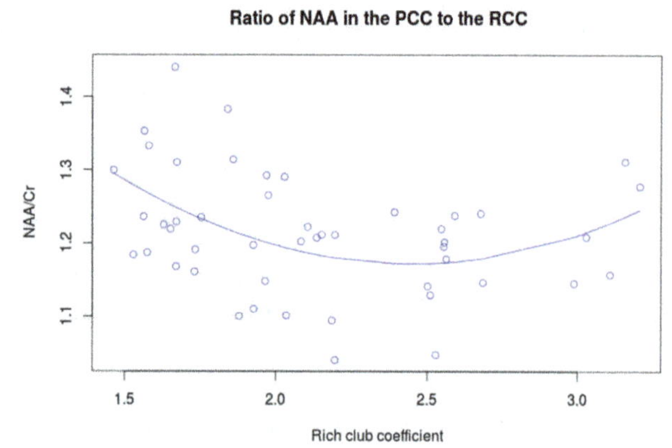

FIGURE 4 | Quadratic relationship between RCC and NAA/Cr. The equation for this curve is: $y = 1.933 - 0.621x + 0.127x^2$ where x is the rich club coefficient.

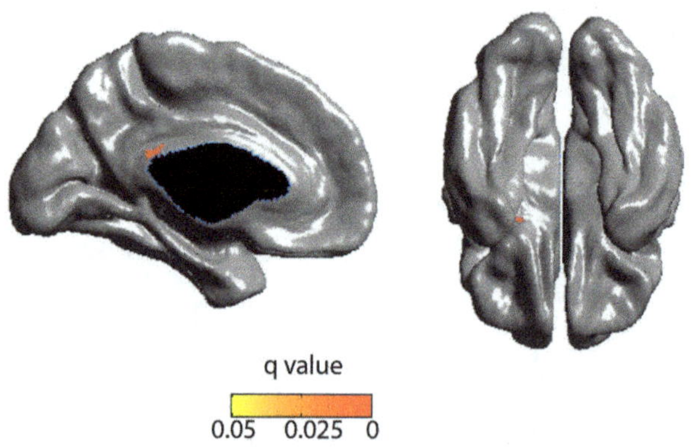

FIGURE 5 | Positive correlation between RCC and CTh (FDR corrected) incorporating age and NAA as covariates. Blue represents FDR corrected significant differences. Red/yellow represent FWE corrected significant differences.

club surrounding the inter-hemispheric fissure. Furthermore, we observe many areas of the cingulate cortex as members of the rich club, suggesting a high level of communication both within the cingulate cortex as well as to other regions of the brain. This result speaks to the central role of the cingulate cortex in information transfer at a whole brain level. Indeed, one third of all rich club members were subregions of the cingulate cortex, including pregenual and rostal parts of the ACC, posterior MCC, dorsal and ventral PCC and Brodman area 23d. During preprocessing we regressed out global signal from out resting state data. This procedure has met with criticism as it can introduce spurious relationships within the data. We observed no relationship between fRCC and GSR, suggesting our results are not driven by the global signal.

The quadratic relationship between the functional rich club and NAA/Cr initially declines linearly, then increases at higher RCC levels. This suggests that other factors, in addition to the NAA/Cr concentration in the PCC, influence the functional rich club coefficient. Confirming this, we found a significant reduction of CTh in the PCC related to the RCC, after accounting for age and NAA/Cr. These results show that both the neuronal integrity and cortical thickness affect the richness of the network.

The directionality of correlations will require further in depth analysis, at best including suitable behavioral parameters. Lower NAA is normally considered indicative of reduced neuronal integrity while its relevance to functional rich club alterations is less clear. Age related whole network changes for example in Alzheimers disease found effects rather in peripheral functional connections leaving the core network rather undisturbed (Daianu et al., 2015) at least for functional connectivity properties. In clinical context, schizophrenia was associated with reduced rich club connections, speaking in favor of a beneficial role of higher functional rich club routing and routing efficiency.

Nodes of the structural rich-club are especially resilient to targeted attacks and enhance global information flow by acting as a "highway" system (van den Heuvel and Sporns, 2011; van den Heuvel et al., 2012; Xia et al., 2016). Nevertheless, the structural rich-club is a relatively high-cost component of brain networks because the wiring cost is greater between members of the rich club than between less well-connected nodes in the periphery (Collin et al., 2014b). Also, structural rich-club nodes have higher levels of metabolic energy consumption than peripheral nodes (Collin et al., 2014b). Structural rich clubs were shown to connect early and are maintained through in maturation ("rich-get-richer"), suggesting that these nodes may have a key developmental role (Schroeter et al., 2015). Thus, it has been argued that maintenance of such a costly network component should offer advantages to the brain's computational performance. In line with this thought, mature rich-clubs were indeed shown to be of great importance for routing of spontaneous activity flow in the network frequently acting as brokers for spontaneous multi-unit activity, suggesting a role of rich-clubs for orchestrating coordinated activity in the network, for example switching between different network states (Crossley et al., 2013; Leech and Sharp, 2014; Senden et al., 2014; Schroeter et al., 2015).

In our case we found lower fRCC associated with higher NAA, thus a direct interpretation in terms of functional relevance will be difficult, particularly since we only investigated healthy subjects.

Our results are in line with previous accounts for the influence of local metabolism within a node on brain network configuration. Horn et al. reported that functional resting state connectivity between pgACC and anterior insula was correlated with Glx concentrations in pgACC (Horn et al., 2010). This effect was localized in that insula MRS did not show similar influences on this connectivity. More recently, Demenescu et al. (2016) show that anterior insula MRS predicted long range resting state connectivity, however toward temporo-parietal and visual cortices. Importantly, these findings of glutamatergic modulations were found explicitly for depressed patients, while healthy controls did not show the same correlation (Horn et al., 2010). This was interpreted as a reflection of a primary glutamatergic deficit in MDD, as supported by respective meta-analyses (Taylor, 2014) while in the absence of a direct

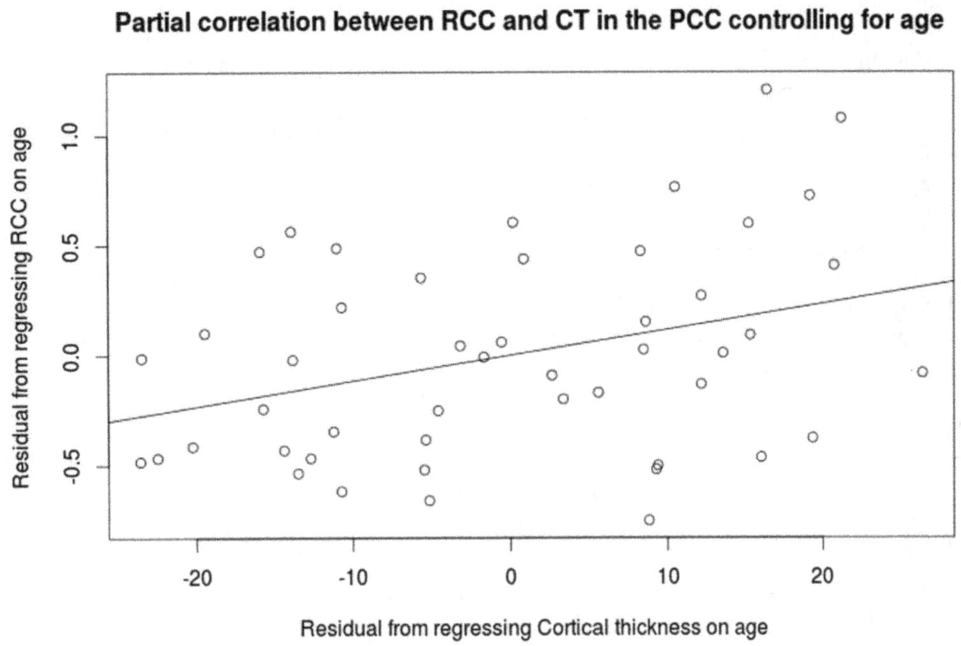

FIGURE 6 | Partial correlation between the rich club coefficient and mean cortical thickness in the PCC ($r = 0.339$, $p = 0.015$, $t = 2.519$).

metabolic deficit variance of the metabolite was considered to be too low.

In contrast, work on PCC MRS in healthy subjects reported an interrelation of both glutamate and GABA on PCC functional connectivity, at least when investigating the default mode network as a whole via independent component analysis (Kapogiannis et al., 2013). Therefore, it is plausible that also in healthy conditions, variance of both functional connectivity and brain metabolites as acquired in MRS is large enough to detect covariations in healthy cohorts. Such covariations should then reflect a common biological mechanism and the most prominent mechanism in healthy cohorts would be that of aging.

Age related brain changes have been investigated in greater extent and prominent effect have ben postulated for NAA (Block et al., 2002). Indeed we found NAA to be correlated with age and RCC however there was no direct correlation between RCC and age. Furthermore, the relationship of PCC cortical thickness was controlled for potential age effects, thus pointing toward a second, age independent mechanism, which relates PCC functional integrity as evident in cortical thickness and NAA levels toward RCC. It must also be stated that the sample included in our study is of rather young age and thus neurodegenerative effects, previously investigated may not be the main driver.

Although Grayson et al. (2014) found an enriched rich club in adolescents, we did not see a significant correlation between age and fRCC ($p = 0.1068$), which may be explained by the vast developmental changes in the brain during the adolescent period (Giedd, 2004) in comparison the putative effects in our sample.

An alternative interpretation would consider the mild apparent, if not statistically significant increase of fRCC with age as a subtle counterpart to the significant age dependent NAA decrease. As such MRS would be considered a very sensitive age marker while secondary effects of age on whole brain organization would be more subtle and not yet detectable in the observed age range between early twenties and mid-fifties. This would then be reflected by the linear component fRCC increase with decreasing NAA, and may, in a far stretch, be interpreted as a sign of age related "hyper-efficiency."

However, such interpretation would not work for the observed quadratic relationship, which for brains with very high RCC's rather found the inverse relationship of increasing fRCC with higher NAA. This suggests that other factors, in addition to the NAA/Cr concentration in the PCC, influence the rich club coefficient. In support of this interpretation, one may add that we found linear negative relationship of CTh in the PCC and fRCC. However, we found this after accounting for age and NAA/Cr, therefore results at this stage should best be appreciated in that we found evidence that both the neuronal integrity and cortical thickness affect the richness of the network and the parallel, potentially driving, or counteracting effects of age and other sources of inter-individual variation will be subject to future investigations in larger cohorts.

Within the context of these considerations, our results in a comparably large, young adult population point toward an effect of local neuronal integrity or at least neurobiological constitution on resting state network configuration.

The new advance in our finding is first the extension to NAA, after previous reports mainly focused on neurotransmitters GABA and Glutamate. Secondly after previous research as investigated metabolite influence on direct connections of a region, either in terms of seed based edges or in terms of the independent component which hosts the location of the single

MRS voxel, we extend the view toward a much more global effect on network constitution. This effect is very likely due to the central role of the PCC within the rich club. While we cannot test this explicitly at this stage, we would assume that the relationship found here is mainly representative of the central role of the PCC within a backbone of small network organization rather than due to the specific impact of NAA in comparison to GABA or glutamate. Ideally, to test such claim, one would request MRS sequences which allow assessment of all mentioned metabolites within the scope of a single session along a number of regions and further leave time for additional resting state assessments. Such methods are available for higher field strengths, making explicit use of the improve line separation (Dou et al., 2013; Li et al, 2016).

LIMITATIONS

Only 13 out of 48 subjects included in this study were female. Due to the small sample of females included, gender effects have not been discussed. However, future work would benefit from investigating gender specific variation in the context of NAA, CTh and RCC.

CONCLUSION

The rich club in fMRI is an area of growing interest, with implications in neurological development (Grayson et al., 2014) and psychiatric disease (van den Heuvel et al., 2013; Collin et al., 2014a). Our findings add evidence to this growing avenue of research, progressing our understanding of the impact of metabolic and structural factors on the rich club. To our knowledge, this is the first study identifying the impact of these factors targeted to the PCC, showing a relationship between CT and NAA/Cr neurotransmitter levels and its effects on this core subnetwork of resting state functional connectivity via the PCC.

AUTHOR CONTRIBUTIONS

MW and HH designed the experiment. AK, MW, and ML acquired the data. AL, ML, MW, Jv, LRD, and VB analyzed the data. AL, VB, MW, and MB interpreted the results. AL drafted the manuscript. AL, VB, MW, ML, Jv, and LRD revised the manuscript. All authors approved the final version of the manuscript.

FUNDING

This study was supported by funding from the following grants: SFB 779/A6 (German Research Foundation) to MW and FP7 MC-ITN R'Birth (Marie Curie) to AL and MW.

ACKNOWLEDGMENTS

The authors would like to thank Claus Tempelmann, Denise Scheermann, Renate Blobel, Carina Födisch, Berit Wiegmann, and Maya Nathan for their help and assistance during data collection and subject testing.

REFERENCES

Block, W., Träber, F., Flacke, S., Jessen, F., Pohl, C., and Schild, H. (2002). *In-vivo* proton MR-spectroscopy of the human brain: assessment of N-acetylaspartate (NAA) reduction as a marker for neurodegeneration. *Amino Acids* 23, 317–323. doi: 10.1007/s00726-001-0144-0

Borchardt, V., Krause, A. L., Starck, T., Nissilä, J., Timonen, M., Kiviniemi, V., et al. (2015). Graph theory reveals hyper-functionality in visual cortices of seasonal affective disorder patients. *World J. Biol. Psychiatry* 16, 123–134. doi: 10.3109/15622975.2014.966144

Buckner, R. L., Bandettini, P. A., O'Craven, K. M., Savoy, R. L., Petersen, S. E., Raichle, M. E., et al. (1996). Detection of cortical activation during averaged single trials of a cognitive task using functional magnetic resonance imaging. *Proc. Natl. Acad. Sci. U.S.A.* 93, 14878–14883. doi: 10.1073/pnas.93.25.14878

Calhoun, V. D., Adali, T., McGinty, V. B., Pekar, J. J., Watson, T. D., and Pearlson, G. D. (2001). fMRI activation in a visual-perception task: network of areas detected using the general linear model and independent components analysis. *Neuroimage* 14, 1080–1088. doi: 10.1006/nimg.2001.0921

Cavassila, S., Deval, S., Huegen, C., van Ormondt, D., and Graveron-Demilly, D. (2001). Cramér-Rao bounds: an evaluation tool for quantitation. *NMR Biomed.* 14, 278–283. doi: 10.1002/nbm.701

Colizza, V., Flammini, A., Serrano, M. A., and Vespignani, A. (2006). Detecting rich-club ordering in complex networks. *Nat. Phys.* 2, 110–115. doi: 10.1038/nphys209

Collin, G., Kahn, R. S., de Reus, M. A., Cahn, W., and van den Heuvel, M. P. (2014a). Impaired rich club connectivity in unaffected siblings of schizophrenia patients. *Schizophr. Bull.* 40, 438–448. doi: 10.1093/schbul/sbt162

Collin, G., Sporns, O., Mandl, R. C. W., and van den Heuvel, M. P. (2014b). Structural and functional aspects relating to cost and benefit of rich club organization in the human cerebral cortex. *Cereb. Cortex.* 24, 2258–2267. doi: 10.1093/cercor/bht064

Crossley, N. A., Mechelli, A., Vértes, P. E., Winton-Brown, T. T., Patel, A. X., Ginestet, C. E., et al. (2013). Cognitive relevance of the community structure of the human brain functional coactivation network. *Proc. Natl. Acad. Sci. U.S.A.* 110, 11583–11588. doi: 10.1073/pnas.1220826110

Daianu, M., Jahanshad, N., Mendez, M. F., Bartzokis, G., Jimenez, E. E., and Thompson, P. M. (2015). Communication of brain network core connections altered in behavioral variant frontotemporal dementia but possibly preserved in early-onset Alzheimer's disease. *Proc. SPIE Int. Soc. Opt. Eng.* 9413:941322. doi: 10.1117/12.2082352

Damoiseaux, J. S., Rombouts, S. A. R. B., Barkhof, F., Scheltens, P., Stam, C. J., Smith, S. M., et al. (2006). Consistent resting-state networks across healthy subjects. *Proc. Natl. Acad. Sci. U.S.A.* 103, 13848–13853. doi: 10.1073/pnas.0601417103

Dautry, C., Vaufrey, F., Brouillet, E., Bizat, N., Henry, P. G., Condé, F., et al. (2000). Early N-acetylaspartate depletion is a marker of neuronal dysfunction in rats and primates chronically treated with the mitochondrial toxin 3-nitropropionic acid. *J. Cereb. Blood Flow Metab.* 20, 789–799. doi: 10.1097/00004647-200005000-00005

Demenescu, L. R., Colic, L., Li, M., Safron, A., Biswal, B., Metzger, C. D., et al. (2016). A spectroscopic approach toward depression diagnosis: local metabolism meets functional connectivity. *Eur. Arch. Psychiatry Clin. Neurosci.* 267, 95–105. doi: 10.1007/s00406-016-0726-1

Demougeot, C., Garnier, P., Mossiat, C., Bertrand, N., Giroud, M., Beley, A., et al. (2001). N-Acetylaspartate, a marker of both cellular dysfunction and neuronal loss: its relevance to studies of acute brain injury. *J. Neurochem.* 77, 408–415. doi: 10.1046/j.1471-4159.2001.00285.x

Dou, W., Palomero-Gallagher, N., van Tol, M.-J., Kaufmann, J., Zhong, K., Bernstein, H.-G., et al. (2013). Systematic regional variations of GABA, glutamine, and glutamate concentrations follow receptor fingerprints of human cingulate cortex. *J. Neurosci.* 33, 12698–12704. doi: 10.1523/JNEUROSCI.1758-13.2013

Duncan, J. S. (1996). Magnetic resonance spectroscopy. *Epilepsia* 37, 598–605. doi: 10.1111/j.1528-1157.1996.tb00622.x

Giedd, J. N. (2004). Structural magnetic resonance imaging of the adolescent brain. *Ann. N.Y. Acad. Sci.* 1021, 77–85. doi: 10.1196/annals.1308.009

Grayson, D. S., Ray, S., Carpenter, S., Iyer, S., Dias, T. G. C., Stevens, C., et al. (2014). Structural and functional rich club organization of the brain in children and adults. *PLoS ONE* 9:e88297. doi: 10.1371/journal.pone.0088297

Greicius, M. D., Krasnow, B., Reiss, A. L., and Menon, V. (2003). Functional connectivity in the resting brain: a network analysis of the default mode hypothesis. *Proc. Natl. Acad. Sci. U.S.A.* 100, 253–258. doi: 10.1073/pnas.0135058100

Greicius, M. D., Supekar, K., Menon, V., and Dougherty, R. F. (2009). Resting-state functional connectivity reflects structural connectivity in the default mode network. *Cereb. Cortex* 19, 72–78. doi: 10.1093/cercor/bhn059

Horn, D. I., Yu, C., Steiner, J., Buchmann, J., Kaufmann, J., Osoba, A., et al. (2010). Glutamatergic and resting-state functional connectivity correlates of severity in major depression - the role of pregenual anterior cingulate cortex and anterior insula. *Front. Syst. Neurosci.* 4:33. doi: 10.3389/fnsys.2010.00033

June, S. K., Singh, V., Jun, K. L., Lerch, J., Ad-Dab'bagh, Y., MacDonald, D., et al. (2005). Automated 3-D extraction and evaluation of the inner and outer cortical surfaces using a Laplacian map and partial volume effect classification. *Neuroimage* 27, 210–221. doi: 10.1016/j.neuroimage.2005.03.036

Kapogiannis, D., Reiter, D. A., Willette, A. A., and Mattson, M. P. (2013). Posteromedial cortex glutamate and GABA predict intrinsic functional connectivity of the default mode network. *Neuroimage* 64, 112–119. doi: 10.1016/j.neuroimage.2012.09.029

Karni, A., Meyer, G., Jezzard, P., Adams, M. M., Turner, R., and Ungerleider, L. G. (1995). Functional MRI evidence for adult motor cortex plasticity during motor skill learning. *Nature* 377, 155–158. doi: 10.1038/377155a0

Langford, E., Schwertman, N., Owens, M., Langford, E., Schwertman, N., and Owens, M. (2001). Is the property of being positively correlated transitive? *Am. Stat.* 55, 322–325. doi: 10.1198/000313001753272286

Leech, R., and Sharp, D. J. (2014). The role of the posterior cingulate cortex in cognition and disease. *Brain* 137, 12–32. doi: 10.1093/brain/awt162

Li, M., Demenescu, L. R., Colic, L., Metzger, C. D., Heinze, H. J., Steiner, J., et al. (2016). Temporal dynamics of antidepressant ketamine effects on glutamine cycling follow regional fingerprints of AMPA and NMDA receptor densities. *Neuropsychopharmacology* doi: 10.1038/npp.2016.184. [Epub ahead of print].

Li, M., Metzger, C. D., Li, W., Safron, A., van Tol, M.-J., Lord, A., et al. (2014). Dissociation of glutamate and cortical thickness is restricted to regions subserving trait but not state markers in major depressive disorder. *J. Affect. Disord.* 169C, 91–100. doi: 10.1016/j.jad.2014.08.001

Lim, H. K., Jung, W. S., Ahn, K. J., Won, W. Y., Hahn, C., Lee, S. Y., et al. (2012). Regional cortical thickness and subcortical volume changes are associated with cognitive impairments in the drug-naive patients with late-onset depression. *Neuropsychopharmacology* 37, 838–849. doi: 10.1038/npp.2011.264

Lord, A., Horn, D., Breakspear, M., and Walter, M. (2012). Changes in community structure of resting state functional connectivity in unipolar depression. *PLoS ONE* 7:e41282. doi: 10.1371/journal.pone.0041282

Lyttelton, O., Boucher, M., Robbins, S., and Evans, A. (2007). An unbiased iterative group registration template for cortical surface analysis. *Neuroimage* 34, 1535–1544. doi: 10.1016/j.neuroimage.2006.10.041

Maslov, S., and Sneppen, K. (2002). Specificity and stability in topology of protein networks. *Science* 296, 910–913. doi: 10.1126/science.1065103

Mayberg, H. S. (2003). Modulating dysfunctional limbic-cortical circuits in depression: towards development of brain-based algorithms for diagnosis and optimised treatment. *Br. Med. Bull.* 65, 193–207. doi: 10.1093/bmb/65.1.193

Meunier, D., Lambiotte, R., and Bullmore, E. T. (2010). Modular and hierarchically modular organization of brain networks. *Front. Neurosci.* 4:200. doi: 10.3389/fnins.2010.00200

Meunier, D., Lambiotte, R., Fornito, A., Ersche, K. D., and Bullmore, E. T. (2009). Hierarchical modularity in human brain functional networks. *Front. Neuroinformatics* 3:37. doi: 10.3389/neuro.11.037.2009

Provencher, S. W. (2001). Automatic quantitation of localized *in vivo* 1H spectra with LCModel. *NMR Biomed.* 14, 260–264. doi: 10.1002/nbm.698

Rubinov, M., Knock, S. A., Stam, C. J., Micheloyannis, S., Harris, A. W., Williams, L. M., et al. (2009). Small-world properties of nonlinear brain activity in schizophrenia. *Hum. Brain Mapp.* 30, 403–416. doi: 10.1002/hbm.20517

Salat, D. H., Buckner, R. L., Snyder, A. Z., Greve, D. N., Desikan, R. S. R., Busa, E., et al. (2004). Thinning of the cerebral cortex in aging. *Cereb. Cortex* 14, 721–730. doi: 10.1093/cercor/bhh032

Schroeter, M. S., Charlesworth, P., Kitzbichler, M. G., Paulsen, O., and Bullmore, E. T. (2015). Emergence of rich-club topology and coordinated dynamics in development of hippocampal functional networks *in vitro*. *J. Neurosci.* 35, 5459–5470. doi: 10.1523/JNEUROSCI.4259-14.2015

Senden, M., Deco, G., De Reus, M. A., Goebel, R., and Van Den Heuvel, M. P. (2014). Rich club organization supports a diverse set of functional network configurations. *Neuroimage* 96, 174–182. doi: 10.1016/j.neuroimage.2014.03.066

Sled, J. G., Zijdenbos, A. P., and Evans, A. C. (1998). A nonparametric method for automatic correction of intensity nonuniformity in MRI data. *IEEE Trans. Med. Imaging* 17, 87–97. doi: 10.1109/42.668698

Sporns, O., Honey, C. J., and Kotter, R. (2007). Identification and classification of hubs in brain networks. *PLoS ONE* 2:e1049. doi: 10.1371/journal.pone.0001049

Taylor, M. J. (2014). Could glutamate spectroscopy differentiate bipolar depression from unipolar? *J. Affect. Disord.* 167, 80–84. doi: 10.1016/j.jad.2014.05.019

Tzourio-Mazoyer, N., Landeau, B., Papathanassiou, D., Crivello, F., Etard, O., Delcroix, N., et al. (2002). Automated anatomical labeling of activations in SPM using a macroscopic anatomical parcellation of the MNI MRI single-subject brain. *Neuroimage* 15, 273–289. doi: 10.1006/nimg.2001.0978

van den Heuvel, M. P., Kahn, R. S., Goi, J., and Sporns, O. (2012). High-cost, high-capacity backbone for global brain communication. *Proc. Natl. Acad. Sci. U.S.A.* 109, 11372–11377. doi: 10.1073/pnas.1203593109

van den Heuvel, M. P., Mandl, R. C. W., Kahn, R. S., and Hulshoff Pol, H. E. (2009). Functionally linked resting-state networks reflect the underlying structural connectivity architecture of the human brain. *Hum. Brain Mapp.* 30, 3127–3141. doi: 10.1002/hbm.20737

van den Heuvel, M. P., and Sporns, O. (2011). Rich-club organization of the human connectome. *J. Neurosci.* 31, 15775–15786. doi: 10.1523/JNEUROSCI.3539-11.2011

van den Heuvel, M. P., Sporns, O., Collin, G., Scheewe, T., Mandl, R. C. W., Cahn, W., et al. (2013). Abnormal rich club organization and functional brain dynamics in schizophrenia. *JAMA Psychiatry* 70, 783–792. doi: 10.1001/jamapsychiatry.2013.1328

Xia, M., Lin, Q., Bi, Y., and He, Y. (2016). Connectomic insights into topologically centralized network edges and relevant motifs in the human brain. *Front. Hum. Neurosci.* 10:158. doi: 10.3389/fnhum.2016.00158

Yan, C.-G., and Zang, Y.-F. (2010). DPARSF: a MATLAB toolbox for pipeline" data analysis of resting-state fMRI. *Front. Syst. Neurosci.* 4:13. doi: 10.3389/fnsys.2010.00013

Yildiz-Yesiloglu, A., and Ankerst, D. P. (2006). Review of 1H magnetic resonance spectroscopy findings in major depressive disorder: a meta-analysis. *Psychiatry Res.* 147, 1–25. doi: 10.1016/j.pscychresns.2005.12.004

Zhang, D. Y., and Raichle, M. E. (2010). Disease and the brain's dark energy. *Nat. Rev. Neurol.* 6, 15–28. doi: 10.1038/nrneurol.2009.198

Zijdenbos, A. P., Forghani, R., and Evans, A. C. (2002). Automatic "pipeline" analysis of 3-D MRI data for clinical trials: application to multiple sclerosis. *IEEE Trans. Med. Imaging* 21, 1280–1291. doi: 10.1109/TMI.2002.806283

12

Genomic Editing of Non-Coding RNA Genes with CRISPR/Cas9 Ushers in a Potential Novel Approach to Study and Treat Schizophrenia

Chuanjun Zhuo [1,2,3*†], *Weihong Hou* [4†], *Lirong Hu* [1], *Chongguang Lin* [1], *Ce Chen* [1] *and Xiaodong Lin* [1]

[1]*Department of Psychiatry, Wenzhou Seventh People's Hospital, Wenzhou, China,* [2]*Department of Psychiatry, Tianjin Mental Health Center, Tianjin Anding Hospital, Tianjin, China,* [3]*Department of Psychiatry, Tianjin Anning Hospital, Tianjin, China,* [4]*Department of Biology, University of North Carolina at Charlotte, Charlotte, NC, USA*

Edited by:
Andrew Harkin, Trinity College, Dublin, Ireland

Reviewed by:
Daniela Tropea, Trinity College, Dublin, Ireland
Hyunsoo Shawn J. E., Duke NUS Graduate Medical School, Singapore
Yingjie Sun, Harvard University, USA

***Correspondence:**
Chuanjun Zhuo
chuanjunzhuotjmh@163.com

These authors have contributed equally to this work.

†

Schizophrenia is a genetically related mental illness, in which the majority of genetic alterations occur in the non-coding regions of the human genome. In the past decade, a growing number of regulatory non-coding RNAs (ncRNAs) including microRNAs (miRNAs) and long non-coding RNAs (lncRNAs) have been identified to be strongly associated with schizophrenia. However, the studies of these ncRNAs in the pathophysiology of schizophrenia and the reverting of their genetic defects in restoration of the normal phenotype have been hampered by insufficient technology to manipulate these ncRNA genes effectively as well as a lack of appropriate animal models. Most recently, a revolutionary gene editing technology known as Clustered Regularly Interspaced Short Palindromic Repeats (CRISPR)/CRISPR-associated nuclease 9 (Cas9; CRISPR/Cas9) has been developed that enable researchers to overcome these challenges. In this review article, we mainly focus on the schizophrenia-related ncRNAs and the use of CRISPR/Cas9-mediated editing on the non-coding regions of the genomic DNA in proving causal relationship between the genetic defects and the pathophysiology of schizophrenia. We subsequently discuss the potential of translating this advanced technology into a clinical therapy for schizophrenia, although the CRISPR/Cas9 technology is currently still in its infancy and immature to put into use in the treatment of diseases. Furthermore, we suggest strategies to accelerate the pace from the bench to the bedside. This review describes the application of the powerful and feasible CRISPR/Cas9 technology to manipulate schizophrenia-associated ncRNA genes. This technology could help researchers tackle this complex health problem and perhaps other genetically related mental disorders due to the overlapping genetic alterations of schizophrenia with other mental illnesses.

Keywords: schizophrenia, non-coding RNAs, lncRNAs, miRNAs, CRISPR/Cas9, gene editing

INTRODUCTION

Schizophrenia is a severe mental illness, in which patients exhibit both mental and behavioral dysfunction mainly associated with neurodevelopmental abnormality. Indeed, schizophrenia is considered as a neurodevelopmental disorder (Marenco and Weinberger, 2000). To date, the pathological causes underlying the onset and progression of schizophrenia remain unclear.

A wealth of science-based evidence has indicated that schizophrenia is a genetically related mental illness that is inherited in approximately 80% of cases (Cardno et al., 1999) and that certain alterations in the genomic DNA inherited from the parents are likely to contribute to disease onset in late adolescence or early adulthood (International Schizophrenia Consortium et al., 2009; Costain et al., 2013; *Human Molecular Genetics*). Decades of research have shown that the interplay between genes and environmental factors largely contribute to the development of schizophrenia (Owen et al., 2016). It has been found that the majority of genetic alterations occur in the non-coding regions of human genome, from which regulatory non-coding RNAs (ncRNAs), mainly microRNAs (miRNAs) and long non-coding RNAs (lncRNAs), are transcribed. miRNAs and lncRNAs are two major regulatory ncRNAs with little capacity to encode proteins and have differences in size, location and biological function. miRNAs play a vital role in the modulation of gene expression, mainly via post-transcriptional destabilization of target mRNAs that harbor one or more complementary sites with miRNAs, translational repression, or a combination of the two molecular mechanisms (Bartel, 2004, 2009). While lncRNAs are defined as regulatory ncRNAs with a size longer than 200 nt in length. In contrast to miRNAs, our knowledge with respect to the molecular mechanism whereby lncRNAs function remains largely unexplored (Ponting et al., 2009; Wilusz et al., 2009). Recently, a growing number of lncRNAs have been reported to be associated with a broad range of diseases, including mental illnesses such as schizophrenia (Barry et al., 2014; Merelo et al., 2015; Rao et al., 2015). miRNAs and lncRNAs as two large groups of regulatory ncRNAs are highly expressed in the brain where they act as important modulators of genes essential for maintaining proper brain development and function. This is of particular importance because it has been well documented that abnormal brain development, maturation and plasticity have been strongly linked to schizophrenia. For instance, manipulation of schizophrenia-associated miRNAs such as miR-132/miR-121 and miR-219 has been reported to alter an activity-dependent neuronal maturation and plasticity at synapse (Nudelman et al., 2010; Tognini et al., 2011; Mellios and Sur, 2012). Further studies have shown that these miRNAs function through either directly regulating synthesis of proteins which are essential for plasticity at the synapse or interacting with transcription factors which are likely to modulate more enduring neuroplastic changes (Smalheiser and Lugli, 2009; Mellios and Sur, 2012). These recent findings of schizophrenia-associated miRNAs suggest that the biological implication of dysregulation of the miRNAs and their targeted genes are profound for schizophrenia. Considering the magnitude of miRNA alterations and their broad effects on target genes in schizophrenia, the schizophrenia-associated miRNAs might be important for the pathogenesis of schizophrenia. Over past years, an increasing number of schizophrenia-associated ncRNAs such as miR-137, lncRNA Gomafu, etc., has been identified, and the correlation of their genetic alterations with the pathogenesis of schizophrenia has been characterized (Sone et al., 2007; International Schizophrenia Consortium et al., 2009; Schizophrenia Psychiatric Genome-Wide Association Study (GWAS) Consortium, 2011; Barry et al., 2014; Ma et al., 2014). However, the exact functional roles of these genetic variations in the development and progression of schizophrenia are less understood. Indeed, the functioning of these ncRNAs in the development of schizophrenia and the correction of their genetic changes in the genomic DNA, the key to develop novel therapies for schizophrenia, have been hampered by insufficient technology to manipulate these ncRNA genes effectively and a lack of appropriate animal models. Apparently, understanding these changes in the genomic DNA, including the coding and non-coding regions in schizophrenia, in combination with the development of novel genetic tools, will undoubtedly enable the mutations to be corrected, which is the key to developing novel therapies for schizophrenia.

In recent years, with a range of advanced technologies, including next-generation sequencing, high-resolution microarrays and genotyping, a great number of miRNAs and lncRNAs associated with schizophrenia have been identified and characterized. The understanding of these ncRNAs and their genetic variations in the development of schizophrenia has relied on the novel tools of advanced technologies in biology and beyond. Clustered regularly interspaced short palindromic repeats (CRISPR)/CRISPR-associated nuclease 9 (Cas9) is a recently developed revolutionary gene editing technology that is able to manipulate effectively the non-coding regions of the genomic DNA in human cell lines and animal models, to create or correct the mutations more easily than ever in living cells and animals, and therefore to overcome obstacles in schizophrenia research and therapy (Bhaya et al., 2011; Jinek et al., 2012; Cho et al., 2013; Cong et al., 2013; Jiang et al., 2013; Mali et al., 2013; Doudna and Charpentier, 2014).

In this review article, we bring together schizophrenia-associated regulatory ncRNAs, mainly miRNAs and lncRNAs, summarize CRISPR/Cas9-mediated editing on the non-coding regions of genomic DNA in human cell lines and animal models, and propose applications of the revolutionary gene editing CRISPR/Cas9 tool in schizophrenia research, especially on the functional study of ncRNAs genes and on the development of animal models to accelerate schizophrenia research, thus proving the causal relationship between genetic defects and the pathophysiology of schizophrenia, and eventually translating the scientific findings into a clinical cure for schizophrenia. The information described in the present review may help researchers to tackle this complex health problem and perhaps other genetically related mental disorders due to the overlapping genetic alterations of schizophrenia with other mental illnesses.

METHODS

A systematic search and review of the recent literature was performed using the main databases, including PubMed, Google Scholar and Wanfang Med Online, by using the following keywords: schizophrenia, mental disorder, gene editing, CRISPR/Cas9, ncRNAs, miRNAs and lncRNAs.

ncRNAs INCLUDING miRNAs AND lncRNAs THAT ARE ASSOCIATED WITH SCHIZOPHRENIA

The involvement of complex genetic components in the etiology of schizophrenia has been well established by a wealth of scientific evidence. Indeed, the heritability of schizophrenia is approximately 80% (Cardno et al., 1999); therefore, novel genomic tools offer hope for insight into the profound etiology of this complicated, genetically related mental illness. Genome-wide association studies have revealed a great number of strong susceptibility loci for schizophrenia, most of which are located in the non-coding regions of the genome, including genetic fragments for the transcription of miRNAs and lncRNAs. In fact, numerous studies have found that the majority of miRNAs and lncRNAs are highly expressed in the brain, where their genetic mutations, abnormal expression and impact on target gene levels may lead to defective development, suppression of synaptic efficacy, and mGluR-dependent synaptic plasticity in the hippocampus (Olde Loohuis et al., 2015; Siegert et al., 2015) as well as other neurological impairment that is largely correlated with schizophrenia and may contribute to its pathogenesis and progression (Krichevsky et al., 2003; Sempere et al., 2004; Giraldez et al., 2005; Vo et al., 2005; Schratt et al., 2006). In the past decade or two, with the help of high-throughput microarray techniques, comparison of differential expression of miRNAs in schizophrenia vs. controls has identified numerous miRNAs that are dysregulated in schizophrenia, which have been summarized previously (Beveridge and Cairns, 2012; Wang J. et al., 2014). In contrast to the above studies with microarray analysis, a genome-wide association study performed in a large-scale population revealed schizophrenia-associated non-coding genes, including miRNA genes, among which miRNA137 stands out (International Schizophrenia Consortium et al., 2009; Schizophrenia Psychiatric Genome-Wide Association Study (GWAS) Consortium, 2011). International Schizophrenia Consortium et al. (2009) reported that the genetic elements for a small ncRNA, the microRNA137 (*MIR137*) gene with chromosomal location 1p21.3, have been the schizophrenia-associated loci, conferring susceptibility to schizophrenia and the discovery has received great attention within the field. In the following large-scale genome-wide association study conducted by Franke et al. (2016) using more than 40,000 recruited participants, the rs1625579 polymorphism in the miRNA137 gene was identified to be strongly linked to schizophrenia (Schizophrenia Psychiatric Genome-Wide Association Study (GWAS) Consortium, 2011; Ma et al., 2014). To date, many further investigations have supported the association between miR137 and schizophrenia as well as the miR-137 variant rs1625579 as a predictor of an earlier age-at-onset of psychosis in schizophrenia (Lett et al., 2013). In a Han Chinese population, analysis of the single nucleotide polymorphism rs1625579 of the miRNA137 gene in a cohort of 1430 individuals with schizophrenia compared with 1570 healthy individuals was performed; rs1625579 showed significant differences in the allele frequencies between those who suffered from schizophrenia and healthy control subjects (Guan et al., 2014), while the single nucleotide polymorphism rs66642155 allelic variant was likely to have an impact on the age-at-onset and the degree of positive symptoms (Wang S. et al., 2014). The molecular mechanism whereby the genetic variants of miR-137 confer a high risk of schizophrenia also has been shown to be related to a declined fronto-striatal brain white and gray matter structure but without changes in the volume of the local brain (Rose et al., 2014; Wright et al., 2016), which may cause symptoms such as poor concentration, low processing speed, cognitive impairment, etc. (Kuswanto et al., 2015); the impact of miR137 genetic alterations on the expression of a set of target neuronal transmission genes and synaptogenesis (Kos et al., 2015; Strazisar et al., 2015; Wright et al., 2015); and involvement of miR137 on a glucocorticoid receptor-dependent signaling pathway (Vallès et al., 2014). A very recent in-depth study in a zebrafish model system by Giacomotto et al. (2016) has reported that a slight change in synaptic function or a defect in the axonal network mediated by schizophrenia-associated suppression of miR-137 is likely responsible for the behavioral phenotype.

Apart from miRNAs, lnRNAs have emerged as one of most important classes of ncRNAs in the regulation of gene expression, and their genetic alterations and dysregulation play an important role in the pathogenesis of various diseases. In contrast to a larger number of schizophrenia-associated miRNAs being studied, only several lncRNAs have been identified to be correlated with this disease, among which myocardial infraction-associated transcript (MIAT), also known as retinal ncRNAs 2, was most recently found to be strongly correlated with schizophrenia. MIAT was originally identified as a new member of the lncRNA family in Blackshaw et al. (2004), and it was initially found to play a role in regulating retinal cell fate differentiation and to be associated with myocardial infraction (Ishii et al., 2006; Rapicavoli et al., 2010; Liao et al., 2016). It is also abundantly expressed in the nucleus of neurons during development through adulthood. In addition, MIAT is known as lncRNA Gomafu (Sone et al., 2007), a Japanese word reflecting its speckled distribution in the nucleoplasm. Despite its chromosomal location of 22q12.1, which has been documented to be associated with schizophrenia, and its expression in the nervous system, the link between this lncRNA and schizophrenia was unveiled in 2014. The Australian research team of Barry et al. (2014) has demonstrated for the first time the strong association of MIAT with schizophrenia, including downregulation of Gomafu in schizophrenic patients, and has provided insight into the mechanisms: acutely declined levels of Gomafu in response to neuronal activation and Gomafu-mediated impaired alternative splicing through its binding directly to the two splicing factors QK1 and serine/arginine-rich splicing factor 1, which ultimately leads to the abnormal regulation of the two schizophrenia genes DISC-1 and ErbB4 (Barry et al., 2014; Liao et al., 2016), causing a decrease in the activity of parvalbumin interneurons (Chung et al., 2016). Soon after the identification of the association between lncRNA Gomafu and schizophrenia, the link of its genetic alterations with schizophrenia in different populations has been subsequently reported. Rao et al. (2015) have conducted an analysis on the genetic variants of lncRNA Gomafu in 1255 patients diagnosed with paranoid schizophrenia, compared to 1209 healthy individuals in a Chinese Han population, and found that the rs1894720 locus was significantly associated with paranoid schizophrenia (Rao et al., 2015). Aside from lncRNA Gomafu, there are other mental disease-related lncRNAs such as Evf2, BDNF-AS and DISC-2 that have been found to be associated with schizophrenia and have been reviewed previously (Merelo et al., 2015).

As the number of new schizophrenia-associated ncRNAs continues to grow and the variants within the ncRNA genes may directly correlate with schizophrenia, there is an urgent need for novel genetic tools that can be used to understand the functional role of these ncRNAs in schizophrenia and to correct the mutations as a novel approach for schizophrenia research and treatment. CRISPR/Cas9 is such a revolutionary technology that can be applied to work especially for this purpose.

CRISPR/Cas9 FOR EDITING GENOMIC ELEMENTS TARGETING NON-CODING RNAs

The CRISPR/Cas9 system, originally well-documented as an adaptive immune defense mechanism in bacteria, is an emerging revolutionary yet feasible technique for precise genome editing of various organisms, including plants, animals, and even humans, so that specific changes in the genomic DNA stretches can be easily and precisely made (Bhaya et al., 2011; Jinek et al., 2012; Cho et al., 2013; Cong et al., 2013; Jiang et al., 2013; Mali et al., 2013; Doudna and Charpentier, 2014). The CRISPR/Cas9 system generally consists of two components: the Cas9 protein and the guide RNA (gRNA). Being guided by the gRNA, the Cas9 protein is recruited to the target site and is able to cut the genomic DNA at a specific site. The past years have witnessed the emergence of this innovative technology as well as dramatic progress in genomic DNA editing with the CRISPR/Cas9 system (Doudna and Charpentier, 2014). The technology has been applied to manipulate the genomic DNA elements targeting not only the coding regions but also the non-coding ones, from which small and long coding ncRNAs such as miRNAs and lncRNAs are encoded. It is particularly important to edit the genomic DNA elements targeting non-coding regions, since silencing these ncRNA genes with the current, conventional RNA interference (RNAi) technology has turned out to be challenging due to their resistance to the RNAi techniques (Zamore et al., 2000; Gilbert et al., 2013; Fatica and Bozzoni, 2014; Hilton et al., 2015). Recently, the obstacles have been overcome by the application of a modified CRISPR/Cas9 system, in which a lentiviral vector expressing two gRNAs are used simultaneously, with which the genomic DNA fragments ranging from 100 to 3000 bp in length have been manipulated and edited (Han et al., 2014; Aparicio-Prat et al., 2015). To date, a number of ncRNA genes in the genomic DNA have been successfully silenced, including miRNAs (miR21, miR29a) and lncRNAs (UCA1, MALAT1), with MALAT1 reduced by up to 98% inside human HCT116, Hela, and HEK293T cell lines after the promoter region of the MALAT1 gene was edited by the Double Excision CRISPR Knockout method (Aparicio-Prat et al., 2015; Ho et al., 2015; Chang et al., 2016). More detailed information about the miRNA and lncRNA genes successfully edited by the CRIPSR/Cas9 system in cell lines and entire animals were summarized in **Tables 1, 2**. This powerful genome-editing tool has brought a wealth of innovative applications and perspectives for both biological research and the treatment of diseases, including the complicated disease of schizophrenia. In the following sections, we offer a review of a number of successful examples of CRISPR/Cas9-mediated editing on the non-coding regions of genomic DNA in human

TABLE 1 | Summary of the miRNA genes successfully edited by the CRISPR/Cas9 system.

miRNA	Chromosomal location	Cells/Animals tested	Results	Reference
miR-21	Chr17	Human HEK293, LNCaP, MCF-7 and HCT-116 cells	The miR-21 gene was knocked out with over 90% reduction of the miR-21 levels	Ho et al. (2015)
miR-29a	Chr7	Human HEK293 cells	Complete knock-out of the miR-29a gene	Ho et al. (2015)
miRNA cluster (miR-17a-1, miR-92a-1)	Chr1	Zebrafish	The deletion of this miRNA cluster gene from dre-miR-17a-1 to dre-miR-92a-2 was obtained in the zebrafish embryos injected with the CRISPR/Cas9 in combination with the gRNAs	Xiao et al. (2013)
miR-17	Chr13	Human HCT-116 and HT-29 cells Mice	The miR-17 expression was decreased by up to 96% and the knock-down phenotype was stable in the human cells and mice	Chang et al. (2016)
miR-141	Chr12	Human HCT-116 and HT-29 cells Mice	Nearly 96% reduction in the miR-141 levels was achieved with long-term stability of the knock-down phenotype and in control of crossing off-target effect on other members in the same family	Chang et al. (2016)

TABLE 2 | Summary of the lncRNA genes successfully edited by the CRISPR/Cas9 system.

miRNA	Chromosomal location	Cells/Animals tested	Results	Reference
UCA1	Chr19	Human HCT-116 cells	After >5.6 kb in length for the UCA1 gene was edited, UCA1 RNA levels were reduced by about 90%	Ho et al. (2015)
MALAT1 or NEAT1	Chr11	Human cell lines: HEK293T, HCT-116, Hela and IMR90	Up to 98%reduction in MALAT1 RNA expression was achieved after the upstream and major promoters in the MALAT1 gene were deleted	Aparicio-Prat et al. (2015)
LncRNA-21A	Chr8	Human HCT-116 cells	475 bp for the lncRNA-21 A gene was targeted, wild-type lncRNA-21A was completely lost	Ho et al. (2015)
AK023948	Chr8	Human MCF-7 cells	The AK023948 gene was knocked out	Ho et al. (2015)
LncRNA Rian	Chr12	Mice	23 kb fragment in the lncRNA *Rian* gene was deleted, and a *Rian* knock-out mouse model with heritability of this large fragment deletion was established	Han et al. (2014)

Abbreviations: UCA1, urothelial cancer associated 1; MALAT1, metastasis associated lung adenocarcinoma transcript 1; NEAT2, noncoding nuclear-enriched abundant transcript 2.

cell lines and animal models as well as comment on the perspectives for both schizophrenia research and an eventual cure for schizophrenia. We also discuss the challenges of translating this advanced technology into a clinical therapy for schizophrenia and suggest strategies for removing the obstacles to accelerate the pace along the path from the bench to the bedside.

PERSPECTIVE OF EDITING ncRNA GENES WITH CRISPR/Cas9 FOR SCHIZOPHRENIA RESEARCH

The application of the novel CRISPR/Cas9 technology in schizophrenia-associated ncRNAs will usher in a new perspective for schizophrenia research to advance our understanding about the biological function for ncRNAs and to facilitate creating animal models with specific mutations or with the original form restored. Silencing or enhancing gene expression to lose or gain function has been well accepted in the study of a gene of interest. RNAi with specific small-interfering RNAs (siRNAs) is a commonly used approach to silence a desired gene encoded by the coding regions of genomic DNA, which usually occurs in the cytoplasm (Zamore et al., 2000). However, siRNAs designed to target ncRNA genes, including lncRNAs and miRNA genes, have been found to be inefficient mainly because many lncRNAs are located in the nucleus (Fatica and Bozzoni, 2014). In fact, it has been difficult to achieve successful knockdown of a desired lncRNA gene. Recently, scientists from independent research groups have applied a modified CRISPR/Cas9 system to target the ncRNA genes in the nucleus that has resulted in robust knockdown of a number of ncRNAs, including miRNAs in the zebrafish genome (Xiao et al., 2013), miRNAs in human cell lines, lncRNAs in a mouse model (Han et al., 2014) and lncRNAs in human cell lines (Ho et al., 2015), allowing the study of the biological roles of schizophrenia-associated ncRNAs in the pathogenesis of schizophrenia. The key feature of the modified CRISPR/Cas9 system is the use of dual gRNAs, which produce two cuts in specific sites and allow deletion of a larger fragment (Ho et al., 2015). With the modified CRISPR/Cas9 system, there is the possibility to manipulate any exon fragment of the ncRNAs and to explore the biological function of these ncRNA genes in schizophrenia. Since schizophrenia is a complex disorder that involves multiple genetic alterations of ncRNAs, the modified CRISPR/Cas9 approach will enable the disruption of these ncRNAs and will test if disruption of these ncRNA genes can cause schizophrenia. Apart from the silencing of ncRNA genes, the CRISPR/Cas9 system can also deliver regulatory components to the target genes and activate or upregulate target gene expression. Together with its silencing of the ncRNA gene, activation of the gene at the transcriptional level also empowers researchers to understand the biological role for a gene in the development and progression of schizophrenia. Apparent knockdown or activation of an ncRNA gene using the modified CRISPR/Cas9 system has couple of advantages: it is more effective than RNAi, and it is able to target multiple genes simultaneously. When it comes to the schizophrenia-associated ncRNAs miR137 and Gomafu, it is possible to target these two ncRNAs simultaneously and investigate if miRNA137 and Gomafu each alone or in combination affect the development and progression of schizophrenia.

The main bottleneck of schizophrenia research has been lack of translatable animal model system to prove causal relationship between genetic defects and pathophysiology of schizophrenia owing to not only difficulties in reproducing its prominent symptoms but also the tedious work required for creating animal models with specific genomic mutations. The CRISPR/Cas9 system brings a novel perspective for developing animal models for schizophrenia research due to a number of advantages. With the help of the CRISPR/Cas9 system, specific mutations of the target ncRNA gene can be introduced into the embryo and the normal form of the ncRNA gene can be restored in a rat or mouse embryo. The rat or mouse as well as its offspring will contain the mutation or restoration of the original form, which allows researchers to compare the symptoms directly, to determine how disruption of these genes affects the development and progression of schizophrenia, and to pinpoint the underlying molecular pathway in those animal models. The generated animal models can also be used to test the efficacy of medications or other potential therapeutic approaches in the treatment of schizophrenia. In fact, the animal model generated by traditional procedures usually takes up to 2 years to get the specific mutations in the offspring because multiple breeding steps are needed, while creating the animal model using the CRISPR/Cas9 approach only requires about 2 months and costs less. Furthermore, in combination with template DNAs and using multiple gRNAs, the CRISPR/Cas9 system is able to introduce a number of desired mutations into the embryo of an animal or their offspring, which is not likely to work out with other previous approaches.

PERSPECTIVE OF EDITING ncRNA GENES WITH CRISPR/Cas9 FOR THE TREATMENT OF SCHIZOPHRENIA

Medications have been the cornerstone therapy for schizophrenia, and medications in combination with psychosocial interventions are widely used to manage schizophrenia. However, medications for schizophrenia usually cause serious adverse side effects; therefore, a large portion of patients with schizophrenia fail to take medications, leading to this devastating mental disease being uncontrolled. As a strong genetic component is involved in the pathogenesis of schizophrenia, multiple alterations in the genomic DNA of neurons have been implicated as causative factors, and fortunately great progress has been recently made in both identifying critical genomic regions and developing advanced genetic technologies, multiple alterations may be manipulated in the genomic DNA of neurons. As we discussed earlier, the genetic mutations in both miRNA and lncRNA genes have been directly linked to schizophrenia. The CRISPR/Cas9 system has provided a valuable tool to correct mutations not only in inheritable genetic diseases but also gene mutations in DNA genomes related to diseases, including ncRNAs genes. The CRISPR/Cas9 system, together with a donor DNA template, is required and delivered together with the CRISPR/Cas9 system into the recipients, and it has been successfully used to replace the mutations with substitutions in cells, plants, and entire animals to correct certain genomic DNA mutations. For example, a research group from Duke University has recently explored the application of the CRISPR/Cas9 system to treat Duchenne muscular dystrophy (DMD), a genetic disease with a debilitating mutation within one of the exons of the dystrophin gene (Nelson C. E. et al., 2016). For the first time, researchers have successfully treated a human disease in a living mouse model (Nelson C. E. et al., 2016) with the CRISPR/Cas9 gene editing technology. Meanwhile, similar results from two other research groups from Harvard University and the University of Texas are exciting as well (Long et al., 2016; Tabebordbar et al., 2016). These three independent research groups have demonstrated that correction of the dystropin gene, the consequential restoration of functional dystrophin, and the enhancement of muscle strength can be achieved after one of the exons in the dystrophin gene was reverted with the CRISPR/Cas9 technique by using different methods to deliver the CRISPR/Cas9 components (Long et al., 2016; Nelson C. E. et al., 2016; Tabebordbar et al., 2016).

In addition to DMD, a variety of other genetic diseases such as sickle-cell anemia and Alzheimer's disease have been treated with the CRISPR/Cas9 technique by correcting the causative mutations and reverting the defect to the original form in the genomic DNA, and functional restoration has been gained (Huang et al., 2015; Sankaran and Weiss, 2015; Paquet et al., 2016). Recently, a research team from Sun-Yatsen University in Guangzhou, China, has explored, for the first time, the utilization of this novel CRISPR/Cas9 system to edit the thalassemia-causing gene in human embryos (Liang et al., 2015; Callaway, 2016). As a result, a number of human embryos have successfully gained the corrected form of the target gene. More recently, the successful application of the CRISPR/Cas9 gene editing technique to human induced pluripotent stem cells (IPSCs) have been reported to generate disease model (Horii et al., 2013) and to treat effectively a number of diseases, including epi-dermolysis bullosa (Osborn et al., 2013), b-thalassemia (Ma et al., 2013), a1-antitrypsin deficiency (Choi et al., 2013), AIDS (Ye et al., 2014), and Niemann-Pick Type C (Maetzel et al., 2014), DMD (Li et al., 2014). Therefore, this novel approach has provided enormous promise for gene therapy of many other forms of diseases including schizophrenia.

Despite the use of genome editing technologies including zinc finger nucleases, TALENS, and CRISPR/Cas9 has opened up the possibility of *in vivo* genome editing therapy. Unlike peripheral nerve disorder such as DMD, brain and mental disorders (i.e., Parkinson's disease and schizophrenia) have a unique challenge in clinical settings. AAVs vectors, which have been recently approved by FDA for a clinical use, have effectively delivered the nucleases and other components to a variety of tissues including brain. Compared to the other genome editing approaches, the gRNA sequence used in the CRISPR/Cas9 system is more easily to be altered than for TALEs, and a much shorter gRNA and multiple gRNAs can be used to result in multiple DNA cuts (Hsu et al., 2014; Cox et al., 2015) suggesting more promising for the use of CRISPR/Cas9 as a potential therapeutic intent. Most recently, Deverman et al. (2016) reported that they developed a harmless virus, namely AAV-PHP.B, to across the blood brain barrier to successfully deliver treatment to the brain.

These exciting results in living mammals and human cells show great potential for treating human diseases by translating this CRISPR/Cas9 system to a novel therapeutic approach to treat genetically related diseases in humans, including schizophrenia and perhaps other genetically related mental disorders due to the overlapping genetic alterations of schizophrenia with other mental illnesses.

CHALLENGES AND FUTURE DIRECTIONS

Despite the remarkable progress, the CRISPR/Cas9 system is still immature and has some limitations and challenges to overcome. Technical improvement is needed, while ethical issues require resolution as well. There are a couple of technical challenges, including specificity, efficiency of the system and penetration of the blood-brain barrier for delivery of the components in the

CRISPR/Cas9 system. When a potential therapeutic approach to treat brain and mental disorders is discovered, the blood-brain barrier always poses an obstacle for the drugs to reach the brain cells. The components themselves in the CRISPR/Cas9 system cannot pass through the blood-brain barrier. In an effort to deliver the CRISPR/Cas9 components, a few inactive genetically engineered viruses have been successfully used as a carrier that can be packed with the CRISPR/Cas9 components, cross the blood-brain barrier, and finally unload those molecules in the brain cells. In spite of having no capacity to cause disease, further improvement of the efficiency and the evaluation of long-term safety are needed. In addition to the above-mentioned technical concerns, there are ethical issues as well for manipulating genomic DNA in human sperm, eggs and embryos, mainly because of limited knowledge regarding the CRISPR/Cas9 system and the long-term impact of genetic disruption and off-targeting on future generations (Krishan et al., 2016). To date, ncRNAs have not been reported to express proteins; Nelson B. R. et al. (2016) have recently reported that a lnRNA encodes a peptide with the ability to enhance SERCA activity in muscle. With the possibility of unidentified proteins being translated by ncRNAs, it is uncertain whether the proteins may exert any unfavorable, even disease-related activity. All of these new questions require answers; therefore, along with other issues, there is still a long way to go before this revolutionary technology is translated into a clinical cure for schizophrenia and possibly other mental diseases as well due to significant overlaps of the risk genes shared by different forms of psychiatric disorders.

AUTHOR CONTRIBUTIONS

CZ: conceptional design and writing of the draft manuscript. WH: conceptional design and writing of the final manuscript. LH, CL, CC and XL collected and examined the enrolled articles in this review.

FUNDING

This review was funded by Jiangsu Haosen pharmaceutical Limited by Share Ltd (2016-Young scholar support project to CZ).

REFERENCES

Aparicio-Prat, E., Arnan, C., Sala, I., Bosch, N., Guigó, R., and Johnson, R. (2015). DECKO: single-oligo, dual-CRISPR deletion of genomic elements including long non-coding RNAs. *BMC Genomics* 16:846. doi: 10.1186/s12864-015-2086-z

Barry, G., Briggs, J. A., Vanichkina, D. P., Poth, E. M., Beveridge, N. J., Ratnu, V. S., et al. (2014). The long non-coding RNA Gomafu is acutely regulated in response to neuronal activation and involved in schizophrenia-associated alternative splicing. *Mol. Psychiatry* 19, 486–494. doi: 10.1038/mp.2013.45

Bartel, D. P. (2004). MicroRNAs: genomics, biogenesis, mechanism and function. *Cell* 116, 281–297. doi: 10.1016/S0092-8674(04)00045-5

Bartel, D. P. (2009). MicroRNAs: target recognition and regulatory functions. *Cell* 136, 215–233. doi: 10.1016/j.cell.2009.01.002

Beveridge, N. J., and Cairns, M. J. (2012). MicroRNA dysregulation in schizophrenia. *Neurobiol. Dis.* 46, 263–271. doi: 10.1016/j.nbd.2011.12.029

Bhaya, D., Davison, M., and Barrangou, R. (2011). CRISPR-Cas systems in bacteria and archaea: versatile small RNAs for adaptive defense and regulation. *Annu. Rev. Genet.* 45, 273–297. doi: 10.1146/annurev-genet-110410-132430

Blackshaw, S., Harpavat, S., Trimarchi, J., Cai, L., Huang, H., Kuo, W. P., et al. (2004). Genomic analysis of mouse retinal development. *PLoS Biol.* 2:E247. doi: 10.1371/journal.pbio.0020247

Callaway, E. (2016). Gene-editing research in human embryos gains momentum. *Nature* 532, 289–290. doi: 10.1038/532289a

Cardno, A. G., Marshall, E. J., Coid, B., Macdonald, A. M., Ribchester, T. R., Davies, N. J., et al. (1999). Heritability estimates for psychotic disorders: the Maudsley twin psychosis series. *Arch. Gen. Psychiatry* 56, 162–168. doi: 10.1001/archpsyc.56.2.162

Chang, H., Yi, B., Ma, R., Zhang, X., Zhao, H., and Xi, Y. (2016). CRISPR/cas9, a novel genomic tool to knock down microRNA *in vitro* and *in vivo*. *Sci. Rep.* 6:22312. doi: 10.1038/srep22312

Cho, S. W., Kim, S., Kim, J. M., and Kim, J. S. (2013). Targeted genome engineering in human cells with the Cas9 RNA-guided endonuclease. *Nat. Biotechnol.* 31, 230–232. doi: 10.1038/nbt.2507

Choi, S. M., Kim, Y., Shim, J. S., Park, J. T., Wang, R. H., Leach, S. D., et al. (2013). Efficient drug screening and gene correction for treating liver disease using patient-specific stem cells. *Hepatology* 57, 2458–2468. doi: 10.1002/hep.26237

Chung, D. W., Volk, D. W., Arion, D., Zhang, Y., Sampson, A. R., and Lewis, D. A. (2016). Dysregulated ErbB4 splicing in schizophrenia: selective effects on parvalbumin expression. *Am. J. Psychiatry* 173, 60–68. doi: 10.1176/appi.ajp.2015.15020150

Cong, L., Ran, F. A., Cox, D., Lin, S., Barretto, R., Habib, N., et al. (2013). Multiplex genome engineering using CRISPR/Cas systems. *Science* 339, 819–823. doi: 10.1126/science.1231143

Costain, G., McDonald-McGinn, D. M., and Bassett, A. S. (2013). Prenatal genetic testing with chromosomal microarray analysis identifies major risk variants for schizophrenia and other later-onset disorders. *Am. J .Psychiatry* 170:1498. doi: 10.1176/appi.ajp.2013.13070880

Cox, D. B. T., Platt, R. J., and Zhang, F. (2015). Therapeutic genome editing: prospects and challenges. *Nat. Med.* 21, 121–131. doi: 10.1038/nm.3793

Deverman, B. E., Pravdo, P. L., Simpson, B. P., Kumar, S. R., Chan, K. Y., Banerjee, A., et al. (2016). Cre-dependent selection yields AAV variants for widespread gene transfer to the adult brain. *Nat. Biotechnol.* 34, 204–209. doi: 10.1038/nbt.3440

Doudna, J. A., and Charpentier, E. (2014). Genome editing. The new frontier of genome engineering with CRISPR-Cas9. *Science* 346:1258096. doi: 10.1126/science.1258096

Fatica, A., and Bozzoni, I. (2014). Long non-coding RNAs: new players in cell differentiation and development. *Nat. Rev. Genet.* 15, 7–21. doi: 10.1038/nrg3606

Franke, B., Stein, J. L., Ripke, S., Anttila, V., Hibar, D. P., van Hulzen, K. J., et al. (2016). Genetic influences on schizophrenia and subcortical brain volumes: large-scale proof of concept. *Nat. Neurosci.* 19, 420–431. doi: 10.1038/nn.4228

Giacomotto, J., Carroll, A. P., Rinkwitz, S., Mowry, B., Cairns, M. J., and Becker, T. S. (2016). Developmental suppression of schizophrenia-associated miR-137 alters sensorimotor function in zebrafish. *Transl. Psychiatry* 6:e818. doi: 10.1038/tp.2016.88

Gilbert, L. A., Larson, M. H., Morsut, L., Liu, Z., Brar, G. A., Torres, S. E., et al. (2013). CRISPR-mediated modular RNA-guided regulation of transcription in eukaryotes. *Cell* 154, 442–451. doi: 10.1016/j.cell.2013.06.044

Giraldez, A. J., Cinalli, R. M., Glasner, M. E., Enright, A. J., Thomson, J. M., Baskerville, S., et al. (2005). MicroRNAs regulate brain morphogenesis in zebrafish. *Science* 308, 833–838. doi: 10.1126/science.1109020

Guan, F., Zhang, B., Yan, T., Li, L., Liu, F., Li, T., et al. (2014). MIR137 gene and target gene CACNA1C of miR-137 contribute to schizophrenia susceptibility in Han Chinese. *Schizophr. Res.* 152, 97–104. doi: 10.1016/j.schres.2013.11.004

Han, J., Zhang, J., Chen, L., Shen, B., Zhou, J., Hu, B., et al. (2014). Efficient *in vivo* deletion of a large imprinted lncRNA by CRISPR/Cas9. *RNA Biol.* 11, 829–835. doi: 10.4161/rna.29624

Hilton, I. B., D'Ippolito, A. M., Vockley, C. M., Thakore, P. I., Crawford, G. E., Reddy, T. E., et al. (2015). Epigenome editing by a CRISPR-Cas9-based acetyltransferase activates genes from promoters and enhancers. *Nat. Biotechnol.* 33, 510–517. doi: 10.1038/nbt.3199

Ho, T. T., Zhou, N., Huang, J., Koirala, P., Xu, M., Fung, R., et al. (2015). Targeting non-coding RNAs with the CRISPR/Cas9 system in human cell lines. *Nucleic Acids Res.* 43:e17. doi: 10.1093/nar/gku1198

Horii, T., Tamura, D., Morita, S., Kimura, M., and Hatada, I. (2013). Generation of an ICF syndrome model by efficient genome editing of human induced pluripotent stem cells using the CRISPR system. *Int. J. Mol. Sci.* 14, 19774–19781. doi: 10.3390/ijms141019774

Hsu, P. D., Lander, E. S., and Zhang, F. (2014). Development and applications of CRISPR-Cas9 for genome engineering. *Cell* 157, 1262–1278. doi: 10.1016/j.cell.2014.05.010

Huang, X., Wang, Y., Yan, W., Smith, C., Ye, Z., Wang, J., et al. (2015). Production of gene-corrected adult beta globin protein in human erythrocytes differentiated from patient iPSCs after genome editing of the sickle point mutation. *Stem Cells* 3, 1470–1479. doi: 10.1002/stem.1969

International Schizophrenia Consortium, Purcell, S. M., Wray, N. R., Stone, J. L., Visscher, P. M., O'Donovan, M. C., et al. (2009). Common polygenic variation contributes to risk of schizophrenia and bipolar disorder. *Nature* 460, 748–752. doi: 10.1038/nature08185

Ishii, N., Ozaki, K., Sato, H., Mizuno, H., Saito, S., Takahashi, A., et al. (2006). Identification of a novel non-coding RNA, MIAT, that confers risk of myocardial infarction. *J. Hum. Genet.* 51, 1087–1099. doi: 10.1007/s10038-006-0070-9

Jiang, W., Bikard, D., Cox, D., Zhang, F., and Marraffini, L. A. (2013). RNA-guided editing of bacterial genomes using CRISPR-Cas systems. *Nat. Biotechnol.* 31, 233–239. doi: 10.1038/nbt.2508

Jinek, M., Chylinski, K., Fonfara, I., Hauer, M., Doudna, J. A., and Charpentier, E. (2012). A programmable dual-RNA-guided DNA endonuclease in adaptive bacterial immunity. *Science* 337, 816–821. doi: 10.1126/science.1225829

Kos, A., Aschrafi, A., and Nadif Kasri, N. (2015). The multifarious hippocampal functions of microRNA-137. *Neuroscientist* 22, 440–446. doi: 10.1177/1073858415608356

Krichevsky, A. M., King, K. S., Donahue, C. P., Khrapko, K., and Kosik, K. S. (2003). A microRNA array reveals extensive regulation of microRNAs during brain development. *RNA* 9, 1274–1281. doi: 10.1261/rna.5980303

Krishan, K., Kanchan, T., and Singh, B. (2016). Human genome editing and ethical considerations. *Sci. Eng. Ethic.* 22, 597–599. doi: 10.1007/s11948-015-9675-8

Kuswanto, C. N., Sum, M. Y., Qiu, A., Sitoh, Y. Y., Liu, J., and Sim, K. (2015). The impact of genome wide supported microRNA-137 (MIR137) risk variants on frontal and striatal white matter integrity, neurocognitive functioning and negative symptoms in schizophrenia. *Am. J. Med. Genet. B Neuropsychiatr. Genet.* 168B, 317–326. doi: 10.1002/ajmg.b.32314

Lett, T. A., Chakravarty, M. M., Felsky, D., Brandl, E. J., Tiwari, A. K., Goncalves, V. F., et al. (2013). The genome-wide supported microRNA-137 variant predicts phenotypic heterogeneity within schizophrenia. *Mol. Psychiatry* 18, 443–450. doi: 10.1038/mp.2013.17

Liang, P., Xu, Y., Zhang, X., Ding, C., Huang, R., Zhang, Z., et al. (2015). CRISPR/Cas9-mediated gene editing in human tripronuclear zygotes. *Protein Cell* 6, 363–372. doi: 10.1007/s13238-015-0153-5

Li, X., Li, Y., Zhao, L., Zhang, D., Yao, X., Zhang, H., et al. (2014). Circulating Muscle-specific miRNAs in Duchenne muscular dystrophy patients. *Mol. Ther. Nucleic Acids.* 3:e177. doi: 10.1038/mtna.2014.29

Liao, J., He, Q., Li, M., Chen, Y., Liu, Y., and Wang, J. (2016). LncRNA MIAT: myocardial infarction associated and more. *Gene* 578, 158–161. doi: 10.1016/j.gene.2015.12.032

Long, C., Amoasii, L., Mireault, A. A., McAnally, J. R., Li, H., Sanchez-Ortiz, E., et al. (2016). Postnatal genome editing partially restores dystrophin expression in a mouse model of muscular dystrophy. *Science* 351, 400–403. doi: 10.1126/science.aad5725

Ma, N., Liao, B., Zhang, H., Wang, L., Shan, Y., Xue, Y., et al. (2013). Transcription activator-like effector nuclease (TALEN)-mediated gene correction in integration-free b-thalassemia induced pluripotent stem cells. *J. Biol. Chem.* 288, 34671–34679. doi: 10.1074/jbc.M113.496174

Ma, G., Yin, J., Fu, J., Luo, X., Zhou, H., Tao, H., et al. (2014). Association of a miRNA-137 polymorphism with schizophrenia in a Southern Chinese Han population. *Biomed Res. Int.* 2014:751267. doi: 10.1016/j.schres.2007.12.348

Maetzel, D., Sarkar, S., Wang, H., Abi-Mosleh, L., Xu, P., Cheng, A. W., et al. (2014). Genetic and chemical correction of cholesterol accumulation and impaired autophagy in hepatic and neural cells derived from Niemann-Pick Type C patient-specific iPS cells. *Stem Cell Reports* 2, 866–880. doi: 10.1016/j.stemcr.2014.03.014

Mali, P., Yang, L., Esvelt, K. M., Aach, J., Guell, M., DiCarlo, J. E., et al. (2013). RNA-guided human genome engineering via Cas9. *Science* 339, 823–826. doi: 10.1126/science.1232033

Marenco, S., and Weinberger, D. R. (2000). The neurodevelopmental hypothesis of schizophrenia: following a trail of evidence from cradle to grave. *Dev. Psychopathol.* 12, 501–527. doi: 10.1017/s0954579400003138

Mellios, M., and Sur, M. (2012). The emerging role of microRNAs in schizophrenia and autism spectrum disorders. *Front. Psychiatry.* 3:39. doi: 10.3389/fpsyt.2012.00039

Merelo, V., Durand, D., Lescallette, A. R., Vrana, K. E., Hong, L. E., Faghihi, M. A., et al. (2015). Associating schizophrenia, long non-coding RNAs and neurostructural dynamics. *Front. Mol. Neurosci.* 8:57. doi: 10.3389/fnmol.2015.00057

Nelson, C. E., Hakim, C. H., Ousterout, D. G., Thakore, P. I., Moreb, E. A., Castellanos Rivera, R. M., et al. (2016). *In vivo* genome editing improves muscle function in a mouse model of Duchenne muscular dystrophy. *Science* 351, 403–407. doi: 10.1126/science.aad5143

Nelson, B. R., Makarewich, C. A., Anderson, D. M., Winders, B. R., Troupes, C. D., Wu, F., et al. (2016). A peptide encoded by a transcript annotated as long noncoding RNA enhances SERCA activity in muscle. *Science* 351, 271–275. doi: 10.1126/science.aad4076

Nudelman, A. S., DiRocco, D. P., Lam-bert, T. J., Garelick, M. G., Le, J., Nathanson, N. M., et al. (2010). Neuronal activity rapidly induces transcription of the CREB- regulated microRNA-132, *in vivo*. *Hippocampus.* 20, 492–498. doi: 10.1002/hipo.20646

Olde Loohuis, N. F., Ba, W., Stoerchel, P. H., Kos, A., Jager, A., Schratt, G., et al. (2015). MicroRNA-137 controls AMPA-receptor-mediated transmission and mGluR-dependent LTD. *Cell Rep.* 11, 1876–1884. doi: 10.1016/j.celrep.2015.05.040

Osborn, M. J., Starker, C. G., McElroy, A. N., Webber, B. R., Riddle, M. J., Xia, L., et al. (2013). TALEN-based gene correction for epidermolysis bullosa. *Mol. Ther.* 21, 1151–1159. doi: 10.1038/mt.2013.56

Owen, M. J., Sawa, A., and Mortensen, P. B. (2016). Schizophrenia. *Lancet* 388, 86–97. doi: 10.1016/S0140-6736(15)01121-6

Paquet, D., Kwart, D., Chen, A., Sproul, A., Jacob, S., Teo, S., et al. (2016). Efficient introduction of specific homozygous and heterozygous mutations using CRISPR/Cas9. *Nature* 533, 125–129. doi: 10.1038/nature17664

Ponting, C. P., Oliver, P. L., and Reik, W. (2009). Evolution and functions of long noncoding RNAs. *Cell* 136, 629–641. doi: 10.1016/j.cell.2009.02.006

Rao, S. Q., Hu, H. L., Ye, N., Shen, Y., and Xu, Q. (2015). Genetic variants in long non-coding RNA MIAT contribute to risk of paranoid schizophrenia in a Chinese Han population. *Schizophr. Res.* 166, 125–130. doi: 10.1016/j.schres.2015.04.032

Rapicavoli, N. A., Poth, E. M., and Blackshaw, S. (2010). The long noncoding RNA RNCR2 directs mouse retinal cell specification. *BMC Dev. Biol.* 10:49. doi: 10.1186/1471-213x-10-49

Rose, E. J., Morris, D. W., Fahey, C., Cannon, D., McDonald, C., Scanlon, C., et al. (2014). The miR-137 schizophrenia susceptibility variant rs1625579 does not predict variability in brain volume in a sample of schizophrenic patients and healthy individuals. *Am. J. Med. Genet. B Neuropsychiatr. Genet.* 165B, 467–471. doi: 10.1002/ajmg.b.32249

Sankaran, V. G., and Weiss, M. J. (2015). Anemia: progress in molecular mechanisms and therapies. *Nat. Med.* 21, 221–230. doi: 10.1038/nm.3814

Schizophrenia Psychiatric Genome-Wide Association Study (GWAS) Consortium. (2011). Genome-wide association study identifies five new schizophrenia loci. *Nat. Genet.* 43, 969–976. doi: 10.1038/ng.940

Schratt, G. M., Tuebing, F., Nigh, E. A., Kane, C. G., Sabatini, M. E., Kiebler, M., et al. (2006). A brain-specific microRNA regulates dendritic spine development. *Nature* 439, 283–289. doi: 10.1038/nature04367

Sempere, L. F., Freemantle, S., Pitha-Rowe, I., Moss, E., Dmitrovsky, E., and Ambros, V. (2004). Expression profiling of mammalian microRNAs uncovers a subset of brain-expressed microRNAs with possible roles in murine and human neuronal differentiation. *Genome Biol.* 5:R13. doi: 10.1186/gb-2004-5-3-r13

Siegert, S., Seo, J., Kwon, E. J., Rudenko, A., Cho, S., Wang, W., et al. (2015). The schizophrenia risk gene product miR-137 alters presynaptic plasticity. *Nat. Neurosci.* 18, 1008–1016. doi: 10.1038/nn.4023

Smalheiser, N. R., and Lugli, G. (2009). microRNA regulation of synaptic plasticity. *Neuromolecular Med.* 11, 133–140. doi: 10.1007/s12017-009-8065-2

Sone, M., Hayashi, T., Tarui, H., Agata, K., Takeichi, M., and Nakagawa, S. (2007). The mRNA-like noncoding RNA Gomafu constitutes a novel nuclear domain in a subset of neurons. *J. Cell Sci.* 120, 2498–2506. doi: 10.1242/jcs.009357

Strazisar, M., Cammaerts, S., van der Ven, K., Forero, D. A., Lenaerts, A. S., Nordin, A., et al. (2015). MIR137 variants identified in psychiatric patients affect synaptogenesis and neuronal transmission gene sets. *Mol. Psychiatry* 20, 472–481. doi: 10.1038/mp.2014.53

Tabebordbar, M., Zhu, K., Cheng, J. K., Chew, W. L., Widrick, J. J., Yan, W. X., et al. (2016). *In vivo* gene editing in dystrophic mouse muscle and muscle stem cells. *Science* 351, 407–411. doi: 10.1126/science.aad5177

Tognini, P., Putignano, E., Coatti, A., and Pizzorusso, T. (2011). Experience-dependent expression of miR-132 regulates ocular dominance plasticity. *Nat. Neurosci.* 14, 1237–1239. doi: 10.1038/nn.2920

Vallès, A., Martens, G. J., De Weerd, P., Poelmans, G., and Aschrafi, A. (2014). MicroRNA-137 regulates a glucocorticoid receptor-dependent signalling network: implications for the etiology of schizophrenia. *J. Psychiatry Neurosci.* 39, 312–320. doi: 10.1503/jpn.130269

Vo, N., Klein, M. E., Varlamova, O., Keller, D. M., Yamamoto, T., Goodman, R. H., et al. (2005). A cAMP-response element binding protein-induced microRNA regulates neuronal morphogenesis. *Proc. Natl. Acad. Sci. U S A* 102, 16426–16431. doi: 10.1073/pnas.0508448102

Wang, S., Li, W., Zhang, H., Wang, X., Yang, G., Zhao, J., et al. (2014). Association of microRNA137 gene polymorphisms with age at onset and positive symptoms of schizophrenia in a Han Chinese population. *Int. J. Psychiatry Med.* 47, 153–168. doi: 10.2190/PM.47.2.f

Wang, J., Wang, Y., Yang, J., and Huang, Y. (2014). microRNAs as novel biomarkers of schizophrenia (Review). *Exp. Ther. Med.* 8, 1671–16766. doi: 10.3892/etm.2014.2014

Wilusz, J. E., Sunwoo, H., and Spector, D. L. (2009). Long noncoding RNAs: functional surprises from the RNA world. *Genes Dev.* 23, 1494–1504. doi: 10.1101/gad.1800909

Wright, C., Calhoun, V. D., Ehrlich, S., Wang, L., Turner, J. A., and Bizzozero, N. I. (2015). Meta gene set enrichment analyses link miR-137-regulated pathways with schizophrenia risk. *Front. Genet.* 6:147. doi: 10.3389/fgene.2015.00147

Wright, C., Gupta, C. N., Chen, J., Patel, V., Calhoun, V. D., Ehrlich, S., et al. (2016). Polymorphisms in MIR137HG and microRNA-137-regulated genes influence gray matter structure in schizophrenia. *Transl. Psychiatry* 6:e724. doi: 10.1038/tp.2015.211

Xiao, A., Wang, Z., Hu, Y., Wu, Y., Luo, Z., Yang, Z., et al. (2013). Chromosomal deletions and inversions mediated by TALENs and CRISPR/Cas in zebrafish. *Nucleic Acids Res.* 41:e141. doi: 10.1093/nar/gkt464

Ye, L., Wang, J., Beyer, A. I., Teque, F., Cradick, T. J., Qi, Z., et al. (2014). Seamless modification of wild-type induced pluripotent stem cells to the natural CCR5Δ32 mutation confers resistance to HIV infection. *Proc. Natl. Acad. Sci. U S A* 111, 9591–9596. doi: 10.1073/pnas.1407473111

Zamore, P. D., Tuschl, T., Sharp, P. A., and Bartel, D. P. (2000). RNAi: double-stranded RNA directs the ATP-dependent cleavage of mRNA at 21 to 23 nucleotide intervals. *Cell* 101, 25–33. doi: 10.1016/S0092-8674(00)80620-0

13

Slitrk Missense Mutations Associated with Neuropsychiatric Disorders Distinctively Impair Slitrk Trafficking and Synapse Formation

*Hyeyeon Kang[1], Kyung Ah Han[1], Seoung Youn Won[2], Ho Min Kim[3], Young-Ho Lee[1], Jaewon Ko[4] and Ji Won Um[1]**

[1] *Department of Physiology and BK21 PLUS Project for Medical Science, Yonsei University College of Medicine, Seoul, Korea,* [2] *Department of Chemistry, Korea Advanced Institute of Science and Technology, Daejeon, Korea,* [3] *Graduate School of Medical Science and Engineering, Korea Advanced Institute of Science and Technology, Daejeon, Korea,* [4] *Department of Biochemistry, College of Life Science and Biotechnology, Yonsei University, Seoul, Korea*

Edited by:
Daniela Tropea, Trinity College, Ireland

Reviewed by:
Chiara Verpelli, Istituto di Neuroscienze (CNR), Italy
Andreas Vlachos, University of Düsseldorf, Germany

***Correspondence:**
Ji Won Um
jiwonum@yuhs.ac

Slit- and Trk-like (Slitrks) are a six-member family of synapse organizers that control excitatory and inhibitory synapse formation by forming *trans*-synaptic adhesions with LAR receptor protein tyrosine phosphatases (PTPs). Intriguingly, genetic mutations of Slitrks have been associated with a multitude of neuropsychiatric disorders. However, nothing is known about the neuronal and synaptic consequences of these mutations. Here, we report the structural and functional effects on synapses of various rare *de novo* mutations identified in patients with schizophrenia or Tourette syndrome. A number of single amino acid substitutions in Slitrk1 (N400I or T418S) or Slitrk4 (V206I or I578V) reduced their surface expression levels. These substitutions impaired glycosylation of Slitrks expressed in HEK293T cells, caused retention of Slitrks in the endoplasmic reticulum and *cis*-Golgi compartment in COS-7 cells and neurons, and abolished Slitrk binding to PTPδ. Furthermore, these substitutions eliminated the synapse-inducing activity of Slitrks, abolishing their functional effects on synapse density in cultured neurons. Strikingly, a valine-to-methionine mutation in Slitrk2 (V89M) compromised synapse formation activity in cultured neuron, without affecting surface transport, expression, or synapse-inducing activity in coculture assays. Similar deleterious effects were observed upon introduction of the corresponding valine-to-methionine mutation into Slitrk1 (V85M), suggesting that this conserved valine residue plays a key role in maintaining the synaptic functions of Slitrks. Collectively, these data indicate that inactivation of distinct cellular mechanisms caused by specific Slitrk dysfunctions may underlie Slitrk-associated neuropsychiatric disorders in humans, and provide a robust cellular readout for the development of knowledge-based therapies.

Keywords: Slitrks, schizophrenia, Tourette's Syndrome, synapse formation, transmembrane protein

INTRODUCTION

Neuropsychiatric disorders such as schizophrenia, autism spectrum disorders (ASDs), and Tourette syndrome usually comprise heterogeneous and complex clinical syndromes with largely unknown etiologies (State, 2011; State and Levitt, 2011). Although epidemiological and descriptive studies have attempted to formulate etiological hypotheses to account for a subset of neuropsychiatric disorders, genetic studies have clearly demonstrated the high heritability of these disorders, albeit with complex inheritance pattern (Heinzen et al., 2015). To further complicate matters, genetic causation can range from a simple point mutation in a single gene to polygenetic causes that enlist an unknown mode of inheritance, incomplete penetrance, variable expressivity, epistasis, and/or etiological heterogeneity (Heinzen et al., 2015). Faced with this daunting challenge, researchers seeking to attain the conceptual advances necessary to design effective and precise therapeutics, critically require a more detailed comprehension of brain function (Insel and Landis, 2013). Rapid advances in human genome sequencing techniques have contributed significantly to the elucidation of candidate genes that are highly associated with a variety of neuropsychiatric disorders (Medland et al., 2014; Heinzen et al., 2015). In particular, large-scale, genome-wide association studies of patients suffering from various neuropsychiatric diseases have identified copy number variants, single-nucleotide polymorphisms and a variety of point mutations (State, 2011; State and Levitt, 2011; Heinzen et al., 2015). Intriguingly, a number of synaptic genes have frequently been identified as susceptibility factors, supporting the well-accepted 'synaptopathy' hypothesis, which posits that distinct synaptic dysfunctions constitute core features of various neuropsychiatric disorders (Brose et al., 2010). Not surprisingly, a host of synaptic adhesion molecules (e.g., neurexins and neuroligins) have been recognized as candidate contributors to various neuropsychiatric disorders, given their central importance in synaptic functions (Sudhof, 2008; Missler et al., 2012; Ko J. et al., 2015). However, how dysfunctions of most synaptic proteins lead to these devastating disorders remains poorly understood. In particular, why identical genetic factors are commonly found in clinically separable neuropsychiatric disorders, a finding that could account for the high comorbidity of a subset of brain disorders (Keezer and Sander, 2016; Keezer et al., 2016), has remained puzzling.

Slit- and Trk-like (Slitrk) proteins constitute a family of leucine-rich repeat (LRR)-containing synaptic adhesion molecules that are highly expressed in the central nervous system (Aruga and Mikoshiba, 2003; Aruga et al., 2003; Beaubien and Cloutier, 2009; de Wit et al., 2011; Ko, 2012). They possess a common structural architecture composed of tandem LRR domains (LRR1 and LRR2), a single transmembrane domain, and a divergent cytoplasmic region (Aruga and Mikoshiba, 2003). Functionally, they control excitatory and inhibitory synapse formation by interacting with LAR-RPTPs (leukocyte common antigen-related receptor protein tyrosine phosphatases, PTP) through the LRR1 domain (Takahashi et al., 2012; Um and Ko, 2013; Yim et al., 2013; Han et al., 2016a; see Um et al., 2014a, for complex structure). Slitrk3 specifically regulates inhibitory synapse development through binding to PTPδ, whereas other Slitrks organize excitatory synapse development through binding to PTPσ (Takahashi et al., 2012; Yim et al., 2013). Like other synaptic adhesion proteins, a subset of Slitrk point mutants have been linked to schizophrenia, ASDs, Tourette syndrome, or obsessive–compulsive disorder (OCD; reviewed in Ko, 2012; Um and Ko, 2013). For example, Slitrk1 has been postulated to be causative for Tourette syndrome (Abelson et al., 2005; Grados and Walkup, 2006), although subsequent studies (Keen-Kim and Freimer, 2006; Chou et al., 2007; Fabbrini et al., 2007; Scharf et al., 2008) have questioned the validity of conclusions reached by these earlier studies (Keen-Kim and Freimer, 2006; Chou et al., 2007; Fabbrini et al., 2007; Scharf et al., 2008). Moreover, several non-synonymous, rare variants of Slitrk1, Slitrk2, and Slitrk4 were recently reported to be associated with schizophrenia or OCD spectrum disorders (Zuchner et al., 2006; Piton et al., 2011; Ozomaro et al., 2013). However, it remains to be determined whether these mutations are functionally significant or represent benign polymorphisms.

Here, we systematically investigated the effects of four Slitrk1, five Slitrk2, and two Slitrk4 missense mutations on biochemical properties, surface transport, ligand-binding activity, and synaptogenic activities in cultured hippocampal neurons. We show that a subset of Slitrk1 (N400I and T418S) and Slitrk4 (V206I and I578V) mutations impair the biochemical and cell-biological properties of the corresponding wild-type (WT) Slitrks, through a common loss-of-function mechanism that basically traps them intracellularly, blocking their surface transport and ligand binding, and abolishing their synapse-promoting activity. By comparison, a Slitrk2 V89M mutation did not alter any of these parameters; instead it acted through a gain-of-function mechanism to compromise the ability of WT Slitrk2 to restore deficits in synapse density observed in Slitrk2-deficient neurons. Intriguingly, the analogous Slitrk1 point mutant (Slitrk1[V85M]) also displayed an impaired ability to rescue synaptogenic deficits in Slitrk1-deficient neurons. Our data reveal the underlying mechanisms by which a subset of Slitrk missense mutations observed in patients with neuropsychiatric disorders induce distinct gain- and loss-of-function phenotypes, and may provide a partial correlation with the clinical phenotypes shown in Slitrk dysfunction-associated disorders.

MATERIALS AND METHODS

In silico Analysis

Previously identified Slitrk missense mutations implicated in neuropsychiatric disorders were analyzed using four different prediction programs. (1) *PolyPhen-2*, available via the Web server[1], predicts the functional significance of an allele replacement from its individual features employing a Naïve Bayes classifier, trained using supervised machine learning. Mutations whose posterior probability scores are associated with estimated false-positive rates (FPR) at or below the first (lower) FPR are predicted to be 'probably damaging'. Mutations with posterior probabilities associated with FPR at or below the second (higher) FPR are predicted to be 'possibly damaging'. Mutations with an estimated FPR above the second (higher) FPR value are classified as 'benign'. (2) *PROVEAN (Protein Variation Effect Analyzer)*, available via the Web server[2], clusters BLAST hits using its CD-HIT module based on a global

[1] http://genetics.bwh.harvard.edu/pph2/

[2] http://provean.jcvi.org/index.php

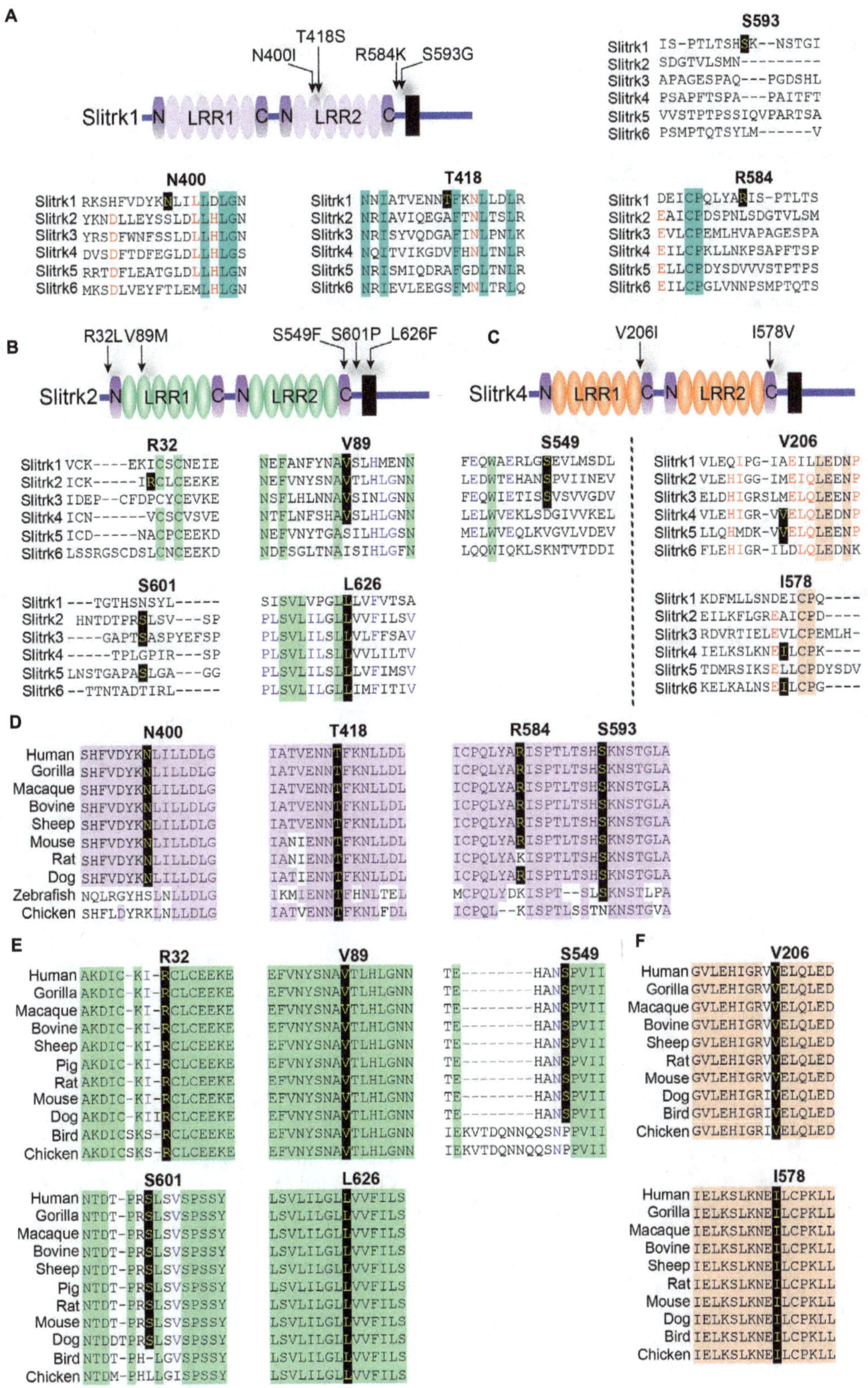

FIGURE 1 | Alignment and conservation across different species of Slitrk1, Slitrk2, and Slitrk4 (Slit- and Trk-like) residues that are mutated in human patients with schizophrenia, Tourette syndrome, or trichotillomania. (A–C) Alignment of human Slitrk amino acids surrounding the mutated residues found in

(Continued)

FIGURE 1 | Continued
human patients with neuropsychiatric disorders. The target mutated resides are indicated in bold. Schematic drawings of the entire domain organization of human Slitrk1 **(A)**, Slitrk2 **(B)**, and Slitrk4 **(C)** are shown. **(D–F)** Similarity or identity of mutated residues investigated in the current study was determined by analyzing the amino acid sequences of human Slitrk1 **(D)**, Slitrk2 **(E)**, and Slitrk4 **(F)** deposited in the National Center for Biotechnology Information (NCBI) database. Identical residues across various species are indicated in yellow letters on a black background. The following GenBank accession numbers were utilized for sequence alignment: Slitrk1/human, NP_443142; Slitrk1/gorilla, XP_004054683; Slitrk1/macaque, NP_001247716; Slitrk1/bovine, XP_002691955; Slitrk1/sheep, XP_004012247; Slitrk1/mouse, EDL00537; Slitrk1/rat, NP_001100753; Slitrk1/dog, XP_542628; Slitrk1/zebrafish, XP_687093; Slitrk1/chicken, XP_416993; Slitrk2/human, NP_001137482; Slitrk2/gorilla, XP_004065021; Slitrk2/macaque, NP_001248149; Slitrk2/bovine, XP_015325702; Slitrk2/sheep, XP_004022343; Slitrk2/pig, XP_013841934; Slitrk2/rat, NP_001101057; Slitrk2/mouse, AAI12407; Slitrk2/dog, XP_013967295; Slitrk2/bird, XP_012428589; Slitrk2/chicken, XP_420364; Slitrk4/human, NP_001171679; Slitrk4/gorilla, XP_004065019; Slitrk4/macaque, XP_001086308; Slitrk4/bovine, XP_005227618; Slitrk4/sheep, XP_004022346; Slitrk4/rat, NP_001100417; Slitrk4/mouse, AAI17892; Slitrk4/dog, XP_005641950; Slitrk4/bird, XP_012428616; and Slitrk4/chicken, XP_015134020.

TABLE 1 | Prediction of functional effect of Slit- and Trk-like (Slitrk) mutations using four different bioinformatics tools.

Gene	amino acid change	Cohort	PolyPhen-2	PROVEAN	Mutation Assessor	PANTHER		Reference
						SubPSEC Score	$P_{deleterious}$	
Slitrk1	V85M	n.a.	Possibly damaging (0.855)	Neutral (−0.968)	Medium (2.31)	n.d.	n.d.	This study
Slitrk1	N400I	TS	Benign (0.162)	Deleterious (−2.943)	Low (1.93)	−2.40948	0.35652	Ozomaro et al., 2013
Slitrk1	T418S	TS	Benign (0.115)	Neutral (−0.274)	Neutral (0.505)	n.d.	n.d.	Ozomaro et al., 2013
Slitrk1	R584K	TTM	Benign (0)	Neutral (0.220)	Neutral (−0.485)	−0.25178	0.06019	Zuchner et al., 2006
Slitrk1	S593G	TTM	Benign (0.014)	Neutral (−1.596)	Medium (2.28)	−1.94135	0.25757	Zuchner et al., 2006
Slitrk2	R32L	SCZ	Benign (0.035)	Neutral (0.487)	Neutral (0.415)	n.d.	n.d.	Piton et al., 2011
Slitrk2	V89M	SCZ	Probably damaging (0.984)	Neutral (−0.932)	Low (1.545)	−2.59958	0.40121	Piton et al., 2011
Slitrk2	S549F	SCZ	Benign (0.203)	Deleterious (−2.957)	Low (0.985)	−3.12094	0.5302	Piton et al., 2011
Slitrk2	S601P	ASD	Benign (0)	Neutral (−0.205)	Neutral (0.5)	−1.47548	0.1788	Piton et al., 2011
Slitrk2	L626F	SCZ	Probably damaging (1)	Deleterious (−2.780)	Medium (1.975)	n.d.	n.d.	Piton et al., 2011
Slitrk4	V206I	SCZ	Probably damaging (0.998)	Neutral (−0.404)	Neutral (0.6)	n.d.	n.d.	Piton et al., 2011
Slitrk4	I578V	SCZ	Benign (0.012)	Neutral (0.173)	Neutral (0.425)	n.d.	n.d.	Piton et al., 2011

ASD, Autism spectrum disorder; n.a., not applicable; n.d., not determined; PANTHER, Protein Analysis Through Evolutionary Relationships; PolyPhen-2, Polymorphism Phenotyping v2; PROVEAN, Protein Variation Effect Analyzer; SCZ, Schizophrenia; SIFT, Sorting Intolerant From Tolerant; TS, Tourette's syndrome; TTM, Trichotillomania.

sequence identity parameter of 75%. The supporting sequence set, representing the top 30 clusters of closely related sequences, is used to generate predictions. For each supporting sequence, a delta alignment score is computed and used to determine the PROVEAN score. If the PROVEAN score is less than or equal to −2.5 (predefined threshold), the protein variant is considered 'deleterious'; variants with scores greater than −2.5 are considered 'neutral'. (3) *MutationAssessor* was automatically run using the Web server[3], as previously described (Reva et al., 2011). (4) *PANTHER (Protein Analysis Through Evolutionary Relationships)*, available through the Web server[4], generates SubPSEC scores, which are continuous values from 0 (neutral) to about −10 (most likely deleterious). A $P_{deleterious}$ value of 0.5 corresponds to a SubPSEC score of −3. The probability that a given variant will cause a deleterious effect on protein function is estimated from $P_{deleterious}$ such that a SubPSEC score of −3 corresponds to a $P_{deleterious}$ of 0.5 (Mi et al., 2016). 'n.d.' in PANTHER indicates that the position does not align to Hidden Markov Model (HMM) libraries.

[3]http://mutationassessor.org/r3/
[4]http://www.pantherdb.org/tools/

Structural Modeling

Structures of human Slitrk2 (LRR1, aa D27–P264; and LRR2, aa S342–P579) and human Slitrk4 (LRR1, aa N28–P64; and LRR2, aa P343–P581) were modeled through the SWISS-MODEL server using human Sltirk1 LRR1 (PDB ID: 4RCA), mouse Slitrk2 LRR1 (PDB ID: 4Y61), and human Slitrk1 LRR2 (PDB ID: 4RCW) as templates. All drawings depicting molecular structures were prepared using PyMOL (PyMOL Molecular Graphics System) (Um et al., 2014a).

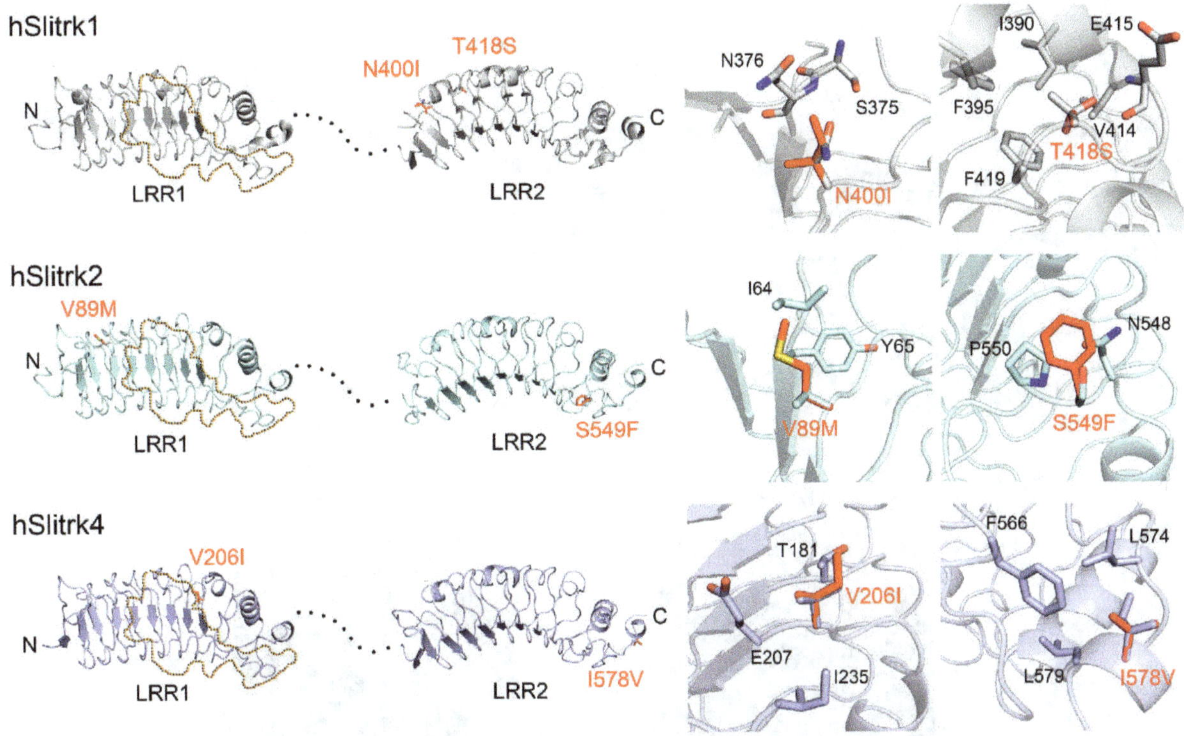

FIGURE 2 | Structural modeling of Slitrk1, Slitrk2, and Slitrk4 residues that are mutated in human patients. Overall structures of LRR1 and LRR2 domains of human Slitrk1, Slitrk2 and Slitrk4 (left). The crystal structure of human Slitrk1 LRR1/human PTPδ Ig1-3 complex (PDB ID: 4RCA) and human Slitrk1 LRR2 (PDB ID: 4RCW) were used for presenting the structures of human Slitrk1 LRR1 and LRR2. The structure of human Slitrk2 and Slitrk4 were modeled with SWISS-MODEL server. The residues corresponding to patients' mutations described in the current study are presented as red sticks in the cartoon presentation. Human Slitrk1, Slitrk2, and Slitrk4 are colored gray, cyan and purple, respectively. Yellow dotted regions in the LRR1 domains of Slitrks indicate the LAR-RPTP binding surfaces based on the 3D structure of the human Slitrk1 LRR1/PTPδ Ig1-3 complex (PDB ID: 4RCA), and black dotted lines represent flexible linkers between LRR1 and LRR2 domains (left). Close-up views of mutated and neighboring residues in LRR domains (right).

Construction of Expression Vectors

pDisplay-Slitrk1 mutants (V85M, N400I, T418S, R584K, S593G), pDisplay-Slitrk2 mutants (R32L, V89M, S549F, S601P, L626F), and pDisplay-Slitrk4 mutants (V206I, I578V) were generated with a site-directed mutagenesis kit (Stratagene) using the corresponding WT pDisplay constructs as templates. The following constructs were previously described: pDisplay-Slitrk1 WT, pDisplay-Slitrk2 WT, pDisplay-Slitrk4 WT, L-315 sh-Slitrk1, L-315 sh-Slitrk2, and L-315 sh-Slitrk4 (Yim et al., 2013); and pVL1393-PTPδ (Um et al., 2014a). The BFP-KDEL vector was purchased from Addgene (construct #49150).

Antibodies

The following antibodies were obtained from the indicated commercial sources: mouse monoclonal anti-HA (clone HA-7; Covance), rabbit polyclonal anti-HA (H6908; Sigma), mouse monoclonal anti-α-tubulin (clone DM1A; Sigma), rabbit polyclonal anti-actin (A2066; Sigma), goat polyclonal anti-EGFP (Rockland), and mouse monoclonal anti-GM130 (clone 35/GM130; BD Transduction Laboratories). The anti-synapsin antibody was previously described (Han et al., 2016b).

Heterologous Synapse-Formation Assay

Heterologous synapse-formation assays were performed using HEK293T cells as previously described (Ko et al., 2009; Um et al., 2014b). In brief, HEK293T cells were cotransfected with EGFP or HA-Slitrk1 WT, HA-Slitrk1 point mutants, HA-Slitrk2 WT, HA-Slitrk2 point mutants, HA-Slitrk4 WT, or HA-Slitrk4 point mutants (described in 'Construction of expression vectors') using the FuGene reagent (Roche). After 48 h, transfected HEK293T cells were trypsinized and seeded onto DIV9 hippocampal neuron cultures. Cells were further cocultured for 72 h and then double-immunostained with anti-HA and anti-synapsin antibodies at DIV12 as described previously (Ko J.S. et al., 2015). All images were acquired with a confocal microscope. For quantifications, the contours of transfected HEK293T cells were chosen as the region of interest. The fluorescence intensity of synapsin puncta normalized to the area of each HEK293T cell was quantified for both red and green channels using MetaMorph Software (Molecular Devices).

Glycosylation Assay

Solubilized proteins from HEK293T cells transfected with expression plasmids for WT or mutant Slitrks, were first denatured by adding 10x denaturing buffer (New England

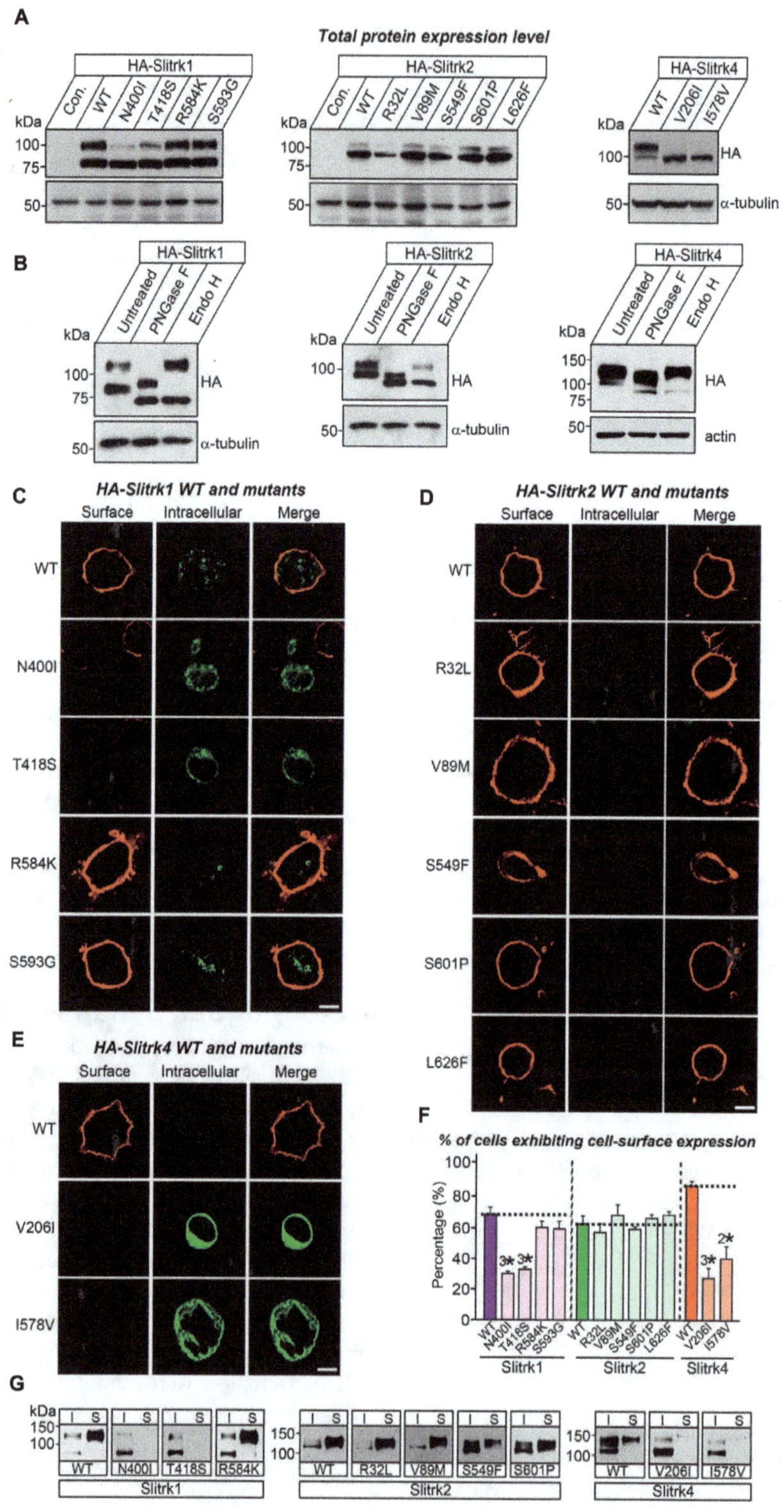

FIGURE 3 | Impaired glycosylation and surface trafficking of a subset of Slitrk mutations. (A) Representative immunoblot images from HEK293T cells transfected with the indicated WT or mutant forms of HA-tagged Slitrk1, Slitrk2, or Slitrk4. Samples containing equal amounts of protein were resolved by SDS-PAGE and immunoblotted using anti-HA antibodies; α-tubulin was used for normalization. Molecular mass markers are labeled in kilodaltons. **(B)** Immunoblot analysis of Endo-H and PNGase F enzyme-digested lysates of HEK293T cells expressing WT HA-tagged Slitrk; α-tubulin or actin was used for normalization. Molecular mass markers are labeled in kilodaltons. **(C–E)** Surface expression analysis of HEK293T cells expressing WT or point mutant forms of HA-tagged Slitrk1

(Continued)

FIGURE 3 | Continued
(C), Slitrk2 **(D)**, or Slitrk4 **(E)**. Transfected cells were immunostained with mouse anti-HA antibodies (red) and detected with Cy3-conjugated anti-mouse secondary antibodies under non-permeabilized conditions, followed by permeabilization of cells. Cells were then stained first with rabbit anti-HA antibodies (green) and then with FITC-conjugated anti-rabbit secondary antibodies. Scale bar, 10 μm (applies to all images). **(F)** Quantification of the proportion of cells exhibiting surface expression of Slitrks. All data are shown as means ± SEMs ($^{2*}p$ < 0.01; $^{3*}p$ < 0.001; ANOVA with *post hoc* Tukey's test; *p*-value of WT Slitrk1 vs Slitrk1[N400I] = 0.000033; *p*-value of WT Slitrk1 vs Slitrk1[T418S] = 0.000065; *p*-value of WT Slitrk1 vs. Slitrk1[R584K] = 0.259; *p*-value of WT Slitrk1 vs. Slitrk1[S593G] = 0.34; *p*-value of WT Slitrk2 vs. Slitrk2[R32L] = 0.941; *p*-value of WT Slitrk2 vs. Slitrk2[V89M] = 0.948; *p*-value of WT Slitrk2 vs. Slitrk2[S549F] = 0.988; *p*-value of WT Slitrk2 vs. Slitrk2[S601P] = 0.997; *p*-value of WT Slitrk2 vs. Slitrk2[L626F] = 0.996; *p*-value of WT Slitrk4 vs. Slitrk4[V206I] = 0.000677; *p*-value of WT Slitrk4 vs. Slitrk4[I578V] = 0.003946). The numbers of cells counted (*n*) were as follows: WT Slitrk1, *n* = 360; Slitrk1[N400I], *n* = 327; Slitrk1[T418S], *n* = 412; Slitrk1[R584K], *n* = 496; Slitrk1[S593G], *n* = 333; WT Slitrk2, *n* = 345; Slitrk2[R32L], *n* = 321; Slitrk2[V89M], *n* = 371; Slitrk2[S549F], *n* = 360; Slitrk2[S601P], *n* = 313; Slitrk2[L626F], *n* = 319; WT Slitrk4, *n* = 256; Slitrk4[V206I], *n* = 181; and Slitrk4[I578V], *n* = 161.
(G) Slitrk surface exposure on transfected HEK293T cells, analyzed by immunoblotting of affinity-purified, surface-biotinylated Slitrk proteins. Biotinylated cell surface proteins (S) and total lysate proteins (I) were assessed by immunoblot with anti-HA antibodies. Input, 5% of total lysates used in biotinylation experiments. Note that mutants of Slitrk1 (N400I and T418S) and Slitrk4 (V206I and I578V) exhibit impaired surface expression, as similarly observed in **(C–F)**.

Biolabs) and heating to 100°C for 10 min. For endoglycosidase H (Endo H) treatment, denatured protein was treated with 1 μl of enzyme and incubated at 37°C for 1 h. For PNGase F treatment, denatured protein was incubated with 1 μl of enzyme in the presence of 2 μl of NP-40 (100%) at 37°C for 1 h. Thereafter, enzyme-treated proteins, together with an equal amount of untreated proteins, were analyzed by immunoblotting with the indicated antibodies followed by enhanced chemiluminescence (ECL) detection.

Biotinylation Assay

Biotinylation experiments in HEK293T cells were performed as previously described (Han et al., 2016b). Briefly, HEK293T cells transfected with the indicated Slitrk plasmids were washed three times with ice-cold PBS containing 1 mM $MgCl_2$ and 1 mM $CaCl_2$. Sulfo-NHS-LC-biotin (1 mg/ml) was then added, and cells were kept at 4°C for 30 min. After incubation, cells were washed three times with PBS plus 100 mM glycine to quench and remove excess biotin. Purified membrane proteins were then incubated with Neutravidin (Thermo Scientific) overnight at 4°C. After three washes with PBS, proteins were eluted with sample buffer and analyzed by immunoblotting.

Primary Neuronal Culture, Transfection, and Immunocytochemistry

Rat hippocampal cultures were prepared from embryonic day 18 (E18) embryos as described previously (Ko et al., 2011; Um et al., 2016). All experimental protocols using pregnant rats were approved by the Institutional Animal Care and Use Committee of Yonsei University College of Medicine. For overexpression, hippocampal neurons were transfected with various Slitrks vector using CalPhos Kit (Clontech) at DIV10 and immunostained at DIV14. For knockdown of Slitrk1, Slitrk2, or Slitrk4, hippocampal neurons were co-transfected with the corresponding L-315 sh-Slitrk vector at DIV8 and immunostained at DIV14, as indicated in the figure legends. For immunocytochemistry, cultured neurons were first fixed with 4% paraformaldehyde/4% sucrose for 10 minutes at room temperature and then permeabilized with 0.2% Triton X-100 in PBS for 5 min at 4°C. Fixed, permeabilized neurons were then blocked by incubating with 3% horse serum/0.1% crystalline grade bovine serum albumin (BSA) in PBS for 30 min at room temperature, and incubated with the indicated primary and secondary antibodies in blocking solution for 1 h each at room temperature.

Neurite Outgrowth Assay

Hippocampal neurons prepared from E18 rat embryo were transfected with WT Slitrk, Slitrk[N400I] or Slitrk[T418S] together with pEGFP-N1 vector at DIV3 and immunostained with anti-EGFP antibodies at DIV6. Fluorescent images of neurons were randomly captured and neurite length was analyzed using MetaMorph software (Molecular Devices).

Confocal Microscopy Image Acquisition and Analysis

Transfected neurons were randomly chosen and acquired at constant imaging settings using a confocal microscope (LSM700; Carl Zeiss) with a 63× objective lens. Z-stack images obtained at 0.1μm intervals by confocal microscopy were converted to maximal projections, and the size and density of presynaptic terminals were analyzed using MetaMorph software. All images were separated into different color channels (red and green), and red-colored images were transformed into an image in grayscale mode using Photoshop (Adobe). After selecting one or two primary dendrites from neurons in a single image frame, dendrite lengths were recorded and dendritic regions of interest were manually traced in MetaMorph software and saved for puncta measurements (in rgn file format). A constant intensity threshold that excluded diffuse nonsynaptic signals but included synaptic signals (90; range, 0–255) was applied to all gray images. The saved dendritic regions were loaded, calibrated, and measured using the 'integrated morphometry analysis' option. The linear density of synapsin clusters was determined from calculated total puncta numbers, normalized to 10 μm length of dendrite. For puncta size and intensity measurements, normalized puncta areas and averaged puncta intensities were calculated and exported automatically to the Excel program (Microsoft). All quantitative analyses were performed in a blinded manner.

Statistics

All data are expressed as means ± SEM. All statistical analyses were performed using SPSS Statistics 23 (IBM, Armonk, NY,

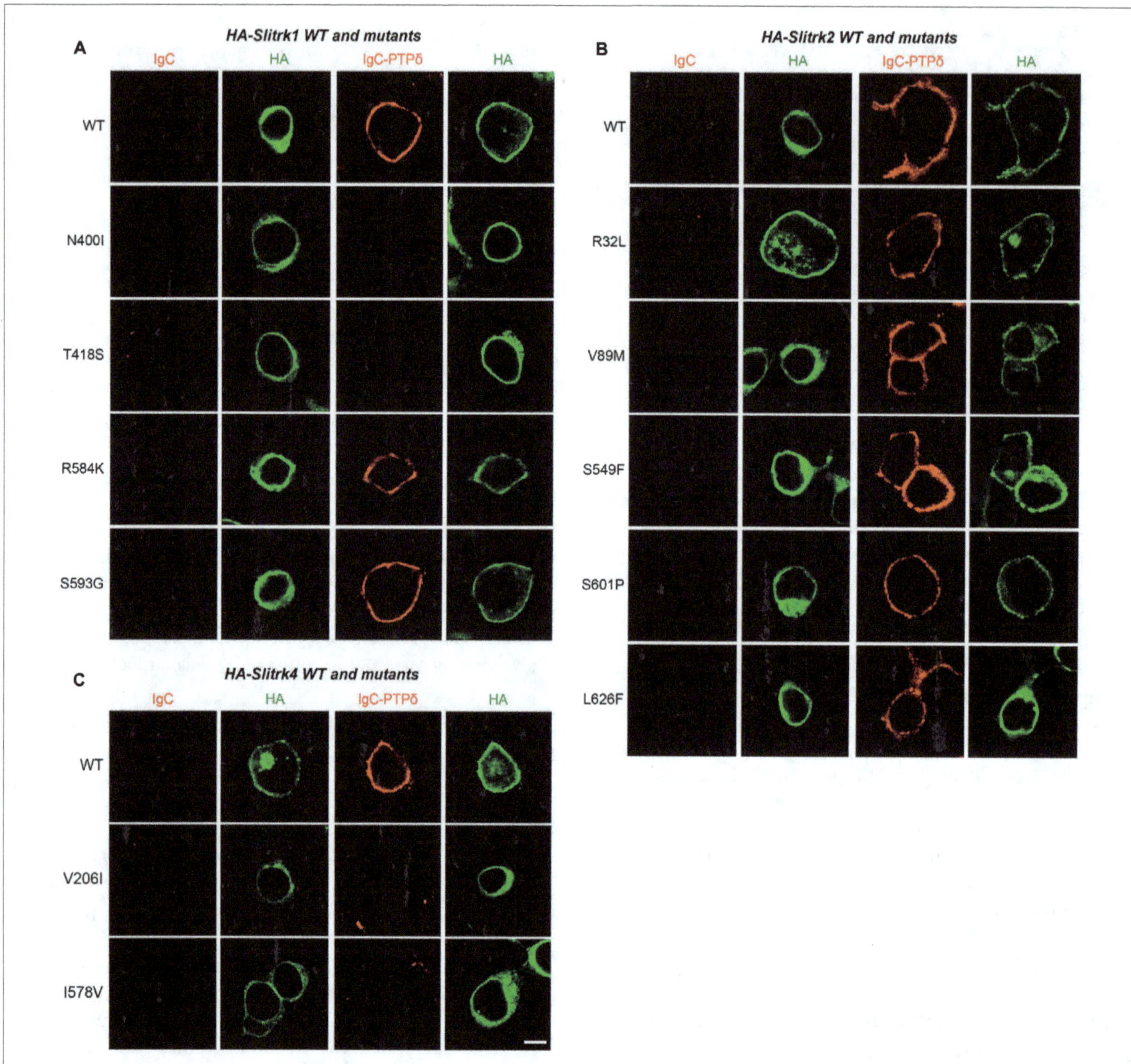

FIGURE 4 | Characterization of LAR-RPTP–binding properties of Slitrk mutations. Representative images of cell-surface–binding assays. HEK293T cells expressing WT or mutant forms of HA-tagged Slitrk1 **(A)**, Slitrk2 **(B)**, or Slitrk4 **(C)** were incubated with 10 μg/ml control IgC or Ig-PTPδ, and then analyzed by immunofluorescence imaging of Ig-fusion proteins (red) and HA antibodies (green). Percentages of the cells exhibiting the binding of Ig-PTPδ were as follows: WT Slitrk1, 66.7%; Slitrk1[N400I], 32%; Slitrk1[T418S], 41%; Slitrk1[R584K], 62%; Slitrk1[S593G], 68.7%; WT Slitrk2, 71%; Slitrk2[R32L], 82%; Slitrk2[V89M], 81%; Slitrk2[S549F], 68.8%; Slitrk2[S601P], 80%; Slitrk2[L626F], 76%; WT Slitrk4, 81%; Slitrk4[V206I], 24%; and Slitrk4[I578V], 22.2%. Note that a subset of Slitrk mutants (Slitrk1[N400I], Slitrk1[T418S], Slitrk4[V206I] and Slitrk4[I578V]) exhibit reduced binding to Ig-PTPδ, paralleling their impaired surface transport (see **Figure 3**). Scale bar, 10 μm (applies to all images).

USA). The normal distribution of the data was investigated by p-values from Kolmogorov-Smirnov test (obtained p-values > 0.05, except the data in **Figures 6C** and **10B**). Thus, these data were statistically evaluated using one-way analysis of variance (ANOVA), using cell numbers (>10) or the number of experiments (>3) as the basis for 'n'. For the **Figures 6C** and **10B,** the data were statistically assessed using a non-parametric Kruskal–Wallis test.

RESULTS

A variety of rare Slitrk point mutations have been found to be associated with schizophrenia or OCD spectrum disorders (Proenca et al., 2011; Ko, 2012; Um and Ko, 2013). Because one of the aims of this study was to evaluate the functional consequences of *SLITRK* gene mutations for neuropsychiatric disorders, we focused on only non-synonymous, missense mutations in this

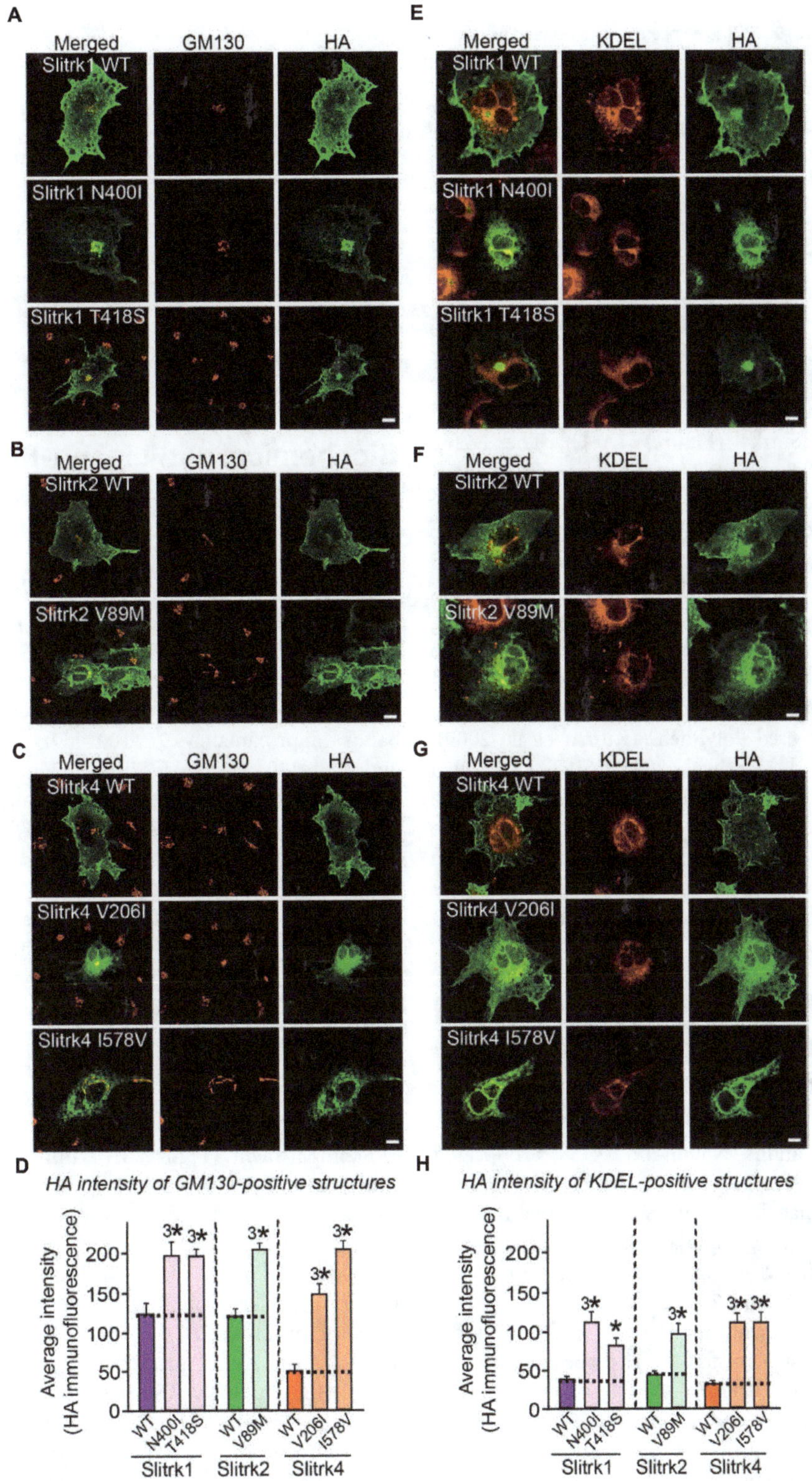

FIGURE 5 | Retention of Slitrk mutant proteins in the *cis*-Golgi and ER in COS-7 cells. (A–C) Immunofluorescence staining of COS-7 cells demonstrates *cis*-Golgi retention of a subset of mutants. COS-7 cells were transfected with WT or mutant forms of HA-tagged Slitrk1 **(A)**, Slitrk2 **(B)**, or Slitrk4 **(C)**, and then stained with anti-HA (green) and anti-GM130 (red) antibodies. Scale bar, 10 μm (applies to all images). **(D)** Quantification of the average intensity of GM130-positive Slitrks. All data are shown as means ± SEMs ($^{3*}p < 0.001$; ANOVA with *post hoc* Tukey's test; *p*-value of WT Slitrk1 vs Slitrk1[N400I] = 0.00053; *p*-value of WT Slitrk1 vs. Slitrk1[T418S] = 0.000383; *p*-value of WT Slitrk2 vs. Slitrk2[V89M] = 1.83943E-7; *p*-value of WT Slitrk4 vs. Slitrk4[V206I] = 8.0637E-9; *p*-value of WT

(Continued)

FIGURE 5 | Continued
Slitrk4 vs. Slitrk4[I578V] = 5.1018E-9). The numbers of cells counted were as follows: WT Slitrk1, $n = 26$; Slitrk1[N400I], $n = 22$; Slitrk1[T418S], $n = 24$; WT Slitrk2, $n = 24$; Slitrk2[V89M], $n = 27$; WT Slitrk4, $n = 19$; Slitrk4[V206I], $n = 22$; and Slitrk4[I578V], $n = 23$. **(E–G)** Immunofluorescence staining of COS-7 cells demonstrates ER retention of mutants. COS-7 cells were transfected with WT or mutant forms of HA-tagged Slitrk1 **(E)**, Slitrk2 **(F)**, or Slitrk4 **(G)**, together with BFP-KDEL (red; pseudo-colored). The cells were then stained with anti-HA (green). Scale bar, 10 μm (applies to all images). **(H)** Quantification of the average intensity of KDEL-positive Slitrks. All data are shown as means ± SEMs (*$p < 0.05$, $^{3*}p < 0.001$; ANOVA with *post hoc* Tukey's test; *p*-value of WT Slitrk1 vs. Slitrk1[N400I] = 0.000093; p-value of WT Slitrk1 vs. Slitrk1[T418S] = 0.036; *p*-value of WT Slitrk2 vs. Slitrk2[V89M] = 0.000712; *p*-value of WT Slitrk4 vs. Slitrk4[V206I] = 0.000257; *p*-value of WT Slitrk4 vs. Slitrk4[I578V] = 0.000458). The numbers of cells counted were as follows: WT Slitrk1, $n = 26$; Slitrk1[N400I], $n = 24$; Slitrk1[T418S], $n = 22$; WT Slitrk2, $n = 17$; Slitrk2[V89M], $n = 23$; WT Slitrk4, $n = 22$; Slitrk4[V206I], $n = 22$; and Slitrk4[I578V], $n = 21$.

study. Eleven missense mutations have previously been reported to be linked to neuropsychiatric disorders (Zuchner et al., 2006; Piton et al., 2011; Ozomaro et al., 2013). These include N400I, T418S, R584K, and S593G in human Slitrk1; R32L, V89M, S549F, S601P, and L626F in human Slitrk2; and V206I and I578V in human Slitrk4 (**Figures 1A–C**). The L626F mutation in human Slitrk2 also exists in other human Slitrks at equivalent positions (**Figure 1B**), but none of the other residues exhibit complete sequence identity across the six Slitrk members (**Figures 1A–C**). Notably, all four mutated residues identified in human Slitrk1 are unique to Slitrk1 (**Figure 1A**). However, most of these residues are quite evolutionarily conserved among various species, implying their possible functional significance (**Figures 1D–F**). To draw inferences regarding the structural and functional importance of these single amino acid substitutions, we employed the widely used PolyPhen2 (Kumar et al., 2009), PANTHER (Thomas and Kejariwal, 2004), SIFT (Adzhubei et al., 2010), and MutationAssessor (Reva et al., 2011) software packages (**Table 1**). Interestingly, none of the Slitrk missense mutations that are the focus of this study were consistently predicted to be either benign or have deleterious impacts on the stability and function of human Slitrks by the four different *in silico* prediction tools (**Table 1**).

Prediction of Structural Phenotypes Produced by Slitrk Missense Mutations, As Reflected in Protein Folding and Three-Dimensional (3D) Structure

Notably, two Slitrk1 mutations (N400I and T418S) are located in the LRR2 domain (**Figure 1A**). Crystal structure of human Slitrk1 LRR2 indicated that the residue N400 of human Slitrk1 forms a weak hydrogen bond with an amino group of the main chain of S375 and a hydroxyl group of the side chain of N376 on the neighboring loop (**Figure 2**). Therefore, mutating N400 to a nonpolar isoleucine (Ile) residue is likely to disrupt these interactions, possibly causing misfolding and aberrant protein trafficking (see below). The side chain of T418 in human Slitrk1 forms a hydrogen bond with a carboxyl group of the main chain of E415 and is involved in hydrophobic interactions with I390, F395, and F419 (**Figure 2**). Thus, a point mutation of T418 to serine (T418S) is also expected to disrupt these hydrophobic interactions. The other Slitrk1 mutations (R584K and S593G) and Slitrk2 mutations (S601P and L626F) are located outside major structural domains, consistent with the results of *in silico* analyses (**Figure 1A; Table 1**). R32L in human Slitrk2 is located immediately preceding the LRR1 domain (i.e., the terminal residue of the signal peptide; **Figure 1A**). Point mutations in human Slitrk2 (V89M or S549F) and human Slitrk4 (V206I or I578V) were predicted to have little effect on the 3D structures of individual Slitrks (**Figure 2**) (Um et al., 2014a).

Biochemical and Ligand-Binding Phenotypes of Disease-Associated Slitrk Missense Mutants

We next investigated the expression levels and intracellular trafficking of Slitrk mutants in non-neuronal cells (**Figure 3**). As is typically observed for numerous glycoproteins (Yim et al., 2013), immunoblot analyses of HEK293T cells transfected with expression vectors for HA-tagged, full-length Slitrks showed that WT Slitrk proteins were detectable as two discrete bands: approximately 75–100 kDa for Slitrk1 and Slitrk2, and 100–110 kDa for Slitrk4 (**Figure 3A**). Total protein expression levels of Slitrk point mutants were comparable to those of the corresponding WT Slitrks (**Figure 3A**). Strikingly, the mature protein levels of a subset of Slitrk1 mutants (N400I and T418S) and Slitrk4 mutants (V206I and I578V) were significantly decreased (**Figure 3A**). The upper band observed in lysates of Slitrk-expressing HEK293T cells represents fully glycosylated mature protein species that are resistant to Endo-H (which cleaves only immature sugars attached in the endoplasmic reticulum, ER) and are presumably presented to the cell surface, whereas the lower band represents glycosylated immature protein species that are sensitive to Endo-H and are undergoing processing in the ER compartment (**Figure 3B**). Immunoblot analyses of WT Slitrks treated with PNGase F, which removes all attached N-linked oligosaccharides, showed a band shift (**Figure 3B**), consistent with a previous report that Slitrks are highly glycosylated (Yim et al., 2013). We next examined the surface and intracellular protein levels of individual WT Slitrks and Slitrk point mutants in HEK293T cells (**Figures 3C–E**). In line with the biochemical data, two Slitrk1 mutants (N400I and T418S) and two Slitrk4 mutants (V206I and I578V), but not the other Slitrk mutants, displayed significantly reduced surface expression levels with complete trapping in intracellular compartment (**Figures 3C–F**). To reaffirm findings of immunofluorescence analyses in HEK293T cells, we performed biotinylation experiments. We found that the same mutations in Slitrk1 (N400I and T418S) and Slitrk4 (V206I and I578V) impaired the surface expression of the corresponding protein (**Figure 3G**). We then performed binding assays between recombinant Ig-fusion proteins of PTPδ (IgC-PTPδ)

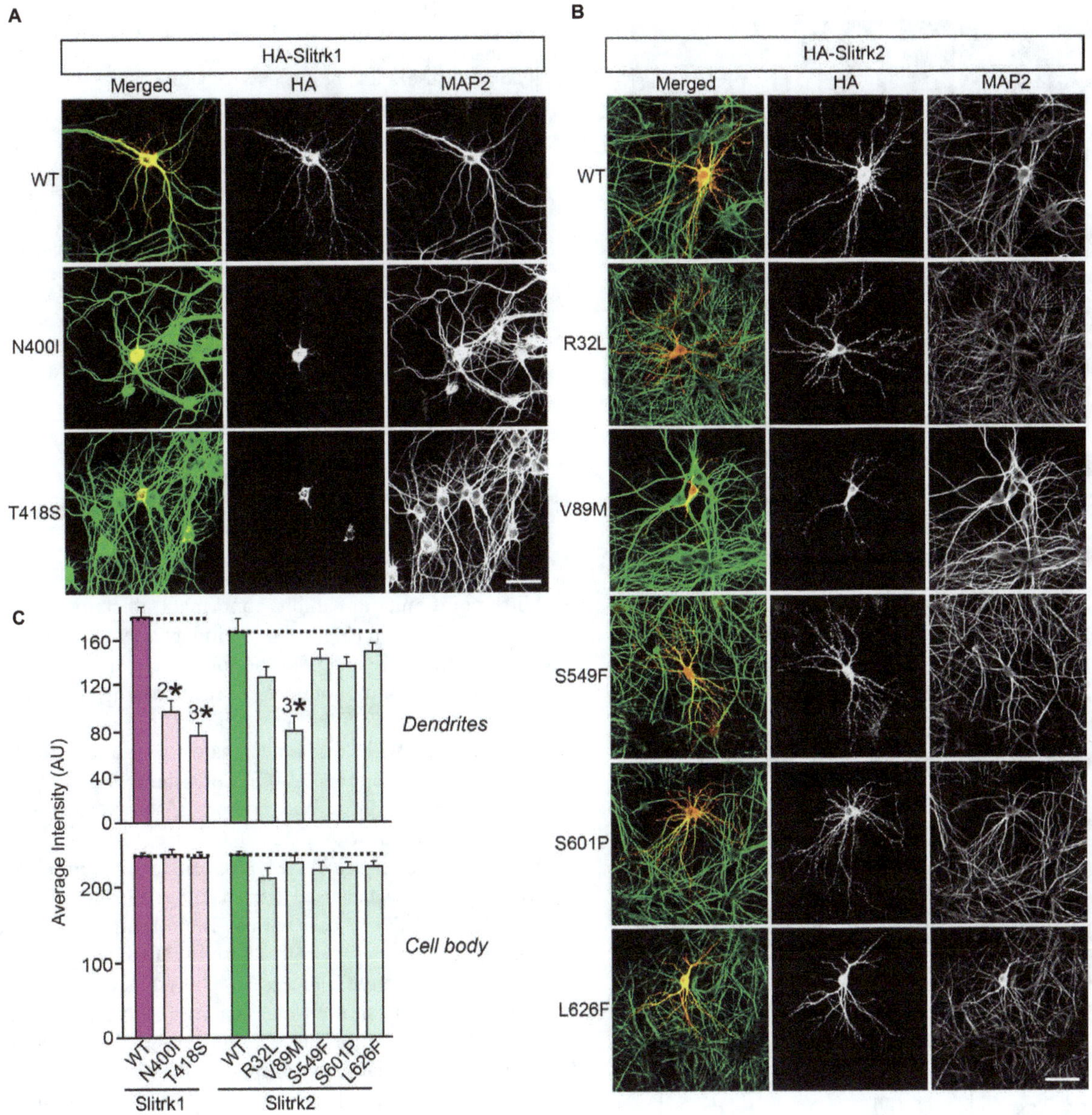

FIGURE 6 | Impaired dendritic targeting of Slitrk1[N400I], Slitrk1[T418S] and Slitrk2[V89M] mutants in cultured hippocampal neurons. **(A–B)** Fluorescence images of hippocampal neurons transfected with wild-type (WT) HA-Slitrk1, HA-Slitrk1[N400I], HA-Slitrk1[T418S], WT HA-Slitrk2, HA-Slitrk2[R32L], HA-Slitrk2[V89M], HA-Slitrk2[S549F], HA-Slitrk2[S601P] or HA-Slitrk2[L626F] at DIV10. The transfected neurons at DIV14 were double-immunostained for antibodies against the somatodendritic marker MAP2 (green) and HA (red). Note that Slitrk1[N400I] and Slitrk1[T418S] are mainly observed in the periphery of soma regions of the transfected neurons, but not in dendritic regions. Meanwhile, Slitrk2[V89M] exhibits decreased dendritic targeting. Scale bar, 50 μm (applies to all images). **(C)** Dendritic targeting of WT HA-Slitrk1, HA-Slitrk1[N400I], HA-Slitrk1[T418S], WT HA-Slitrk2, HA-Slitrk2[R32L], HA-Slitrk2[V89M], HA-Slitrk2[S549F], HA-Slitrk2[S601P], or HA-Slitrk2[L626F] in hippocampal neurons was quantified by measuring average intensity of HA immunofluorescence in primary dendrites. The average intensity of Slitrk WT and mutants in soma region of the transfected neurons was also quantified. All data are shown as means ± SEMs ($^{2*}p < 0.01$; $^{3*}p < 0.001$; a non-parametric Kruskal–Wallis test; *p*-value of WT Slitrk1 vs. Slitrk1[N400I] = 0.001; *p*-value of WT Slitrk1 vs. Slitrk1[T418S] < 0.001; *p*-value of WT Slitrk2 vs. Slitrk2[R32L] = 0.052; *p*-value of WT Slitrk2 vs. Slitrk2[V89M] = 0.000; *p*-value of WT Slitrk2 vs. Slitrk2[S549F] = 0.178; *p*-value of WT Slitrk2 vs. Slitrk2[S601P] = 0.169; *p*-value of WT Slitrk2 vs. Slitrk2[L626F] = 0.284). '*n*' denotes the number of neurons as follows: WT Slitrk1, $n = 16$; Slitrk1[N400I], $n = 19$; Slitrk1[T418S], $n = 16$; WT Slitrk2, $n = 16$; Slitrk2[R32L], $n = 14$; Slitrk2[V89M], $n = 14$; Slitrk2[S549F], $n = 13$; Slitrk2[S601P], $n = 14$; and Slitrk2[L626F], $n = 13$.

and HEK293T cells expressing HA-tagged Slitrks (**Figure 4**). Recombinant IgC-PTPδ robustly bound to HEK293T cells expressing various Slitrk mutants, except those expressing the Slitrk1/4 mutants with impaired surface expression (**Figures 4** and **3C–G**). These data suggest that a subset of Slitrk point mutations observed in neuropsychiatric patients causes improper biochemical processing and abnormal cellular trafficking in non-neuronal cells.

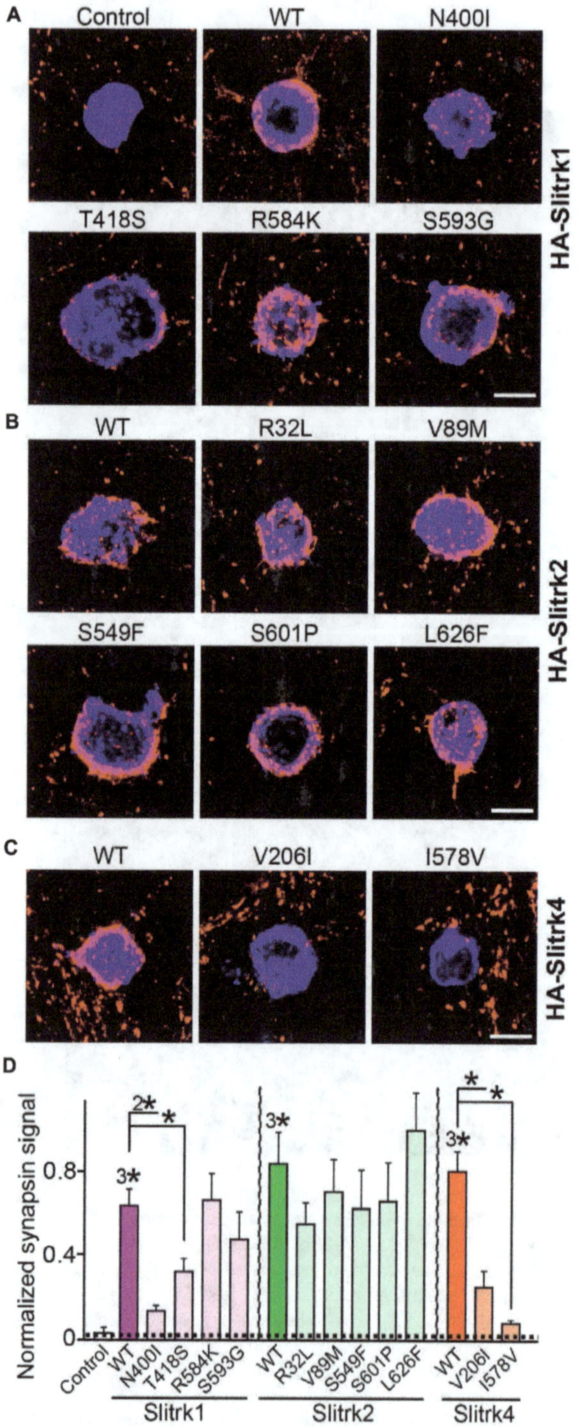

FIGURE 7 | Impaired synaptogenic activity of a subset of Slitrk mutants in cultured hippocampal neurons. (A–C) Representative images of the heterologous synapse-formation activities of WT Slitrk and the indicated point mutants in cultured hippocampal neurons. Neurons were cocultured with HEK293T cells transfected with WT or the indicated mutant forms of HA-Slitrk1 **(A)**, HA-Slitrk2 **(B)**, or HA-Slitrk4 **(C)** at DIV10. Neurons at DIV12 were then immunostained with antibodies against EGFP or HA (blue) and synapsin (red). Scale bar, 10 μm (applies to all images). **(D)** Synapse-formation activity in panels **(A–C)** was quantified by measuring the ratio of synapsin *(Continued)*

FIGURE 7 | Continued
staining intensity (red) to HA/EGFP intensity (blue). All data are shown as means ± SEMs (*$p < 0.05$; 2*$p < 0.01$; 3*$p < 0.001$; ANOVA with *post hoc* Tukey's test; *p*-value of WT Slitrk1 vs. Slitrk1[N400I] = 0.00176; *p*-value of WT Slitrk1 vs. Slitrk1[T418S] = 0.0497; *p*-value of WT Slitrk1 vs. Slitrk1[R584K] = 0.959; *p*-value of WT Slitrk1 vs. Slitrk1[S593G] = 0.434; *p*-value of WT Slitrk2 vs. Slitrk2[R32L] = 0.818; *p*-value of WT Slitrk2 vs. Slitrk2[V89M] = 0.957; *p*-value of WT Slitrk2 vs. Slitrk2[S549F] = 0.956; *p*-value of WT Slitrk2 vs. Slitrk2[S601P] = 0.984; *p*-value of WT Slitrk2 vs. Slitrk2[L626F] = 0.987; *p*-value of WT Slitrk4 vs. Slitrk4[V206I] = 0.00062; and *p*-value of WT Slitrk4 vs. Slitrk4[I578V] = 1.5112E-7). '*n*' denotes the number of HEK293T cells as follows: Control, $n = 14$; WT Slitrk1, $n = 14$; Slitrk1[N400I], $n = 12$; Slitrk1[T418S], $n = 14$; Slitrk1[R584K], $n = 14$; Slitrk1[S593G], $n = 21$; WT Slitrk2, $n = 12$; Slitrk2[R32L], $n = 10$; Slitrk2[V89M], $n = 10$; Slitrk2[S549F], $n = 15$; Slitrk2[S601P], $n = 15$; Slitrk2[L626F], $n = 15$; WT Slitrk4, $n = 17$; Slitrk4[V206I], $n = 13$; and Slitrk4[I578V], $n = 15$.

Cellular Phenotypes of Disease-Associated Slitrk Missense Mutants

The immunocytochemical results clearly indicate that a subset of Slitrk point mutants exhibits abnormal trafficking and decreased surface expression (**Figure 3**). To independently corroborate this interpretation, we analyzed the subcellular distribution of Slitrk mutants using immunofluorescence microscopy (**Figure 5**). First, we transfected COS-7 cells with WT or mutant Slitrks, and stained them with antibodies against HA and GM130 (a *cis*-Golgi marker) (**Figures 5A–C**). Consistent with the biochemical data, a subset of Slitrk mutant proteins showed distinct patterns of colocalization with GM130 (**Figures 5A–C**). The average fluorescence intensity of GM130-positive Slitrk mutant proteins was significantly increased than that of WT (**Figure 5D**). We also cotransfected COS-7 cells with WT and mutant Slitrks, together with a blue fluorescent protein-fused KDEL construct to visualize the ER compartment (**Figures 5E–G**). Again, we found that Slitrk mutant proteins showed overlapping colocalization with BFP-KDEL (**Figure 5H**). These data indicate that Slitrk mutants are in general intracellularly trapped in the *cis*-Golgi and/or ER in non-neuronal cells. To ensure that these Slitrk mutations had a similar effect on the transport of Slitrks out of the ER in neurons, we transfected cultured hippocampal neurons with WT or mutant Slitrks and analyzed them by immunocytochemistry (**Figure 6**). HA-tagged WT Slitrk1 and Slitrk2 were efficiently transported into dendrites, whereas HA-Slitrk1[N400I], HA-Slitrk1[T418S] or HA-Slitrk2[V89M] were either completely retained in the cell body of transfected neurons or displayed markedly impaired trafficking into dendrites (**Figures 6A,B**), as judged by the comparable immunofluorescence signals in the soma of transfected neurons (**Figure 6C**). Notably, other Slitrk2 mutants were targeted to dendrites similarly to Slitrk2 WT (**Figures 6B,C**). These observations suggest that the surface transport deficiency observed in heterologous cells (except for HA-Slitrk2[V89M]) is similarly recapitulated in cultured hippocampal neurons. We were unable to examine the distribution of WT or mutant forms of HA-Slitrk4 because the expression levels of these constructs were too low to be evaluated in this type of analysis.

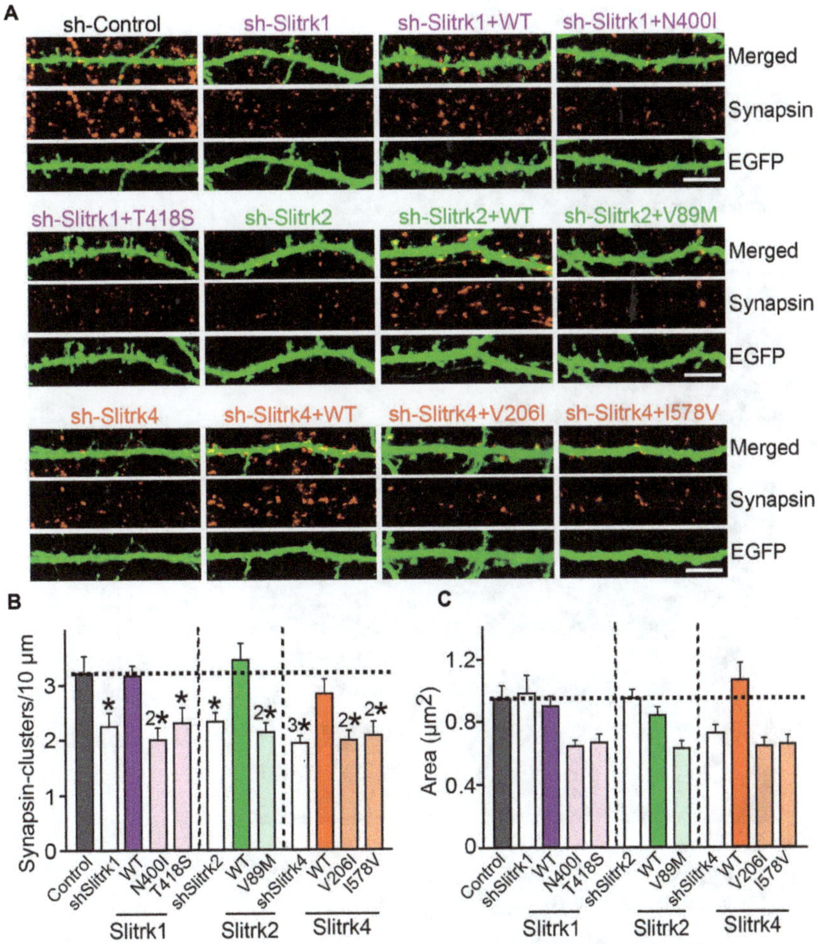

FIGURE 8 | Impaired regulation of synapse density by a subset of Slitrk mutants in cultured hippocampal neurons. (A) Cultured hippocampal neurons were transfected with a lentiviral vector expressing sh-Control, sh-Slitrk1, sh-Slitrk2 or sh-Slitrk4, or coexpressing the indicated sh-Slitrk vector and corresponding shRNA-resistant Slitrk vectors at DIV8 and analyzed at DIV14 by double-immunofluorescence staining with antibodies to EGFP (green) and synapsin (red). Scale bar, 5 μm (applies to all images). **(B,C)** Summary data showing the effects of Slitrk molecular replacement in neurons on synapsin puncta density **(B)** and synapsin puncta size **(C)**. More than three dendrites per transfected neuron were analyzed and group-averaged. All data shown are means ± SEMs ($*p < 0.05$; $^{2*}p < 0.01$; $^{3*}p < 0.001$; ANOVA with *post hoc* Tukey's test; *p*-value of sh-Control vs. sh-Slitrk1 = 0.029; *p*-value of sh-Control vs. sh-Slitrk1+WT Slitrk1 = 0.99; *p*-value of sh-Control vs. sh-Slitrk1+Slitrk1[N400I] = 0.004; *p*-value of sh-Control vs. sh-Slitrk1+Slitrk1[T418S] = 0.049; *p*-value of sh-Control vs. sh-Slitrk2 = 0.039; *p*-value of sh-Control vs. sh-Slitrk2+WT Slitrk2 = 0.99; *p*-value of sh-Control vs. sh-Slitrk2+Slitrk2[V89M] = 0.0093; *p*-value of sh-Control vs. sh-Slitrk4 = 0.00075; *p*-value of sh-Control vs. sh-Slitrk4+WT Slitrk4 = 0.877; *p*-value of sh-Control vs. sh-Slitrk4+Slitrk4[V206I] = 0.003; and *p*-value of sh-Control vs. sh-Slitrk4+Slitrk4[I578V] = 0.008). '*n*' denotes the number of neurons as follows: sh-Control, $n = 16$, sh-Slitrk1, $n = 14$, sh-Slitrk1+WT Slitrk1, $n = 14$; sh-Slitrk1+Slitrk1[N400I], $n = 14$; sh-Slitrk1+Slitrk1[T418S], $n = 14$; sh-Slitrk2, $n = 13$; sh-Slitrk2+WT Slitrk2, $n = 13$; sh-Slitrk2+Slitrk2[V89M], $n = 13$; sh-Slitrk4, $n = 17$; sh-Slitrk4+WT Slitrk4, $n = 15$; sh-Slitrk4+Slitrk4[V206I], $n = 15$; and sh-Slitrk4+Slitrk4[I578V], $n = 15$.

Neuronal Phenotypes of Disease-Associated Slitrk Missense Mutants

Slitrks were previously shown to trigger presynaptic differentiation when expressed in heterologous cells and cocultured in contact with axons (Takahashi et al., 2012; Yim et al., 2013). To test whether the surface transport-deficient Slitrk mutants showed differences in presynaptic differentiation-inducing behavior compared with WT Slitrks, we performed heterologous synapse-formation assays with HEK293T cells expressing WT or mutant Slitrks (**Figure 7**). We found that, whereas WT Slitrk1, Slitrk2, and Slitrk4 robustly recruited synapsin clustering into the corresponding transfected HEK293T cells, Slitrk1[N400I] and Slitrk1[T418S] as well as Slitrk4[V206I] and Slitrk4[I578V] mutants were functionally inactive, as expected by their lack of surface transport (**Figures 7A,C**; see quantification in **Figure 7D**). None of the tested Slitrk2 mutants exhibited altered synapse-inducing activity (**Figures 7B,D**). To determine whether the surface transport-impairing Slitrk mutations also compromised the ability of WT Slitrk proteins to promote synapse formation in cultured neurons, we introduced Slitrk isoform-specific knockdown (KD) vectors into cultured hippocampal neurons at 8 days *in vitro* (DIV8), and stained

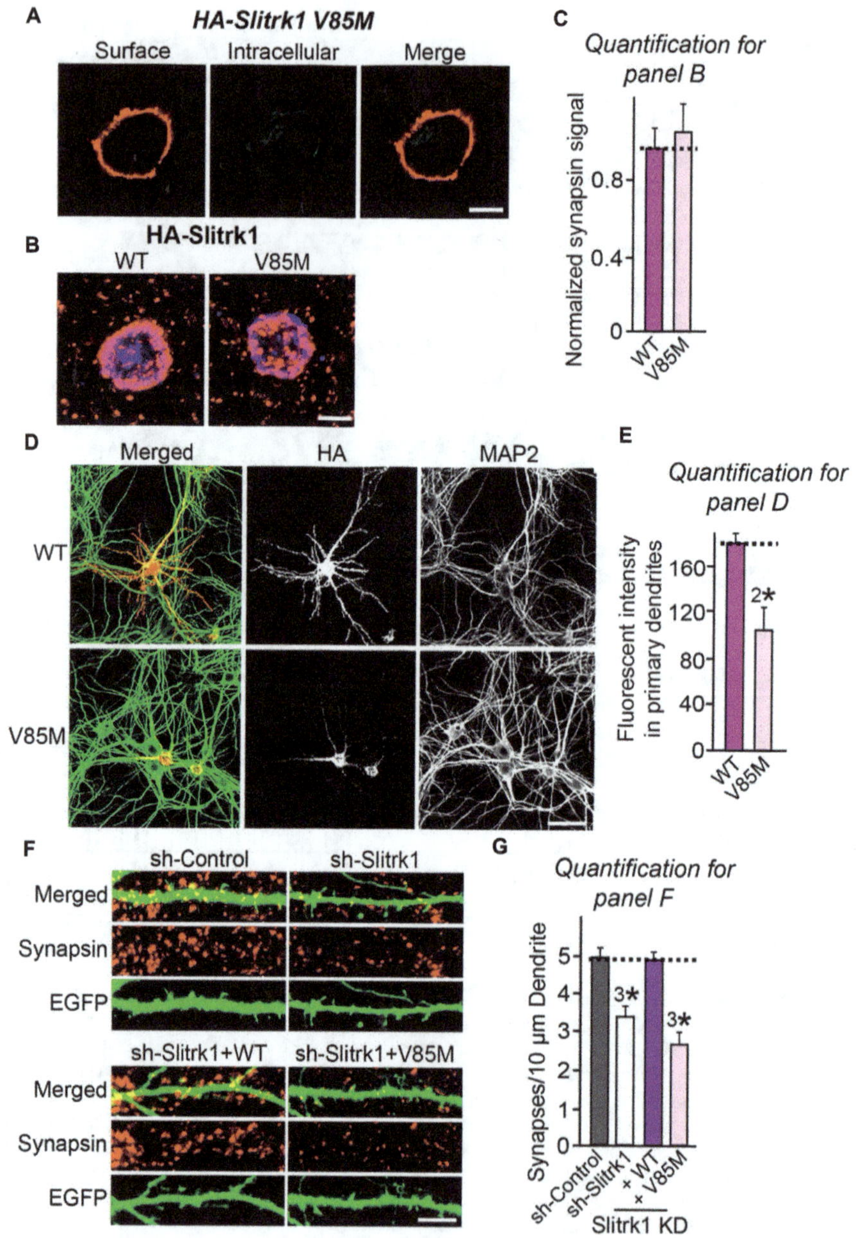

FIGURE 9 | Characterization of the Slitrk1[V85M] mutant in heterologous synapse-formation assays and transfected neurons. (A) Surface expression analysis of HEK293T cells expressing HA-tagged Slitrk1[V85M]. Transfected cells were immunostained with mouse anti-HA antibodies (red) and detected with Cy3-conjugated anti-mouse secondary antibodies under non-permeabilized conditions, followed by permeabilization of cells. Cells were then stained first with rabbit anti-HA antibodies (green) and then with FITC-conjugated anti-rabbit secondary antibodies. Scale bar, 10 μm (applies to all images). **(B,C)** Representative images **(B)** and summary graph **(C)** of heterologous synapse-formation activities of WT Slitrk1 and Slitrk1[V85M]. Neurons were stained with antibodies against HA (blue; pseudo-colored) and synapsin (red). Scale bar, 10 μm (applies to all images). '*n*' denotes the number of HEK293T cells analyzed: WT Slitrk1, $n = 13$; and Slitrk1[V85M], $n = 12$. **(D)** Fluorescence images of hippocampal neurons transfected with WT HA-Slitrk1 or HA-Slitrk1[V85M], at DIV8. After 48 h (DIV10), the transfected neurons were double-immunostained for antibodies against the somatodendritic marker MAP2 (green) and HA (red). Note that Slitrk1[V85M] exhibits decreased dendritic targeting. Scale bar, 50 μm (applies to all images). **(E)** Dendritic targeting of WT HA-Slitrk1 or HA-Slitrk1[V85M] in hippocampal neurons was quantified by measuring fluorescent intensity (HA) in primary dendrites. All data are shown as means ± SEM ($^{2*}p < 0.01$; Student's t-test; p-value = 0.00215). '*n*' denotes the number of neurons as follows: WT Slitrk1, $n = 15$ and Slitrk1[V85M], $n = 13$. **(F,G)** Representative images **(F)** and summary graph **(G)** of neuron transfection assays with a lentiviral vector expressing sh-Control, sh-Slitrk1, or coexpressing sh-Slitrk1 and the indicated shRNA-resistant Slitrk1 vectors at DIV8 and analyzed at DIV14 by double-immunofluorescence staining with antibodies to EGFP (green) and synapsin (red). Scale bar, 5 μm (applies to all images). All data are shown as means ± SEMs ($^{3*}p < 0.001$; ANOVA with *post hoc* Tukey's test; p-value of sh-Control vs. sh-Slitrk1 = 0.000411; p-value of sh-Control vs. sh-Slitrk1+WT Slitrk1 = 0.991; and p-value of sh-Control vs sh-Slitrk1+Slitrk1[V85M] = $2.74E^{-7}$). '*n*' denotes the number of neurons quantified as follows: sh-Control, $n = 15$, sh-Slitrk1, $n = 15$, sh-Slitrk1+WT Slitrk1, $n = 15$; and sh-Slitrk1+Slitrk1[V85M], $n = 17$.

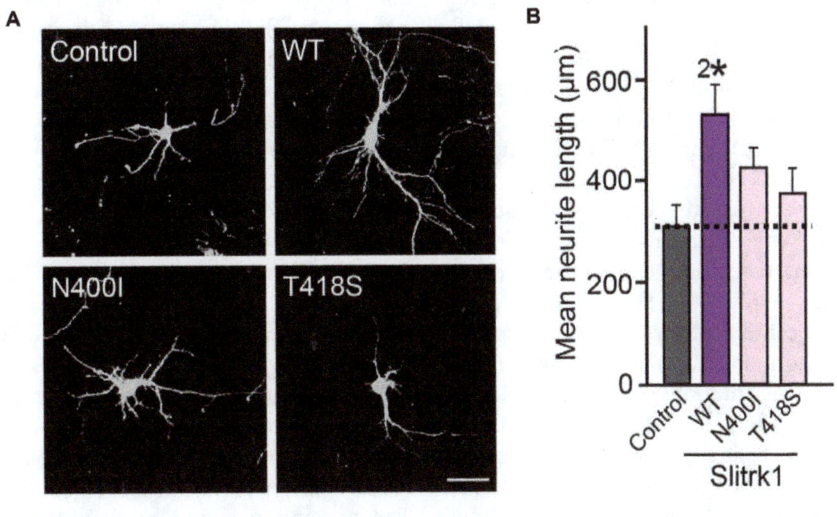

FIGURE 10 | The effect of the Slitrk1[N400I] and Slitrk1[T418S] mutants on neurite outgrowth in cultured hippocampal neurons. (A) Representative images of DIV6 hippocampal neurons transfected with WT HA-Slitrk1, HA-Slitrk1[N400I], or HA-Slitrk1[T418S] at DIV3. Scale bar, 50 μm (applies to all images). **(B)** Quantification of total neurite length per hippocampal neuron at DIV6. All data are shown as means ± SEMs ($^{2*}p < 0.01$; a non-parametric Kruskal–Wallis test; p-value of Control vs. WT Slitrk1 = 0.003; p-value of Control vs. Slitrk1[N400I] = 0.0634; p-value of Control vs. Slitrk1[T418S] = 0.300). 'n' denotes the number of neurons as follows: Control, n = 15, WT Slitrk1, n = 16, Slitrk1[N400I], n = 14; and Slitrk1[T418S], n = 14.

the transfected neurons with anti-EGFP and anti-synapsin antibodies at DIV14 (**Figure 8**). As previously reported (Yim et al., 2013), single KD of Slitrk1, Slitrk2, or Slitrk4 significantly decreased the linear density of synapsin clusters (**Figures 8A,B**). Expression of short hairpin RNA (shRNA)-resistant forms of WT Slitrk1, Slitrk2, or Slitrk4 completely rescued these deficits in the numbers of synapsin clusters (**Figures 8A,B**). Similar to the results of heterologous synapse-formation assays, expression of shRNA-resistant Slitrk1 mutants (N400I or T418S) or Slitrk4 mutants (V206I or I578V) failed to reverse the reduction in the density of synapsin clusters induced by knockdown of Slitrk1 or Slitrk4 (**Figures 8A,B**). Strikingly, expression of the Slitrk2[V89M] mutant, which showed total expression levels, surface transport, and synapse-inducing properties comparable to those of WT Slitrk2, did not rescue the Slitrk2 KD-induced deficit in the numbers of synapsin clusters, likely due to impaired dendritic targeting in neurons (**Figures 8A,B** and **3**). Since the valine residue at position 89 in human Slitrk2 is also found Slitrk1, -3 and -4 (but not Slitrk5 and- 6; **Figure 1B**), we introduced a similar point mutation into human Slitrk1 (Slitrk1[V85M]) and examined whether this artificially generated Slitrk1 mutant behaves similarly to Slitrk2[V89M] (**Figure 9**). We found that Slitrk1[V85M] showed surface expression levels and synaptogenic activity comparable to those of WT Slitrk1 (**Figures 9A–C**), but exhibited decreased dendritic targeting in hippocampal neurons (**Figures 9D,E**). Moreover, Slitrk1[V85M] showed impaired synapse-promoting activity when expressed in Slitrk1-deficient neurons (**Figures 9F,G**). These data suggest that different Slitrk variants found in patients with neuropsychiatric disorders may manifest distinct cellular readouts, compounding the enormous complexity at both cellular and behavioral levels.

DISCUSSION

The 'synaptopathy' hypothesis has been dominant in the neuroscience field since the term was coined, aided in part by the rapid advent of high-resolution human genetic sequencing technologies (Brose et al., 2010). Various classes of synaptic genes have been associated with a range of neuropsychiatric and neurodevelopmental disorders, particularly in the case of ASDs and schizophrenia, although most copy number variants are rarely found in patients with these disorders (Glessner et al., 2012; Malhotra and Sebat, 2012). Surprisingly, similar genetic pathways have often been found to be linked to phenotypically distinct outcomes, confounding the interpretation of genetic approaches (Marshall and Scherer, 2012). Specifically, synaptic adhesion molecules and their associated scaffold proteins, such as neurexin-1α, neuroligin-4 and Shank3, are among the few synaptic genes that are frequently identified as causative factors for ASDs and schizophrenia (Sudhof, 2008; Won et al., 2013; de la Torre-Ubieta et al., 2016). However, how these disease-susceptible genes cause the associated disorders has only recently begun to be understood.

In the present study, we employed a series of functional approaches to ask whether Slitrk mutations identified in schizophrenia, trichotillomania or OCDs alter the biochemical, cellular and synaptic processes that are mediated by WT Slitrk proteins. We found that a subset of Slitrk1, Slitrk2, and Slitrk4 missense mutants exhibit common and distinct phenotypes in a variety of assays, results that often differed from those predicted by algorithm-based *in silico* analyses (**Table 1**). Indeed, many of these mutations did not induce any prominent alterations in the properties of Slitrk proteins, although it is possible that the functional assays employed in the current study were unable to capture all aspects of Slitrk function. Thus, our data underscore the importance of experimentally testing whether candidate mutants identified based on human genetics are physiologically significant. In exploring whether candidate human mutations have distinctive phenotypes at molecular and cellular levels, we focused on two Slitrk1 missense mutations (N400I and T418S), a single Slitrk2 mutation (V89M), and two Slitrk4 mutations (V206I and I578V).

Our data suggest that the respective disorder phenotypes observed in patients with Slitrk mutations are at least partly caused by Slitrk dysfunctions, based on the following evidence: (1) most of the mutated residues in Slitrk1, Slitrk2, and Slitrk4 are evolutionarily conserved across various species, although only a few are also found across all six Slitrk family members; (2) most of the substitutions caused retention in intracellular compartments, such as the ER and *cis*-Golgi, with an accompanying loss of normal Slitrk glycosylation patterns; (3) none of the substitutions perturbed ligand-binding properties, judging from previously determined complex structures; and (4) all but one of the substitutions abolished the effects of Slitrks on synapse formation, with Slitrk2[V89M] uniquely exhibiting the ability to trigger presynaptic differentiation. Notably, none of the Slitrk mutations described here abolished binding to LAR-RPTPs *per se*. However, a majority of Slitrk mutations are positioned in the LRR2 domain of Slitrks (**Figure 1**); thus, the possibility that LRR2 domain-mediated molecular interaction(s) might be influenced by Slitrk mutations cannot be excluded at this point. At present, precisely how Slitrks promote distinct types of synapse development in an isoform-dependent manner remains to be elucidated (Yim et al., 2013), but it would be worthwhile investigating the relationship between altered synapse numbers induced by Slitrk missense mutations and the development of associated neuropsychiatric disorders in follow-up studies. Intriguingly, Slitrk family proteins resemble neuroligin family proteins in many ways (Brose, 2013). For example, the action of Slitrk3 at inhibitory synapses is phenomenologically analogous to that of neuroligin-2, whereas the effects of the other Slitrk family members are related to those of neuroligin-1. However, more rigorous analyses should be undertaken to provide a complete understanding of how synaptogenic adhesion molecules operate cooperatively, competitively, or both.

Most Slitrk substitutions represent loss-of-function mutations that perturb the normal folding and glycosylation of Slitrks, seemingly similar to the situation previously described for the R87W substitution in human neuroligin-4 and D1129H substitution in human CNTNAP2 (Zhang et al., 2009; Falivelli et al., 2012). The V89M substitution is somewhat analogous to previous descriptions of the R451C substitution in human neuroligin-3 (Comoletti et al., 2004; De Jaco et al., 2010) in that Slitrk2[V89M] protein retained WT-like presynapse-inducing activity (**Figure 7**). However, this substitution acted as dominant-negative mutation, abolishing the ability of Slitrk2 to promote synapse formation in transfected neurons because of its ability to alter the synaptic properties of neurons (**Figure 8**). Intriguingly, our preliminary analyses indicate a weak correlation between dendritic spine density and synapsin puncta density in Slitrk-deficient neurons (Data not shown). Further investigation using membrane-anchored GFP plasmid to more accurately visualize the dendritic spines would be required to solve the seemingly discrepancy between postsynaptic spine density and presynaptic marker density.

Currently, we have no insight into how the V89M substitution causes inactivation of Slitrk2 function, but a similar valine-to-methionine mutation was previously described for BDNF (brain-derived neurotrophic factor) (Bath and Lee, 2006; Chen et al., 2006). The human BDNF[V66M] polymorphism, which is associated with altered dendritic trafficking of BDNF mRNA, changes in hippocampal volume, impaired hippocampal-dependent memory and NMDA-receptor dependent synaptic plasticity, and extinction of conditioned aversive memory, has been implicated in anxiety disorders (Chiaruttini et al., 2009; Yu et al., 2009; Ninan et al., 2010). The pathophysiological mechanism postulated for the effect of this BDNF mutation is that sortilin directly interacts with WT BDNF, but not BDNF[V66M], in secretory granules and controls the pathway that regulates its secretion in neurons (Chen et al., 2005). However, Slitrk2[V89M] does not block the transport of Slitrk2 protein to the cell surface; thus, it is conceivable that other mechanism(s) may operate in this case. Slitrk1[N400I] was previously shown to be unable to stimulate neurite outgrowth (Ozomaro et al., 2013), and the current study also found that its glycosylation, surface transport, and synaptogenic activities were impaired (**Figures 3–8**). In contrast, Slitrk1[T418S] was not previously examined, because it was frequently detected in individuals without OCDs and thus was considered to be functionally tolerated in the general population (Ozomaro et al., 2013). However, our data clearly suggested that the T418S mutation also abolishes the surface transport of Slitrk1 proteins, possibly by impairing glycosylation patterns, similar to the biochemical and cellular phenotypes of the N400I mutation. More intriguingly, the Slitrk1[T418S] mutation also compromised the enhanced neurite outgrowth activity shown by Slitrk1 WT (**Figure 10**).

Apart from the unique action of the Slitrk2 V89M mutation, the other Slitrk1, Slitrk2, and Slitrk4 mutations described in the current study have features in common that are typical of loss-of-function mutations, consistent with the phenotypes of Slitrk KD in cultured hippocampal neurons (Yim et al., 2013). Remarkably, Slitrk1-knockout (KO) mice exhibit elevated anxiety-like behaviors that are attributable to increased norepinephrine levels, and administration of the centrally acting adrenergic agonist clonidine has been shown to normalize these behaviors (Katayama et al., 2010). However, the core symptoms of Tourette syndrome and trichotillomania, such as self-grooming, were not reported in Slitrk1-KO mice (Katayama et al., 2010). In the case of neuroligin-3, the R451C mutation exhibits distinct gain-of-function synaptic phenotypes compared with neuroligin-3-KO mice, but both neuroligin-3 R451C knock-in (KI) and KO also impair tonic endocannabinoid signaling in specific interneuron-type synapses (Foldy et al., 2013). Thus, a worthwhile task would be to compare the behavioral, physiological, and circuit phenotypes of Slitrk-KI mice harboring some of the point mutations with altered Slitrk functions described in the current study with those obtained from Slitrk-KO mice. These approaches hold the potential of unveiling more detailed pathophysiological mechanisms underlying Slitrk-associated neuropsychiatric disorders.

AUTHOR CONTRIBUTIONS

JK and JWU conceived and supervised the project; HK, KAH, SYW, and JWU performed the experiments; HK, KAH, HMK, YHL, JK, and JWU analyzed the data; JK and JWU wrote the paper. All authors were involved in drafting the paper and provided final approval of the version to be submitted.

FUNDING

This study was supported by a grant from the National Research Foundation of Korea (NRF) funded by the Ministry of Science, ICT and Future Planning (2016R1A2B2006821 to JK), a faculty research grant from Yonsei University College of Medicine (6-2016-0032 to JWU); and a grant from the Korean Healthcare Technology R&D Project, Ministry for Health & Welfare Affairs, Republic of Korea (HI15C3026 to JWU).

ACKNOWLEDGMENTS

We thank the members of Ko and Um laboratories for critical comments on the manuscript.

REFERENCES

Abelson, J. F., Kwan, K. Y., O'Roak, B. J., Baek, D. Y., Stillman, A. A., Morgan, T. M., et al. (2005). Sequence variants in SLITRK1 are associated with Tourette's syndrome. *Science* 310, 317–320. doi: 10.1126/science.1116502

Adzhubei, I. A., Schmidt, S., Peshkin, L., Ramensky, V. E., Gerasimova, A., Bork, P., et al. (2010). A method and server for predicting damaging missense mutations. *Nat. Methods* 7, 248–249. doi: 10.1038/nmeth0410-248

Aruga, J., and Mikoshiba, K. (2003). Identification and characterization of Slitrk, a novel neuronal transmembrane protein family controlling neurite outgrowth. *Mol. Cell. Neurosci.* 24, 117–129. doi: 10.1016/S1044-7431(03)00129-5

Aruga, J., Yokota, N., and Mikoshiba, K. (2003). Human SLITRK family genes: genomic organization and expression profiling in normal brain and brain tumor tissue. *Gene* 315, 87–94. doi: 10.1016/S0378-1119(03)00715-7

Bath, K. G., and Lee, F. S. (2006). Variant BDNF (Val66Met) impact on brain structure and function. *Cogn. Affect. Behav. Neurosci.* 6, 79–85. doi: 10.3758/CABN.6.1.79

Beaubien, F., and Cloutier, J. F. (2009). Differential expression of Slitrk family members in the mouse nervous system. *Dev. Dyn.* 238, 3285–3296. doi: 10.1002/dvdy.22160

Brose, N. (2013). Why we need more synaptogenic cell-adhesion proteins. *Proc. Natl. Acad. Sci. U.S.A.* 110, 3717–3718. doi: 10.1073/pnas.1300505110

Brose, N., O'Connor, V., and Skehel, P. (2010). Synaptopathy: dysfunction of synaptic function? *Biochem. Soc. Trans.* 38, 443–444. doi: 10.1042/BST0380443

Chen, Z. Y., Ieraci, A., Teng, H., Dall, H., Meng, C. X., Herrera, D. G., et al. (2005). Sortilin controls intracellular sorting of brain-derived neurotrophic factor to the regulated secretory pathway. *J. Neurosci.* 25, 6156–6166. doi: 10.1523/JNEUROSCI.1017-05.2005

Chen, Z. Y., Jing, D., Bath, K. G., Ieraci, A., Khan, T., Siao, C. J., et al. (2006). Genetic variant BDNF (Val66Met) polymorphism alters anxiety-related behavior. *Science* 314, 140–143. doi: 10.1126/science.1129663

Chiaruttini, C., Vicario, A., Li, Z., Baj, G., Braiuca, P., Wu, Y., et al. (2009). Dendritic trafficking of BDNF mRNA is mediated by translin and blocked by the G196A (Val66Met) mutation. *Proc. Natl. Acad. Sci. U.S.A.* 106, 16481–16486. doi: 10.1073/pnas.0902833106

Chou, I. C., Wan, L., Liu, S. C., Tsai, C. H., and Tsai, F. J. (2007). Association of the Slit and Trk-like 1 gene in Taiwanese patients with Tourette syndrome. *Pediatr. Neurol.* 37, 404–406. doi: 10.1016/j.pediatrneurol.2007.06.017

Comoletti, D., De Jaco, A., Jennings, L. L., Flynn, R. E., Gaietta, G., Tsigelny, I., et al. (2004). The Arg451Cys-neuroligin-3 mutation associated with autism reveals a defect in protein processing. *J. Neurosci.* 24, 4889–4893. doi: 10.1523/JNEUROSCI.0468-04.2004

De Jaco, A., Lin, M. Z., Dubi, N., Comoletti, D., Miller, M. T., Camp, S., et al. (2010). Neuroligin trafficking deficiencies arising from mutations in the alpha/beta-hydrolase fold protein family. *J. Biol. Chem.* 285, 28674–28682. doi: 10.1074/jbc.M110.139519

de la Torre-Ubieta, L., Won, H., Stein, J. L., and Geschwind, D. H. (2016). Advancing the understanding of autism disease mechanisms through genetics. *Nat. Med.* 22, 345–361. doi: 10.1038/nm.4071

de Wit, J., Hong, W., Luo, L., and Ghosh, A. (2011). Role of leucine-rich repeat proteins in the development and function of neural circuits. *Annu. Rev. Cell. Dev. Biol.* 27, 697–729. doi: 10.1146/annurev-cellbio-092910-154111

Fabbrini, G., Pasquini, M., Aurilia, C., Berardelli, I., Breedveld, G., Oostra, B. A., et al. (2007). A large Italian family with Gilles de la Tourette syndrome: clinical study and analysis of the SLITRK1 gene. *Mov. Disord.* 22, 2229–2234. doi: 10.1002/mds.21697

Falivelli, G., De Jaco, A., Favaloro, F. L., Kim, H., Wilson, J., Dubi, N., et al. (2012). Inherited genetic variants in autism-related CNTNAP2 show perturbed trafficking and ATF6 activation. *Hum. Mol. Genet.* 21, 4761–4773. doi: 10.1093/hmg/dds320

Foldy, C., Malenka, R. C., and Sudhof, T. C. (2013). Autism-associated neuroligin-3 mutations commonly disrupt tonic endocannabinoid signaling. *Neuron* 78, 498–509. doi: 10.1016/j.neuron.2013.02.036

Glessner, J. T., Connolly, J. J., and Hakonarson, H. (2012). Rare genomic deletions and duplications and their role in neurodevelopmental disorders. *Curr. Top. Behav. Neurosci.* 12, 345–360. doi: 10.1007/7854_2011_179

Grados, M. A., and Walkup, J. T. (2006). A new gene for Tourette's syndrome: a window into causal mechanisms? *Trends Genet.* 22, 291–293. doi: 10.1016/j.tig.2006.04.003

Han, K. A., Jeon, S., Um, J. W., and Ko, J. (2016a). Emergent synapse organizers: LAR-RPTPs and their companions. *Int. Rev. Cell. Mol. Biol.* 324, 39–65. doi: 10.1016/bs.ircmb.2016.01.002

Han, K. A., Woo, D., Kim, S., Choii, G., Jeon, S., Won, S. Y., et al. (2016b). Neurotrophin-3 regulates synapse development by modulating TrkC-PTPsigma synaptic adhesion and intracellular signaling pathways. *J. Neurosci.* 36, 4816–4831. doi: 10.1523/JNEUROSCI.4024-15.2016

Heinzen, E. L., Neale, B. M., Traynelis, S. F., Allen, A. S., and Goldstein, D. B. (2015). The genetics of neuropsychiatric diseases: looking in and beyond the exome. *Annu. Rev. Neurosci.* 38, 47–68. doi: 10.1146/annurev-neuro-071714-034136

Insel, T. R., and Landis, S. C. (2013). Twenty-five years of progress: the view from NIMH and NINDS. *Neuron* 80, 561–567. doi: 10.1016/j.neuron.2013.09.041

Katayama, K., Yamada, K., Ornthanalai, V. G., Inoue, T., Ota, M., Murphy, N. P., et al. (2010). Slitrk1-deficient mice display elevated anxiety-like behavior and noradrenergic abnormalities. *Mol. Psychiatry* 15, 177–184. doi: 10.1038/mp.2008.97

Keen-Kim, D., and Freimer, N. B. (2006). Genetics and epidemiology of Tourette syndrome. *J. Child Neurol.* 21, 665–671. doi: 10.1177/08830738060210081101

Keezer, M. R., and Sander, J. W. (2016). Comorbidity as an epidemiological construct. *Lancet Neurol.* 15, 32. doi: 10.1016/S1474-4422(15)00352-X

Keezer, M. R., Sisodiya, S. M., and Sander, J. W. (2016). Comorbidities of epilepsy: current concepts and future perspectives. *Lancet Neurol.* 15, 106–115. doi: 10.1016/S1474-4422(15)00225-2

Ko, J. (2012). The leucine-rich repeat superfamily of synaptic adhesion molecules: LRRTMs and Slitrks. *Mol. Cells* 34, 335–340. doi: 10.1007/s10059-012-0113-3

Ko, J., Choii, G., and Um, J. W. (2015). The balancing act of GABAergic synapse organizers. *Trends Mol. Med.* 21, 256–268. doi: 10.1016/j.molmed.2015.01.004

Ko, J., Fuccillo, M. V., Malenka, R. C., and Sudhof, T. C. (2009). LRRTM2 functions as a neurexin ligand in promoting excitatory synapse formation. *Neuron* 64, 791–798. doi: 10.1016/j.neuron.2009.12.012

Ko, J. S., Pramanik, G., Um, J. W., Shim, J. S., Lee, D., Kim, K. H., et al. (2015). PTPsigma functions as a presynaptic receptor for the glypican-4/LRRTM4 complex and is essential for excitatory synaptic transmission. *Proc. Natl. Acad. Sci. U.S.A.* 112, 1874–1879. doi: 10.1073/pnas.1410138112

Ko, J., Soler-Llavina, G. J., Fuccillo, M. V., Malenka, R. C., and Sudhof, T. C. (2011). Neuroligins/LRRTMs prevent activity- and Ca2+/calmodulin-dependent synapse elimination in cultured neurons. *J. Cell Biol.* 194, 323–334. doi: 10.1083/jcb.201101072

Kumar, P., Henikoff, S., and Ng, P. C. (2009). Predicting the effects of coding non-synonymous variants on protein function using the SIFT algorithm. *Nat. Protoc.* 4, 1073–1081. doi: 10.1038/nprot.2009.86

Malhotra, D., and Sebat, J. (2012). CNVs: harbingers of a rare variant revolution in psychiatric genetics. *Cell* 148, 1223–1241. doi: 10.1016/j.cell.2012.02.039

Marshall, C. R., and Scherer, S. W. (2012). Detection and characterization of copy number variation in autism spectrum disorder. *Methods Mol. Biol.* 838, 115–135. doi: 10.1007/978-1-61779-507-7_5

Medland, S. E., Jahanshad, N., Neale, B. M., and Thompson, P. M. (2014). Whole-genome analyses of whole-brain data: working within an expanded search space. *Nat. Neurosci.* 17, 791–800. doi: 10.1038/nn.3718

Mi, H., Poudel, S., Muruganujan, A., Casagrande, J. T., and Thomas, P. D. (2016). PANTHER version 10: expanded protein families and functions, and analysis tools. *Nucleic Acids Res.* 44, D336–D342. doi: 10.1093/nar/gkv1194

Missler, M., Sudhof, T. C., and Biederer, T. (2012). Synaptic cell adhesion. *Cold Spring Harb. Perspect. Biol.* 4:a005694. doi: 10.1101/cshperspect.a005694

Ninan, I., Bath, K. G., Dagar, K., Perez-Castro, R., Plummer, M. R., Lee, F. S., et al. (2010). The BDNF Val66Met polymorphism impairs NMDA receptor-dependent synaptic plasticity in the hippocampus. *J. Neurosci.* 30, 8866–8870. doi: 10.1523/JNEUROSCI.1405-10.2010

Ozomaro, U., Cai, G., Kajiwara, Y., Yoon, S., Makarov, V., Delorme, R., et al. (2013). Characterization of SLITRK1 variation in obsessive-compulsive disorder. *PLoS ONE* 8:e70376. doi: 10.1371/journal.pone.0070376

Piton, A., Gauthier, J., Hamdan, F. F., Lafreniere, R. G., Yang, Y., Henrion, E., et al. (2011). Systematic resequencing of X-chromosome synaptic genes in autism spectrum disorder and schizophrenia. *Mol. Psychiatry* 16, 867–880. doi: 10.1038/mp.2010.54

Proenca, C. C., Gao, K. P., Shmelkov, S. V., Rafii, S., and Lee, F. S. (2011). Slitrks as emerging candidate genes involved in neuropsychiatric disorders. *Trends Neurosci.* 34, 143–153. doi: 10.1016/j.tins.2011.01.001

Reva, B., Antipin, Y., and Sander, C. (2011). Predicting the functional impact of protein mutations: application to cancer genomics. *Nucleic Acids Res.* 39, e118. doi: 10.1093/nar/gkr407

Scharf, J. M., Moorjani, P., Fagerness, J., Platko, J. V., Illmann, C., Galloway, B., et al. (2008). Lack of association between SLITRK1var321 and Tourette syndrome in a large family-based sample. *Neurology* 70, 1495–1496. doi: 10.1212/01.wnl.0000296833.25484.bb

State, M. W. (2011). The genetics of Tourette disorder. *Curr. Opin. Genet. Dev.* 21, 302–309. doi: 10.1016/j.gde.2011.01.007

State, M. W., and Levitt, P. (2011). The conundrums of understanding genetic risks for autism spectrum disorders. *Nat. Neurosci.* 14, 1499–1506. doi: 10.1038/nn.2924

Sudhof, T. C. (2008). Neuroligins and neurexins link synaptic function to cognitive disease. *Nature* 455, 903–911. doi: 10.1038/nature07456

Takahashi, H., Katayama, K., Sohya, K., Miyamoto, H., Prasad, T., Matsumoto, Y., et al. (2012). Selective control of inhibitory synapse development by Slitrk3-PTPdelta trans-synaptic interaction. *Nat. Neurosci.* 15, S381–S382. doi: 10.1038/nn.3040

Thomas, P. D., and Kejariwal, A. (2004). Coding single-nucleotide polymorphisms associated with complex vs. Mendelian disease: evolutionary evidence for differences in molecular effects. *Proc. Natl. Acad. Sci. U.S.A.* 101, 15398–15403. doi: 10.1073/pnas.0404380101

Um, J. W., Choii, G., Park, D., Kim, D., Jeon, S., Kang, H., et al. (2016). IQ Motif and SEC7 Domain-containing Protein 3 (IQSEC3) interacts with gephyrin to promote inhibitory synapse formation. *J. Biol. Chem.* 291, 10119–10130. doi: 10.1074/jbc.M115.712893

Um, J. W., Kim, K. H., Park, B. S., Choi, Y., Kim, D., Kim, C. Y., et al. (2014a). Structural basis for LAR-RPTP/Slitrk complex-mediated synaptic adhesion. *Nat. Commun.* 5:5423. doi: 10.1038/ncomms6423

Um, J. W., Pramanik, G., Ko, J. S., Song, M. Y., Lee, D., Kim, H., et al. (2014b). Calsyntenins function as synaptogenic adhesion molecules in concert with neurexins. *Cell Rep.* 6, 1096–1109. doi: 10.1016/j.celrep.2014.02.010

Um, J. W., and Ko, J. (2013). LAR-RPTPs: synaptic adhesion molecules that shape synapse development. *Trends Cell Biol.* 23, 465–475. doi: 10.1016/j.tcb.2013.07.004

Won, H., Mah, W., and Kim, E. (2013). Autism spectrum disorder causes, mechanisms, and treatments: focus on neuronal synapses. *Front. Mol. Neurosci.* 6:19. doi: 10.3389/fnmol.2013.00019

Yim, Y. S., Kwon, Y., Nam, J., Yoon, H. I., Lee, K., Kim, D. G., et al. (2013). Slitrks control excitatory and inhibitory synapse formation with LAR receptor protein tyrosine phosphatases. *Proc. Natl. Acad. Sci. U.S.A.* 110, 4057–4062. doi: 10.1073/pnas.1209881110

Yu, H., Wang, Y., Pattwell, S., Jing, D., Liu, T., Zhang, Y., et al. (2009). Variant BDNF Val66Met polymorphism affects extinction of conditioned aversive memory. *J. Neurosci.* 29, 4056–4064. doi: 10.1523/JNEUROSCI.5539-08.2009

Zhang, C., Milunsky, J. M., Newton, S., Ko, J., Zhao, G., Maher, T. A., et al. (2009). A neuroligin-4 missense mutation associated with autism impairs neuroligin-4 folding and endoplasmic reticulum export. *J. Neurosci.* 29, 10843–10854. doi: 10.1523/JNEUROSCI.1248-09.2009

Zuchner, S., Cuccaro, M. L., Tran-Viet, K. N., Cope, H., Krishnan, R. R., Pericak-Vance, M. A., et al. (2006). SLITRK1 mutations in trichotillomania. *Mol. Psychiatry* 11, 887–889. doi: 10.1038/sj.mp.4001865

14

MPTP Impairs Dopamine D1 Receptor-Mediated Survival of Newborn Neurons in Ventral Hippocampus to Cause Depressive-Like Behaviors in Adult Mice

*Tingting Zhang[1,2], Juan Hong[1,2], Tingting Di[2] and Ling Chen[1,2]**

[1] State Key Lab of Reproductive Medicine, Nanjing Medical University, Nanjing, China, [2] Department of Physiology, Nanjing Medical University, Nanjing, China

Edited by:
Andrew Harkin,
Trinity College Dublin, Ireland

Reviewed by:
Subhabrata Sanyal,
Biogen Idec, USA
Sungjin Park,
University of Utah, USA

***Correspondence:**
Ling Chen
lingchen@njmu.edu.cn

Parkinson's disease (PD) is characterized by motor symptoms with depression. We evaluated the influence of dopaminergic depletion on hippocampal neurogenesis process to explore mechanisms of depression production. Five consecutive days of 1-Methyl-4-phenyl-1,2,3,6-tetrahydropyridine (MPTP) injection in mice (MPTP-mice) reduced dopaminergic fibers in hippocampal dentate gyrus (DG). MPTP-mice exhibited depressive-like behaviors later for 2–3 weeks. BrdU was injected 4 h after last-injection of MPTP. BrdU-positive (BrdU$^+$) cells in dorsal (d-DG) and ventral (v-DG) DG were examined on day 1 (D1), 7 (D7), 14 (D14) and 21 (D21) after BrdU injection. Fewer D7-, D14- and D21-BrdU$^+$ cells or BrdU$^+$/NeuN$^+$ cells, but not D1-BrdU$^+$ cells, were found in v-DG of MPTP-mice than in controls. However, the number of BrdU$^+$ cells in d-DG did not differ between the both. Loss of doublecortin-positive (DCX$^+$) cells was observed in v-DG of MPTP-mice. Protein kinase A (PKA) and Ca^{2+}/cAMP-response element binding protein (CREB) phosphorylation were reduced in v-DG of MPTP-mice, which were reversed by D1-like receptor (D1R) agonist SKF38393, but not D2R agonist quinpirole. The treatment of MPTP-mice with SKF38393 on days 2–7 after BrdU-injection reduced the loss of D7- and D21-BrdU$^+$ cells in v-DG and improved the depressive-like behaviors; these changes were sensitive to PKA inhibitor H89. Moreover, the v-DG injection of SKF38393 in MPTP-mice could reduce the loss of D21-BrdU$^+$ cells and relieve the depressive-like behaviors. In control mice, the blockade of D1R by SCH23390 caused the reduction of D21-BrdU$^+$ cells in v-DG and the depressive-like behaviors. Our results indicate that MPTP-reduced dopaminergic depletion impairs the D1R-mediated early survival of newborn neurons in v-DG, producing depressive-like behaviors.

Keywords: Parkinson's disease (PD), dopaminergic receptor (DR), depression, neurogenesis, hippocampal dentate gyrus (DG)

INTRODUCTION

Parkinson's disease (PD) is a neurodegenerative disorder characterized by motor symptoms and a progressive loss of dopaminergic neurons (Rodriguez-Oroz et al., 2009). Major depression is present in approximately 30–50% of PD patients (Bower et al., 2010; Nègre-Pagès et al., 2010). However, the underlying mechanisms remain unclear.

The hippocampal volume is smaller in patients with depression than in normal subjects of the same-age (Videbech and Ravnkilde, 2015). Electroconvulsive therapy in refractory depression can increase hippocampal volume. Growing evidence suggests that neurogenesis continues throughout adulthood within the hippocampal dentate gyrus (DG; Toni et al., 2008). The newly generated neurons can integrate into hippocampal circuitry, thereby maintaining a functional structure, which is required for mood control and antidepressant efficacy (Petrik et al., 2012). The deficits in adult neurogenesis in the postmortem brains of PD patients have recently attracted much attention. For example, Höglinger et al. (2004) have reported the deficits in the hippocampal neurogenesis of PD patients. The hippocampal cell proliferation capacity is decreased in PD patients (Guiard et al., 2009). A reduction in neuronal precursor cells has been observed in the subgranular zone (SGZ) of patients with PD (Borta and Höglinger, 2007).

The hippocampus and the midbrain dopaminergic neurons of the ventral tegmental area (VTA) form a functional loop (Lisman and Grace, 2005). Dopaminergic fibers, originating mainly from VTA (Gasbarri et al., 1997), directly contact the newborn cells in DG, but are sparse in the granule cell layer or adjacent hilus (Höglinger et al., 2004). Neuronal precursor cells in the hippocampal DG of adult mammals express all dopaminergic receptors (DRs), which receive dopaminergic afferents (Takamura et al., 2014). Dopamine (DA) has been reported to play an important role in the regulation of endogenous neurogenesis in the adult mammalian brain. The activation of D1-like receptors (D1R) promotes the survival of newborn cells in the adult hippocampus (Takamura et al., 2014). Winner et al. (2009) have observed that a D2-like receptor (D2R) agonist in DA-depleted rats increases the proliferation of neural precursor cells in the subventricular zone (SVZ) but not in SGZ. A large body of evidence has established that the DA depletion in rodents decreases the cell proliferation and survival of neuronal precursor cells in DG (Höglinger et al., 2004; Khaindrava et al., 2011). However, other data have revealed that the DA depletion increases or has no effect on cell proliferation (Oizumi et al., 2008; Park and Enikolopov, 2010).

In rodents and primates, the changes in afferent and efferent connectivity along the longitudinal axis of the hippocampus suggest distinct functions of the dorsal and ventral hippocampus. The dorsal DG (d-DG) receives projections arising in the lateral and caudomedial portion of entorhinal cortex, whereas the ventral DG (v-DG) receives inputs from the rostromedial region of the entorhinal cortex (Dolorfo and Amaral, 1998). The innervation density of dopaminergic plexuses is very high in the ventral hippocampus, but is low in the dorsal portion (Bjarkam et al., 2003). 1-Methyl-4-phenyl-1,2,3,6-tetrahydropyridine (MPTP) is commonly used to prepare an animal model of PD as it selectively induces cell death of dopaminergic neurons (Schober, 2004). The MPTP lesion can be used for behavioral studies of affective disorders in C57BL/6 mice (Gorton et al., 2010). To investigate whether the DA depletion in PD brain impairs the hippocampal neurogenesis to cause the depression, we in this study examined the affective behaviors and the neurogenesis process of d-DG and v-DG (including the proliferation of stem cells, the differentiation of progenitor cells and the survival of newborn neurons) in mice treated with MPTP (MPTP-mice), and explored the correlation between hippocampal neurogenesis deficits and depressive-like behaviors. The present study provides evidence that MPTP-reduced dopaminergic afferents impairs the D1R-mediated early survival of newly generated neurons in v-DG, which may be responsible for the production of depressive-like behaviors.

MATERIALS AND METHODS

Mice

The use of animals was approved by Institutional Animal Care and Use Committee of Nanjing Medical University and was performed in accordance with the experimental animal guidelines of Laboratory Animal Research Institute. Eight-week-old male C57BL/6 mice (24–26 g; Oriental Bio Service Inc., Nanjing, China) were used at the beginning of the experiment. The mice were maintained under constant environmental conditions (temperature 23 ± 2°C, humidity 55 ± 5% and 12:12 h light/dark cycle) in Animal Research Center of Nanjing Medical University with free access to food and water.

Drug Administration

The mice received an intraperitoneal (i.p.) injection of MPTP (25 mg/kg, measured as free base; Sigma-Aldrich, St. Louis, MO, USA) once a day for five consecutive days (Crocker et al., 2003). BrdU (Sigma-Aldrich) was dissolved freshly in 0.9% saline to make 10 mg/ml solution just before injection. Mice were given three injections of BrdU (50 mg/kg, i.p.) at intervals of 6 h. SKF38393 (Tocris, UK), SCH23390 and quinpirole (Sigma-Aldrich) were dissolved in sterile saline; L-sulpiride and H89 (Sigma-Aldrich) were dissolved in 1.0% DMSO (Sutton and Caron, 2015). The mice were treated daily with the injection (i.p.) of SKF38393 (10 mg/kg), H89 (1 mg/kg; Seyedi et al., 2014), quinpirole (2 mg/kg), SCH23390 (0.5 mg/kg) or L-sulpiride (15 mg/kg). For the v-DG injection of drugs, the mice were anesthetized with chloral hydrate (400 mg/kg, i.p.) and placed in a stereotaxic instrument (Stoelting, Wood Dale, IL, USA). The scalp was incised and a small hole (2 mm diameter) was drilled in the skull using a dental drill. Guide cannulas (26-Gauge, Plastics One, Roanoke, VA, USA) were implanted into the bilateral v-DG (2.3 mm posterior, 1.3 mm lateral and 2.0 mm ventral to Bregma; Zhou et al., 2011b). On day 2 after surgery, the dummy cannulas were removed from the guide cannula, and then replaced by infusion cannulas (30 Gauge). The infusion cannula was connected by polyethylene tubing (PE 10; Becton Dickinson, Sparks, MD, USA) with a stepper-motorized micro-syringe (Stoelting, Wood Dale, IL, USA). SKF38393 (4.8 nmol), SCH23390 (0.6 nmol) and H89 (0.8 nmol) were diluted with ACSF and infused daily in a volume of 0.2 μl/side (Lai et al., 2008; Nasehi et al., 2011). After 2% Evans-blue (2.5 μl) was injected, the mice were killed by an overdose of chloral hydrate, and coronal sections (100 μm) were cut using a cryostat to validate the injection-site. Control mice were given an equal volume of vehicle.

Behavioral Examination

A single cohort of animals was used for the following test sequence: open-field test (OFT) → Forced swim test (FST) → Tail suspension test (TST; Zhou et al., 2014). All behavioral data were captured by a video-monitor and analyzed using TopScan Lite 2.0 (Clever Sys., Reston, VA, USA).

OFT was performed in a cuboid Plexiglass box (60 cm × 60 cm × 40 cm). Total distance traveled (mm/6 min) was recorded.

FST was performed in a glass cylinder (300 mm high, 280 mm in diameter) that was filled with water (25 ± 1°C) to a height of 20 cm. Total immobility time during a 6 min test was scored. Mice were considered to be immobile when they stopped struggling and moved only to remain floating in the water, while keeping their heads above water.

TST was performed by using adhesive tape to attach the tail to a rod that was 60 cm above the floor. Trials were conducted for a period of 6 min, during which the immobility time was recorded.

Morris water maze task (MWM) was performed in a black-colored plastic pool (diameter = 120 cm) at 20 ± 1°C. A cylindrical platform (diameter = 7 cm) was placed 0.5 cm below the surface of water. Each mouse was randomly released from four different quadrants and allowed to swim for 90 s. Four trials were conducted each day with an intertrial interval of 30 min. Average swimming speed (m/s) and latency (s) to reach the platform were scored for all trials. If a mouse could not reach the platform within 90 s, the experimenter gently assisted the mouse onto the platform and allowed it to remain there for 15 s.

Immuno-Staining and Quantification

BrdU Immuno-Staining

Mice were anesthetized with chloral hydrate (400 mg/kg, i.p.) and perfused transcardially with 4% paraformaldehyde on day 1 (D1), day 7 (D7) , day 14 (D14) and day 21 (D21) after the last-injection of BrdU. Coronal hippocampal slices (40 μm) were cut using a vibrating microtome (Microslicer DTK 1500; Dousaka EM Co, Japan). The d-DG (AP: −0.94 to −2.30) and the v-DG (AP: −2.46 to AP: −3.80) were each harvested on the basis of the coordinates of the Paxinos and Franklin atlas of the mouse brain (O'Leary et al., 2012). The free-floating sections were treated with 3% normal goat serum, and then incubated with mouse anti-BrdU antibody (1:1000, Millipore, Billerica, MA, USA) at 4°C overnight. The sections were incubated in biotin-labeled goat anti-mouse IgG antibody (1:500, Bioworld Technology, Inc., St. Louis Park, MN, USA) for 2 h. Immunoreactivities were visualized using an avidin-biotin horseradish peroxidase complex (Vector Laboratories, Inc., Burlingame, CA, USA). BrdU-positive ($BrdU^+$) cells in SGZ and granule cell layer of every 5th section (200 μm apart) were counted using a conventional light microscope (DP70, Olympus Optical, Tokyo, Japan). The number of $BrdU^+$ cells per section was multiplied by five to obtain the total number per DG (Sha et al., 2015).

BrdU and NeuN or GFAP Double Immuno-Staining

The sections were incubated with rat anti-BrdU antibody (1:200, Abcam, Cambridge, UK), which was detected using CY3-labeled anti-rat IgG antibody (1:200, Millipore) and mouse anti-neuronal nuclei (NeuN) antibody (1:500, Millipore), which was detected using fluorescein-labeled anti-mouse antibody (1:50, Millipore) or mouse anti-GFAP antibody (1:200, Millipore), which was detected using a FITC-labeled anti-mouse antibody (1:50, Millipore). $BrdU^+$/$NeuN^+$ or $GFAP^+$ cells were observed using a confocal laser-scanning microscope (Leica, Heidelberg, Germany). The number of $BrdU^+$/$NeuN^+$ or $GFAP^+$ cells per section (200 μm apart) was multiplied by 5 to obtain the total number.

Doublecortin (DCX) or Tyrosine Hydroxylase (TH) Immuno-Staining

The free-floating sections (40 μm) were incubated with goat anti-DCX antibody (1:500, Santa Cruz, CA, USA) or chicken anti-TH (1:1000, Abcam) at 4°C overnight, and then in biotin-labeled rabbit anti-goat IgG antibody (1:500, Bioworld) or goat anti-chicken IgG antibody (1:500, Santa Cruz) for 2 h at room temperature. Density of doublecortin positive (DCX^+) cells was expressed as the number per mm length along SGZ (Sha et al., 2015). Tyrosine hydroxylase positive (TH^+) cells were counted using a stereological system, which consisted of a light microscope with a CCD camera (DP70), a motorized specimen stage for automatic sampling and a computer running Microbrightfield Stereo Investigator software (Microbrightfield, Williston, VT, USA; Hong et al., 2015).

Western Blot Analysis

After the dorsal and ventral hippocampal slices were harvested, the DG regions were micro-dissected and stored at −80°C until assayed. Protein was extracted and the concentration of protein was determined using a bicinchoninic acid (BCA) protein assay kit (Pierce, IL, USA). Protein (40 μg) was separated by 10% acrylamide denaturing gels (SDS-PAGE) and transferred to membranes. The membranes were incubated with rabbit anti-protein kinase A (PKA) phosphorylation (1:1000, Millipore) and rabbit anti-cyclic AMP-response element binding protein (CREB) phosphorylation (1:1000, Santa Cruz, CA, USA). Then, the membranes were incubated with horseradish peroxidase-labeled goat anti-rabbit antibody (1:5000, Santa Cruz, CA, USA), and developed using an enhanced chemiluminescence detection kit (Millipore). After visualization, the blots were stripped by incubation in stripping buffer for 15 min, and then incubated with rabbit anti-PKA antibody (1:1000, Millipore) and rabbit anti-CREB antibody

(1:1000, Santa Cruz, CA, USA). An internal control was performed using mouse anti-β-actin antibody (1:2000, Cell Signaling, Danvers, MA, USA). Western blot bands were scanned and analyzed with the ImageJ analysis software package (NIH).

Reverse Transcription-Polymerase Chain Reaction (RT-PCR)

Total RNA of v-DG and d-DG was isolated using TRIzol reagent (Invitrogen, Camarillo, CA, USA) and reverse-transcribed into cDNA using a PrimeScript RT reagent kit (Takara, China) for quantitative PCR (ABI Step One Plus, Foster City, CA, USA) in the presence of a fluorescent dye (SYBR Green I; Takara). The relative expression of genes was determined using the $2^{-\Delta\Delta ct}$ method with normalization to the GAPDH expression. The primer sequences of *D1R* and *D2R* mRNA were designed as described in a previous publication (Kim et al., 2010).

Statistical Analysis

The group data were expressed as the means ± standard error (SEM). All statistical analyses were performed using SPSS software, version 16.0 (SPSS Inc., Chicago, IL, USA). Differences among means were analyzed using the Student's *t*-tests or one/two-factor analysis of variance (ANOVA) or repeated-measures ANOVA, followed by a *post hoc* Bonferroni test. Differences of $p < 0.05$ were considered statistically significant.

RESULTS

MPTP Causes Depression-Like Behaviors in Mice

MPTP injection had a marked effect on the dopaminergic neurons in VTA ($F_{(4,49)} = 6.767$, $p < 0.001$; **Figure 1A**). In comparison with the control values, the number of TH^+ cells on day 1 (D1, $p < 0.05$), day 7 (D7, $p < 0.01$), day 14 (D14, $p < 0.01$) and day 21 (D21, $p < 0.01$) after the last-injection of MPTP (post-MPTP) was significantly reduced.

The affective behaviors were examined on days 5–7, days 12–14 and days 19–21 post-MPTP (**Figure 1B**). MPTP-mice had a tendency to travel a shorter total distance in the OFT (**Figure 1C**), but the group comparison with control mice failed to reach statistical difference ($F_{(1,54)} = 0.825$, $p = 0.368$). Depression-like behaviors were examined by FST and TST. There was a main effect of MPTP-injection for the immobility time in FST ($F_{(1,54)} = 16.130$, $p < 0.001$; **Figure 1D**) and TST ($F_{(1,54)} = 15.360$, $p < 0.001$; **Figure 1E**). Notably, MPTP-mice showed a progressive prolongation of immobility time in FST and TST from day 13–14 (FST: $p < 0.05$; TST: $p < 0.05$) to day 20–21 (FST: $p < 0.01$; TST: $p < 0.01$) post-MPTP.

The spatial memory was further examined using the place learning of the MWM on days 22–26 post-MPTP. Repeated-measures ANOVA revealed that the escape latency of hidden platform progressively decreased with training days in all groups ($F_{(4,72)} = 59.308$, $p < 0.001$; **Figure 1F**), which was not affected by the MPTP-injection ($F_{(1,18)} = 0.049$, $p = 0.828$).

MPTP Impairs the Survival of Newborn Neurons in Ventral DG

To investigate the mechanisms underlying the MPTP-induced depression-like behaviors, we examined the dopaminergic innervations and the hippocampal neurogenesis in d-DG and v-DG (**Figure 2A**). In control mice, the density of TH positive (TH^+) fibers in v-DG was higher than that in d-DG (**Figure 2B**). In comparison with those of controls, the TH^+ fibers in v-DG were clearly decreased on day 7 post-MPTP. The BrdU was injected starting from 4 h post-MPTP. $BrdU^+$ cells were examined on day 1 (D1), day 7 (D7), day 14 (D14) and day 21 (D21) after the BrdU-injection (**Figure 2C**). The number of $BrdU^+$ cells (D1→D7→D14→D21) in either d-DG ($F_{(3,72)} = 57.836$, $p < 0.001$; **Figure 2D**) or v-DG ($F_{(3,72)} = 64.856$, $p < 0.001$; **Figure 2E**) were decreased progressively in all groups. MPTP injection markedly reduced the number of $BrdU^+$ cells in v-DG ($F_{(1,72)} = 7.800$, $p = 0.007$), but not in d-DG ($F_{(1,72)} = 3.497$, $p = 0.066$). In comparison with controls, the MPTP-mice had significantly fewer D7-$BrdU^+$ cells ($p < 0.01$), D14-$BrdU^+$ cells ($p < 0.01$) and D21-$BrdU^+$ cells ($p < 0.01$), but not D1-$BrdU^+$ cells ($p > 0.05$), in v-DG. However, the numbers of D1-$BrdU^+$ cells ($p > 0.05$), D7-$BrdU^+$ cells ($p > 0.05$), D14-$BrdU^+$ cells ($p > 0.05$) and D21-$BrdU^+$ cells ($p > 0.05$) in d-DG had no significant difference between MPTP-mice and control mice.

Doublecortin (DCX), a microtubule-associated protein, is specifically expressed in immature neuroblasts and progenitor cells (Francis et al., 1999). To evaluate the survival of young newborn neurons, we examined the number of DCX^+ cells in the hippocampal DG on day 7 post-MPTP. The results showed that the number of DCX^+ cells was significantly reduced in v-DG ($p < 0.01$, $n = 10$; **Figure 2F**), but not in d-DG ($p > 0.05$, $n = 10$), compared with those in control mice.

To examine the differentiation of precursor cells, we further examined the number and relative proportions of D21-$BrdU^+$ cells expressing NeuN, a mature neuron marker, or glial fibrillary acidic protein (GFAP), a glial marker. The number of D21-$BrdU^+$/$NeuN^+$ cells in v-DG of MPTP-mice was less than that in control mice ($p < 0.01$, $n = 10$; **Figure 2G**), whereas there was no difference in d-DG between the both ($p > 0.05$, $n = 10$). In contrast, the number of D21-$BrdU^+$/$GFAP^+$ cells in v-DG ($p > 0.05$, $n = 10$; **Figure 2H**) or d-DG ($p > 0.05$, $n = 10$) did not differ between MPTP-mice and control mice. In v-DG of MPTP-mice, the ratio of $BrdU^+$/$NeuN^+$ cells to total D21-$BrdU^+$ cells (53.79 ± 5.02%) was lower than that in control mice (76.60 ± 5.48%, $p < 0.01$, $n = 10$), whereas the ratio of $BrdU^+$/$GFAP^+$ cells (15.06 ± 1.09%) was higher than the ratio in control mice (10.54 ± 0.74%, $p < 0.01$, $n = 10$).

MPTP Reduces D1R-Activated PKA-CREB Signaling

The RT-PCR analysis showed that the levels of *D1R* (v-DG: $p > 0.05$; d-DG: $p > 0.05$, $n = 8$; **Figure 3A**) and *D2R* mRNA (v-DG: $p > 0.05$; d-DG: $p > 0.05$, $n = 8$; **Figure 3B**) were

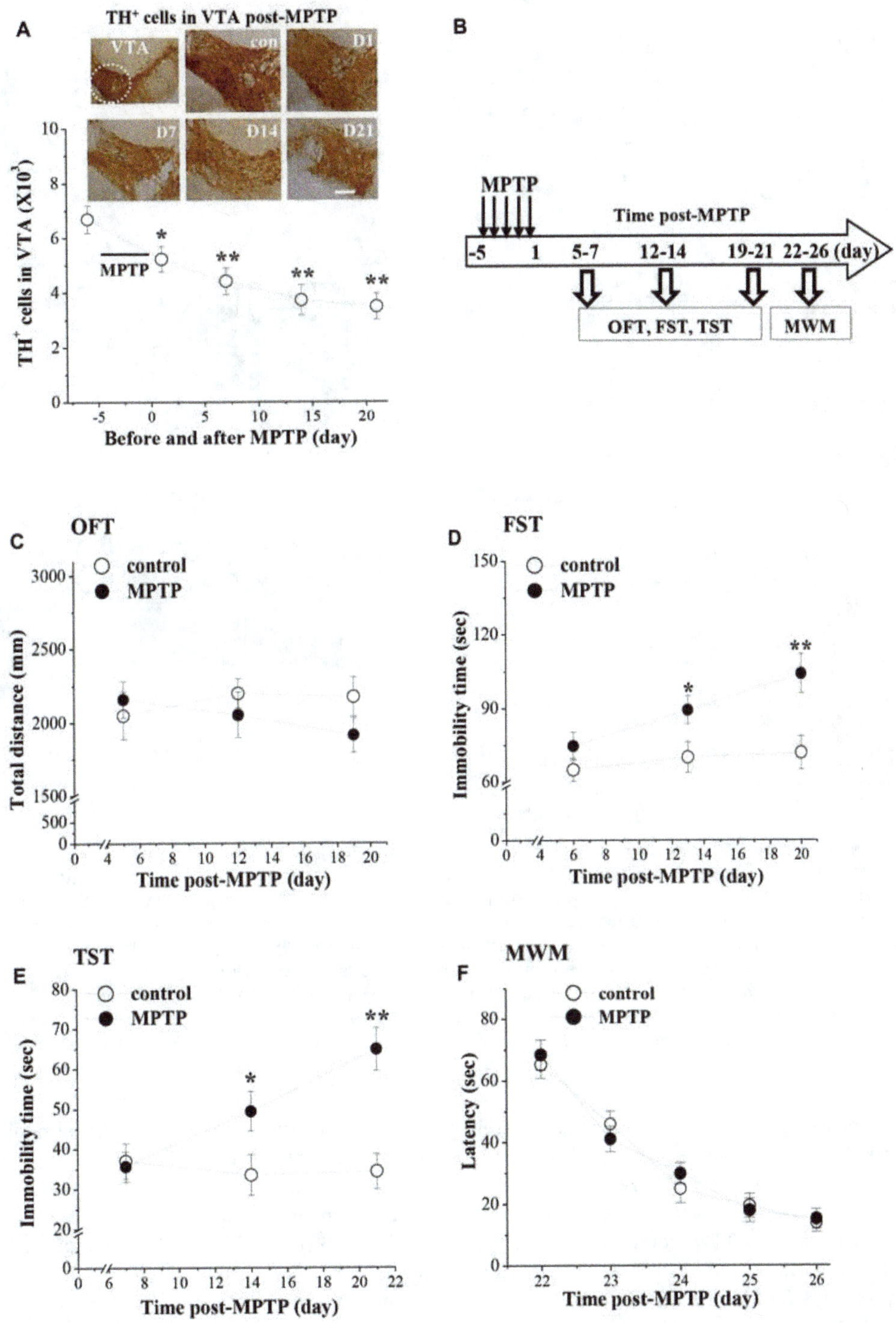

FIGURE 1 | Influence of 1-Methyl-4-phenyl-1,2,3,6-tetrahydropyridine (MPTP)-induced dopamine (DA) depletion on affective behaviors in mice. **(A)** Representative photomicrographs of tyrosine hydroxylase (TH) immuno-staining in ventral tegmental area (VTA; a circular area is indicated by white line). Scale bars = 40 μm. Stereological counts of TH+ cells throughout VTA on day 1 (D1), 7 (D7), 14 (D14) and 21 (D21) after the last-injection of MPTP (post-MPTP). *$p < 0.05$ and **$p < 0.01$ vs. control mice (one-way ANOVA). **(B)** Time chart of the experimental procedure. Horizontal open arrow indicates the time post-MPTP (day). Vertical open arrows indicate the time of open-field test (OFT), forced swim test (FST) and tail suspension test (TST) and Morris water maze task (MWM). **(C)** Each point represents the total distance traveled within 6 min in OFT on day 5, 12 and 19 post-MPTP, respectively. **(D,E)** The points indicate the immobility time in FST and TST on days 6–7, days 13–14 and days 20–21 post-MPTP, respectively. *$p < 0.05$ and **$p < 0.01$ vs. control mice (two-way ANOVA). **(F)** Each point represents the mean latencies (sec) to reach the hidden platforms on days 22–26 post-MPTP.

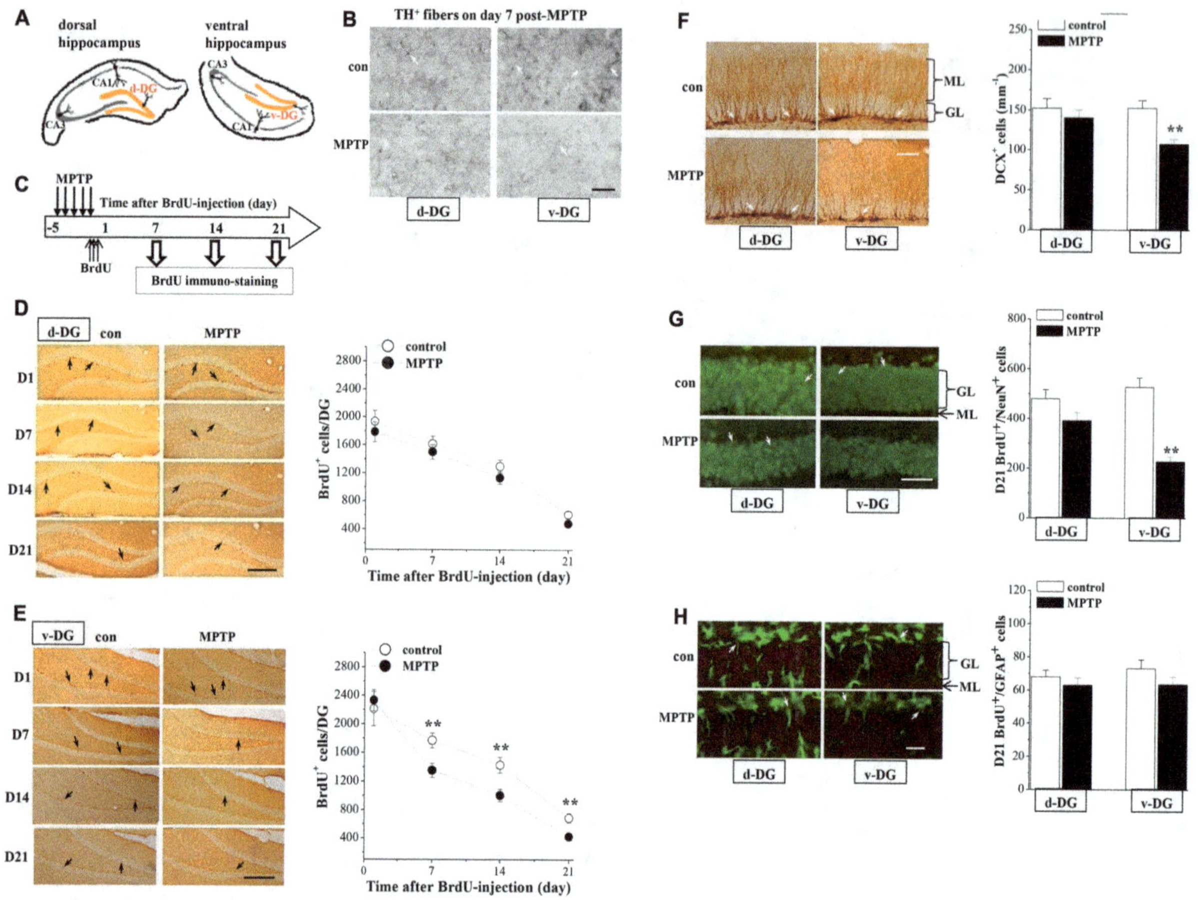

FIGURE 2 | Influence of MPTP-induced DA depletion on neurogenesis in dentate gyrus (DG). (A) Schematic diagram of dorsal DG (d-DG) and ventral DG (v-DG; orange area). **(B)** Representative pictures of TH$^+$ fibers (white arrows) in d-DG and v-DG on day 7 post-MPTP. Scale bars = 50 μm. **(C)** Time chart of the experimental procedure. Horizontal open arrow indicates the time after BrdU-injection (day). Vertical open arrows indicate the time of BrdU immuno-staining. **(D,E)** Representative images of BrdU-positive (BrdU$^+$) cells (black arrows) in d-DG **(D)** and v-DG **(E)**. Scale bar = 100 μm. The points represent the mean number of D1-, D7-, D14- and D21-BrdU$^+$ cells in d-DG and v-DG. $^{**}p < 0.01$ vs. control mice (two-way ANOVA). **(F)** Bar graph shows the mean number of DCX-positive (DCX$^+$) cells in d-DG and v-DG on day 7 post-MPTP. $^{**}p < 0.01$ vs. control mice (Student's *t*-tests). Representative images of DCX$^+$ cells (white arrows). ML: molecular layer; GL: granular cell layer. Scale bar = 50 μm. **(G,H)** Bar graph shows the mean number of D21-BrdU$^+$/NeuN$^+$ cells and D21-BrdU$^+$/GFAP$^+$ cells in d-DG and v-DG. $^{**}p < 0.01$ vs. control mice. Representative images of BrdU$^+$/NeuN$^+$ cells **(G)** and BrdU$^+$/GFAP$^+$ **(H)** cells (white arrows). Neuronal nuclei (NeuN) and glial fibrillary acidic protein (GFAP) are shown in green and BrdU is shown in red, newborn cells are shown in yellow. Scale bars = 50 μm.

not altered on day 7 post-MPTP. Compared with the control levels, the phosphorylation of PKA (p-PKA: $p < 0.01$; **Figure 3C**) or CREB (p-CREB: $p < 0.01$, $n = 8$; **Figure 3D**) in v-DG was reduced on day 7 post-MPTP, which was reversed by the administration of D1R agonist SKF38393 for 2 days ($p < 0.01$, $n = 8$). The PKA inhibitor H89 could block the D1R-reversed CREB phosphorylation in v-DG of MPTP-mice ($p < 0.05$, $n = 8$). The administration of D1R antagonist SCH23390 for 2 days to control mice decreased the phosphorylation of PKA ($p < 0.01$) and CREB ($p < 0.01$, $n = 8$) in v-DG. Consistently with the results of a report by Zhao et al. (2013), the activation of D2R by quinpirole led to a decline in the phosphorylation of PKA ($p < 0.05$) and CREB ($p < 0.05$, $n = 8$) in v-DG of control mice, whereas the D2R antagonist L-sulpiride had no effects ($p > 0.05$, $n = 8$). The treatment of MPTP-mice with quinpirole showed a tendency to decrease the phosphorylation of PKA and CREB in v-DG, but the difference had no statistical significance ($p > 0.05$, $n = 8$). In contrast, MPTP-mice did not show the changes in the levels of the PKA and CREB phosphorylation ($p > 0.05$, $n = 8$) in d-DG compared with those of controls, which was not affected by SKF38393 ($p > 0.05$, $n = 8$) or quinpirole ($p > 0.05$, $n = 8$). Furthermore, the phosphorylation of PKA or CREB in d-DG of control mice was not altered by the application of SCH23390 ($p > 0.05$, $n = 8$) or L-sulpiride ($p > 0.05$, $n = 8$).

MPTP Reduces the D1R-Mediated Survival of Newborn Neurons

The newborn cells in the adult hippocampal DG express functional D1R and D2R (Takamura et al., 2014). To test whether the down-regulation of D1R-activated PKA-CREB signaling affects the survival of young newborn neurons, MPTP-

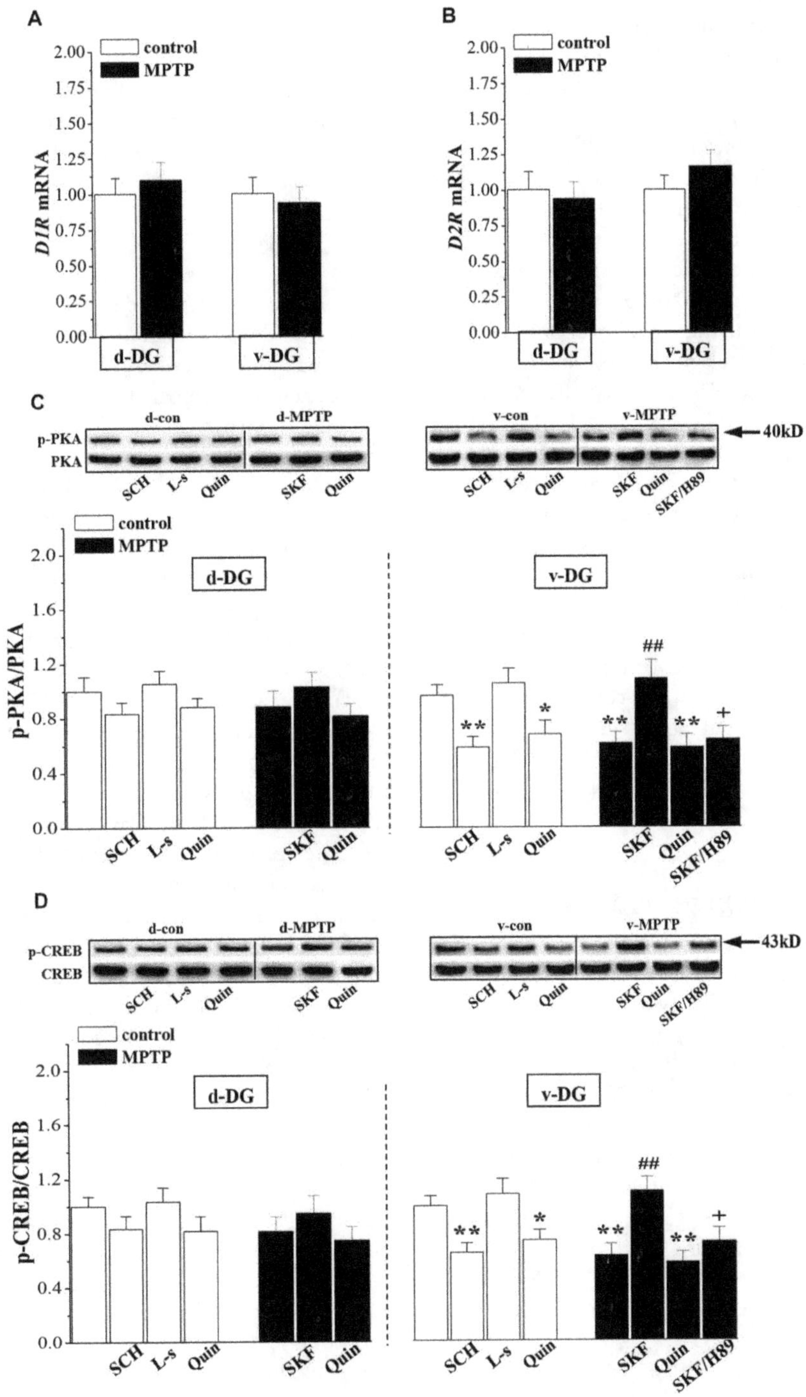

FIGURE 3 | Influence of MPTP-induced DA depletion on phosphorylation of PKA and CREB. (A,B) Levels of D1-like receptors (*D1R*) and *D2R* mRNA in d-DG and v-DG on day 7 post-MPTP. **(C,D)** Bar graphs show the mean levels of PKA and CREB phosphorylation in d-DG and v-DG of MPTP-mice untreated or treated with SKF38393 (SKF, 10 mg/kg, i.p.), H89 (1 mg/kg, i.p.) or quinpirole (Quin, 2 mg/kg, i.p.) for 2 days and control mice untreated or treated with SCH23390 (SCH, 0.5 mg/kg, i.p.) or L-sulpiride (L-s, 15 mg/kg. i.p.) for 2 days. $^{*}p < 0.05$ and $^{**}p < 0.01$ vs. control mice; $^{\#\#}p < 0.01$ vs. MPTP-mice; $^{+}p < 0.05$ vs. MPTP-mice treated with SKF.

mice were treated with SKF38393 or quinpirole daily on days 2–7 after the BrdU-injection, and control mice received the treatment with SCH23390, L-sulpiride or quinpirole. Then, we examined the number of D7- and D21-BrdU^{+} cells, respectively (**Figure 4A**). As shown in **Figures 4B,C**, the treatment with SKF38393 in MPTP-mice not only rescued the loss of D7-BrdU$^+$ cells ($p < 0.01$, $n = 10$), but also corrected the reduction of D21-BrdU$^+$ cells ($p < 0.01$, $n = 10$) in v-DG, which was sensitive to H89 ($p < 0.05$, $n = 10$). However, the administration of quinpirole to MPTP-mice had no effects on the reduced D7- or D21-BrdU$^+$ cells in v-DG ($p > 0.05$, $n = 10$). Interestingly, the treatment of control mice with either SCH23390 ($p < 0.01$, $n = 10$) or quinpirole ($p < 0.05$, $n = 10$), but not L-sulpiride ($p > 0.05$, $n = 10$), caused a decrease in the number of D7-BrdU$^+$ cells in v-DG, which was associated with the reduction of D21-BrdU$^+$ cells (SCH23390: $p < 0.01$, $n = 10$; quinpirole: $p < 0.05$, $n = 10$). In contrast, the number of D7- or D21-BrdU$^+$ cells in d-DG of control mice was not affected by SCH23390, quinpirole or L-sulpiride ($p > 0.05$, $n = 10$). However, the application of SKF38393 on days 16–21 after the BrdU-injection had no effect on the reduced D21-BrdU$^+$ cells in v-DG of MPTP-mice ($p > 0.05$, $n = 10$; **Figure 4D**). At the same time, the treatment of control mice with SCH23390 did not change the number of D21-BrdU$^+$ cells in v-DG ($p > 0.05$, $n = 10$). Additionally, the administration of SKF38393 for 6 days post-MPTP could increase the number of DCX$^+$ cells in v-DG ($p < 0.01$, $n = 10$; **Figure 4E**), while the activation of D2R by quinpirole could not ($p > 0.05$, $n = 10$). Similarly, the treatment of control mice with SCH23390 ($p < 0.01$, $n = 10$), but not L-sulpiride ($p > 0.05$, $n = 10$), caused a reduction in the number of DCX$^+$ cells in v-DG.

Association of MPTP-Impaired Neurogenesis With Depressive-Like Behaviors

To explore whether the impaired neurogenesis in MPTP-mice is related to their depressive-like behaviors, MPTP-mice were treated with SKF38393 or quinpirole for 18 days starting from the first-injection of MPTP, and control mice received SCH23390 and quinpirole for 18 days (**Figure 5A**). To avoid the direct effects of drugs, the affective behavioral tests were performed on days 6–7 after the end of the drugs administration. The results showed that the treatment of MPTP-mice with SKF38393, but not quinpirole, corrected the prolongation of the immobility time in FST ($p < 0.05$, $n = 10$; **Figure 5B**) and TST ($p < 0.01$, $n = 10$; **Figure 5C**), which was blocked by H89 (FST: $p < 0.05$; TST: $p < 0.05$, $n = 10$). In addition, the administration of SCH23390 (FST: $p < 0.01$; TST: $p < 0.01$, $n = 10$) or quinpirole (FST: $p < 0.05$; TST: $p < 0.05$, $n = 10$) to control mice caused an increase in the immobility time of FST and TST.

To determine further the relationship between the MPTP-impaired neurogenesis and the depressive-like behaviors, MPTP-mice were treated with the v-DG injection of SKF38393 (**Figure 5E**), and control mice received the v-DG injection of SCH23390 and H89 for 18 days (**Figure 5D**). Similarly, the v-DG injection of SKF38393 in MPTP-mice could prevent the prolongation of the immobility time in FST ($p < 0.05$, $n = 10$; **Figure 5F**) and TST ($p < 0.01$, $n = 10$; **Figure 5G**) and the reduction of D21-BrdU$^+$ cells in v-DG ($p < 0.01$, $n = 10$; **Figure 5H**). The v-DG injection of SCH23390 and H89 in control mice caused the prolongation of the immobility time in FST (SCH23390: $p < 0.01$, $n = 10$; H89: $p < 0.05$, $n = 10$) and TST (SCH23390: $p < 0.05$, $n = 10$; H89: $p < 0.05$, $n = 10$) and the loss of D21-BrdU$^+$ cells in v-DG (SCH23390: $p < 0.01$, $n = 10$; H89: $p < 0.05$, $n = 10$).

DISCUSSION

The present study provides evidence that the MPTP-induced decline of dopaminergic afferents in v-DG impairs the D1R-mediated early survival of newly generated neurons, and this deficit in hippocampal neurogenesis is associated with depressive-like behaviors.

The adult DG contains at least two types of proliferating immature cells: GFAP$^+$ radial glia-like cell (B-cell) and GFAP$^-$ cell (C-cells). The B-cells, as stem cells, generate frequently dividing transit-amplifying C-cells. Asymmetrically divided C-cells are more likely to be progenitor cells and can differentiate into neural precursors or DCX$^+$ neuroblasts (A-cells; Zhao et al., 2008). D2R is predominantly expressed in C-cells, while A-cells express both D1R and D2R (Höglinger et al., 2004). The activation of D2R has been reported to stimulate C-cell proliferation (Yang et al., 2008). The number of D1-BrdU$^+$ cells in v-DG or d-DG of MPTP-mice was not altered, although the dopaminergic neurons in VTA were reduced by approximately 25% on day 1 post-MPTP. The microtubule-associated protein DCX expression is specific to newly generated neurons, but not to glial cells and undifferentiated cells, which reaches a peak during the second week and is down-regulated concomitantly with the appearance of NeuN (Rao and Shetty, 2004). DCX, as an immature neuron marker, is used to evaluate the survival of young newborn neurons (Kim et al., 2009). MPTP-mice had a significant decrease in the DCX$^+$ cells in v-DG, which could be rescued by the activation of D1R rather than D2R. In addition, the blockade of D1R caused a decrease of the DCX$^+$ cells in v-DG of control mice. The number of D7-BrdU$^+$ cells in v-DG of MPTP-mice was reduced. Although fewer D14- or D21-BrdU$^+$ cells were found in v-DG of MPTP-mice than those in control mice, the percentage of reduced BrdU$^+$ cells (D7 → −25% D14 → −57% D21) in MPTP-mice did not differ from control mice (D7 → −20% D14; D14→ −52% D21). Therefore, it is likely that the MPTP-induced DA depletion mainly impairs the early survival of newborn neurons in v-DG. Khaindrava et al. (2011) have reported that DA depletion causes deficits in the survival of newborn cells in DG. Our pharmacological experiments support this idea by showing that in MPTP-mice, the D1R agonist when administered on days 2–7 after BrdU-injection rescued the loss of D7- or D21-BrdU$^+$ cells, but when administered on days 16–21 after BrdU-injection, it failed to alter the reduced D21-BrdU$^+$ cells in MPTP-mice. Moreover, the blockade of D1R on days 2–7 after BrdU-injection reduced the number of D7- and D21-BrdU$^+$ cells in control mice. The absolute number of D21-BrdU$^+$/NeuN$^+$ cells and proportion of these

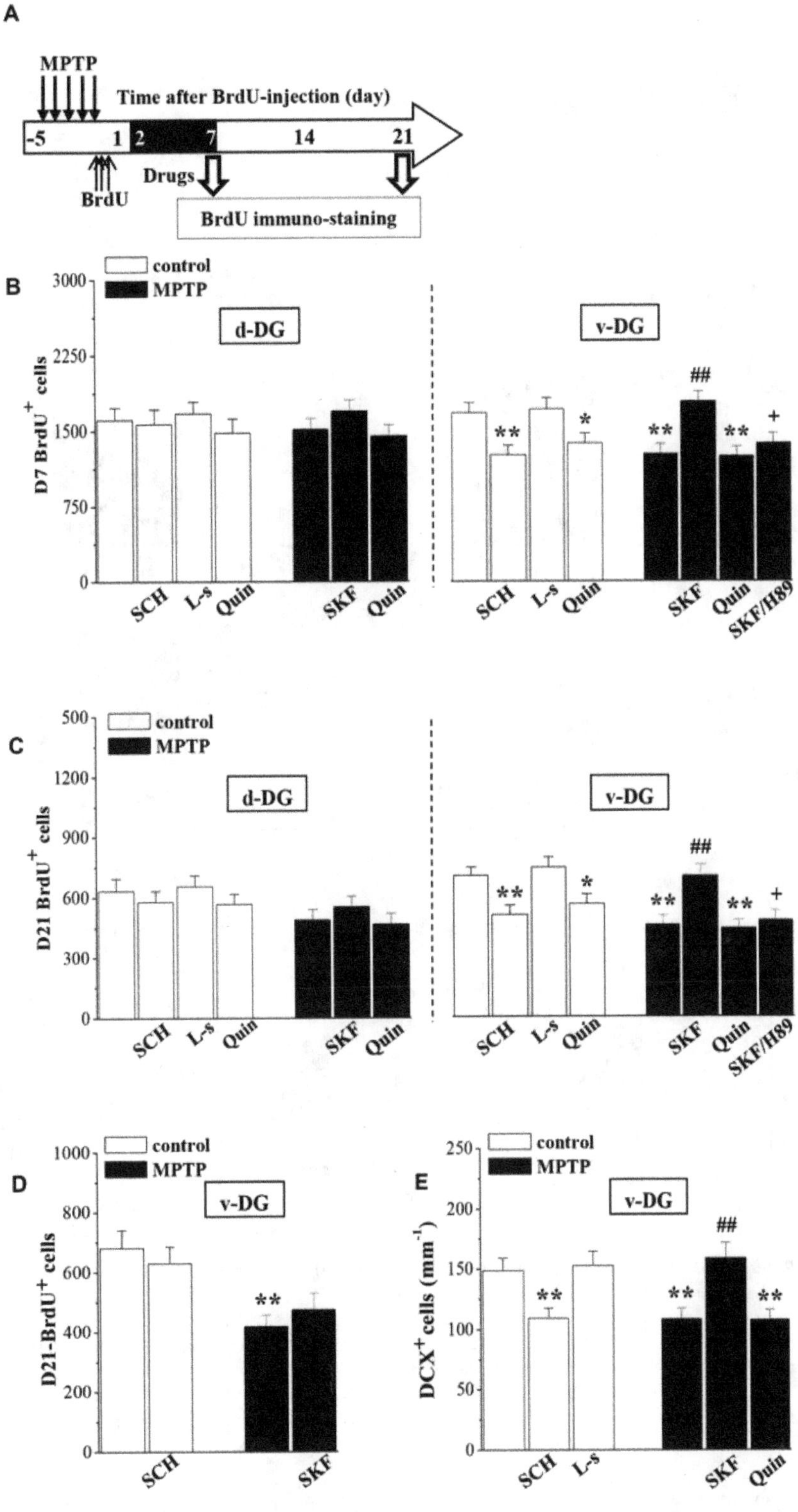

FIGURE 4 | Involvement of D1R and D2R in MPTP-impaired survival of newborn neurons. (A) Time chart of the experimental procedure. The drugs were administered on days 2–7 after the BrdU-injection (black part). **(B,C)** Bar graph shows the mean number of D7-BrdU$^+$ cells and D21-BrdU$^+$ cells in d-DG and v-DG of MPTP-mice treated with SKF38393 (SKF), H89 or quinpirole (Quin) or control mice treated with SCH23390 (SCH), L-sulpiride (L-s) or Quin. $^*p < 0.05$ and $^{**}p < 0.01$ vs. control mice; $^{\#\#}p < 0.01$ vs. MPTP-mice; $^+p < 0.05$ vs. MPTP-mice treated with SKF. **(D)** Bar graph shows the mean number of D21-BrdU$^+$ cells in v-DG when the drugs were administered on days 16–21 after the BrdU-injection. $^{**}p < 0.01$ vs. control mice. **(E)** Bar graph shows the mean number of DCX$^+$ cells in v-DG when the drugs were administered on days 2–7 post-MPTP. $^{**}p < 0.01$ vs. control mice; $^{\#\#}p < 0.01$ vs. MPTP-mice.

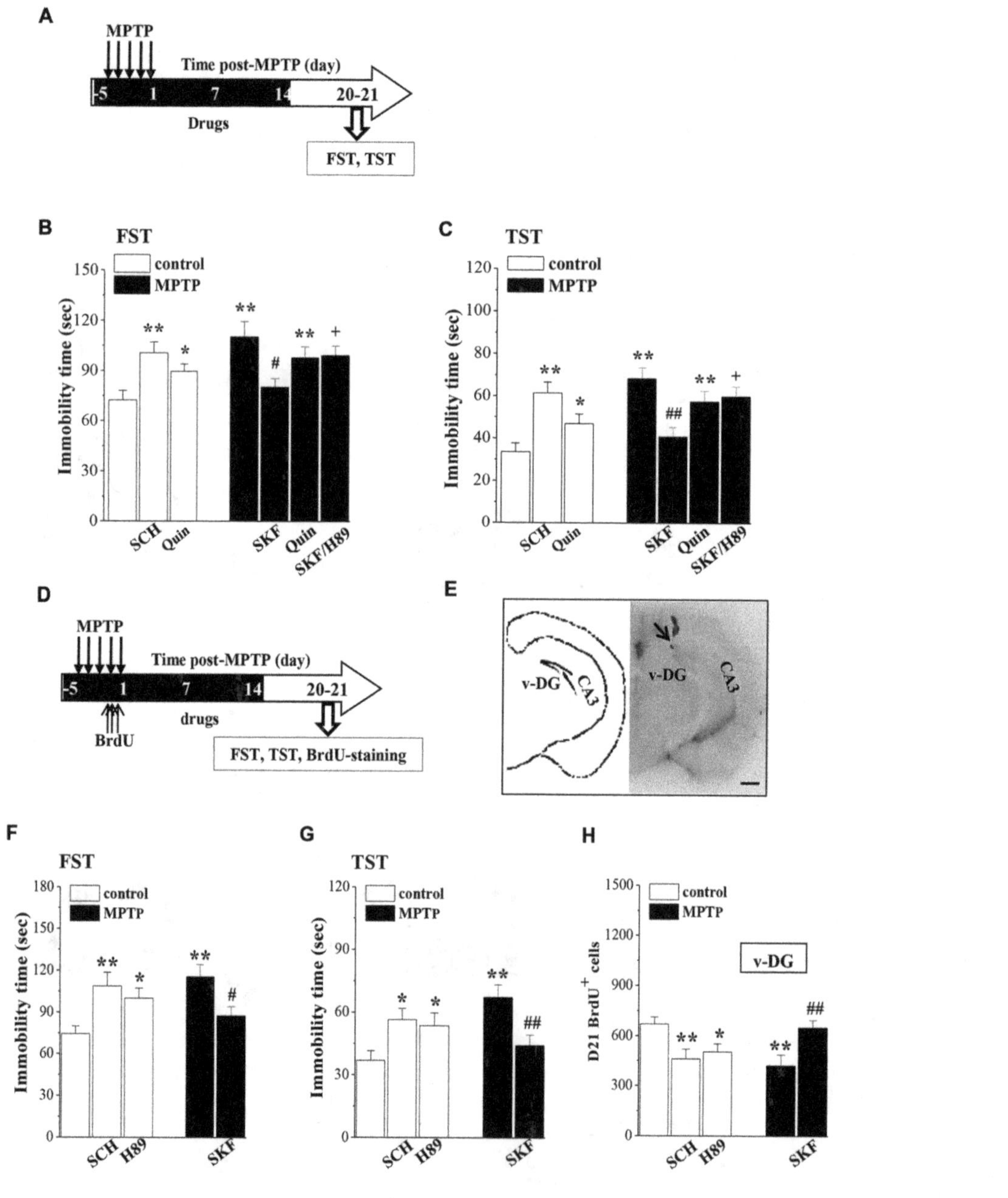

FIGURE 5 | Influence of MPTP-induced DA depletion on depressive-like behaviors. (A) Time chart of SKF38393 (SKF), quinpirole (Quin), SCH23390 (SCH) and H89 injection (i.p.) for 18 days (black part). **(B,C)** Bar graphs show the immobility time in FST and TST on days 6–7 after the last-administration of drugs. $^*p < 0.05$ and $^{**}p < 0.01$ vs. control mice. $^{\#}p < 0.05$ and $^{\#\#}p < 0.01$ vs. MPTP-mice.$^{+}p < 0.05$ vs. MPTP-mice treated with SKF. **(D)** Time chart of v-DG injection of SKF38393 (SKF), SCH23390 (SCH) and H89 for 18 days (black part). **(E)** The representative Evans-blue image of v-DG injection (right panel) and schematic diagram of v-DG (left panel). Scale bar = 1.0 mm. Black arrow indicates the site of the v-DG injection (black spot). CA3: hippocampal CA3 region. **(F,G)** Bar graphs show the immobility time in FST and TST on days 6–7 after the v-DG last-injection of drugs. $^*p < 0.05$ and $^{**}p < 0.01$ vs. control mice. $^{\#}p < 0.05$ and $^{\#\#}p < 0.01$ vs. MPTP-mice. **(H)** Bar graph shows the mean number of D21-BrdU$^+$ cells in v-DG. $^*p < 0.05$ and $^{**}p < 0.01$ vs. control mice. $^{\#\#}p < 0.01$ vs. MPTP-mice.

cells relative to the total D21-BrdU$^+$ cells were reduced in v-DG of MPTP-mice. The number of BrdU$^+$/GFAP$^+$ cells in v-DG of MPTP-mice did not differ from control mice, and the ratio of BrdU$^+$/GFAP$^+$ cells was higher than the ratio in control mice. Thus, it is conceivable that the MPTP-induced DA depletion does not affect the differentiation of precursor cells. On the other hand, the number of BrdU$^+$ cells, DCX$^+$ cells, BrdU$^+$/NeuN$^+$ cells or BrdU$^+$/GFAP$^+$ cells in d-DG did not differ between control and MPTP-mice, which was not affected by the activation or blockade of D1R and D2R. Consistently with the report by Bjarkam et al. (2003), there was few dopaminergic projections in d-DG, indicating that the neurogenesis process in d-DG may be insensitive to the dopaminergic regulation.

The administration of D1R agonist to MPTP-mice could rescue the loss of D7-BrdU$^+$ cells in a PKA-dependent manner, but the D2R agonist did not. The major signaling cascaded by D1R activation is the cAMP-PKA pathway in the hippocampus (Arnsten and Dudley, 2005). PKA-CREB signaling is one of the most important pathways for promoting neuron regeneration in DG (Miyamoto et al., 2009). The activation of PKA induces the phosphorylation of CREB at Ser-133, thereby facilitating the gene transcription of key molecules such as *c-Fos*, Jun-B, Bcl-2, GDNF and neurotrophins to regulate neuronal survival and regeneration. Inhibition of phosphodiesterase-4, an enzyme that catalyzes the hydrolysis of cAMP, stimulates the activation of CREB and increases the survival of newborn cells (Nakagawa et al., 2002). In this study, we observed the decline of PKA and CREB phosphorylation in v-DG of MPTP-mice without changes in the expression of D1R. In v-DG of MPTP-mice, the decrease of PKA and CREB phosphorylation could be corrected by the D1R agonist and the protection of D1R agonist on the D7-BrdU$^+$ cells was blocked by the inhibition of PKA. The blockade of D1R caused the loss of D7-BrdU$^+$ cells and decline of PKA and CREB phosphorylation in v-DG of control mice. The D2R antagonist haloperidol has been shown to decrease (Wakade et al., 2002), increase (Kippin et al., 2005) or not affect (Malberg et al., 2000) hippocampal neurogenesis. Our results showed that the activation of D2R reduced the PKA and CREB phosphorylation and the D7-BrdU$^+$ cells in v-DG of control mice. Therefore, it is proposed that the MPTP-induced DA depletion through the down-regulation of D1R-induced PKA-CREB signaling impairs the early survival of newborn neurons in v-DG.

It is widely accepted that the hippocampal neurogenesis is required for mood control (Petrik et al., 2012) and cognitive performance (Rola et al., 2004). Selectively impairing the adult neurogenesis by telomerase inhibitor could cause the depression-like behaviors in mice (Zhou et al., 2011a). Irradiation of young animals impairs hippocampal neurogenesis that is associated with cognitive deficits (Rola et al., 2004). The newly generated neurons are integrated into the neuronal circuitry within 3–4 weeks after birth (Zhao et al., 2006) to regulate hippocampal output (Ming and Song, 2011). Importantly, we have observed the depressive-like behaviors in MPTP-mice for 2–3 weeks later after DA depletion. The timing of depressive-like behaviors in MPTP-mice seems to be coincident with the loss of mature newborn neurons. Interestingly, MPTP-mice did not appear affected by the spatial cognitive deficits, although they showed depressive-like behaviors. One possible explanation may be a difference in the regions of impaired neurogenesis in hippocampal DG. The idea may be supported by the facts that the lesions in the dorsal hippocampus affect spatial learning and memory (Moser et al., 1995), while lesions of the ventral hippocampus lead to anxiety and depressive-like behaviors (McHugh et al., 2004). The antidepressants may exert their behavioral effects by increasing neurogenesis in v-DG (Banasr et al., 2006). In particular, the v-DG injection of SKF38393 in MPTP-mice not only reduced the loss of D21-BrdU$^+$ cells but also relieved the depressive-like behaviors. In control mice, the v-DG injection of either SCH23390 or H89 caused the reduction of D21-BrdU$^+$ cells in v-DG, which was companied by the production of depressive-like behaviors. These results indicate a possible cause-and-effect relationship between the MPTP-impaired neurogenesis and the MPTP-induced affective disorder. In addition, the ventral hippocampus is involved in regulation of the hypothalamic-pituitary-adrenal axis (Herman et al., 1995), buffering the stress response (Snyder et al., 2011). The basolateral amygdaloid complex receives the hippocampal afferents (Supcun et al., 2012). Hippocampal dysfunction affects the synaptic plasticity of the basolateral amygdaloid complex, which is important for the acquisition and consolidation of fear memories (Goosens and Maren, 2002) and the extinction of learned fear (Dalton et al., 2012).

Forebrain DA circuitry has been studied by two largely independent researchers: a nigrostriatal DA system that originates in the substantia nigra (SN) and a mesolimbic DA system that originate in the VTA. MPTP selectively destroys the dopaminergic neurons in the SN and VTA (Lu et al., 2014; Hong et al., 2015; the present study). Target neurons in the primary terminal field of the SN are striatal medium spiny neurons. It is well known that the MPTP-induced loss of dopaminergic neurons in SN pars compacta through the striatal DA depletion impairs the motor functions including slowness, rigidity, resting tremor and postural instability (Fahn, 2003). The projection fields of VTA DA neurons are the hippocampus or medial prefrontal cortex, which contributes to the emotional regulation (Russo and Nestler, 2013). Tye et al. (2013) have reported that the selective inhibition of VTA DA neurons acutely induces multiple distinct depression-like behaviors. Furthermore, the dopaminergic fibers from VTA dopaminergic neurons have been reported to contact directly with the newborn cells in DG (Höglinger et al., 2004). Taken together, the results in the present study give an indication that the MPTP-impaired VTA dopaminergic neurons leading to the dopaminergic deficiency in v-DG, impairs the D1R-mediated early survival of newborn neurons.

The present study provides evidence that the MPTP-induced dopaminergic depletion impairs the D1R-mediated early survival of newly generated neurons in v-DG; this impairment of hippocampal neurogenesis is associated with the production of the depressive-like behaviors. Thus, D1R agonists may be candidate substrates for treating PD depression.

AUTHOR CONTRIBUTIONS

In this study, TZ performed the immuno-staining, western blotting and all statistical analysis. JH finished the behavioral examination and RT-PCR analysis. TD carried out the animal care. LC designed the experiment and finished the manuscript.

FUNDING

This study was supported by the National 973 Basic Research Program of China (2014CB943303) and the National Natural Science Foundation of China (81471157; 81671253).

REFERENCES

Arnsten, A. F., and Dudley, A. G. (2005). Methylphenidate improves prefrontal cortical cognitive function through α2 adrenoceptor and dopamine D1 receptor actions: relevance to therapeutic effects in attention deficit hyperactivity disorder. *Behav. Brain Funct.* 1:2. doi: 10.1186/1744-9081-1-2

Banasr, M., Soumier, A., Hery, M., Mocaër, E., and Daszuta, A. (2006). Agomelatine, a new antidepressant, induces regional changes in hippocampal neurogenesis. *Biol. Psychiatry* 59, 1087–1096. doi: 10.1016/j.biopsych.2005.11.025

Bjarkam, C. R., Sørensen, J. C., and Geneser, F. A. (2003). Distribution and morphology of serotonin-immunoreactive axons in the hippocampal region of the New Zealand white rabbit. I. Area dentata and hippocampus. *Hippocampus* 13, 21–37. doi: 10.1002/hipo.10042

Borta, A., and Höglinger, G. U. (2007). Dopamine and adult neurogenesis. *J. Neurochem.* 100, 587–595. doi: 10.1111/j.1471-4159.2006.04241.x

Bower, J. H., Grossardt, B. R., Maraganore, D. M., Ahlskog, J. E., Colligan, R. C., Geda, Y. E., et al. (2010). Anxious personality predicts an increased risk of Parkinson's disease. *Mov. Disord.* 25, 2105–2113. doi: 10.1002/mds.23230

Crocker, S. J., Smith, P. D., Jackson-Lewis, V., Lamba, W. R., Hayley, S. P., Grimm, E., et al. (2003). Inhibition of calpains prevents neuronal and behavioral deficits in an MPTP mouse model of Parkinson's disease. *J. Neurosci.* 23, 4081–4091.

Dalton, G. L., Wu, D. C., Wang, Y. T., Floresco, S. B., and Phillips, A. G. (2012). NMDA GluN2A and GluN2B receptors play separate roles in the induction of LTP and LTD in the amygdala and in the acquisition and extinction of conditioned fear. *Neuropharmacology* 62, 797–806. doi: 10.1016/j.neuropharm.2011.09.001

Dolorfo, C. L., and Amaral, D. G. (1998). Entorhinal cortex of the rat: topographic organization of the cells of origin of the perforant path projection to the dentate gyrus. *J. Comp. Neurol.* 398, 25–48. doi: 10.1002/(SICI)1096-9861(19980817)398:1<25::AID-CNE3>3.0.CO;2-B

Fahn, S. (2003). Description of Parkinson's disease as a clinical syndrome. *Ann. N Y Acad. Sci.* 991, 1–14. doi: 10.1111/j.1749-6632.2003.tb07458.x

Francis, F., Koulakoff, A., Boucher, D., Chafey, P., Schaar, B., Vinet, M. C., et al. (1999). Doublecortin is a developmentally regulated, microtubule-associated protein expressed in migrating and differentiating neurons. *Neuron* 23, 247–256. doi: 10.1016/s0896-6273(00)80777-1

Gasbarri, A., Sulli, A., and Packard, M. G. (1997). The dopaminergic mesencephalic projections to the hippocampal formation in the rat. *Prog. Neuropsychopharmacol. Biol. Psychiatry* 21, 1–22. doi: 10.1016/s0278-5846(96)00157-1

Goosens, K. A., and Maren, S. (2002). Long-term potentiation as a substrate for memory: evidence from studies of amygdaloid plasticity and Pavlovian fear conditioning. *Hippocampus* 12, 592–599. doi: 10.1002/hipo.10099

Gorton, L. M., Vuckovic, M. G., Vertelkina, N., Petzinger, G. M., Jakowec, M. W., and Wood, R. I. (2010). Exercise effects on motor and affective behavior and catecholamine neurochemistry in the MPTP-lesioned mouse. *Behav. Brain Res.* 213, 253–262. doi: 10.1016/j.bbr.2010.05.009

Guiard, B. P., Ei Mansari, M., and Blier, P. (2009). Prospect of a dopamine contribution in the next generation of antidepressant drugs: the triple reuptake inhibitors. *Curr. Drug Targets* 10, 1069–1084. doi: 10.2174/138945009789735156

Herman, J. P., Cullinan, W. E., Morano, M. L., Aki, H., and Watson, S. J. (1995). Contribution of the ventral subiculum to inhibitory regulation of the hypothalamo-pituitary-adrenocortical axis. *J. Neuroendocrinol.* 7, 475–482. doi: 10.1111/j.1365-2826.1995.tb00784.x

Höglinger, G. U., Rizk, P., Muriel, M. P., Duyckaerts, C., Oertel, W. H., Caille, I., et al. (2004). Dopamine depletion impairs precursor cell proliferation in Parkinson disease. *Nat. Neurosci.* 7, 726–735. doi: 10.1038/nn1265

Hong, J., Sha, S., Zhou, L., Wang, C., Yin, J., and Chen, L. (2015). Sigma-1 receptor deficiency reduces MPTP-induced parkinsonism and death of dopaminergic neurons. *Cell Death Dis.* 6:e1832. doi: 10.1038/cddis.2015.194

Khaindrava, V., Salin, P., Melon, C., Ugrumov, M., Kerkerian-Le-Goff, L., and Daszuta, A. (2011). High frequency stimulation of the subthalamic nucleus impacts adult neurogenesis in a rat model of Parkinson's disease. *Neurobiol. Dis.* 42, 284–291. doi: 10.1016/j.nbd.2011.01.018

Kim, J. S., Jung, J., Lee, H. J., Kim, J. C., Wang, H., Kim, S. H., et al. (2009). Differences in immunoreactivities of Ki-67 and doublecortin in the adult hippocampus in three strains of mice. *Acta Histochemica* 111, 150–156. doi: 10.1016/j.acthis.2008.05.002

Kim, Y., Wang, W. Z., Comte, I., Pastrana, E., Tran, P. B., Brown, J., et al. (2010). Dopamine stimulation of postnatal murine subventricular zone neurogenesis via the D3 receptor. *J. Neurochem.* 114, 750–760. doi: 10.1111/j.1471-4159.2010.06799.x

Kippin, T. E., Kapur, S., and van der Kooy, D. (2005). Dopamine specifically inhibits forebrain neural stem cell proliferation, suggesting a novel effect of antipsychotic drugs. *J. Neurosci.* 25, 5815–5823. doi: 10.1523/JNEUROSCI.1120-05.2005

Lai, Y.-T., Fan, H.-Y., Cherng, C. G., Chiang, C.-Y., Kao, G.-S., and Yu, L. (2008). Activation of amygdaloid PKC pathway is necessary for conditioned cues-provoked cocaine memory performance. *Neurobiol. Learn. Mem.* 90, 164–170. doi: 10.1016/j.nlm.2008.03.006

Lisman, J. E., and Grace, A. A. (2005). The hippocampal-VTA loop: controlling the entry of information into long-term memory. *Neuron* 46, 703–713. doi: 10.1016/j.neuron.2005.05.002

Lu, M., Sun, X. L., Qiao, C., Liu, Y., Ding, J. H., and Hu, G. (2014). Uncoupling protein 2 deficiency aggravates astrocytic endoplasmic reticulum stress and nod-like receptor protein 3 inflammasome activation. *Neurobiol. Aging* 35, 421–430. doi: 10.1016/j.neurobiolaging.2013.08.015

Malberg, J. E., Eisch, A. J., Nestler, E. J., and Duman, R. S. (2000). Chronic antidepressant treatment increases neurogenesis in adult rat hippocampus. *J. Neurosci.* 20, 9104–9110.

McHugh, S., Deacon, R., Rawlins, J., and Bannerman, D. M. (2004). Amygdala and ventral hippocampus contribute differentially to mechanisms of fear and anxiety. *Behav. Neurosci.* 118, 63–78. doi: 10.1037/0735-7044.118.1.63

Ming, G. L., and Song, H. (2011). Adult neurogenesis in the mammalian brain: significant answers and significant questions. *Neuron* 70, 687–702. doi: 10.1016/j.neuron.2011.05.001

Miyamoto, N., Tanaka, R., Zhang, N., Shimura, H., Onodera, M., Mochizuki, H., et al. (2009). Crucial role for Ser133-phosphorylated form of cyclic AMP-responsive element binding protein signaling in the differentiation and survival of neural progenitors under chronic cerebral hypoperfusion. *Neuroscience* 162, 525–536. doi: 10.1016/j.neuroscience.2009.05.004

Moser, M. B., Moser, E. I., Forrest, E., Andersen, P., and Morris, R. (1995). Spatial learning with a minislab in the dorsal hippocampus. *Proc. Natl. Acad. Sci. U S A* 92, 9697–9701. doi: 10.1073/pnas.92.21.9697

Nakagawa, S., Kim, J. E., Lee, R., Malberg, J. E., Chen, J., Steffen, C., et al. (2002). Regulation of neurogenesis in adult mouse hippocampus by cAMP and the cAMP response element-binding protein. *J. Neurosci.* 22, 3673–3682.

Nasehi, M., Mafi, F., Oryan, S., Nasri, S., and Zarrindast, M. R. (2011). The effects of dopaminergic drugs in the dorsal hippocampus of mice in the nicotine-induced anxiogenic-like response. *Pharmacol. Biochem. Behav.* 98, 468–473. doi: 10.1016/j.pbb.2011.02.011

Nègre-Pagès, L., Grandjean, H., Lapeyre-Mestre, M., Montastruc, J. L., Fourrier, A., Lépine, J. P., et al. (2010). Anxious and depressive symptoms in Parkinson's disease: the French cross-sectionnal DoPaMiP study. *Mov. Disord.* 25, 157–166. doi: 10.1002/mds.22760

Oizumi, H., Hayashita-Kinoh, H., Hayakawa, H., Arai, H., Furuya, T., Ren, Y. R., et al. (2008). Alteration in the differentiation-related molecular expression in the subventricular zone in a mouse model of Parkinson's disease. *Neurosci. Res.* 60, 15–21. doi: 10.1016/j.neures.2007.09.004

O'Leary, O. F., O'Connor, R. M., and Cryan, J. F. (2012). Lithium-induced effects on adult hippocampal neurogenesis are topographically segregated along the dorso-ventral axis of stressed mice. *Neuropharmacology* 62, 247–255. doi: 10.1016/j.neuropharm.2011.07.015

Park, J. H., and Enikolopov, G. (2010). Transient elevation of adult hippocampal neurogenesis after dopamine depletion. *Exp. Neurol.* 222, 267–276. doi: 10.1016/j.expneurol.2010.01.004

Petrik, D., Lagace, D. C., and Eisch, A. J. (2012). The neurogenesis hypothesis of affective and anxiety disorders: are we mistaking the scaffolding for the building? *Neuropharmacology* 62, 21–34. doi: 10.1016/j.neuropharm.2011.09.003

Rao, M. S., and Shetty, A. K. (2004). Efficacy of doublecortin as a marker to analyse the absolute number anddendritic growth of newly generated neurons in the adult dentate gyrus. *Eur. J. Neurosci.* 19, 234–246. doi: 10.1111/j.0953-816x.2003.03123.x

Rodriguez-Oroz, M. C., Jahanshahi, M., Krack, P., Litvan, I., Macias, R., Bezard, E., et al. (2009). Initial clinical manifestations of Parkinson's disease: features and pathophysiological mechanisms. *Lancet Neurol.* 8, 1128–1139. doi: 10.1016/s1474-4422(09)70293-5

Rola, R., Raber, J., Rizk, A., Otsuka, S., VandenBerg, S. R., Morhardt, D. R., et al. (2004). Radiation-induced impairment of hippocampal neurogenesis is associated with cognitive deficits in young mice. *Exp. Neurol.* 188, 316–330. doi: 10.1016/j.expneurol.2004.05.005

Russo, S. J., and Nestler, E. J. (2013). The brain reward circuitry in mood disorders. *Nat. Rev. Neurosci.* 14, 609–625. doi: 10.1038/nrn3381

Schober, A. (2004). Classic toxin-induced animal models of Parkinson's disease: 6-OHDA and MPTP. *Cell Tissue Res.* 318, 215–224. doi: 10.1007/s00441-004-0938-y

Seyedi, S. Y., Salehi, F., Payandemehr, B., Hossein, S., Hosseini-Zare, M. S., Nassireslami, E., et al. (2014). Dual effect of cAMP agonist on ameliorative function of PKA inhibitor in morphine-dependent mice. *Fundam. Clin. Pharmacol.* 28, 445–454. doi: 10.1111/fcp.12045

Sha, S., Hong, J., Qu, W. J., Lu, Z. H., Li, L., Yu, W. F., et al. (2015). Sex-related neurogenesis decrease in hippocampal dentate gyrus with depressive-like behaviors in sigma-1 receptor knockout mice. *Eur. Neuropsychopharmacol.* 25, 1275–1286. doi: 10.1016/j.euroneuro.2015.04.021

Snyder, J. S., Soumier, A., Brewer, M., Pickel, J., and Cameron, H. A. (2011). Adult hippocampal neurogenesis buffers stress responses and depressive behaviour. *Nature* 476, 458–461. doi: 10.1038/nature10287

Supcun, B., Ghadiri, M. K., Zeraati, M., Stummer, W., Speckmann, E. J., and Gorji, A. (2012). The effects of tetanic stimulation on plasticity of remote synapses in the hippocampus-perirhinal cortex-amygdala network. *Synapse* 66, 965–974. doi: 10.1002/syn.21591

Sutton, L. P., and Caron, M. G. (2015). Essential role of D1R in the regulation of mTOR complex1 signaling induced by cocaine. *Neuropharmacology* 99, 610–619. doi: 10.1016/j.neuropharm.2015.08.024

Takamura, N., Nakagawa, S., Masuda, T., Boku, S., Kato, A., Song, N., et al. (2014). The effect of dopamine on adult hippocampal neurogenesis. *Prog. Neuropsychopharmacol. Biol. Psychiatry* 50, 116–124. doi: 10.1016/j.pnpbp.2013.12.011

Toni, N., Laplagne, D. A., Zhao, C., Lombardi, G., Ribak, C. E., Gage, F. H., et al. (2008). Neurons born in the adult dentate gyrus form functional synapses with target cells. *Nat. Neurosci.* 11, 901–907. doi: 10.1038/nn.2156

Tye, K. M., Mirzabekov, J. J., Warden, M. R., Ferenczi, E. A., Tsai, H. C., Finkelstein, J., et al. (2013). Dopamine neurons modulate neural encoding and expression of depression-related behaviour. *Nature* 493, 537–541. doi: 10.1038/nature11740

Videbech, P., and Ravnkilde, B. (2015). Hippocampal volume and depression: a meta-analysis of MRI studies. *Am. J. Psychiatry* 161, 1957–1966. doi: 10.1176/appi.ajp.161.11.1957

Wakade, C. G., Mahadik, S. P., Waller, J. L., and Chiu, F. C. (2002). Atypical neuroleptics stimulate neurogenesis in adult rat brain. *J. Neurosci. Res.* 69, 72–79. doi: 10.1002/jnr.10281

Winner, B., Desplats, P., Hagl, C., Klucken, J., Aigner, R., Ploetz, S., et al. (2009). Dopamine receptor activation promotes adult neurogenesis in an acute Parkinson model. *Exp. Neurol.* 219, 543–552. doi: 10.1016/j.expneurol.2009.07.013

Yang, P., Arnold, S. A., Habas, A., Hetman, M., and Hagg, T. (2008). Ciliary neurotrophic factor mediates dopamine D2 receptor-induced CNS neurogenesis in adult mice. *J. Neurosci.* 28, 2231–2241. doi: 10.1523/JNEUROSCI.3574-07.2008

Zhao, C., Deng, W., and Gage, F. H. (2008). Mechanisms and functional implications of adult neurogenesis. *Cell* 132, 645–660. doi: 10.1016/j.cell.2008.01.033

Zhao, W., Huang, Y., Liu, Z., Cao, B. B., Peng, Y. P., and Qiu, Y. H. (2013). Dopamine receptors modulate cytotoxicity of natural killer cells via cAMP-PKA-CREB signaling pathway. *PloS One* 8:e65860. doi: 10.1371/journal.pone.0065860

Zhao, C., Teng, E. M., Summers, R. G., Ming, G.-L., and Gage, F. H. (2006). Distinct morphological stages of dentate granule neuron maturation in the adult mouse hippocampus. *J. Neurosci.* 26, 3–11. doi: 10.1523/JNEUROSCI.3648-05.2006

Zhou, Q. G., Hu, Y., Wu, D. L., Zhu, L. J., Chen, C., Jin, X., et al. (2011a). Hippocampal telomerase is involved in the modulation of depressive behaviors. *J. Neurosci.* 31, 12258–12269. doi: 10.1523/JNEUROSCI.0805-11.2011

Zhou, Q. G., Zhu, L. J., Chen, C., Wu, H. Y., Luo, C. X., Chang, L., et al. (2011b). Hippocampal neuronal nitric oxide synthase mediates the stress-related depressive behaviors of glucocorticoids by downregulating glucocorticoid receptor. *J. Neurosci.* 31, 7579–7590. doi: 10.1523/JNEUROSCI.0004-11.2011

Zhou, L., Yin, J., Wang, C., Liao, J., Liu, G., and Chen, L. (2014). Lack of seipin in neurons results in anxiety- and depression-like behaviors via down regulation of PPARgamma. *Hum. Mol. Genet.* 23, 4094–4102. doi: 10.1093/hmg/ddu126

15

Genetic Determinants of Parkinson's Disease: Can They Help to Stratify the Patients Based on the Underlying Molecular Defect?

Sara Redenšek[1], *Maja Trošt*[2] *and Vita Dolžan*[1*]

[1] *Pharmacogenetics Laboratory, Institute of Biochemistry, Faculty of Medicine, University of Ljubljana, Ljubljana, Slovenia,*
[2] *Department of Neurology, University Medical Centre Ljubljana, Ljubljana, Slovenia*

Edited by:
Daniela Tropea,
Trinity College, Ireland

Reviewed by:
Robert Petersen,
Case Western Reserve University, USA
Anelyssa D'Abreu,
Brown University, USA

***Correspondence:**
Vita Dolžan
vita.dolzan@mf.uni-lj.si

Parkinson's disease (PD) is a sporadic progressive neurodegenerative brain disorder with a relatively strong genetic background. We have reviewed the current literature about the genetic factors that could be indicative of pathophysiological pathways of PD and their applications in everyday clinical practice. Information on novel risk genes is coming from several genome-wide association studies (GWASs) and their meta-analyses. GWASs that have been performed so far enabled the identification of 24 loci as PD risk factors. These loci take part in numerous cellular processes that may contribute to PD pathology: protein aggregation, protein, and membrane trafficking, lysosomal autophagy, immune response, synaptic function, endocytosis, inflammation, and metabolic pathways are among the most important ones. The identified single nucleotide polymorphisms are usually located in the non-coding regions and their functionality remains to be determined, although they presumably influence gene expression. It is important to be aware of a very low contribution of a single genetic risk factor to PD development; therefore, novel prognostic indices need to account for the cumulative nature of genetic risk factors. A better understanding of PD pathophysiology and its genetic background will help to elucidate the underlying pathological processes. Such knowledge may help physicians to recognize subjects with the highest risk for the development of PD, and provide an opportunity for the identification of novel potential targets for neuroprotective treatment. Moreover, it may enable stratification of the PD patients according to their genetic fingerprint to properly personalize their treatment as well as supportive measures.

Keywords: Parkinson's disease, genetic risk factors, genome-wide association studies, single nucleotide polymorphisms, personalized medicine

INTRODUCTION

Parkinson's disease (PD) is the second most common neurodegenerative brain disease after Alzheimer's disease. It is believed that both genetic and environmental factors contribute to the development of PD. It is a chronic, progressive and incurable disease (Pringsheim et al., 2014). Two pathological hallmarks characterize PD: the formation of cytoplasmic inclusions termed Lewy bodies and Lewy neurites and the loss of dopaminergic neurons in the substantia nigra pars compacta (Gallegos et al., 2015). The disease manifests as bradykinesia, muscular rigidity, rest tremor and postural and gait impairment (Postuma et al., 2015), which can be accompanied by several other nonmotor symptoms (Gallegos et al., 2015). At the present time, there is unfortunately no cure for PD except for the symptomatic treatment and supportive measures (Connolly and Lang, 2014).

Two different forms of PD have been identified, i.e., sporadic and familial. The familial form starts at an earlier stage of life (<50 years), is usually more severe and progresses more quickly (Klein and Westenberger, 2012). At early stages of research on genetics of PD, only linkage studies were performed, which means that families with PD history were included in the study. These studies identified mutations in six genes that conclusively cause monogenic PD—*SNCA*, *LRRK2*, *Parkin*, *PINK1*, *DJ-1*, *ATP13A2* (Klein and Westenberger, 2012).

In this review, we focus mainly on the sporadic form of the disease. However, there is some overlap between genes associated with familial and sporadic disease; in particular, *SNCA* and *LRRK2* are involved in both forms (Verstraeten et al., 2015; van der Brug et al., 2015). Recently, genome-wide association studies (GWASs) that compared single nucleotide polymorphisms' (SNPs) frequencies between sporadic PD patients and healthy individuals have identified several loci as Parkinson's disease susceptibility genes (Klein and Westenberger, 2012; Nalls et al., 2014). A few of these loci, 24 in particular, harboring SNPs that were found to be associated with PD were validated in the replication phase of the latest and largest meta-analysis of GWASs performed by Nalls et al. in 2014. In the discovery phase, they performed a meta-analysis of GWASs including 13,708 cases and 95,282 controls chosen from the populations of European descent (the USA, France, Germany, Iceland, the Netherlands, the UK; 23 and Me), while the replication phase of the study included 5,353 cases and 5,551 controls (Nalls et al., 2014). The identified loci segregate with numerous cellular pathways that may contribute to PD pathology: protein aggregation, protein, and membrane trafficking, lysosomal autophagy, immune response, synaptic function, endocytosis, inflammation, and metabolic pathways being among the most important ones (Kumaran and Cookson, 2015). Each locus identified as a risk factor has a rather low contribution to PD development; therefore, a combination of molecular defects rather than a single event probably plays a role in PD risk, hence the idea of a cumulative nature of genetic risk factors (Pihlstrom et al., 2016).

This review summarizes the latest knowledge on genetics and genomics of PD susceptibility, obtained by GWASs and their meta-analyses. We focus on the largest meta-analysis of GWASs on PD risk so far (Nalls et al., 2014), but we also searched the PubMed database and GWAS catalog (Welter et al., 2014) for studies that pointed out the same loci as the above-mentioned meta-analysis. We identified 13 GWASs and their meta-analyses (summarized in **Table 1**), which we included in this review. We compiled the available data on the 24 loci that were found to be associated with the risk of sporadic form of PD. To obtain the information about gene functions, we searched the PubMed database and collected the available data on genes' functions with the help of the following words: "Parkinson's disease and *gene name*" or "Parkinson's disease and polymorphisms and *gene name*." We divided the susceptibility genes into seven groups according to their physiological functions: protein aggregation; protein, and membrane trafficking; lysosomal autophagy; immune system; neurodevelopment, neuron cell differentiation, and survival; mitochondrial homeostasis; and genes involved in other processes. This review highlights the main functions of these genes' products and their role in the PD pathogenesis.

GENETIC DETERMINANTS OF RISK FOR SPORADIC PD AND THEIR IMPLICATED PATHWAYS

Protein Aggregation

The products of the genes listed below, i.e., SNCA and tau, are both constituents of the protein aggregates typical of PD called Lewy bodies. PD is often thought to be a prion-like disease because of the presence of these bodies (Hasegawa et al., 2016).

SNCA

SNCA codes for α-synuclein (SNCA), which is a small, acidic protein of 14.5 kDA and 140 amino acids (Gallegos et al., 2015). It is the main component of aggregates called Lewy bodies, a hallmark of PD pathology. Lewy bodies are formed because a mutated protein usually adopts the β-sheet structure, which is harder to degrade than α-helixes, the main conformation of native proteins (Gallegos et al., 2015; Inoshita and Imai, 2015). Different variants of the gene have been connected to both familial and sporadic forms of PD. Several studies on families with positive PD history have reported the association of *SNCA* with PD, the first one being published in 1997 by Polymeropoulos et al. (1997). The association with sporadic PD was first described by Kruger et al. who compared the allelic frequences of *REP1* polymorphism in the promoter region of *SNCA* between cases and controls (Kruger et al., 1999). This association was later confirmed on a larger set of data (Maraganore et al., 2006). The majority of GWASs performed also confirmed *SNCA* as a susceptibility gene (Satake et al., 2009; Simon-Sanchez et al., 2009; Edwards et al., 2010; Hamza et al., 2010; Do et al., 2011; Nalls et al., 2011, 2014; Saad et al., 2011; Spencer et al., 2011; Lill et al., 2012; Pankratz et al., 2012; Hill-Burns et al., 2014). To date, over 800 SNPs within *SNCA* have been reported, with nearly half of them showing a positive association with PD (Kumaran and Cookson, 2015). SNPs within *SNCA* recognized as PD susceptibility factors by GWASs are listed in **Table 2**. The most replicated SNP rs256220 was confirmed as a risk factor in six studies, whereas several others were found in only one or two studies. Some *SNCA* mutations can cause both sporadic and familial forms of PD. These are usually more penetrant (Singleton et al., 2013). Besides point mutations—Ala53Thr, Ala30Pro, and Glu46Lys in the amino-terminal sequence, whole locus multiplications (duplications and triplications) were also found in both forms (Bisaglia et al., 2009).

SNCA is widely expressed in the central nervous system, especially in the presynaptic terminals of neurons (Inoshita and Imai, 2015). It has two main physiological roles, the first being

TABLE 1 | GWAS studies and their meta-analyses that identified 24 risk loci included in this review.

Study	Ancestry	Number of cases	
		Initial phase (cases vs. controls)	Replication phase (cases vs. controls)
Nalls et al., 2014#	European Initial phase—*USA, *France, *Germany, *Iceland, *Netherlands, *UK, *23andMe Replication phase—*US, *UK, *France, *Germany, *Greece, *Netherlands, *NeuroX	13,708 vs. 95,282	5,353 vs. 5,551
Vacic et al., 2014	Ashkenazi Jewish Initial phase—*Israel, *US Replication phase—*Israel, *US	1,130 vs. 2,611	306 vs. 2,583
Hill-Burns et al., 2014	European Initial phase—*US Replication phase—not reported	1,565 sporadic cases + 435 familial cases vs. 1,986 controls	1,528 sporadic cases + 707 familial cases vs. 796 controls
Lill et al., 2012#	Initial phase—*US Replication phase—European and Asian	2,197 vs. 2,061	Up to 98,080
Pankratz et al., 2012#	European	4,238 vs. 4,239	3,738 vs. 2,111
Do et al., 2011	European	3,426 vs. 29,624	Not applicable
Nalls et al., 2011#	Initial phase—*France, *Germany, *UK, *US Replication phase—*US, *France, *Germany, *Netherlands, *Iceland, *UK	5,333 vs. 12,019	7,053 vs. 9,007
Hamza et al., 2010	European	2,000 vs. 1,986	Up to 1,447 vs. 1,468
Saad et al., 2011	European	1,039 vs. 1,984	3,232 vs. 7,064
Spencer et al., 2011	Initial phase—*UK Replication phase—*France	1,705 vs. 5,175	1,039 vs. 1,984
Edwards et al., 2010	European	1,752 vs. 1,745	Not applicable
Satake et al., 2009	Japanese	988 vs. 2,521	933 vs. 15,753
Simon-Sanchez et al., 2009	European	1,713 vs. 3,978	3,361 vs. 4,573

**country of recruitment, if specified.*
#meta-analysis.
Data compiled from the GWAS catalog database and PDgene (Lill et al., 2012; Nalls et al., 2014; Welter et al., 2014).

the control of synaptic membrane processes and the second being the control of neurotransmitter release via interactions with members of the SNARE family (Bellucci et al., 2012; Tsigelny et al., 2012). It promotes SNARE-complex assembly through a non-enzymatic mechanism, binding to phospholipids via its N-terminal and to synaptobrevin-2 via its C-terminal (Burre et al., 2010). SNCA is deeply involved in the synaptic vesicle cycle, including trafficking, docking, fusion, and recycling after exocytosis. It was also suggested that SNCA is a negative regulator of neurotransmitter release, including dopamine, with traffic restriction of synaptic vesicles from the resting pool to the sites of release (Emanuele and Chieregatti, 2015).

Wild-type SNCA is translocated to the lysosomes for degradation via chaperone-mediated autophagy via the lysosomal membrane receptor LAMP2A (Gan-Or et al., 2015). Lysosomal enzyme β-glucocerebrosidase (GBA) then modulates SNCA levels (Klein and Westenberger, 2012). Mutant SNCA somehow inhibits chaperone-mediated autophagy, presumably by attaching to the LAMP2A and preventing its internalization of wild-type and mutant SNCA. Recently, it has been shown that GBA and SNCA form a positive feedback loop that leads to the accumulation of SNCA. The loss of GBA function results in the accumulation of SNCA, whereas SNCA inhibits the lysosomal activity of GBA (Mazzulli et al., 2011).

SNCA is presumably also involved in dopamine release and in the synaptic vesicle dynamics, especially in the recycling pathway. The excess of SNCA reduces the recycling of synaptic vesicles and their motility (Inoshita and Imai, 2015). Furthermore, it has been confirmed that dopamine can interact with the SNCA molecule via the C-terminal residues which can induce and/or modulate its structure and oligomerization. As a result dopamine blocks chaperone-mediated autophagy of SNCA. This may explain why dopaminergic neurons are more prone to SNCA accumulation (Bellucci et al., 2012; Lashuel et al., 2013; Gan-Or et al., 2015).

SNCA also modulates dopamine vesicle trafficking by other mechanisms. According to Ahn et al. SNCA binds and consequently inhibits phospholipase D2 (PLD2), which is involved in vesicle trafficking in terms of endo- and exocytosis (Ahn et al., 2002). SNCA's interacting partner is also actin which is essential for synaptic vesicle mobilization between different functional pools. SNCA binding modulates actin's polymerization in a manner dependent on Ca^{2+} concentration (Bellani et al., 2010). Intracellular Ca^{2+} concentration may also change due to the formation of pore-like structures in the cell membranes by mutant SNCA (Lashuel et al., 2002). Furthermore, SNCA's interacting partner is also a rate-limiting enzyme in the dopamine synthesis, tyrosine hydroxylase (TH), responsible for the conversion of tyrosine to L-3,4-dihydroxyphenylalanine

TABLE 2 | SNPs within loci associated with protein aggregation recognized as PD susceptibility factors by GWASs.

Gene/locus Chromosome	SNP	MAF (1000 genomes project)	Risk allele: OR	Study
SNCA Ch 4	rs356182 g.90626111G>A (intron variant)	G = 0.4044	G: OR = 1.32	Nalls et al., 2014
	rs356219 g.90637601G>A (intron variant)	A = 0.4892	OR = 1.29	Lill et al., 2012
			G: OR = 1.29	Nalls et al., 2011
	rs356220 g.90641340T>C (intron variant)	C = 0.4834	OR = 1.38	Pankratz et al., 2012
			T: OR = 1.29	Do et al., 2011
			T: OR = 1.27	Spencer et al., 2011
			T: OR = 1.38	Hamza et al., 2010
			T: OR = 1.38	Hill-Burns et al., 2014
			T: OR = 1.37	Saad et al., 2011
	rs11931074 g.90639515G>T (intron variant)	T = 0.3806	OR = 1.37	Satake et al., 2009
	rs2736990 g.90678541G>A c.307-28113C>T (intron variant)	A = 0.3934	G: OR = 1.23	Simon-Sanchez et al., 2009
			OR = 1.29	Edwards et al., 2010
	rs6532194 g.90780902C>T (intergenic variant)	T = 0.3694	OR = 1.29	Lill et al., 2012
MAPT Ch 8	rs17649553 g.43994648C>T (intron variant)	T = 0.0865	C: OR = 1.3	Nalls et al., 2014
	900 kb inversion	H1/H2		Lill et al., 2012
	rs2942168 g.43714850C>T (intron variant)	A = 0.0863	G: OR = 1.27	Nalls et al., 2011
	rs393152 g.43719143A>G (intron variant)	G = 0.2476	A: OR = 1.3	Simon-Sanchez et al., 2009
	rs12185268 g.43923683A>G p.Ile471Val (missense variant)	G = 0.0863	A: OR = 1.3	Do et al., 2011
	rs8070723 g.44081064A>G c.1828-6612A>G (intron variant)	G = 0.1190	OR = 1.3	Spencer et al., 2011
	rs17577094 g.44187492A>G c.1290-15425T>C (intron variant)	G = 0.0865	OR = 1.56	Vacic et al., 2014
	rs11012 g.43513441C>T c.*1783G>A	T = 0.0807	T: OR = 1.43	Edwards et al., 2010
	rs199498 g.46788237T>C c.81-14328A>G (intron variant)	C = 0.2578	T: OR = 1.35	Hill-Burns et al., 2014
	rs199533 g.44828931G>A p.Lys702 = (synonimous variant)	A = 0.0791	C: OR = 1.35	Hamza et al., 2010

Ch, Chromosome. Data compiled from the GWAS catalog database, the dbSNP and the e!Ensembl (Sherry et al., 2001; Welter et al., 2014; Yates et al., 2016).
**Denotes SNPs in 3'-UTR.*

(L-DOPA). This interaction inhibits the phosphorylation of TH and thus also its action (Venda et al., 2010).

SNCA is also linked to neuroinflammation. In mice with aggregated SNCA, MHCII expression is induced in microglia. Moreover, SNCA as a danger-associated molecular pattern (DAMP) stimulates toll-like receptors (TLR). Misfolded and fibrillar SNCA activates microglia via TLR2 and TLR4 and activation of NLRP3 inflammasome (Gustot et al., 2015). These processes contribute to dopaminergic neuronal death (Dzamko et al., 2015; Kumaran and Cookson, 2015).

In addition, *SNCA* mutations can lead to dysfunctions in several other cellular pathways, such as mitochondrial function, oxidative stress, cytochrome c release, ER stress, apoptosis (Gallegos et al., 2015).

MAPT

MAPT encodes a microtubule-associated protein tau, which has a role in stabilizing microtubules in the neurons. The gene was first recognized as a PD risk factor by Pastor et al. (2000). It has been repeatedly confirmed as a risk factor for sporadic PD by GWASs and their meta-analyses (Simon-Sanchez et al., 2009; Edwards et al., 2010; Hamza et al., 2010; Do et al., 2011; Nalls et al., 2011, 2014; Spencer et al., 2011; Lill et al., 2012; Hill-Burns et al., 2014; Vacic et al., 2014), but each variant has only been pointed out once and has not been replicated in other studies. More than 40 mutations have been discovered to date. They are either coding mutations, that affect the binding activity of the tau or its susceptibility to aggregation, or mutations that alter the splicing of exon 10 which encodes the fourth microtubule binding repeat (4R tau isoforms) (Wray and Lewis, 2010). Mutations within *MAPT* locus recognized as PD susceptibility factors by GWASs are listed in **Table 2**. The *MAPT* locus is the longest region of linkage disequilibrium in Caucasians. There are two variants of the locus resulting from an inversion of a 900 kb long portion of the sequence, which leads to two haplotypes—H1 and H2. *MAPT* H1 haplotype increases the transcription of the gene, whereas *MAPT* H2 haplotype decreases it (Golpich et al., 2015). The inversion is present in the H2 haplotype, which has a 20% frequency in the Caucasians, but is almost not present in the Asian population (Wider et al., 2010; Schulte and Gasser, 2011; Soto-Ortolaza and Ross, 2016). *MAPT* association was not replicated in the Japanese population probably due to inter-population heterogeneity at this locus (Satake et al., 2009; Labbé and Ross, 2014). H1 haplotype is more dynamic and can be subdivided into subhaplotypes. Homozygous *MAPT* H1/H1 genotype is a biomarker of dementia in PD (Lin and Wu, 2015). As H1 haplotype is associated with a greater risk of PD and other neurodegenerative diseases, it may be assumed that H2 haplotype is under positive selection (Schulte and Gasser, 2011). Polymorphisms in the *MAPT* gene are also involved in the pathologies of Alzheimer's disease (AD), progressive supranuclear palsy (PSP), and corticobasal degeneration (CBD) (Vandrovcova et al., 2009).

MAPT encoded protein tau is a potential component of Lewy bodies. In PD patients with a more pronounced cognitive decline, neurofibrillary tangles, more typical of AD, can also be found besides Lewy bodies. These tangles consist of hyperphosphorylated tau (Horvath et al., 2013; Lin and Wu, 2015). Physiologically, phosphorylation of the tau protein regulates its propensity to interact with microtubules (Wray and Lewis, 2010). According to some studies, SNCA also promotes tau fibrillization and influences tau phosphorylation (Giasson et al., 2003). The interplay between the two genes was also confirmed by the study of Goris et al., reporting nearly a double risk of PD in carriers of the combined *MAPT* H1/H1 and *SNCA* rs356219 G/G genotype (Goris et al., 2007). Most of the pathological changes in the *MAPT* sequence disrupt the ability of tau to interact with microtubules (Wray and Lewis, 2010). Tau is also fundamental for the maintenance of cytoskeletal network via the regulation of axonal transport by interactions with kinesin and dynein (Kumaran and Cookson, 2015).

Mutated MAPT may also affect the function of lysosomes and its role in autophagy, since it is degraded with this process (Gan-Or et al., 2015).

MAPT gene lies in a block of nearly complete linkage disequilibrium that extends over nearly 2 Mb, therefore it is possible that other genes from this region are also associated with PD risk (Charlesworth et al., 2012). For example, a variant in the *CRHR1* gene coding for the corticotropin-releasing hormone receptor has recently been recognized as a factor that decreases the PD susceptibility (Davis et al., 2016).

Protein and Membrane Trafficking

SNPs within loci associated with protein and membrane trafficking recognized as PD susceptibility factors by GWASs are listed in **Table 3**. The genes within this group are involved in processes, such as clathrin-mediated vesicular transport, trafficking, and fusing of synaptic vesicles, clearance of Golgi-derived vesicles, endo- and exocytosis and protein sorting.

TMEM175/GAK/DGKQ

A haplotype block *TMEM175/GAK/DGKQ* (transmembrane protein 175/cyclin G associated kinase/theta diacylglicerol kinase) was first associated with sporadic PD in the GWAS performed by Hamza et al. after it was already confirmed to be associated with the familial form of the disease (Pankratz et al., 2009; Hamza et al., 2010). This locus was reevaluated several times by different research groups and also showed positive results in other GWASs and meta-analyses of GWASs. The most replicated SNP is an intron variant rs11248060, others were found in individual studies only (Edwards et al., 2010; Do et al., 2011; Nalls et al., 2011, 2014; Lill et al., 2012; Pankratz et al., 2012).

GAK is a particularly promising candidate for a risk gene, because it is differentially expressed in the substantia nigra pars compacta of PD patients as compared to controls (Pankratz et al., 2009). *GAK* gene product participates in multiple steps of clathrin-mediated vesicular transport. For example, together with the heat-shock cognate protein 70 (Hsc70), it promotes the uncoating of endocytosed clathrin-coated vesicles. Probably it has also some other functions related to its serine/threonine kinase domain. It also directly interacts with LRRK2 and participates in the clearance of Golgi-derived vesicles via the lysosomal autophagy pathway as a part of LRRK2/RAB7L1/GAK trans-Golgi complex (Kumaran and Cookson, 2015; Perrett et al., 2015). Recently, depletion of GAK has been shown to influence lysosomal sorting of cathepsin D, the main lysosomal enzyme involved in SNCA degradation (Latourelle et al., 2009). Knockdown of GAK in primary rat neurons increased SNCA toxicity (Perrett et al., 2015). GAK also takes part in cell cycle regulation (Labbé and Ross, 2014).

Less is known about *DGKQ*; however, it is expressed in the brain where it may be involved in the phosphatidylinositol and lipid signaling (Pankratz et al., 2009). DGK proteins are also known to affect Ca^{2+} signaling as well as the trafficking and fusing of synaptic vesicles at nerve terminals in the central nervous system (Ran and Belin, 2014).

NUCKS1/RAB7L1

A haplotype block NUCKS1/RAB7L1 (nuclear casein kinase and cyclin-dependent kinase substrate 1/RAB7, member RAS oncogene family-like 1) is in linkage disequilibrium and is also known by the name PARK16 locus. This locus contains five genes—*SLC45A3*, *NUCKS1*, *RAB7L1*, *SLC41A1*, and *PM20D1*. The association between PD and *NUCKS1* was first described in the GWAS conducted by Simon-Sanchez et al. (2009), whereas the association with *RAB7L1* was first shown in Satake et al. GWAS (Satake et al., 2009). The implication of this locus in PD was then again confirmed in meta-analysis of GWASs by Nalls et al. and in the GWAS by Vacic et al. (Nalls et al., 2014; Vacic et al., 2014). Four SNPs were pointed out by genome-wide studies in this locus but none of them was replicated.

RAB7L1, also named RAB29, is a cytoplasmic GTP-binding protein, which plays an important role in endo- and exocytosis. Exocytosis is relevant in PD because dopamine is released via exocytotic vesicles and because it has been shown that vesicle abnormalities occur in SNCA knock-out mice (Plagnol et al., 2011). RAB7L1 is one of the LRRK2 interacting partners in the process of removal of Golgi derived vesicles by autophagy-dependent mechanisms. RAB7L1 deficiency caused neurodegeneration in mammalian or *Drosophila* dopaminergic neurons having a human *LRRK2* mutation, while *RAB7L1* overexpression restored the function of *LRRK2* mutant neurons. MacLeod et al. showed that expressing mutant LRRK2 or reducing the expression of RAB7L1 in a cell line led to the loss of components of the retromer complex, which regulates protein sorting from the lysosome to the Golgi apparatus.

TABLE 3 | SNPs within loci associated with protein and membrane trafficking recognized as PD susceptibility factors by GWASs.

Gene/locus	SNP	MAF (1000 genomes project)	Risk allele: OR	Study
TMEM175/GAK/DGKQ Ch 4	rs34311866 g.951947T>C p.Met311Thr (missense variant)	C = 0.1400	C: OR = 1.27	Nalls et al., 2014
	rs11248060 g.964359C>T (intron variant)	T = 0.1066	OR = 1.21	Lill et al., 2012
			OR = 1.26	Pankratz et al., 2012
			NA	Edwards et al., 2010
	rs6599388 g.939087C>T (intron variant)	T = 0.3243	T: OR = 1.16	Nalls et al., 2011
	rs11248051 g.858332C>T (intron variant)	T = 0.0966	T: OR = 1.46	Hamza et al., 2010
	rs6599389 g.939113G>A (intron variant)	A = 0.1092	A: OR = 1.31	Do et al., 2011
NUCKS1/RAB7L1 Ch 1	rs823118 g.205723572C>T (upstream gene variant)	T = 0.4111	T: OR = 1.122	Nalls et al., 2014
	rs947211 g.205752665A>G (intergenic variant)	A = 0.4613	OR = 1.3	Satake et al., 2009
	rs823128 g.205713378G>A (intron variant)	G = 0.1765	A: OR = 1.52	Simon-Sanchez et al., 2009
	rs823114 g.205719532G>A c.-431C>T (upstream gene variant)	A = 0.4073	OR = 1.33	Vacic et al., 2014
LRRK2 Ch 12	rs76904798 g.40614434C>T (intron variant)	T = 0.1318	T: OR = 1.155	Nalls et al., 2014
	rs34637584 g.40734202G>A p.Gly2019Ser (missense variant)	A = 0.0002	A: OR = 9.62	Do et al., 2011
	rs1442190 g.41365640G>A c.*325G>A	A = 0.0747	OR = 3.72	Vacic et al., 2014
	rs34778348 g.40757328G>A p.Gly2385Arg (missense variant)	A = 0.0048	OR = 2.23	Lill et al., 2012
	rs1491942 g.40620808C>G c.237+1366C>G (intron variant)	G = 0.2979	OR = 1.17	Lill et al., 2012
			G: OR = 1.27	Nalls et al., 2011
	rs1994090 g.40428561G>T c.717-6250C>A (intron variant)	G = 0.1472	OR = 1.39	Satake et al., 2009
INPP5F Ch 10	rs117896735 g.121536327G>A c.179-4820G>A (intron variant)	A = 0.0040	A: OR = 1.624	Nalls et al., 2014
BCKDK/STX1B Ch 16	rs14235 g.31110472G>A c.615G>A p.Thr205 = (synonymous variant)	A = 0.3592	A: OR = 1.103	Nalls et al., 2014
VPS13C Ch 15	rs2414739 g.61701935G>A (intron variant)	G = 0.3209	A: OR = 1.113	Nalls et al., 2014

NA, data not available; Ch, Chromosome. Data compiled from the GWAS catalog database, the dbSNP and the e!Ensembl (Sherry et al., 2001; Welter et al., 2014; Yates et al., 2016).
**Denotes SNPs in 3'-UTR.*

Secondary to these changes, the swelling of lysosomes and the reduction of lysosomal mannose 6-phosphate receptor (M6PR) accumulation occur (MacLeod et al., 2013; Perrett et al., 2015). M6PRs are needed for the recruitment and transport of lysosomal hydrolases to the lysosome; therefore, the disruption of this function may lead to lysosomal dysfunction (Gan-Or et al., 2015). RAB7L1 thus functions downstream of GAK in the retromer sorting process (Hoang, 2014). The authors also suggested an epistatic effect, with nonlinear increase in PD susceptibility when both risk alleles are present in the patient's DNA sequence (MacLeod et al., 2013).

Less is known about NUCKS1 and its involvement in PD pathogenesis. NUCKS1 is a nuclear protein containing several consensus phosphorylation sites for casein kinase II and cyclin-dependent kinases of unknown function (Satake et al., 2009). According to some studies, NUCKS1 might also be involved in inflammation and immunity (Dzamko et al., 2015). The recent GWAS meta-analysis has reported that rs823118 was tagged an expression quantitative trait locus and also a methylation quantitative trait locus for both RAB7L1 and NUCKS1 (Wang et al., 2016).

LRRK2

LRRK2 (leucine-rich repeat kinase 2) gene was first described as a risk factor for the familial form of PD, but was later also confirmed as sporadic PD susceptibility gene by GWASs. It encompasses rare highly penetrant variants as well as more common variants with a lower effect (van der Brug et al., 2015). *LRRK2* mutations are the most common gene defect in sporadic PD (Perrett et al., 2015). The first GWAS that confirmed *LRRK2* as a risk factor for sporadic PD was performed by Satake et al. (2009). Later, its association with PD was also confirmed in other GWASs and their meta-analyses (Do et al., 2011; Nalls et al., 2011, 2014; Lill et al., 2012; Vacic et al., 2014). Six different SNPs were found by GWASs as risk factors, but only one (rs1491942) was also replicated in a later study (Lill et al., 2012). *LRRK2* accounts for a large part of risk for sporadic PD in some populations—Ashkenazi Jews, Arabs, East Asians. Coding variability at the *LRRK2* locus explains 10% of PD risk in these populations. In the outbred Europeans, *LRRK2* and *GBA* account for around 8% of risk. Carriers of *LRRK2* mutations usually have Lewy bodies, the minority has also tangles, but some of them have neither (Hardy, 2010).

LRRK2 is a multidomain protein that has a GTPase and kinase function as well as many protein/protein interaction motifs. It is expressed in axons and dendrites in the striatum and the cortex, but expression is low in nigral cell bodies. LRRK2 seems to regulate actin complexes, vesicle trafficking, endosome maturation, cytoskeletal dynamics, and protein translation (Volta et al., 2015). It was detected as a binding partner of the late-endosomal marker Rab7 and also as a binding partner of the lysosomal marker LAMP2A, which generated the idea that it has an important function in the endo-lysosomal pathway. Mutant LRRK2-RAB7 colocalization can lead to a reduced RAB7 function and impaired late endosomal trafficking events. LRRK2 also interacts with RAB7L1 to modify protein sorting. It also binds the PD susceptibility factor GAK in a complex that promotes removal of Golgi derived vesicles by autophagy-dependent mechanisms (Perrett et al., 2015). It is tightly linked to endocytotic and exocytotic processes required for rapid synaptic vesicles and receptor recycling via interaction with clathrin (Volta et al., 2015). It regulates endophilin association to clathrin-coated vesicles through phosphorylation (Drouet and Lesage, 2014). Furthermore, it influences the action of EndoA via phosphorylation, a protein important for endocytic synaptic vesicles recycling (Inoshita and Imai, 2015). Moreover, LRRK2 is involved in mitochondrial membrane maintenance via fusion/fission processes and in lysosomal autophagy and recycling of V-ATPase required for lysosomal acidification (Ryan et al., 2015; Volta et al., 2015). The dysregulation of mitochondrial function can also be caused by the inhibition of the endogenous peroxidase phosphorylation by mutant LRRK2 (Saiki et al., 2012). LRRK2 also has a role in neuroinflammation by increasing the cytokine release from activated primary microglial cells, which results in neurotoxicitiy (Russo et al., 2014; Blesa et al., 2015). Moreover, it interferes with the translation machinery by phosphorylation of several proteins, for example translation repressor protein 4E-BP (Taymans et al., 2015).

Among PD patients having the LRRK2 mutation, the most common one is p.Gly2019Ser (rs34637584). The penetrance is high—50% at the age of 50 and 74% at the age of 79. This mutation is located in the kinase domain resulting in an increase in the activity (Wallings et al., 2015). 1.6% of sporadic PD patients possess this mutation (Satake et al., 2009). Mutated LRRK2 (p.Gly2019Ser) actually binds to outer mitochondrial membrane, which leads to a decrease in mitochondrial membrane potential and to a decrease in the intracellular ATP level. On the contrary, mitochondrial elongation and interconnectivity were elevated (Subramaniam and Chesselet, 2013).

INPP5F

Inositol polyphosphate-5-phosphatase F (*INPP5F*), one of the polyphosphoinositide phosphatases, was first described as a PD risk factor in a meta-analysis carried out by Nalls et al. in 2014 (Nalls et al., 2014), which means that only one SNP was found to be associated with PD susceptibility so far. The gene's product is supposed to be involved in the endocytic pathways. It contains a Sac domain, which is involved in the endocytosis of synaptic vesicles (Inoshita and Imai, 2015; Nakatsu et al., 2015). The knowledge about the gene's function is limited and on the basis of only one study pointing out the association, we cannot reach any conclusions as to the main role of the gene in PD pathology and the actual association.

BCKDK/STX1B

BCKDK/STX1B (branched chain ketoacid dehydrogenase kinase/syntaxin 1B) locus was established as a PD risk factor in GWAS meta-analysis by Nalls et al. Only one SNP (rs14235) is known to be associated with PD, thus replication studies are needed to confirm the actual association (Nalls et al., 2014).

BCKDK is located in the mitochondrial matrix and plays a major role in valine, leucine and isoleucine catabolism. Its function is phosphorylation and thus inactivation of the BCKD. BCKD concentration is the same in all tissues, whereas BCKDK concentration varies. BCKD's level of function is thus regulated by BCKDK (García-Cazorla et al., 2014).

STX1B codes for syntaxin 1B, which functions as a synaptic receptor for vesicle transport. It was previously shown to be directly implicated in the process of calcium-dependent synaptic transmission in rat brain, having been suggested to play a role in the excitatory pathway of synaptic transmission (Plagnol et al., 2011). It plays a role in dopamine neurotransmission (Kalia and Lang, 2015).

VPS13C

Vacuolar protein sorting 13 homolog C (VPS13C) was shown to be associated with PD as a risk factor only in the meta-analysis by Nalls et al. (2014). First, it was considered only as a risk factor for sporadic PD, but it has recently been discovered that it could also cause the familial autosomal-recessive early-onset form of PD with a very severe course of the disease (Lesage et al., 2016). The gene has two variants, variant 2 being specific to brain tissue (Velayos-Baeza et al., 2004). It functions in the vesicular transport, more specifically endosomal transport pathway (Inoshita and Imai, 2015). Functional studies of the protein are lacking, but a very recent one also suggests a protein quality control function (Yang et al., 2016). More association and functional studies will have to be conducted to be completely confident of the gene's role in PD susceptibility and pathology.

Lysosomal Autophagy

SNPs within loci associated with lysosomal autophagy recognized as PD susceptibility factors by GWASs are listed in **Table 4**. These genes are playing their part in general lysosomal functions, especially lysosomal autophagy.

GBA/SYT11

GBA (beta acid glucosidase) is associated with PD susceptibility according to several GWASs and their meta-analyses, but the first association was found in 2011 by Do et al. (Do et al., 2011;

TABLE 4 | SNPs within loci associated with lysosomal autophagy recognized as PD susceptibility factors by GWASs.

Gene/locus	SNP	MAF (1000 genomes project)	Risk allele: OR	Study
GBA/SYT11 Ch 1	rs35749011 g.155135036G>A (intergenic variant)	A = 0.0054	A: OR = 1.824	Nalls et al., 2014
	i4000416 g.155205634T>C c.1226A>C p.Asn409Ser (missense variant)	C = 0.0006	C: OR = 4.05	Do et al., 2011
	rs1630500 g.154855055G>A (intergenic variant)	A = 0.0559	OR = 1.75	Vacic et al., 2014
	rs12726330 g.155108167G>A c.-262G>A (splice region variant)	A = 0.0052	OR = 1.71	Pankratz et al., 2012
	rs34372695 g.156030037C>T c.-1155C>T (upstream gene variant)	T = 0.0088	T: OR = 1.47	Nalls et al., 2011
SCARB2/FAM47E Ch 4	rs6812193 g.77198986C>T c.871-236C>T (intron variant)	T = 0.3133	C: OR = 1.1	Nalls et al., 2014
			C: OR = 1.19	Do et al., 2011
			C: OR = 1.12	Simon-Sanchez et al., 2009

Ch, Chromosome. Data compiled from the GWAS catalog database, the dbSNP and the e!Ensembl (Sherry et al., 2001; Welter et al., 2014; Yates et al., 2016).

Pankratz et al., 2012; Nalls et al., 2014; Vacic et al., 2014). On the other hand, *SYT11* (synaptotagmin XI) was confirmed as a PD risk gene by Nalls et al. in 2011 (Nalls et al., 2011, 2014). No SNP has been replicated in a later study.

GBA is located within the inner lysosomal membrane, where it cleaves membrane glucocerebrosides into ceramide and glucose. Functional studies have shown that any kind of reduction in GBA enzymatic activity leads to the accumulation of SNCA which, in turn, inhibits the function of normal GBA, causing the additional aggregation of SNCA. The authors hypothesize that the reduction of GBA function, either caused by *GBA* mutations or impaired GBA trafficking from ER and Golgi to lysosomes, increases the glucocerebrosides concentration in lipid rafts. This change in membrane composition may lead to the reduced formation of LAMP2A (chaperone-mediated autophagy receptor) protein-complexes, which could result in diminished autophagy of SNCA and its accumulation. GBA dysfunction may also lead to general disruption in lysosomal function and autophagy. Furthermore, it can also be the reason for defective mitophagy and mitochondrial damage. It was also shown that PD patients with no mutation in the *GBA* may have a lower enzyme activity. This implies that other factors may also affect the GBA function, for example environmental factors (Gan-Or et al., 2015).

SYT11 encodes a calcium-sensing protein involved in membrane trafficking in synaptic transmision and is also a substrate of Parkin, which is a risk factor for the familial form of PD. Due to its ability of calcium-dependent phospholipid binding, it is important in the regulation of vesicle fusion and endocytosis at synaptic terminals (Ran and Belin, 2014). More studies will have to be performed in order to properly determine the function of the gene.

SCARB2/FAM47E

SCARB2/FAM47E (scavenger receptor class B member 2) locus was first found to be associated with PD in 2009 by Simon-Sanchez et al.; this was later confirmed by two other GWASs—Do et al. and Nalls et al. The same SNP (rs6812193) was pointed out in all three studies (Simon-Sanchez et al., 2009; Do et al., 2011; Nalls et al., 2014).

SCARB2 encodes the lysosomal membrane protein type 2 (LIMP-2), which is a GCase receptor. It directs GBA to lysosomes. The reduced function of SCARB2 can lead to a reduced GBA activity and decreased SNCA degradation (Gan-Or et al., 2015). The receptor, being an enterovirus 71 receptor, also plays a role in the neuroinflammation process (Dzamko et al., 2015). *FAM47E* lies in close proximity to *SCARB2* and the most frequently associated SNP (rs6812193) is situated between the two genes. However, among the two, SCARB2 seems to be a more promising candidate for a PD risk factor (Do et al., 2011; Ran and Belin, 2014).

Immune System

SNPs within loci associated with the immune system recognized as PD susceptibility factors by GWASs are listed in **Table 5**. The genes' function in PD susceptibility and pathology should be tested in a more targeted way with the help of cell and animal models. There are some indications that genes mentioned below play a role in the immune system, but we do not know to what extent and if this is their main purpose, except for *HLA-DQB1* whose function is quite well determined. There is also a need for more association studies especially for *STK39, HLA-DQB1* and *DDRGK1*.

BST1

BST1 (bone marrow stromal cell antigen-1) was recognized as a PD risk factor in the Satake et al. GWAS in 2009 and after that in several other GWASs. Three intron variants were found to be associated with PD risk. Two of them (rs11724635 and rs4698412) were replicated in a later study (Satake et al., 2009; Nalls et al., 2011, 2014; Saad et al., 2011; Pankratz et al., 2012). BST1, a member of the CD38 gene family, is a cell surface protein bound to the membrane by glycosylphosphatidylinositol linkage; it possesses both ADP ribosyl cyclase and cyclic ADP ribose hydrolase enzymatic activities. It produces cyclic ADP-ribose, which as a second messenger releases calcium from intracellular

TABLE 5 | SNPs within loci associated with immune system recognized as PD susceptibility factors by GWASs.

Gene/locus	SNP	MAF (1000 genomes project)	Risk allele: OR	Study
BST1 Ch 4	rs11724635 g.15737101C>A (intron variant)	A = 0.4079	A: OR = 1.126	Nalls et al., 2014
			A: OR = 1.15	Nalls et al., 2011
	rs4538475 g.15737937A>G c.*195A>G (intron variant)	G = 0.3089	OR = 1.24	Satake et al., 2009
	rs4698412 g.15737348G>A c.852-328G>A (intron variant)	A = 0.4077	OR = 1.14	Pankratz et al., 2012
			A: OR = 1.14	Saad et al., 2011
STK39 Ch 2	rs1474055 g.169110394C>T (intergenic variant)	T = 0.2007	T: OR = 1.214	Nalls et al., 2014
	rs2102808 g.169117025G>T (intergenic variant)	T = 0.2083	C: OR = 1.18	Nalls et al., 2011
HLA-DQB1 Ch 6	rs9275326 g.32666660C>T (intergenic variant)	T = 0.0843	C: OR = 1.21	Nalls et al., 2014
DDRGK1 Ch 20	rs8118008 g.3168166A>G (downstream gene variant)	G = 0.4597	A: OR = 1.111	Nalls et al., 2014

Ch, Chromosome. Data compiled from the GWAS catalog database, the dbSNP and the e!Ensembl (Sherry et al., 2001; Welter et al., 2014; Yates et al., 2016).
**Denotes SNPs in 3'-UTR.*

ER stores, leading to calcium influx. Calcium is a great regulator of neurotransmitter release from presynaptic terminals; therefore, a disruption in neuronal calcium homeostasis could lead to selective death of dopaminergic neurons. Interestingly, BST1 seems to be an important factor in the immune system, since it is highly expressed in bone marrow cells in patients with rheumatoid arthritis and facilitates immature B-cell proliferation and growth (Chen et al., 2014; Ran and Belin, 2014).

STK39

STK39 (serine threonine kinase 39) is highly expressed in the brain and pancreas (Wang et al., 2014). It codes for a SPAK protein (Ste20-related proline/alanine rich-kinase) (Kumaran and Cookson, 2015). As a PD risk factor, it was first described by Nalls et al. in 2011 and then again confirmed three years later by the same group. Two different intergenic variants were pointed out in these studies (Nalls et al., 2011, 2014). It is a serine/threonine kinase, which is activated under cellular stress and plays a role in stress signals, ion homeostasis and inflammation (Li et al., 2013; Ran and Belin, 2014). It has been shown that its overexpression alters intestinal inflammatory levels in mouse models of colitis, whereas its knockout attenuates intestinal inflammation (Dzamko et al., 2015; Kumaran and Cookson, 2015). Apart from PD, it has been associated with hypertension, autism and early-stage non-small-cell lung cancer (Li et al., 2013).

HLA-DQB1

HLA-DQB1 (major histocompatibility complex, class II, DQ beta 1) was shown to be associated with the risk for PD in the Nalls et al. study in 2014 (Nalls et al., 2014). Only one intergenic variant was shown to be associated with a PD risk, which means that more association studies confirming the association need to be conducted. It plays a key role in the immune system by presenting peptides to the antigen presenting cells. The HLA region is one of the most complex regions in the genome. It encompasses a high number of closely packed genes, with numerous polymorphisms and complicated patterns of linkage disequilibrium. As part of immune response HLA genes, are involved in many pathologies, such as autoimmune diseases, infections and malignant and neurological disorders. The HLA region is divided into classes, I and II, but they both code for proteins that present antigens to T cell receptors as part of the adaptive immune system. HLA class II molecules are expressed in antigen presenting cells—macrophages, B lymphocytes and dendritic cells. They consist of two chains, alpha (DQA) and beta (DQB) (Lampe et al., 2003; Wissemann et al., 2013; Chang et al., 2015). Several *HLA* genes (Hill-Burns et al., 2011) are thought to be associated with PD, besides *HLA-DQB1* also *HLA-DRA* (Hamza et al., 2010; Pankratz et al., 2012; Hill-Burns et al., 2014) and *HLA-DRB* (Ahmed et al., 2012).

DDRGK1

DDRGK1 (DDRGK domain containing 1) gene was found to be associated with PD in the meta-analysis of GWASs performed by Nalls et al. (2014), but the association has not been confirmed yet. DDRGK1 regulates the nuclear factor-κB (NF-κB) activity (Dzamko et al., 2015). NF-κB is a group of inducible nuclear transcription factors; it is largely expressed in a wide variety of cells and regulates the expression of a lot of genes in response to different stimuli. It plays an important role in inflammation, immune system as well as in tumorigenesis (Mitchell et al., 2016). DDRGK1 is localized in the endoplasmic reticulum (ER) and its expression is induced by ER stress (Xi et al., 2013).

Neurodevelopment, Neuron Cell Differentiation and Survival

SNPs within loci associated with neurodevelopment, neuron cell differentiation and survival recognized as PD susceptibility factors by GWASs are listed in **Table 6**.

CCDC62

CCDC62 (coiled-coil domain containing 62) was found to be related to PD susceptibility in the Nalls et al. studies conducted in 2011 and 2014 (Nalls et al., 2011, 2014) pointing out two different intron variants. The gene has a role in cell growth, estrogen receptor transactivation, cyclin D1 expression in prostate cancer cells as well as in other varieties of cancer, since its antibodies are

TABLE 6 | SNPs within loci associated with neurodevelopment, neuron cell differentiation and survival recognized as PD susceptibility factors by GWASs.

Gene/locus	SNP	MAF (1000 genomes project)	Risk allele: OR	Study
CCDC62 Ch 12	rs11060180 g.123303586A>G c.2002-4327A>G (intron variant)	G = 0.2516	A: OR = 1.105	Nalls et al., 2014
	rs12817488 g.123296294G>A c.1852-1523G>A (intron variant)	A = 0.4159	T: OR = 1.14	Nalls et al., 2011
RIT2 Ch 18	rs12456492 g.43093415A>G c.103+22002T>C (intron variant)	G = 0.3297	G: OR = 1.11	Nalls et al., 2014
			OR = 1.19	Pankratz et al., 2012
	rs4130047 g.43098270T>C c.103+17147A>G (intron variant)	C = 0.3237	C: OR = 1.16	Do et al., 2011
FGF20 Ch 8	rs591323 g.16697091G>A (intron variant)	A = 0.3652	G: OR = 1.09	Nalls et al., 2014
GCH1 Ch 14	rs11158026 g.55348869C>T c.344-16715G>A (intron variant)	C = 0.4898	C: OR = 1.11	Nalls et al., 2014
GPNMB Ch 2	rs199347 g.23293746A>G c.224-42A>G (intron variant)	A = 0.4832	A: OR = 1.11	Nalls et al., 2014

Ch, Chromosome. Data compiled from the GWAS catalog database, the dbSNP and the e!Ensembl (Sherry et al., 2001; Welter et al., 2014; Yates et al., 2016).

often produced and thus detected (Li et al., 2013; Lu et al., 2016). Until recently, it was mainly reported as related to cancer (Yu et al., 2015). In order to define the gene's function more precisely, more functional studies are required.

RIT2

RIT2 (ras-like without CAAX 2) was first described as a PD susceptibility factor in the GWAS performed by Do et al. in 2011 and after that confirmed in two meta-analyses (Pankratz et al., 2012; Nalls et al., 2014). Two variants within the gene were found to be associated with the PD risk. One of them (rs12456492) was replicated, while the other (rs4130047) was significant in only one study (Do et al., 2011; Pankratz et al., 2012; Nalls et al., 2014). RIT2 is a small GTPase of the Ras family. It is neuron-specific and preferentially expressed in dopaminergic neurons in substantia nigra (Ran and Belin, 2014). Accumulating reports suggest its important role in neuronal differentiation and function. It promotes neurite outgrowth through Rac/Cdc42 activation and calmodulin association (Zhang et al., 2013). It binds calmodulin 1, a phosphorylase kinase, in a calcium-dependent manner and regulates certain signaling pathways and cellular processes (Do et al., 2011). It interacts with SNCA and tau via calmodulin (Lu et al., 2015). RIT2 is also a specific interacting partner of the dopamine transporter (DAT). DAT is a transmembrane protein which can be internalized by protein kinase C-mediated endocytosis and thus downregulated. It was proposed that extracellular dopamine concentrations and half-life are regulated in this manner. This process presumably depends on RIT2 GTPase activity (Zhang et al., 2013; Ran and Belin, 2014). A reduced production of RIT2 was detected in postmortem samples of PD patients when compared to controls (Bossers et al., 2009). In another postmortem study, a possible regulation of INF-γ signaling by RIT2 was discovered (Liscovitch and French, 2014).

FGF20

FGF20 (fibroblast growth factor 20) was proved to be associated with PD in the Nalls et al. meta-analysis (Nalls et al., 2014), in which one intron variant within the gene with a positive association was found. More studies will have to be done to confirm this association. FGF20 is a neurotrophic factor preferentially expressed in substantia nigra pars compacta. It acts in an autocrine/paracrine manner. FGF20 regulates central nervous development and function (Plagnol et al., 2011). It plays a major role in dopaminergic neurons differentiation and survival (Itoh and Ohta, 2013). According to some studies, FGF20 also increases SNCA levels in dopaminergic neurons, but there is a huge discrepancy among studies (Wang et al., 2008; Wider et al., 2009; Sekiyama et al., 2014; Tarazi et al., 2014).

GCH1

GCH1 (GTP cyclohydrolase 1) was found to be associated with PD pathology only in the Nalls et al. meta-analysis of GWASs (Nalls et al., 2014), which means that more studies whose results will show a positive association are required to claim that the association is in fact true. GCH1 is an essential enzyme in dopamine synthesis in the nigrostriatal nervous cells. Mutations in this gene can result in the degeneration of nigral neurons. Loss of function leads to severe depletion of dopamine levels and is the most frequent cause of DOPA-responsive dystonia (DRD), a rare disease that classically occurs during the childhood and is manifested as generalized dystonia and an excellent sustained response to low doses of levodopa, usually without motor fluctuations. DRD is often associated with PD. Mutations in the gene might cause striatal cell death and thus evolve into PD. The enzyme controls the first and rate-limiting step in the biosynthesis of tetrahydrobiopterin (BH_4), which is a cofactor of tyrosine hydroxylase, which converts tyrosine to levodopa (Mencacci et al., 2014; Rengmark et al., 2016). It may also have some role in inflammation (Dzamko et al., 2015). The debate on whether this gene is related to the familial or sporadic form is still ongoing. Some say that PD-like symptoms in adulthood could also be a different phenotype of DRD.

GPNMB

GPNMB (glycoprotein nonmetastatic melanoma protein B) was recognized as associated with a PD risk in the Nalls et al. meta-analysis in 2014. As the association was found in one study only, we cannot conclude that the association is definite (Nalls et al., 2014). It presumably plays an important role in

TABLE 7 | SNPs within loci associated with mitochondrial homeostasis recognized as PD susceptibility factors by GWASs.

Gene/locus	SNP	MAF (1000 genomes project)	Risk allele: OR	Study
SREBF1/RAI1 Ch 17	rs11868035 g.17715101G>A c.*835C>T (splice region variant)	G = 0.4876	G: OR = 1.18	Do et al., 2011
MCCC1 Ch 3	rs12637471 g.182762437G>A c.732+764C>T (intron variant)	A = 0.3375	G: OR = 1.1876	Nalls et al., 2014
	rs11711441 g.182821275G>A (intron variant)	A = 0.1406	G: OR = 1.19	Nalls et al., 2011
	rs10513789 g.182760073T>G c.733-535A>C (intron variant)	G = 0.3115	T: OR = 1.25	Do et al., 2011

Ch, Chromosome. Data compiled from the GWAS catalog database, the dbSNP and the e!Ensembl (Sherry et al., 2001; Welter et al., 2014; Yates et al., 2016).
**Denotes SNPs in 3′-UTR.*

neuronal survival and neuroprotection (Xu et al., 2016). It is also known as osteoactivin, dendritic cell-heparin integrin ligand or haematopoietic growth factor inducible neurokinin-1 type. It is important for the differentiation and functioning of osteoclasts and osteoblasts, the impairment T-cell activation, the invasion, and metastasis of many cancers and the regulation of degeneration/regeneration of extracellular matrix in skeletal muscles. The gene was also associated with amyotrophic lateral sclerosis as another type of a neurodegenerative disease (Tanaka et al., 2012). The protein mostly localizes in lysosomes. It is also involved in phagocytosis and helps to recruit an autophagy protein LC3-II to the phagosome. It is essential for the fusion of phagosome and lysosome to degrade the phagosome content (Gan-Or et al., 2015). GPNMB is somehow involved in innate and adaptive immunity along with many PD susceptibility factors. It may play a role in regulating microglial inflammation downstream of LPS activation (Dzamko et al., 2015; Herrero et al., 2015).

Mitochondrial Homeostasis

SNPs within loci associated with mitochondrial homeostasis recognized as PD susceptibility factors by GWASs are listed in **Table 7**.

SREBF1/RAI1

SREBF1/RAI1 (sterol regulatory element binding transcription factor 1/retinoic acid induced 1) locus was associated with PD susceptibility for the first time by Do et al. GWAS (Do et al., 2011). In 2014, it was again confirmed by the meta-analysis of GWASs (Nalls et al., 2014). The same SNP (rs11868035) was pointed out in both studies.

SREBF1 encodes SREBP-1 (sterol regulatory element-binding protein 1), a transcriptional activator (Do et al., 2011). The connection of mitophagy pathway and familial PD has been firmly established via two genes—*PINK1* and *Parkin*, but also GWASs and functional studies found the association between this pathway and sporadic PD through *SREBF1*. It is involved in the mitophagy as well as in the regulation of lysosomal lipid accumulation. Mitochondria and lipid metabolism have complementary functions via Krebs cycle. Knockdown of SREBF1 blocks the translocation of Parkin into the mitochondria and consequently decreases mitophagy (Gan-Or et al., 2015). This process can be restored by the addition of exogenous lipids, both fatty acids and cholesterol. Downregulation of *SREBF1* may also decrease mitophagy by blocking the stabilization of PINK1 on the outer mitochondrial membrane of injured mitochondria, which can also be repaired by additional exogenous lipids (Ivatt and Whitworth, 2014). It regulates cholesterol synthesis and its cellular uptake from plasma LDL. A reduced expression of SREBF1 also downregulates the *NPC1* gene, which may lead to the accumulation of cholesterol within late endosomes and lysosomes (Gan-Or et al., 2015). Autophagic turnover of mitochondria needs to be balanced with its biogenesis, which heavily relies upon SREBP pathway for membrane synthesis (Ivatt et al., 2014). Some studies also suggest that SREBP-1 is an important mediator of NMDA-induced excitotoxicity (Do et al., 2011). It may also be involved in the innate immune response via lipid metabolism (Jeon and Osborne, 2012).

RAI1 is a part of transcription regulation mechanism, beacuse it has the ability to remodel chromatin and interacts with the basic transcriptional machinery (Do et al., 2011).

MCCC1

MCCC1 [methylcrotonyl-CoA carboxylase 1 (alpha)] was shown to be associated with sporadic PD in 2011 with two GWASs and after that again confirmed with the meta-analysis. In all three studies, a different intron variant was implicated as a risk factor (Do et al., 2011; Nalls et al., 2011, 2014). Its product, a biotin-requiring enzyme, functions within the mitochondria as a part of leucine catabolism pathway (Wang et al., 2014). It is currently not known if this enzyme has a role in the mitophagy or mitochondrial quality control. Researchers are also debating on whether this gene or rather *LAMP3* located on the same locus is involved in PD pathogenesis (Gan-Or et al., 2015).

Other Processes

SNPs within loci associated with other processes recognized as PD susceptibility factors by GWASs are listed in **Table 8**. More association and functional studies will have to be performed to discover a clear connection between a PD risk and genes mentioned below.

ACMSD/TMEM163

ACMSD/TMEM 163 (aminocarboxymuconate semialdehyde decarboxylase-transmembrane protein 163) was shown to be associated with PD by Nalls et al. studies as well as by Pankratz et al. meta-analysis of GWASs. Two variants were found in these three studies, which means that one of them (rs6430538) was also replicated (Nalls et al., 2011, 2014; Pankratz et al., 2012). This gene is expressed at very low but significant levels

TABLE 8 | SNPs within loci associated with other processes recognized as PD susceptibility factors by GWASs.

Gene/locus	SNP	MAF (1000 genomes project)	Risk allele: OR	Study
ACMSD/TMEM163 Ch 2	rs6430538 g.135539967C>T (intron variant)	C = 0.1891	C: OR = 1.1429	Nalls et al., 2014
			OR = 1.15	Pankratz et al., 2012
	rs6710823 g.135592381G>A (intron variant)	NA	G: OR = 1.1	Nalls et al., 2011
MIR4697 Ch 11	rs329648 g.133895472T>C (downstream gene variant)	T = 0.4645	T: OR = 1.105	Nalls et al., 2014
SIPA1L2 Ch 1	rs10797576 g.232664611C>T (intron variant)	T = 0.1274	T: OR = 1.131	Nalls et al., 2014

NA, data not available; Ch, Chromosome. Data compiled from the GWAS catalog database, the dbSNP and the e!Ensembl (Sherry et al., 2001; Welter et al., 2014; Yates et al., 2016).

in the brain and encodes a cytosolic enzyme (Martí-Massó et al., 2013). ACMSD is involved in the picolinic and quinolinic acid homeostasis and is thus a possible therapeutic target for many central nervous system disorders (Plagnol et al., 2011). ACMSD is also categorized as a detoxifying enzyme because of its ability to prevent the accumulation of neurotoxic metabolite quinolinate, which is one of the tryptophan catabolites (Ran and Belin, 2014). It also participates in the kynurenine pathway of tryptophan catabolism. Mutations in the gene presumably result in a decreased enzymatic activity, which means that the conversion of tryptophan to picolinic acid is blocked. Consequently, quinolinic acid levels in the brain are elevated. Quinolinat is also an intermediate of the de novo synthesis of NAD from tryptophan (Martí-Massó et al., 2013).

MIR4697

MIR4697 is a non-protein coding sequence that was shown to be associated with PD in the Nalls et al. meta-analysis in 2014 (Nalls et al., 2014) in which one SNP with a positive association was found. The function of the microRNA in general is not known, much less its function in PD pathology (Chen et al., 2016).

SIPA1L2

SIPA1L2 (signal-induced proliferation-associated 1 like 2) is a gene related to PD pathogenesis according to the Nalls et al. study conducted in 2014, but the function of the gene has to be determined yet. Only one SNP has been pointed out as a risk factor so far (Nalls et al., 2014).

APPLICABILITY OF THE KNOWLEDGE ABOUT GENETIC SUSCEPTIBILITY FACTORS FOR PD

The knowledge about the genetic factors of PD risk or pathogenesis related to a specific pathway could be applied in the clinical setting to support early diagnosis and to predict disease prognosis as suggested by the study of Nalls et al. (2015). Furthermore, the information on susceptibility genes could be easily integrated in composite diagnostic and/or prognostic algorithms that at present include clinical characteristics and imaging data (Siderowf et al., 2012; Gaenslen et al., 2014; Noyce et al., 2014). These genetic factors could also help to stratify the patients on the basis of underlying molecular defect into respective groups that would benefit from targeting a specific pathway with novel or existing treatment approaches, which would enable personalized treatment planning. The latter also indicates an opportunity to identify novel potential targets for innovative treatment approaches and supportive measures.

First, described genetic factors could support early diagnosis. This is an important goal for clinicians dealing with PD, because it is important to start treatment early in the disease course (Olanow and Schapira, 2013). It would be ideal to identify patients in the prodromal phase of the disease (Berg et al., 2015). By the time motor symptoms occur, more than half of dopaminergic neurons are already lost. The time of the prediagnostic phase, which can last for up to 20 years, thus presents the window of opportunity for searching for and for the application of neuroprotective treatment (Salat et al., 2016). For the purpose of early diagnosis, a panel of genes should be tested for different mutations and polymorphisms to check the cumulative effect of the genetic defects as a single mutation or polymorphism has a very low contribution to disease risk. The combined assessment of early non-motor symptoms with a genetic predisposition could be an ideal method to identify the patients in the earliest phases of the disease. Only genetic testing for diagnosis of sporadic PD or for the prediction of developing sporadic PD is not specific and sensitive enough at the moment. There is no known genetic factor or combination of genetic factors that could conclusively predict the development of sporadic PD. Therefore, genetic testing would probably be more suitable for high risk families with positive PD history or for people with manifestations of early non-motor symptoms and not for general population. Furthermore, a cumulative score and not individual genetic factors should be considered, jointly with clinical and imaging data. Nalls et al. developed an algorithm for early diagnosis of PD on the basis of clinical and genetic classification. Their model included several clinical factors, such as age, gender, olfactory function and family history of PD. They combined clinical factors with a genetic risk score, that accounted for 28 genetic variants identified and replicated in the most recent large-scale meta-analysis of PD GWASs data plus two other rare risk variants, a *GBA* (rs76763715) and a *LRRK2* (rs34637584) mutation. The model correctly distinguished between patients with PD and controls with an area under curve of 0.923 with both high sensitivity (0.834) and specificity (0.903). They also validated the model on five other cohorts and AUC was never lower than 0.894 (Nalls et al., 2015). There are a few prospective longitudinal studies running (PARS, TREND, PREDICT-PD), which are looking for biomarkers to identify PD and predict the way of disease progression before a diagnosis based on motor symptoms can be made, and assessing combinations of risk factors and early features of PD. Among these studies, PARS included a cohort of elderly patients with olfactory dysfunction, TREND included people older than 50 years with one of prodromal symptoms of PD (olfactory dysfunction, REM sleep behavior disorder or depression), while PREDICT-PD included general population from 60 to 80 years of age irrespective of PD prodromal symptoms (Salat et al., 2016).

Furthermore, the impact of genetic susceptibility factors on the disease prognosis could be evaluated. It would be interesting to explore the association between the course of the disease and the genetic defect in genes involved in certain pathways. For example, *GBA* mutations or *MAPT* H1 allele status might be independent risk factors for cognitive impairment in PD patients and the knowledge of these allele statuses in patients could have an impact on the treatment plan (Clarimón and Kulisevsky, 2013).

Moreover, genetic susceptibility factors segregating in different pathways could help to stratify PD patients into distinct groups according to the differences in the main molecular cause of the disease. So far, the stratification of patients has only been made based on different phenotypes (van Rooden et al., 2010, 2011; Fereshtehnejad et al., 2015), but our main idea is to group them on the basis of the main molecular cause of the disease rather than on the basis of different ways of manifestation. The stratification should be based on cumulative effects of genetic susceptibility factors within a particular pathway as well as across pathways, so different combinations of genetic defects should be tested to find a way to stratify the PD patients. This approach was already addressed in a review written by Schapira et al. (Schapira, 2013), where the problem of aetiologically heterogeneous cohorts of PD patients evaluated in different studies was exposed. The latter makes it difficult to seek for different genetic biomarkers as there may be different ones in distinct groups. The stratification of PD patients based on underlying genetic defects could also be beneficial in a clinical setting as patients with different genetic defects may need different treatment plans. This kind of personalized treatment could become the treatment of choice in PD in the future, as we could stratify patients into groups according to their compromised pathway and treat them according to their underlying pathogenic processes. The treatment could be adjusted for each group to obtain the best possible response.

Last but not least, the disease genes or the products of the genes involved in the aethiopathogenesis could serve as novel targets for neuroprotective or disease-modifying drugs to delay or prevent disease progression. However, the problem of a very modest impact of the above-mentioned mutations and polymorphisms on the PD pathology occurs. If the impact of a single mutation is very low, there is probably no point in developing a new active pharmaceutical agent specific for that target, because the effect on the disease course would probably not be satisfactory. A more feasible way of incorporating means of personalized medicine and patient startification into PD management is to target a corrupted pathway as a whole instead of focusing only on the compromised gene and its product. The goal would be to strengthen or improve the function of a compromised pathway, such as protein aggregation; protein and membrane trafficking; lysosomal autophagy; immune system; neurodevelopment, neuron cell differentiation and survival; mitochondrial homeostasis; and genes involved in other processes. Although this is a less specific approach, it focuses on the putative main cause of the disease occurrence in a particular patient. In the light of this, there is a possibility of the repurposing of drugs already used for other indications, for example ursodeoxycholic acid, nicotine, caffeine, isradipine, exenatide, statins (Salat et al., 2016). In order to establish such a pathway-oriented approach, clinical trials must focus on PD patients with the same underlying molecular defect. As long as heterogenous cohorts are evaluated in these studies, no such treatment will be available (Korczyn and Hassin-Baer, 2015).

FUTURE PERSPECTIVES

With the emergence of GWASs, researchers believed that the discovery of the exact genetic background of PD is at their fingertips, but more questions arose afterwards. GWASs are a type of studies with no hypothesis at the time of their performance, so the results must be critically evaluated and supported by functional studies of genes recognized to be involved in the pathogenesis of a certain disease. Apart from functional studies of not yet known genes' functions, animal disease models should also be investigated to check and validate the results of GWASs. We also have to be aware of the fact, that GWAS usually detect common SNPs that most probably have a modest impact only. Rare but highly penetrant SNPs are often overlooked. Hence, in terms of susceptibility prediction or early diagnosis, physicians should check several genetic biomarkers (SNPs) and their cumulative impact on the prognosis along with clinical and imaging data. Additionally, SNPs associated with a certain disease are often not located within the disease gene, but are rather in linkage disequlibrium with it.

The main goal of searching for genetic biomarkers of PD susceptibility is early diagnosis or more optimistically, a chance to slow down or even prevent the development of the disease. Furthermore, with better characterization of risk genes' functions, we could stratify the PD patients into groups according to the main route of pathogenesis. Prospective monitoring is needed to compare the symptomatology as well as the rate of progression between the groups in order to get a chance of tailoring the therapy to each group. To take this idea to the next level, one could also find new drug targets based on the susceptibility genes or their products if the impact of the susceptibility gene is high enough. A personalized approach would allow to treat each group of patients with the most effective and safest drug and adopt optimal supportive measures, e.g., antiinflammatory therapy for patients with an increased inflammatory response.

CONCLUSIONS

In conclusion, the newest GWASs have identified top hit susceptibility genes with emerging information on their physiological functions and involvement in PD pathology. These susceptibility genes belong to specific pathways that are already known to be compromised in PD and could thus serve as a genetic tool for the stratification of patients. In our opinion, this would allow the treatment of patients according to the underlying cause of their clinical signs to choose the most beneficial treatment with minimal side effects. This knowledge gives the opportunity to personalize the treatment of PD patients, but more studies need to be carried out on cell models, animal models and patients before new knowledge can be translated into the everyday clinical practice of PD treatment.

AUTHOR CONTRIBUTIONS

All authors have made a substantial intellectual contribution to this work and approved its final version for submission. VD and SR formed the review focus. SR conducted the literature review and summarized and wrote the first draft of the manuscript under the supervision of VD. VD and MT evaluated the manuscript and contributed to the final version.

FUNDING

This work was partially funded by the Horizon 2020 Artemida 664536 Grant and the Slovenian Research Agency (ARRS) Grant P1-0170.

REFERENCES

Ahmed, I., Tamouza, R., Delord, M., Krishnamoorthy, R., Tzourio, C., Mulot, C., et al. (2012). Association between Parkinson's disease and the HLA-DRB1 locus. *Mov. Disord.* 27, 1104–1110. doi: 10.1002/mds.25035

Ahn, B. H., Rhim, H., Kim, S. Y., Sung, Y. M., Lee, M. Y., Choi, J. Y., et al. (2002). α-Synuclein interacts with phospholipase D isozymes and inhibits pervanadate-induced phospholipase D activation in human embryonic kidney-293 cells. *J. Biol. Chem.* 277, 12334–12342. doi: 10.1074/jbc.M110414200

Bellani, S., Sousa, V. L., Ronzitti, G., Valtorta, F., Meldolesi, J., and Chieregatti, E. (2010). The regulation of synaptic function by α-synuclein. *Commun. Integr. Biol.* 3, 106–109. doi: 10.4161/cib.3.2.10964

Bellucci, A., Zaltieri, M., Navarria, L., Grigoletto, J., Missale, C., and Spano, P. (2012). From α-synuclein to synaptic dysfunctions: new insights into the pathophysiology of Parkinson's disease. *Brain Res.* 2, 183–202. doi: 10.1016/j.brainres.2012.04.014

Berg, D., Postuma, R. B., Adler, C. H., Bloem, B. R., Chan, P., Dubois, B., et al. (2015). MDS research criteria for prodromal Parkinson's disease. *Mov. Disord.* 30, 1600–1611. doi: 10.1002/mds.26431

Bisaglia, M., Mammi, S., and Bubacco, L. (2009). Structural insights on physiological functions and pathological effects of α-synuclein. *FASEB J.* 23, 329–340. doi: 10.1096/fj.08-119784

Blesa, J., Trigo-Damas, I., Quiroga-Varela, A., and Jackson-Lewis, V. R. (2015). Oxidative stress and Parkinson's disease. *Front. Neuroanat.* 9:91. doi: 10.3389/fnana.2015.00091

Bossers, K., Meerhoff, G., Balesar, R., van Dongen, J. W., Kruse, C. G., Swaab, D. F., et al. (2009). Analysis of gene expression in Parkinson's disease: possible involvement of neurotrophic support and axon guidance in dopaminergic cell death. *Brain Pathol.* 19, 91–107. doi: 10.1111/j.1750-3639.2008.00171.x

Burre, J., Sharma, M., Tsetsenis, T., Buchman, V., Etherton, M. R., and Sudhof, T. C. (2010). α-synuclein promotes SNARE-complex assembly *in vivo* and *in vitro*. *Science* 329, 1663–1667. doi: 10.1126/science.1195227

Chang, K. H., Wu, Y. R., Chen, Y. C., Fung, H. C., Lee-Chen, G. J., and Chen, C. M. (2015). STK39, But Not BST1, HLA-DQB1, and SPPL2B polymorphism, is associated with han-chinese parkinson's disease in taiwan. *Medicine* 94:e1690. doi: 10.1097/MD.0000000000001690

Charlesworth, G., Gandhi, S., Bras, J. M., Barker, R. A., Burn, D. J., Chinnery, P. F., et al. (2012). Tau acts as an independent genetic risk factor in pathologically proven PD. *Neurobiol. Aging* 33, 4. doi: 10.1016/j.neurobiolaging.2011.11.001

Chen, C.-M., Chen, Y.-C., Chiang, M.-C., Fung, H.-C., Chang, K.-H., Lee-Chen, G.-J., et al. (2016). Association of GCH1 and MIR4697, but not SIPA1L2 and VPS13C polymorphisms, with Parkinson's disease in Taiwan. *Neurobiol. Aging* 39, 221. e1–5. doi: 10.1016/j.neurobiolaging.2015.12.016

Chen, M.-L., Lin, C.-H., Lee, M.-J., and Wu, R.-M. (2014). BST1 rs11724635 interacts with environmental factors to increase the risk of Parkinson's disease in a Taiwanese population. *Parkinsonism Relat. Disord.* 20, 280–283. doi: 10.1016/j.parkreldis.2013.11.009

Clarimón, J., and Kulisevsky, J. (2013). Parkinson's disease: from genetics to clinical practice. *Curr. Genomics* 14, 560–567. doi: 10.2174/1389202914666131210212305

Connolly, B. S., and Lang, A. E. (2014). Pharmacological treatment of Parkinson disease: a review. *JAMA* 311, 1670–1683. doi: 10.1001/jama.2014.3654

Davis, A. A., Andruska, K. M., Benitez, B. A., Racette, B. A., Perlmutter, J. S., and Cruchaga, C. (2016). Variants in GBA, SNCA, and MAPT influence Parkinson disease risk, age at onset, and progression. *Neurobiol. Aging* 37, 30. doi: 10.1016/j.neurobiolaging.2015.09.014

Do, C. B., Tung, J. Y., Dorfman, E., Kiefer, A. K., Drabant, E. M., Francke, U., et al. (2011). Web-based genome-wide association study identifies two novel loci and a substantial genetic component for Parkinson's disease. *PLoS Genet.* 7, 23. doi: 10.1371/journal.pgen.1002141

Drouet, V., and Lesage, S. (2014). Synaptojanin 1 mutation in Parkinson's disease brings further insight into the neuropathological mechanisms. *Biomed Res. Int.* 2014:289728. doi: 10.1155/2014/289728

Dzamko, N., Geczy, C. L., and Halliday, G. M. (2015). Inflammation is genetically implicated in Parkinson's disease. *Neuroscience* 302, 89–102. doi: 10.1016/j.neuroscience.2014.10.028

Edwards, T. L., Scott, W. K., Almonte, C., Burt, A., Powell, E. H., Beecham, G. W., et al. (2010). Genome-wide association study confirms SNPs in SNCA and the MAPT region as common risk factors for Parkinson disease. *Ann. Hum. Genet.* 74, 97–109. doi: 10.1111/j.1469-1809.2009.00560.x

Emanuele, M., and Chieregatti, E. (2015). Mechanisms of α-synuclein action on neurotransmission: cell-autonomous and non-cell autonomous role. *Biomolecules* 5, 865–892. doi: 10.3390/biom5020865

Fereshtehnejad, S. M., Romenets, S. R., Anang, J. B., Latreille, V., Gagnon, J. F., and Postuma, R. B. (2015). New Clinical Subtypes of Parkinson Disease and their longitudinal progression: a prospective cohort comparison with other phenotypes. *JAMA Neurol.* 72, 863–873. doi: 10.1001/jamaneurol.2015.0703

Gaenslen, A., Wurster, I., Brockmann, K., Huber, H., Godau, J., Faust, B., et al. (2014). Prodromal features for Parkinson's disease–baseline data from the TREND study. *Eur. J. Neurol.* 21, 766–772. doi: 10.1111/ene.12382

Gallegos, S., Pacheco, C., Peters, C., Opazo, C. M., and Aguayo, L. G. (2015). Features of α-synuclein that could explain the progression and irreversibility of Parkinson's disease. *Front. Neurosci.* 9:59. doi: 10.3389/fnins.2015.00059

Gan-Or, Z., Dion, P. A., and Rouleau, G. A. (2015). Genetic perspective on the role of the autophagy-lysosome pathway in Parkinson disease. *Autophagy* 11, 1443–1457. doi: 10.1080/15548627.2015.1067364

García-Cazorla, A., Oyarzabal, A., Fort, J., Robles, C., Castejon, E., Ruiz-Sala, P., et al. (2014). Two novel mutations in the BCKDK (branched-chain keto-acid dehydrogenase kinase) gene are responsible for a neurobehavioral deficit in two pediatric unrelated patients. *Hum. Mutat.* 35, 470–477. doi: 10.1002/humu.22513

Giasson, B. I., Forman, M. S., Higuchi, M., Golbe, L. I., Graves, C. L., Kotzbauer, P. T., et al. (2003). Initiation and synergistic fibrillization of tau and α-synuclein. *Science* 300, 636–640. doi: 10.1126/science.1082324

Golpich, M., Amini, E., Hemmati, F., Ibrahim, N. M., Rahmani, B., Mohamed, Z., et al. (2015). Glycogen synthase kinase-3 β (GSK-3β) signaling: implications for Parkinson's disease. *Pharmacol. Res.* 97, 16–26. doi: 10.1016/j.phrs.2015.03.010

Goris, A., Williams-Gray, C. H., Clark, G. R., Foltynie, T., Lewis, S. J., Brown, J., et al. (2007). Tau and α-synuclein in susceptibility to, and dementia in, Parkinson's disease. *Ann. Neurol.* 62, 145–153. doi: 10.1002/ana.21192

Gustot, A., Gallea, J. I., Sarroukh, R., Celej, M. S., Ruysschaert, J. M., and Raussens, V. (2015). Amyloid fibrils are the molecular trigger of inflammation in Parkinson's disease. *Biochem. J.* 471, 323–333. doi: 10.1042/BJ20150617

Hamza, T. H., Zabetian, C. P., Tenesa, A., Laederach, A., Montimurro, J., Yearout, D., et al. (2010). Common genetic variation in the HLA region is associated with late-onset sporadic Parkinson's disease. *Nat. Genet.* 42, 781–785. doi: 10.1038/ng.642

Hardy, J. (2010). Genetic analysis of pathways to Parkinson disease. *Neuron* 68, 201–206. doi: 10.1016/j.neuron.2010.10.014

Hasegawa, M., Nonaka, T., and Masuda-Suzukake, M. (2016). Prion-like mechanisms and potential therapeutic targets in neurodegenerative disorders. *Pharmacol. Ther.* 1, 30236–30234. doi: 10.1016/j.pharmthera.2016.11.010

Herrero, M. T., Estrada, C., Maatouk, L., and Vyas, S. (2015). Inflammation in Parkinson's disease: role of glucocorticoids. *Front. Neuroanat.* 9:32. doi: 10.3389/fnana.2015.00032

Hill-Burns, E. M., Factor, S. A., Zabetian, C. P., Thomson, G., and Payami, H. (2011). Evidence for more than one Parkinson's disease-associated variant within the HLA region. *PLoS ONE* 6:e27109. doi: 10.1371/journal.pone.0027109

Hill-Burns, E. M., Wissemann, W. T., Hamza, T. H., Factor, S. A., Zabetian, C. P., and Payami, H. (2014). Identification of a novel Parkinson's disease locus via stratified genome-wide association study. *BMC Genomics* 15:118. doi: 10.1186/1471-2164-15-118

Hoang, Q. Q. (2014). Pathway for Parkinson disease. *Proc. Natl. Acad. Sci. U.S.A.* 111, 2402–2403. doi: 10.1073/pnas.1324284111

Horvath, J., Herrmann, F. R., Burkhard, P. R., Bouras, C., and Kovari, E. (2013). Neuropathology of dementia in a large cohort of patients with Parkinson's disease. *Parkinsonism Relat. Disord.* 19, 864–868. doi: 10.1016/j.parkreldis.2013.05.010

Inoshita, T., and Imai, Y. (2015). Regulation of vesicular trafficking by Parkinson's disease-associated genes. *AIMS Mol. Sci.* 2, 461–475. doi: 10.3934/molsci.2015.4.461

Itoh, N., and Ohta, H. (2013). Roles of FGF20 in dopaminergic neurons and Parkinson's disease. *Front. Mol. Neurosci.* 6:15. doi: 10.3389/fnmol.2013.00015

Ivatt, R. M., Sanchez-Martinez, A., Godena, V. K., Brown, S., Ziviani, E., and Whitworth, A. J. (2014). Genome-wide RNAi screen identifies the Parkinson disease GWAS risk locus SREBF1 as a regulator of mitophagy. *Proc. Natl. Acad. Sci. U.S.A.* 111, 8494–8499. doi: 10.1073/pnas.1321207111

Ivatt, R. M., and Whitworth, A. J. (2014). SREBF1 links lipogenesis to mitophagy and sporadic Parkinson disease. *Autophagy* 10, 1476–1477. doi: 10.4161/auto.29642

Jeon, T. I., and Osborne, T. F. (2012). SREBPs: metabolic integrators in physiology and metabolism. *Trends Endocrinol. Metab.* 23, 65–72. doi: 10.1016/j.tem.2011.10.004

Kalia, L. V., and Lang, A. E. (2015). Parkinson's disease. *Lancet* 386, 896–912. doi: 10.1016/S0140-6736(14)61393-3

Klein, C., and Westenberger, A. (2012). Genetics of Parkinson's disease. *Cold Spring Harb. Perspect. Med.* 2:a008888. doi: 10.1101/cshperspect.a008888

Korczyn, A. D., and Hassin-Baer, S. (2015). Can the disease course in Parkinson's disease be slowed? *BMC Med.* 13, 295. doi: 10.1186/s12916-015-0534-x

Kruger, R., Vieira-Saecker, A. M., Kuhn, W., Berg, D., Muller, T., Kuhnl, N., et al. (1999). Increased susceptibility to sporadic Parkinson's disease by a certain combined α-synuclein/apolipoprotein E genotype. *Ann. Neurol.* 45, 611–617.

Kumaran, R., and Cookson, M. R. (2015). Pathways to Parkinsonism Redux: convergent pathobiological mechanisms in genetics of Parkinson's disease. *Hum. Mol. Genet.* 24, 22. doi: 10.1093/hmg/ddv236

Labbé, C., and Ross, O. A. (2014). Association studies of sporadic Parkinson's Disease in the genomic era. *Curr. Genomics* 15, 2–10. doi: 10.2174/1389202914666131210212745

Lampe, J. B., Gossrau, G., Herting, B., Kempe, A., Sommer, U., Fussel, M., et al. (2003). HLA typing and Parkinson's disease. *Eur. Neurol.* 50, 64–68. doi: 10.1159/000072500

Lashuel, H. A., Overk, C. R., Oueslati, A., and Masliah, E. (2013). The many faces of α-synuclein: from structure and toxicity to therapeutic target. *Nat. Rev. Neurosci.* 14, 38–48. doi: 10.1038/nrn3406

Lashuel, H. A., Petre, B. M., Wall, J., Simon, M., Nowak, R. J., Walz, T., et al. (2002). α-synuclein, especially the Parkinson's disease-associated mutants, forms pore-like annular and tubular protofibrils. *J. Mol. Biol.* 322, 1089–1102. doi: 10.1016/S0022-2836(02)00735-0

Latourelle, J. C., Pankratz, N., Dumitriu, A., Wilk, J. B., Goldwurm, S., Pezzoli, G., et al. (2009). Genomewide association study for onset age in Parkinson disease. *BMC Med. Genet.* 10:98. doi: 10.1186/1471-2350-10-98

Lesage, S., Drouet, V., Majounie, E., Deramecourt, V., Jacoupy, M., Nicolas, A., et al. (2016). Loss of VPS13C Function in autosomal-recessive parkinsonism causes mitochondrial dysfunction and increases pinkl/parkin-dependent mitophagy. *Am. J. Hum. Genet.* 98, 500–513. doi: 10.1016/j.ajhg.2016.01.014

Li, N. N., Tan, E. K., Chang, X. L., Mao, X. Y., Zhang, J. H., Zhao, D. M., et al. (2013). Genetic association study between STK39 and CCDC62/HIP1R and Parkinson's disease. *PLoS ONE* 8:e79211. doi: 10.1371/journal.pone.0079211

Lill, C. M., Roehr, J. T., McQueen, M. B., Kavvoura, F. K., Bagade, S., Schjeide, B. M., et al. (2012). Comprehensive research synopsis and systematic meta-analyses in Parkinson's disease genetics: the PDGene database. *PLoS Genet.* 8:e1002548. doi: 10.1371/journal.pgen.1002548.

Lin, C. H., and Wu, R. M. (2015). Biomarkers of cognitive decline in Parkinson's disease. *Parkinsonism Relat. Disord.* 21, 431–443. doi: 10.1016/j.parkreldis.2015.02.010

Liscovitch, N., and French, L. (2014). Differential co-expression between α-Synuclein and IFN-gamma signaling genes across development and in Parkinson's disease. *PLoS ONE* 9:e115029.. doi: 10.1371/journal.pone.0115029

Lu, Y., Liu, W., Tan, K., Peng, J., Zhu, Y., and Wang, X. (2015). Genetic association of RIT2 rs12456492 polymorphism and Parkinson's disease susceptibility in Asian populations: a meta-analysis. *Sci. Rep.* 5:13805. doi: 10.1038/srep13805

Lu, Y., Tan, L., Shen, N., Peng, J., Wang, C., Zhu, Y., et al. (2016). Possible association of CCDC62 rs12817488 polymorphism and Parkinson's disease risk in Chinese population: a meta-analysis. *Sci. Rep.* 6:23991. doi: 10.1038/srep23991

MacLeod, D. A., Rhinn, H., Kuwahara, T., Zolin, A., Di Paolo, G., McCabe, B. D., et al. (2013). RAB7L1 interacts with LRRK2 to modify intraneuronal protein sorting and Parkinson's disease risk. *Neuron* 77, 425–439. doi: 10.1016/j.neuron.2012.11.033

Maraganore, D. M., de Andrade, M., Elbaz, A., Farrer, M. J., Ioannidis, J. P., Kruger, R., et al. (2006). Collaborative analysis of α-synuclein gene promoter variability and Parkinson disease. *JAMA* 296, 661–670. doi: 10.1001/jama.296.6.661

Martí-Massó, J. F., Bergareche, A., Makarov, V., Ruiz-Martinez, J., Gorostidi, A., de Munain, A. L., et al. (2013). The ACMSD gene, involved in tryptophan metabolism, is mutated in a family with cortical myoclonus, epilepsy, and parkinsonism. *J. Mol. Med.* 91, 1399–1406. doi: 10.1007/s00109-013-1075-4

Mazzulli, J. R., Xu, Y. H., Sun, Y., Knight, A. L., McLean, P. J., Caldwell, G. A., et al. (2011). Gaucher disease glucocerebrosidase and α-synuclein form a bidirectional pathogenic loop in synucleinopathies. *Cell* 146, 37–52. doi: 10.1016/j.cell.2011.06.001

Mencacci, N. E., Isaias, I. U., Reich, M. M., Ganos, C., Plagnol, V., Polke, J. M., et al. (2014). Parkinson's disease in GTP cyclohydrolase 1 mutation carriers. *Brain* 137(Pt 9), 2480–2492. doi: 10.1093/brain/awu179

Mitchell, S., Vargas, J., and Hoffmann, A. (2016). Signaling via the NFkappaB system. *Wiley Interdiscip. Rev. Syst. Biol. Med.* 8, 227–241. doi: 10.1002/wsbm.1331

Nakatsu, F., Messa, M., Nandez, R., Czapla, H., Zou, Y. X., Strittmatter, S. M., et al. (2015). Sac2/INPP5F is an inositol 4-phosphatase that functions in the endocytic pathway. *J. Cell Biol.* 209, 85–95. doi: 10.1083/jcb.201409064

Nalls, M. A., McLean, C. Y., Rick, J., Eberly, S., Hutten, S. J., Gwinn, K., et al. (2015). Diagnosis of Parkinson's disease on the basis of clinical and genetic classification: a population-based modelling study. *Lancet Neurol.* 14, 1002–1009. doi: 10.1016/S1474-4422(15)00178-7

Nalls, M. A., Pankratz, N., Lill, C. M., Do, C. B., Hernandez, D. G., Saad, M., et al. (2014). Large-scale meta-analysis of genome-wide association data identifies six new risk loci for Parkinson's disease. *Nat. Genet.* 46, 989–993. doi: 10.1038/ng.3043

Nalls, M. A., Plagnol, V., Hernandez, D. G., Sharma, M., Sheerin, U. M., Saad, M., et al. (2011). Imputation of sequence variants for identification of genetic risks for Parkinson's disease: a meta-analysis of genome-wide association studies. *Lancet* 377, 641–649. doi: 10.1016/S0140-6736(10)62345-8

Noyce, A. J., Bestwick, J. P., Silveira-Moriyama, L., Hawkes, C. H., Knowles, C. H., Hardy, J., et al. (2014). PREDICT-PD: identifying risk of Parkinson's disease in the community: methods and baseline results. *J. Neurol. Neurosurg. Psychiatr.* 85, 31–37. doi: 10.1136/jnnp-2013-305420

Olanow, C. W., and Schapira, A. H. (2013). Therapeutic prospects for Parkinson disease. *Ann. Neurol.* 74, 337–347. doi: 10.1002/ana.24011

Pankratz, N., Beecham, G. W., DeStefano, A. L., Dawson, T. M., Doheny, K. F., Factor, S. A., et al. (2012). Meta-analysis of Parkinson's disease: identification of a novel locus, RIT2. *Ann. Neurol.* 71, 370–384. doi: 10.1002/ana.22687

Pankratz, N., Wilk, J. B., Latourelle, J. C., DeStefano, A. L., Halter, C., Pugh, E. W., et al. (2009). Genomewide association study for susceptibility genes contributing to familial Parkinson disease. *Hum. Genet.* 124, 593–605. doi: 10.1007/s00439-008-0582-9

Pastor, P., Ezquerra, M., Munoz, E., Marti, M. J., Blesa, R., Tolosa, E., et al. (2000). Significant association between the tau gene A0/A0 genotype and Parkinson's disease. *Ann. Neurol.* 47, 242–245. doi: 10.1002/1531-8249(200002)47:2<242::AID-ANA16>3.0.CO;2-L

Perrett, R. M., Alexopoulou, Z., and Tofaris, G. K. (2015). The endosomal pathway in Parkinson's disease. *Mol. Cell Neurosci.* 66(Pt A), 21–28. doi: 10.1016/j.mcn.2015.02.009

Pihlstrom, L., Morset, K. R., Grimstad, E., Vitelli, V., and Toft, M. (2016). A cumulative genetic risk score predicts progression in Parkinson's disease. *Mov. Disord.* 8:26505. doi: 10.1002/mds.26505

Plagnol, V., Nalls, M. A., Bras, J. M., Hernandez, D. G., Sharma, M., Sheerin, U. M., et al. (2011). A two-stage meta-analysis identifies several new loci for parkinson's disease. *PLoS Genet.* 7:e1002142. doi: 10.1371/journal.pgen.1002142

Polymeropoulos, M. H., Lavedan, C., Leroy, E., Ide, S. E., Dehejia, A., Dutra, A., et al. (1997). Mutation in the α-synuclein gene identified in families with Parkinson's disease. *Science* 276, 2045–2047. doi: 10.1126/science.276.5321.2045

Postuma, R. B., Berg, D., Stern, M., Poewe, W., Olanow, C. W., Oertel, W., et al. (2015). MDS clinical diagnostic criteria for Parkinson's disease. *Mov. Disord.* 30, 1591–1601. doi: 10.1002/mds.26424

Pringsheim, T., Jette, N., Frolkis, A., and Steeves, T. D. (2014). The prevalence of Parkinson's disease: a systematic review and meta-analysis. *Mov. Disord.* 29, 1583–1590. doi: 10.1002/mds.25945

Ran, C., and Belin, A. C. (2014). The genetics of Parkinson's disease: review of current and emerging candidates. *J. Parkinsonism Restless Legs Syndrome* 4, 63–75. doi: 10.2147/JPRLS.S38954

Rengmark, A., Pihlstrom, L., Linder, J., Forsgren, L., and Toft, M. (2016). Low frequency of GCH1 and TH mutations in Parkinson's disease. *Parkinsonism Relat. Disord.* 29, 109–111. doi: 10.1016/j.parkreldis.2016.05.010

Russo, I., Bubacco, L., and Greggio, E. (2014). LRRK2 and neuroinflammation: partners in crime in Parkinson's disease? *J. Neuroinflammation* 11, 1742–2094. doi: 10.1186/1742-2094-11-52

Ryan, B. J., Hoek, S., Fon, E. A., and Wade-Martins, R. (2015). Mitochondrial dysfunction and mitophagy in Parkinson's: from familial to sporadic disease. *Trends Biochem. Sci.* 40, 200–210. doi: 10.1016/j.tibs.2015.02.003

Saad, M., Lesage, S., Saint-Pierre, A., Corvol, J. C., Zelenika, D., Lambert, J. C., et al. (2011). Genome-wide association study confirms BST1 and suggests a locus on 12q24 as the risk loci for Parkinson's disease in the european population. *Hum. Mol. Genet.* 20, 615–627. doi: 10.1093/hmg/ddq497

Saiki, S., Sato, S., and Hattori, N. (2012). Molecular pathogenesis of Parkinson's disease: update. *J. Neurol. Neurosurg. Psychiatr.* 83, 430–436. doi: 10.1136/jnnp-2011-301205

Salat, D., Noyce, A. J., Schrag, A., and Tolosa, E. (2016). Challenges of modifying disease progression in prediagnostic Parkinson's disease. *Lancet Neurol.* 15, 637–648. doi: 10.1016/S1474-4422(16)00060-0

Satake, W., Nakabayashi, Y., Mizuta, I., Hirota, Y., Ito, C., Kubo, M., et al. (2009). Genome-wide association study identifies common variants at four loci as genetic risk factors for Parkinson's disease. *Nat. Genet.* 41, 1303–1307. doi: 10.1038/ng.485

Schapira, A. H. (2013). Recent developments in biomarkers in Parkinson disease. *Curr. Opin. Neurol.* 26, 395–400. doi: 10.1097/WCO.0b013e3283633741

Schulte, C., and Gasser, T. (2011). Genetic basis of Parkinson's disease: inheritance, penetrance, and expression. *Appl. Clin. Genet.* 4, 67–80. doi: 10.2147/TACG.S11639

Sekiyama, K., Takamatsu, Y., Waragai, M., and Hashimoto, M. (2014). Role of genomics in translational research for Parkinson's disease. *Biochem. Biophys. Res. Commun.* 452, 226–235. doi: 10.1016/j.bbrc.2014.06.028

Sherry, S. T., Ward, M.-H., Kholodov, M., Baker, J., Phan, L., Smigielski, E. M., et al. (2001). dbSNP: the NCBI database of genetic variation. *Nucleic Acids Res.* 29, 308–311. doi: 10.1093/nar/29.1.308

Siderowf, A., Jennings, D., Eberly, S., Oakes, D., Hawkins, K. A., Ascherio, A., et al. (2012). Impaired olfaction and other prodromal features in the Parkinson at-risk syndrome study. *Mov. Disord.* 27, 406–412. doi: 10.1002/mds.24892

Simon-Sanchez, J., Schulte, C., Bras, J. M., Sharma, M., Gibbs, J. R., Berg, D., et al. (2009). Genome-wide association study reveals genetic risk underlying Parkinson's disease. *Nat. Genet.* 41, 1308–1312. doi: 10.1038/ng.487

Singleton, A. B., Farrer, M. J., and Bonifati, V. (2013). The genetics of Parkinson's disease: progress and therapeutic implications. *Mov. Disord.* 28, 14–23. doi: 10.1002/mds.25249

Soto-Ortolaza, A. I., and Ross, O. A. (2016). Genetic susceptibility variants in parkinsonism. *Parkinsonism Relat. Disord.* 22, 7. doi: 10.1016/j.parkreldis.2015.09.011

Spencer, C. C., Plagnol, V., Strange, A., Gardner, M., Paisan-Ruiz, C., Band, G., et al. (2011). Dissection of the genetics of Parkinson's disease identifies an additional association 5′ of SNCA and multiple associated haplotypes at 17q21. *Hum. Mol. Genet.* 20, 345–353. doi: 10.1093/hmg/ddq469

Subramaniam, S. R., and Chesselet, M. F. (2013). Mitochondrial dysfunction and oxidative stress in Parkinson's disease. *Prog. Neurobiol.* 107, 17–32. doi: 10.1016/j.pneurobio.2013.04.004

Tanaka, H., Shimazawa, M., Kimura, M., Takata, M., Tsuruma, K., Yamada, M., et al. (2012). The potential of GPNMB as novel neuroprotective factor in amyotrophic lateral sclerosis. *Sci. Rep.* 2:573. doi: 10.1038/srep00573

Tarazi, F. I., Sahli, Z. T., Wolny, M., and Mousa, S. A. (2014). Emerging therapies for Parkinson's disease: from bench to bedside. *Pharmacol. Ther.* 144, 123–133. doi: 10.1016/j.pharmthera.2014.05.010

Taymans, J. M., Nkiliza, A., and Chartier-Harlin, M. C. (2015). Deregulation of protein translation control, a potential game-changing hypothesis for Parkinson's disease pathogenesis. *Trends Mol. Med.* 21, 466–472. doi: 10.1016/j.molmed.2015.05.004

Tsigelny, I. F., Sharikov, Y., Wrasidlo, W., Gonzalez, T., Desplats, P. A., Crews, L., et al. (2012). Role of α-synuclein penetration into the membrane in the mechanisms of oligomer pore formation. *FEBS J.* 279, 1000–1013. doi: 10.1111/j.1742-4658.2012.08489.x

Vacic, V., Ozelius, L. J., Clark, L. N., Bar-Shira, A., Gana-Weisz, M., Gurevich, T., et al. (2014). Genome-wide mapping of IBD segments in an Ashkenazi PD cohort identifies associated haplotypes. *Hum. Mol. Genet.* 23, 4693–4702. doi: 10.1093/hmg/ddu158

van der Brug, M. P., Singleton, A., Gasser, T., and Lewis, P. A. (2015). Parkinson's disease: from human genetics to clinical trials. *Sci. Transl. Med.* 7, 305ps20. doi: 10.1126/scitranslmed.aaa8280

Vandrovcova, J., Pittman, A. M., Malzer, E., Abou-Sleiman, P. M., Lees, A. J., Wood, N. W., et al. (2009). Association of MAPT haplotype-tagging SNPs with sporadic Parkinson's disease. *Neurobiol. Aging* 30, 1477–1482. doi: 10.1016/j.neurobiolaging.2007.11.019

van Rooden, S. M., Colas, F., Martinez-Martin, P., Visser, M., Verbaan, D., Marinus, J., et al. (2011). Clinical subtypes of Parkinson's disease. *Mov. Disord.* 26, 51–58. doi: 10.1002/mds.23346

van Rooden, S. M., Heiser, W. J., Kok, J. N., Verbaan, D., van Hilten, J. J., and Marinus, J. (2010). The identification of Parkinson's disease subtypes using cluster analysis: a systematic review. *Mov. Disord.* 25, 969–978. doi: 10.1002/mds.23116

Velayos-Baeza, A., Vettori, A., Copley, R. R., Dobson-Stone, C., and Monaco, A. P. (2004). Analysis of the human VPS13 gene family. *Genomics* 84, 536–549. doi: 10.1016/j.ygeno.2004.04.012

Venda, L. L., Cragg, S. J., Buchman, V. L., and Wade-Martins, R. (2010). α-Synuclein and dopamine at the crossroads of Parkinson's disease. *Trends Neurosci.* 33, 559–568. doi: 10.1016/j.tins.2010.09.004

Verstraeten, A., Theuns, J., and Van Broeckhoven, C. (2015). Progress in unraveling the genetic etiology of Parkinson disease in a genomic era. *Trends Genet.* 31, 140–149. doi: 10.1016/j.tig.2015.01.004

Volta, M., Milnerwood, A. J., and Farrer, M. J. (2015). Insights from late-onset familial parkinsonism on the pathogenesis of idiopathic Parkinson's disease. *Lancet Neurol.* 14, 1054–1064. doi: 10.1016/S1474-4422(15) 00186-6

Wallings, R., Manzoni, C., and Bandopadhyay, R. (2015). Cellular processes associated with LRRK2 function and dysfunction. *FEBS J.* 282, 2806–2826. doi: 10.1111/febs.13305

Wang, G., van der Walt, J. M., Mayhew, G., Li, Y.-J., Züchner, S., Scott, W. K., et al. (2008). Variation in the miRNA-433 binding site of fgf20 confers risk for parkinson disease by overexpression of α-synuclein. *Am. J. Hum. Genet.* 82, 283–289. doi: 10.1016/j.ajhg.2007.09.021

Wang, L., Cheng, L., Lu, Z. J., Sun, X. Y., Li, J. Y., and Peng, R. (2016). Association of three candidate genetic variants in RAB7L1/NUCKS1, MCCC1 and STK39 with sporadic Parkinson's disease in Han Chinese. *J. Neural Transm.* 123, 425–430. doi: 10.1007/s00702-016-1526-5

Wang, Y. Q., Tang, B. S., Yu, R. L., Li, K., Liu, Z. H., Xu, Q., et al. (2014). Association analysis of STK39, MCCC1/LAMP3 and sporadic PD in the Chinese Han population. *Neurosci. Lett.* 566, 206–209. doi: 10.1016/j.neulet.2014.03.007

Welter, D., MacArthur, J., Morales, J., Burdett, T., Hall, P., Junkins, H., et al. (2014). The NHGRI GWAS Catalog, a curated resource of SNP-trait associations. *Nucleic Acids Res.* 42(Database issue):6. doi: 10.1093/nar/gkt1229

Wider, C., Dachsel, J. C., Soto, A. I., Heckman, M. G., Diehl, N. N., Yue, M., et al. (2009). FGF20 and parkinson's disease: no evidence of association or pathogenicity via α-synuclein expression. *Mov. Disord.* 24, 455–459. doi: 10.1002/mds.22442

Wider, C., Vilarino-Guell, C., Jasinska-Myga, B., Heckman, M. G., Soto-Ortolaza, A. I., Cobb, S. A., et al. (2010). Association of the MAPT locus with Parkinson's disease. *Eur. J. Neurol.* 17, 483–486. doi: 10.1111/j.1468-1331.2009.02847.x

Wissemann, W. T., Hill-Burns, E. M., Zabetian, C. P., Factor, S. A., Patsopoulos, N., Hoglund, B., et al. (2013). Association of Parkinson disease with structural and regulatory variants in the HLA region. *Am. J. Hum. Genet.* 93, 984–993. doi: 10.1016/j.ajhg.2013.10.009

Wray, S., and Lewis, P. A. (2010). A tangled web - tau and sporadic Parkinson's disease. *Front. Psychiatry* 1:150. doi: 10.3389/fpsyt.2010.00150

Xi, P., Ding, D., Zhou, J., Wang, M., and Cong, Y. S. (2013). DDRGK1 regulates NF-κB activity by modulating IκBα stability. *PLoS ONE* 8:e64231. doi: 10.1371/journal.pone.0064231

Xu, Y., Chen, Y., Ou, R., Wei, Q.-Q., Cao, B., Chen, K., et al. (2016). No association of GPNMB rs156429 polymorphism with Parkinson's disease, amyotrophic lateral sclerosis and multiple system atrophy in Chinese population. *Neurosci. Lett.* 622, 113–117. doi: 10.1016/j.neulet.2016.04.060

Yang, R.-Y., Xue, H., Yu, L., Velayos-Baeza, A., Monaco, A. P., and Liu, F.-T. (2016). Identification of VPS13C as a Galectin-12-Binding Protein That Regulates Galectin-12 Protein Stability and Adipogenesis. *PLoS ONE* 11:e0153534. doi: 10.1371/journal.pone.0153534

Yates, A., Akanni, W., Amode, M. R., Barrell, D., Billis, K., Carvalho-Silva, D., et al. (2016). Ensembl 2016. *Nucleic Acids Res.* 44, D710–D716. doi: 10.1093/nar/gkv1157

Yu, R.-l., Guo, J.-f., Wang, Y.-q., Liu, Z.-h., Sun, Z.-f., Su, L., et al. (2015). The single nucleotide polymorphism Rs12817488 is associated with Parkinson's disease in the Chinese population. *J. Clin. Neurosci.* 22, 1002–1004. doi: 10.1016/j.jocn.2014.11.024

Zhang, L., Wahlin, K., Li, Y. Y., Masuda, T., Yang, Z. Y., Zack, D. J., et al. (2013). RIT2, a neuron-specific small guanosine triphosphatase, is expressed in retinal neuronal cells and its promoter is modulated by the POU4 transcription factors. *Mol. Vis.* 19, 1371–1386.

16

Influence of Aerobic Training and Combinations of Interventions on Cognition and Neuroplasticity after Stroke

Annabelle Constans[1†], Caroline Pin-barre[1,2†], Jean-Jacques Temprado[1], Patrick Decherchi[1] and Jérôme Laurin[1]*

[1] *Aix-Marseille Université, CNRS, ISM, UMR 7287, Marseille, France,* [2] *Université Nice Sophia Antipolis, LAMHESS, UPRES EA 6309, Nice, France*

Edited by:
Daniela Tropea,
Trinity College Dublin, Ireland

Reviewed by:
In Koo Hwang,
Seoul National University, South Korea
Ramesh Kandimalla,
Emory University, USA

***Correspondence:**
Jérôme Laurin
jerome.laurin@univ-amu.fr

†These authors have equally contributed to this work and should be considered both as first authors.

Stroke often aggravated age-related cognitive impairments that strongly affect several aspects of quality of life. However, few studies are, to date, focused on rehabilitation strategies that could improve cognition. Among possible interventions, aerobic training is well known to enhance cardiovascular and motor functions but may also induce beneficial effects on cognitive functions. To assess the effectiveness of aerobic training on cognition, it seems necessary to know whether training promotes the neuroplasticity in brain areas involved in cognitive functions. In the present review, we first explore in both human and animal how aerobic training could improve cognition after stroke by highlighting the neuroplasticity mechanisms. Then, we address the potential effect of combinations between aerobic training with other interventions, including resistance exercises and pharmacological treatments. In addition, we postulate that classic recommendations for aerobic training need to be reconsidered to target both cognition and motor recovery because the current guidelines are only focused on cardiovascular and motor recovery. Finally, methodological limitations of training programs and cognitive function assessment are also developed in this review to clarify their effectiveness in stroke patients.

Keywords: aging neuroscience, stroke rehabilitation, cerebral ischemia, angiogenesis, cognitive disorders, exercise intensity, neurotrophic factors, rat and human model

INTRODUCTION

Sedentary older adults are prone to cardiovascular diseases, such as stroke (Bherer et al., 2013), which occurs when blood flow is interrupted to a part of the brain. This trauma leads to severe motor dysfunctions and it may also aggravate cognitive impairments resulting from normal aging (Rafnsson et al., 2007, 2009; Deary et al., 2009; Waldstein and Wendell, 2010). Indeed, stroke survivors have more than twice the risk of subsequently developing dementia compared with people who have never had a stroke (Tatemichi et al., 1992; Patel et al., 2002). For instance, a stroke situated on the left hemisphere might disturb language and comprehension, which reduce the ability to communicate (Karbe et al., 1990; Pirmoradi et al., 2016). When the right hemisphere is affected, the intuitive thinking, reasoning, solving problems as well as the perception, judgment and the visual-spatial functions could be impaired (Tatemichi et al., 1994; Patel et al., 2002; Cumming et al., 2012; Sun et al., 2014b; Harris et al., 2015; Tiozzo et al., 2015; Save-Pédebos et al., 2016). It makes thus difficult for patients to locate objects, walk up or down stairs or get dressed. Consequently, cognitive disorders are one of the strongest predictor of the inability to return to work, that contribute to the socioeconomic burden of stroke (Kauranen et al., 2013). However, stroke-induced cognitive disorders are often underestimated relative to motor impairments because they are confused with pre-existing symptoms of age-related mild cognitive impairments or Alzheimer's Disease (AD; **Figure 1**; Sun et al., 2014b; Corriveau et al., 2016). Furthermore, cognitive impairments are frequently associated with poor motor recovery (Patel et al., 2002; Leśniak et al., 2008; Rand et al., 2010). It suggests that stroke-induced cognitive dysfunctions and brain plasticity might also affect the stability, flexibility and learning of complex movements (e.g., locomotion, unimanual aiming, bimanual coordination), in which cognitive resources are highly involved as it was already observed in older adults (Temprado et al., 1999, 2013; Sleimen-Malkoun et al., 2012, 2013; Cohen et al., 2016).

It is thus of great importance to find effective interventions to induce both motor and cognitive improvement after stroke. In this respect, it is now widely established that aerobic training enhances cardiorespiratory fitness, muscular endurance and functional recovery of stroke patients resulting in a higher quality of life (Ivey et al., 2005; Macko et al., 2005; Marsden et al., 2013). Over the past few years, few studies have also shown that aerobic training could improve cognitive functions and promotes neuroplasticity in stroke patients (Quaney et al., 2009; Rand et al., 2010; Wogensen et al., 2015). In support of these observations, animal studies have revealed that such training effects on cognitive functions might be partially mediated by the release of neurotrophic factors that promotes angiogenesis, neurogenesis, synaptogenesis and synthesis of neurotransmitters that could not be directly investigated at central level in humans (Churchill et al., 2002; Cotman et al., 2007; Lövdén et al., 2010). However, despite firm evidence supporting the use of aerobic exercise for stroke patients, the mechanisms underlying neuroplasticity that is at origin of cognitive and motor recovery in stroke patients remain unknown.

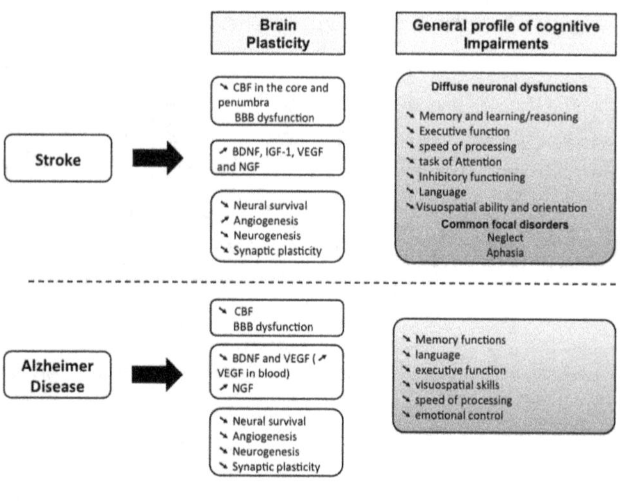

FIGURE 1 | Comparison of the main cognitive impairments between stroke patient and people with Alzheimer Disease (AD). Both AD and cerebrovascular disease increase with age. Although the cause of stroke and AD are distinct, we can observe that the cognitive impairments can be confused because these two brain disturbances could lead to dementia. The hypothesis of vascular contributions to cognitive impairment and dementia (VCID) is that cognitive impairments result from cerebrovascular damages and thus cover the effect of AD, cerebrovascular diseases, including stroke, on cognition (Corriveau et al., 2016). It can be added that more stroke is severe, more the risk of dementia is high. Micro-infarct, silent stroke or small vessel insults are often related to mild cognitive impairments (see also McDonnell et al., 2011; Cumming et al., 2012). However, the outcomes on brain plasticity is specific to each brain disorders (Sopova et al., 2014).

In the present review, we first examine how aerobic training might play a beneficial role on cognition after stroke. In particular, we highlight the influence of aerobic training on neuroplasticity in both human and animal. We also discuss whether additional rehabilitation strategies and/or pharmacological treatments could accentuate neuroplasticity and consequently, the recovery of cognitive functions. In addition, we present the different exercise parameters that should be taken into account in aerobic training, namely: intensity, duration, frequency (number of session per week) and types of exercise as well as timing of training initiation after stroke onset. Indeed, they might differ in their effectiveness to improve cognition and motor functions. Therefore, classic recommendations for aerobic exercise are reconsidered to target cognition as well as motor and cardiovascular functions. Finally, we discuss about the methodological limitations that may hamper the understanding of aerobic training effects on cognition both in human and animal studies.

INFLUENCE OF AEROBIC TRAINING ON NEUROPLASTICITY AND COGNITIVE FUNCTIONS

Cognitive disorders (i.e., executive function and/or information processing speed), motor dysfunctions (i.e., locomotion, balance and strength impairments) and cardiorespiratory fitness weakness are frequently observed in both elderly and stroke people. However, the severity of these impairments is exacerbated due to ischemia in older stroke patients (Gordon et al., 2008; Billinger et al., 2012; Cumming et al., 2013; Harada et al., 2013). Moreover, some neural mechanisms involved in cognitive disorders appear to be close between aging and cerebral ischemia. Specifically, a decrease of neurotrophic factor release (Ang et al., 2003; Silhol et al., 2005; Chae and Kim, 2009) or an abnormal level of oxidative stress and inflammation in hippocampus have been observed in both population (Joseph et al., 2005; Wang et al., 2007). In addition, cerebral blood flow decreases in ischemic region (Cupini et al., 2001; Zhang et al., 2013a) while the reduced vessel density in aging brain leads to an overall reduced blood flow and oxygenation into the brain (Petcu et al., 2010). Therefore, promoting angiogenesis might be critical for these two populations.

In numerous studies, it was demonstrated that aerobic training could induce beneficial effects on brain plasticity and associated cognitive functions as well as motor and cardiorespiratory functions in aging population (Patel et al., 2002; McAuley et al., 2004; Kramer and Erickson, 2007; Leśniak et al., 2008; Erickson and Kramer, 2009). Thus, it can be hypothesized that such training could lead to similar positive effects on cognitive functions in stroke patients. In the following, we present evidence supporting this hypothesis in both older adults and animal studies. Then, on the basis of the few available studies in the literature, we made an overview of the effects of aerobic training on cognitive functions in people and animal with cerebral ischemia.

Studies on Healthy Older Adults

It is now recognized that aerobic training stimulates the positive plasticity of the aging brain. Such exercise-related plasticity mediates the maintenance, or even the increase, of cognitive performance as indicated by the improvement of executive functions and long-term memory. Such enhancements were observed in spite of the heterogeneity of methods, subject characteristics, training parameters or cognitive tasks used in the related studies (Colcombe and Kramer, 2003). Thanks to the use of sophisticated brain imaging technologies, cerebral modifications induced by aerobic training has been observed at both structural (i.e., increase in white and gray matter volumes and changes in synaptic connections) and functional (i.e., changes in brain activation patterns) levels (Churchill et al., 2002; Cotman and Berchtold, 2002; Colcombe and Kramer, 2003; Colcombe et al., 2004a,b, 2006; McAuley et al., 2004; Erickson and Kramer, 2009; Greenwood and Parasuraman, 2010; Voss et al., 2010a,b). For instance, using functional magnetic resonance imagery (fMRI), it was shown that elderly people aerobically trained displayed a higher activation of brain areas involved in attentional control and inhibitory functioning, while a reduced activation is observed in brain areas involved in behavioral conflict (Colcombe et al., 2004a). Additionally, 12-week of both bike and treadmill aerobic training increases the hippocampal and anterior cingulate cortex cerebral blood flow and also an immediate and delayed verbal memory. Such increase is closely related to neuroregeneration (Petcu et al., 2010; Chapman et al., 2013; Duzel et al., 2016). This result was recently reinforced by showing with the use of gadolinium-based perfusion imaging (3 Tesla MRI) that aerobic fitness improvement in healthy older adults is correlated with changes in hippocampal perfusion and volume that were positively related to changes in recognition memory and early recall for complex spatial objects (Maass et al., 2015).

Circulating neurotrophic factor measurements such as brain-derived neurotrophic factor (BDNF), insulin-like growth factor-1 (IGF-1) and vascular endothelial growth factor (VEGF; see below for details) might also explain the influence of aerobic training on neuroplasticity and cognition in Human but this point remains controversial (Cotman et al., 2007). In the one hand, few studies have observed an increase in serum BDNF level in older adults after 1-year of aerobic training that was correlated with an increase in hippocampal volume and improvement in spatial memory performance as well as in executive function (Erickson et al., 2012; Leckie et al., 2014). Specifically, Leckie et al. (2014), revealed that the oldest subjects exhibited the greatest increase in circulating BDNF levels and improvement in task performance after training. This observation suggests that age affects BDNF serum levels (Leckie et al., 2014). On the other hand, numerous studies did not provide robust evidence for enhancement of these neurotrophic factors after several weeks of training in aging people (Voss et al., 2013; Maass et al., 2015). For instance, serum BDNF, VEGF and IGF-1 level did not increase after 12-month of aerobic or non-aerobic (stretching exercises) training despite an increase of connectivity in the temporal lobe between the bilateral parahippocampus and the bilateral middle temporal gyrus (Voss et al., 2013). Recently, Maass et al. (2015), confirmed these results by showing that no difference in changes of circulating BDNF, VEGF and IGF-1 was observed after 3-month of treadmill (training group) or progressive-muscle relaxation/stretching (control group) despite an increase of hippocampal perfusion and volume (Maass et al., 2015). On the basis of these results, it was suggested that the training-related improvement of cerebral perfusion could lead to beneficial effects on neural function without any contribution of growth factors.

These contradictory findings might result from limitations associated with the circulating serum growth factor measurements and training protocols. For instance, nutritional status and changes in energy balance inducing by exercise interventions might affect growth factor levels (Monteleone et al., 2004). Moreover, as it was previously mentioned (Coelho et al., 2013), studies presented different training durations and exercise intensity and heterogeneous samples. Authors also included a different proportion of females and/or males in their studies. Such imbalance in gender composition of experimental groups could have an effect of baseline serum BDNF that might hide possible influence of aerobic training (Komulainen et al., 2008; Driscoll et al., 2012). It has also been suggested that the variable time-windows of circulating growth factor measurements and the analysis techniques used for quantifying blood growth factor levels could also affect the results and need to be clarified (Maass et al., 2015). Finally, data from circulating growth factor assessment should be interpreted with caution since no direct relationships between circulating and brain growth factor levels has been found in human. Studies on human only demonstrated that peripheral BDNF was associated with cognitive performance and cerebral structure integrity (Ventriglia et al., 2013). However, it was also established in animal model that BDNF, VEGF and IGF-1 might have the potential to cross the blood-brain barrier (BBB) in both directions in the central nervous system (CNS; Pan et al., 1998; Cotman et al., 2007). As an illustration, Karege et al. (2002), demonstrated that serum BDNF was positively correlated with cortical BDNF in rat model. In addition, blocking the peripheral IGF-1 or VEGF access to the brain impeded exercise-induced plasticity in the hippocampus (Karege et al., 2002; Cotman et al., 2007). However, other studies have shown in neurological disorders such as stroke and depression that changes in regional brain BDNF levels are not associated with changes of BDNF levels in peripheral blood (Elfving et al., 2010; Béjot et al., 2011). To date, it thus remains difficult to clearly determine the real role of circulating growth factors on cognitive function in older subjects.

Studies on Healthy Animals

Animal experiments could provide information about neuroplasticity mechanisms at cellular level in brain areas involved in cognitive functions. To date, three main neurotrophic factors have been identified to contribute to increase neuroplasticity after aerobic training: (i) the VEGF, which is a protein whose main role is to stimulate angiogenesis; (ii) the BDNF, which is a critical protein involved in brain plasticity. Indeed, this neurotrophin mediates numerous proteins expressions and molecular pathways, i.e., synapsin-I and synpatophysin, both involved in synaptic transmission and neurotransmitter release, C-AMP response element-binding protein (CREB) and beta calcium/calmodulinedependent kinase II (β-CaMKII) both contributing in long-term potentiation (LTP). BDNF thus promotes synaptic plasticity, neurogenesis and neuronal survival within the hippocampus (Vaynman et al., 2004; Cassilhas et al., 2012); and (iii) the IGF-1, which is a peptide that crosses the BBB and stimulates neurogenesis and angiogenesis. These growth factors act together to promote training-related benefits in brain plasticity and associated cognitive functions.

It was found in adult rats that aerobic training induced-angiogenesis is associated with an increase in brain VEGF mRNA and protein (Ding et al., 2006; Cotman et al., 2007). Moreover, Swain et al. (2003), have proved that prolonged voluntary exercise induced an increase of blood volume in the motor cortex of 19% greater than control animals (Swain et al., 2003). Angiogenesis needs to be promoted because some animal studies have suggested that angiogenesis was closely linked to adult neurogenesis and other neuroplasticity mechanisms (Pereira et al., 2007).

It was demonstrated that 8-week of aerobic training on treadmill induced an improvement in learning speed and spatial learning. Authors suggested that these results could be explained by an increase of hippocampal BDNF and IGF-1 and more precisely by the activation of BDNF/TrkB/β-CaMKII pathway and to a lesser extent to IGF-1/IGF-1R/Akt (also known as protein kinase B) pathway (Cassilhas et al., 2012). Radák et al. (2001, 2006) indicated that short- and long-term memory was improved after 8 weeks of regular swimming exercise in middle-aged rats (14-month-old). BDNF and nerve growth factor (NGF) expressions were up-regulated as well as a reduction of accumulation of reactive carbonyl derivatives that are known to damage proteins, nucleic acids ad lipids (Radák et al., 2001, 2006). Similarly, one study on aging rat model, induced by D-galactose injection, has shown that 8-week of moderate aerobic training treadmill could importantly increase both level of NGF and his receptor, the tyrosine kinase A (TrkA) in the hippocampus. NGF/TrkA actives the phosphoinositide 3-kinase (PI3-K)/Akt pathway that decreases apoptosis (Wiesmann and de Vos, 2001; Chae and Kim, 2009). Excessive reactive oxygen species (ROS) production can also trigger apoptosis in brain areas such as the hippocampus that contribute to neurodegenerative disorders and cognitive function impairments in aging people. However, moderate intensity training on treadmill (18 m/min, 30 min/day during 15 weeks) in middle-age female rats (12-month-old) could enhance antioxidant defense system and thus induced a neuroprotective effect in the hippocampus (Marosi et al., 2012). Training also facilitated the release of metabolic proteins in the hippocampus such as mitochondrial precursor of ornithine aminotransferase and isocitrate deshydrogenase subunit alpha. However, these results remain difficult to interpret because authors suggested that alteration of mitochondrial proteins may be either reflecting mitochondrial damage or adaptation to mitochondrial dysfunction (Kirchner et al., 2008).

Studies on Stroke Patients

Only three studies investigated the role of aerobic training on cognition in stroke patients (**Table 1**). Two of them indicated that aerobic training might reduce cognitive disorders by improving functional outcomes as well as motor learning by the increase of information processing speed and implicit memory while executive functions remain affected (Quaney et al., 2009; El-Tamawy et al., 2014). However, patients did not preserve long-term beneficial effects 8 weeks after the end of aerobic training (Quaney et al., 2009). Contrary to what was observed in healthy subject, an acute and short aerobic exercise on treadmill (20 min; 70% of the heart rate reserve) did not induce cognitive improvement in stroke patient while a slightly improvement of the movement of upper-extremity was observed (Ploughman et al., 2008).

Studies on Animal with Cerebral Ischemia

Consistent with healthy older animals, neuroplasticity can be partially promoted by aerobic training through up-regulation of the expression of BDNF, synapsin-I and post-synpatic density protein 95 (PSD-95), also involved in LTP within hippocampus (dentate gyrus, CA1 and CA3 areas) and by increase of both CREB phosphorylation and newborn cell survival (Luo et al., 2007; Shih et al., 2013). The beneficial effect of training was reinforced when the activation of the high affinity BDNF receptor, the TrkB, was blocked because the function of BDNF was reduced and the exercise-induced spatial learning enhancement was impeded (Griesbach et al., 2009). Thus, consistent with data collected within aging rodents, it is supposed that BDNF-mediated pathway contributed to explain the improvement of spatial memory performances after cerebral ischemia. Furthermore, spatial memory performances were positively correlated with an increase of both newborn cell survival in bilateral dentate gyrus and restored microtubule-associated protein 2 (MAP2) density after cerebral ischemia (Luo et al., 2007; Shimada et al., 2013). Treadmill training might also protect against cognitive impairments in rats with bilateral common carotid artery occlusion (CCAO) by reducing the lipoperoxidation in the hippocampus through an increase of antioxidant capacity and by improving the acquisition of a spatial task as well as the performance for both retention and working memory (**Figure 2**; Cechetti et al., 2012). In addition, few weeks of treadmill training in rat with cerebral ischemia increases the VEGF, and its regulatory protein, caveolin-1, and improves the cerebral blood flow in ischemic region (Zhang et al., 2013a; Gao et al., 2014). However, no study has directly shown that vascular changes could contribute to explaining the cognitive disorders.

TABLE 1 | Summary of aerobic training protocols with or without combination (pharmacological agents or other types of exercise) and their effects on cognition in stroke patient.

Studies	Participants	Aerobic training	Combination	Cognitive assessments	Results
Ploughman et al. (2008)	$n = 21$; (61.4 ± 10.2 years old); 6 months to 5 years post-stroke.	- AEX: single bout of 20 min on BWSTT at 70% of THR or 13 on The Borg RPE Scale. - Control condition: 20 min review of home exercises.	none	- TMT-A and B - Symbol digit substitution test - Paced auditory serial addition test	No significant improvement observed No relationship between exercise intensity and cognitive tests.
Quaney et al. (2009)	$n = 38$ (58.96 ± 14.68 and 64.10 ± 12.30 years old); > 6 months post-stroke.	- AEX: 45 min on cyclo-ergometer 3 times/week for 8 weeks at 70% HRmax ($n = 19$). - Control group: Upper- and lower-extremities stretching activities 45 min on cyclo-ergometer 3 times/week for 8 weeks at home ($n = 19$).	none	- WCST - Stroop task - TMT-A and B - SRTT test - PGFM	↗ VO_{2peak} ↗ Complex motor learning tasks No significant improvement observed of executive function measures
Rand et al. (2010)	$n = 11$ (67 ± 10.8 years old); > 4 years post-stroke.	AEX: 1 h composed of stretching, balance, task specifics exercises and 20 min of moderate exercise on The Borg RPE Scale (somewhat hard), 2 times/week for 6 months.	1 h of recreation time, 2 times/week for 6 months.	- Digit backwards - TMT - RAVLT - WWT - Digit symbol - Stroop test	↗ Dual task, response inhibition and memory at 3 months ↗ Executive functions ↗ Response inhibition at 6 months ↗ VO_2 max at 3 and 6 months
Kluding et al. (2011)	$n = 9$ (63.7 ± 9.1 years old); > 6 months post-stroke.	AEX: 1 h on TBRS, 3 times/week for 12 weeks.	Lower extremity muscle strengthening exercises: 1 h, 3 times/week for 12 weeks.	- Digit span backwards task - Flancker test - Memory component of the SIS	↗ Digit span backwards task ↗ SIS total score (including memory subscale) Significant relationship between improvement of aerobic and Flancker tests

(Continued)

TABLE 1 | (Continued).

Studies	Participants	Aerobic training	Combination	Cognitive assessments	Results
Marzolini et al. (2013)	$n = 41$ (63.6 ± 13.5 years old); 10 weeks post-stroke (74 ± 135 days).	AEX: treadmill or cyclo-ergometer depending on patient ability, 20–60 min, 5 times/week for 6 months at 40–70% of HRR or VO_{2peak}, HR achieved at the ATge and/or 11–6 on the RPE of the Borg Scale. Intensity was progressively increased.	Resistance training during 6 months: - 50% to 60% of 1RM for non-affected limb; - ≥ 50% of 1RM and/or 13–14 RPE on the last repetition on the affected limb. - Intensity from 10–15 repetitions.	MoCA (7 different cognitive domains): - Visuo-spatial and executive function - Attention and concentration - Language - Delayed recall - Orientation - Abstraction - Naming	↗ VO_{2peak} ↗ VO_2 at the ATge ↗ Upper- and lower-muscular strength ↗ Attention and concentration ↗ Visuo-spatial and executive function
El-Tamawy et al. (2014)	$n = 30$ (49.67 ± 6.98 and 48.4 ± 6.39 years old); 3–18 months post-stroke.	AEX: 30 min, 3 times/week for 8 weeks of physiotherapy program + 45 min cyclo-ergometer Control group: 30 min, 3 times/week for 8 weeks of physiotherapy program	none	- ACER test	↗ serum BDNF level ↗ ACER for AEX group Significant correlation between changes in serum BDNF level and in ACER test
Bartolo et al. (2015)	$n = 47$ (64.5–67 years old); Within the previous 2 weeks post-stroke.	L-deprenyl ($n = 23$) Placebo group ($n = 24$) Both group: 1 h of physiotherapy (6 days/week) + 30 min of cyclo/arm-ergometer training (5 days/week) + 1 h of occupational therapy (3 days/week) during 6 weeks.	L-deprenyl: 10 mg/day once day during 6 weeks.	- TMT-A and B - MoCA and RAVLT - Logical memory - Digit Span - Corsi's test - Attentive matrices - Stroop test - Symbol digit - PM-47 and FAB - Phonological fluency - Semantic fluency	↗ Logical memory ↗ Attentive matrices ↗ TMT-A and B ↗ PM-47 ↗ MoCA ↗ Digit Span ↗ Stroop test

↗ indicate an increase, ↘ a decrease respectively; BWSTT: Body-Weight-Supported Treadmill Training; THR: Target Heart Rates; RPE: Rating of Perceived Exertion; TMT: Trail making tests parts A and B; AEX: Aerobic Exercise; HRR: Heart Rate Reserve; HRmax: Heart Rate Maximal; WCST: Wisconsin Card Sorting test; SRTT: Serial Reaction Time Task; PGFM: Predictive Grip Force Modulation; RAVLT: Rey Auditory Verbal Learning Test; WWT: Walking While Talking; SIS: Stroke Impact Scale; ATge: Gas Exchange Anaerobic threshold; RM: Repetition Maximum; ACER: Addenbrooke's cognitive examination-revised; TBRS: Total Body Recumbent Stepper; MoCA: Montreal Cognitive Assessment ; PM-47: Raven's Coloured Progressive Matrices 47; FAB: Frontal Assessment Battery; BDNF: Brain Derived Neurotrophic Factor.

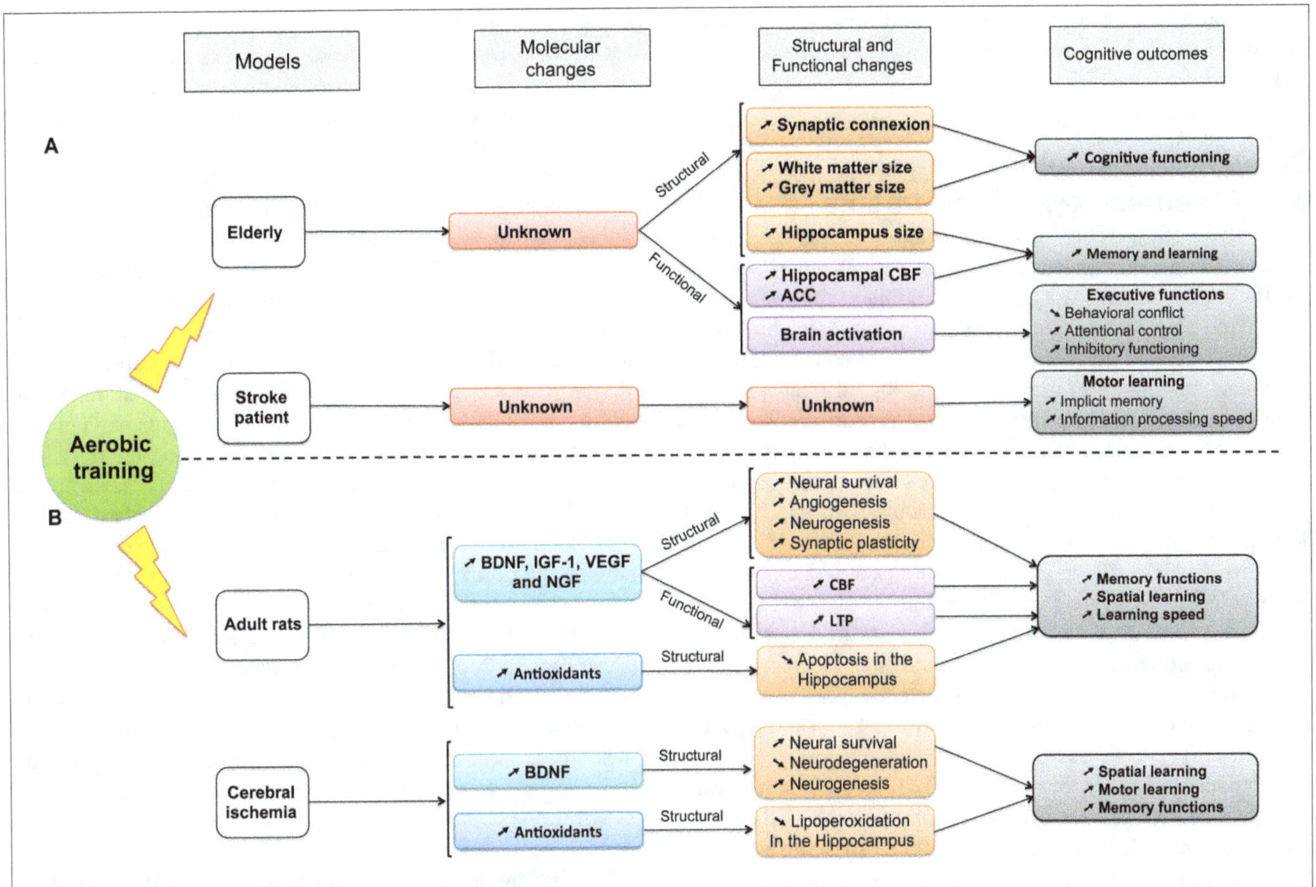

FIGURE 2 | A summary of the established effects of aerobic training on molecular, structural and functional changes and their consequences on cognitive functions (see details in the text). Different models are compared: aging and stroke in both **(A)** human and **(B)** animal populations. ACC, Anterior Cingulate Cortex; BDNF, Brain-Derived Neurotrophic Factor; CBF, Cerebral Blood Flow; IGF-1, Insulin Growth Factor-1; LTP, Long-term potentiation; NGF, Nerve Growth Factor; VEGF, Vascular Endothelial Growth Factor.

IS THE COMBINATION OF AEROBIC TRAINING WITH OTHER TYPES OF THERAPIES EFFECTIVE FOR IMPROVING COGNITION RECOVERY AFTER STROKE?

Combination with Other Rehabilitation Exercises

The question arises of whether different types of exercise could be combined to improve the effects that they could have separately. As reviewed by Chang et al. (2012), resistance exercise alone could positively impact selective cognitive functions in older adult such as information-processing speed, attention and several aspects of memory and executive functions (Chang et al., 2012). It was postulated that the main potential underlying mechanism for these benefits is based on resistance training-induced IGF-1 both in brain and blood circulation. Moreover, growing evidence have shown that the combination of aerobic and resistance training induced superior beneficial effect on cognition than aerobic exercise alone in aging population (Colcombe and Kramer, 2003). In this way, the association between resistance and aerobic training might be a potential strategy to further facilitate the cognitive function recovery in stroke population. However, few studies have been conducted to test this attractive hypothesis (Rand et al., 2010; Kluding et al., 2011; Marzolini et al., 2013). Results indicated that combination of aerobic training and lower extremity muscle strengthening improved executive functions, attention and voluntary motor control (Kluding et al., 2011). This is consistent with the study carried out by Marzolini et al. (2013), in which 6 months of both aerobic training at moderate intensity associated with resistance exercises induced improvements in the Montreal Cognitive Assessment (MoCA) scores in subdomain of attention/concentration and visuospatial/executive functioning (Marzolini et al., 2013). Another study on chronic stroke patients combining aerobic training with stretching, balance and task-specific exercises as well as sessions of recreation time has shown an improvement in verbal memory and cognitive flexibility but did not promote executive function (Rand et al., 2010). However, since the isolated effects of resistance and aerobic training were not compared with the combination of both of them, it remains difficult to ensure that such combination induces superior beneficial effects on cognition than aerobic intervention alone after stroke. It should also be noticed that the neuroplasticity associated with cognition recovery after combination of aerobic and other rehabilitation strategies has not been investigated in both human and animal stroke studies.

Combination of Aerobic Training with Pharmacological Treatments

Currently, both aerobic and behavioral training have been shown to improve cognition on stroke patient but it remains insufficient to induce total recovery (Quaney et al., 2009; Cherry et al., 2014). Thus, it seems crucial to find new strategy combinations including aerobic exercise to amplify the effects on cognition. Many pharmacological treatments are possible candidates to improve cognitive function after stroke by stimulating brain plasticity. For instance, the drug memantine, used for the treatment of moderate to severe dementia of the Alzheimer's type, could increase synaptic plasticity and LTP and decrease overactivation of N-methyl-D-aspartate-type glutamate receptors (NMDA-r) in order to limit excitotoxic neuronal death (Martin and Wang, 2010; Berthier et al., 2011). Other substances, like citicoline, an intermediate in the generation of phosphatidylcholine from choline, could increase the level of acetylcholine and dopamine as well as decrease infarct volume in animal model with cerebral ischemia (Alvarez-Sabín and Román, 2011).

To date, only the intravenous (IV) recombinant tissue plasminogen activator (rt-PA) was approval by the USA Food and Drug Administration for the treatment of acute ischemic stroke in human (Marshall, 2015). The rt-PA is focused on thrombolytic events and could reduce the infarct volume (Nys et al., 2006) by restoring cerebral blood flow and oxygen supply to ischemic brain tissue (Thompson and Ronaldson, 2014). When rt-PA is administrated within the first 3 h after stroke, it could improve clinical outcomes and activities of daily life from 3, 6 and 12 months (Kwiatkowski et al., 1999; Nys et al., 2006; Murao et al., 2014). However, the effects of rt-PA administration during the first 24 h on cognitive functions are limited to aphasia that is explained by the reperfusion of language areas (only for one-third of patient; Nys et al., 2006; Hajjar et al., 2013; Kremer et al., 2013). Only one study used rt-PA in combination with physical activity during leisure-time. Results showed that combination of the 2 strategies did not accentuate the cognitive and physical improvements compared to rt-PA alone after 3 months (Decourcelle et al., 2015).

In preclinical study, L-deprenyl is a pharmacological treatment used to decrease ROS known to contribute to neuronal cell death in the ischemic core following permanent middle cerebral artery occlusion in mice (Unal et al., 2001). This substance has already shown the clinical effectiveness on cognitive functions in the elderly human with AD (Wilcock et al., 2002). L-deprenyl generates an amphetamine-like effect by acting on the release of dopamine and hampering its reuptake that contribute to the modulation of both attention and executive functions (**Table 1;** Bartolo et al., 2015). After stroke, combination of both L-deprenyl and standard rehabilitation including physiotherapy, cycle arm-ergometer training and occupational therapy during 6 weeks showed an improvement of logical memory, visual selective attention and non-verbal reasoning (Bartolo et al., 2015). However, this study did not compare the effect of such combination with the L-deprenyl treatment effect or the standard rehabilitation alone. Therefore, it remains difficult to postulate that the combination of these two strategies reinforced the cognitive recovery. In rat model, D-amphetamine administration combined to locomotor training enhances locomotor recovery after cortical injury (Feeney et al., 1982; Ramic et al., 2006). Moreover, other study assessed the effect of D-amphetamine administration combined with functional rehabilitation and physical therapy alone on cognitive memory performance and motor recovery after embolic stroke. Results showed that D-amphetamine with functional rehabilitation was more effective to improve cognitive performance than training alone, especially for memory, but the latter could improve fine motor performance (Rasmussen et al., 2006). By contrast, it was found in stroke patient that the combination of unique training session of—lower-extremity stability platform task, upper-extremity simulated feeding task and declarative learning—with D-cycloserine treatment did not accentuate the effect of motor and cognitive training (Cherry et al., 2014). This agent is already known to improve both motor and cognitive functions through increasing LTP in the hippocampus by regulating NMDA-r (Yaka et al., 2007). Cherry et al. (2014) postulated that an unique training session is not enough to amplify pharmacological treatment and that D-cycloserine could not act on the reduced NMDA-r function, and thus, on the motor task learning after stroke.

Finally, the review of literature suggests that no efficient combination between pharmacological treatments and training has yet found to improve recovery on cognitive functions. However, several combinations of pharmacological treatments and aerobic training have proven effectiveness on motor recovery after cerebral ischemia (Pin-Barre and Laurin, 2015). For example, the combination of both S-nitrosoglutathione and training accentuated neuroplasticity (reduce excitotoxicity, inflammation and protect BBB integrity) and motor recovery (Sakakima et al., 2012). Future studies should investigate the effects of these types of associations on cognitive recovery.

MOTOR VS. COGNITIVE FUNCTION RECOVERY: CAN AEROBIC TRAINING SIMILARLY FACILITATE BOTH?

Currently, the recommendations for the use of aerobic training after stroke were only established according to the effectiveness of endurance programs on cardiovascular and motor functions (Pang et al., 2013; Billinger et al., 2014). The cognitive outcomes are thus not taken into account for prescribing physical exercise. However, several findings arising from rodent studies indicate that the most appropriate intensity, the optimal timing to initiate training and the exercise mode (type of exercise) for improving motor performance might be different to improve cognitive function and motor recovery.

Cognitive Performance Improvement by Aerobic Training

Exercise Intensity

Low-intensity aerobic training seems to be more effective than high-intensity training to promote cognitive health. Indeed, animal studies have shown that low-intensity training induced superior positive effects on spatial learning task in a water maze test and on both object recognition and location tasks than intense training (Shih et al., 2013; Shimada et al., 2013). Such cognitive task improvements were concomitant with an increase in plasticity-related proteins such as the increase of hippocampal BDNF level, synapsin-I as well as the number of dendritic spines and the number of neurons in the ipsilateral dentate gyrus (Shen et al., 2013; Shih et al., 2013; Shimada et al., 2013). It was mainly explained by the fact that, compared to low-intensity exercise, the high-intensity exercise induced higher levels of stress-hormone, which might downregulate BDNF level in hippocampus (Schaaf et al., 1999; Soya et al., 2007). Nevertheless, caution is required concerning the chosen running intensity. Indeed, the speed, fixed to 20–22 m/min, was considered as "high" intensity in Shih and Shimada's studies (Shih et al., 2013; Shimada et al., 2013) while others have classified such range of speed as moderate intensity (Sun et al., 2008; Ni et al., 2012). Therefore, the real influence of exercise intensity based on physiological parameters (for example, lactate threshold or VO_{2peak}) on cognitive recovery remains to be further investigated (see "Methodological Considerations" Section).

Timing of Training Initiation

Late exercise, beginning after the first week post-brain injury, is more effective than early exercise (starting during the first week) to improve cognitive functions. Indeed, spatial learning and retention were better improved with the late training and was associated with the upregulation of BDNF (Griesbach et al., 2004; Clark et al., 2008). Voluntary running wheel training, starting 1 week after transient focal cerebral ischemia in mice, promoted neurogenesis in the adult dentate gyrus and spatial memory rebuilding (Luo et al., 2007). Interestingly, the Schmidt meta-analysis indicated that a start of skilled forelimb training from days 1 to 5 post-injury was more effective to improve cognitive function compared to late training (Bland et al., 2000; Wurm et al., 2007; Schmidt et al., 2014). It might be suggested that motor skilled training might start before aerobic training to improve cognitive functions.

Forced vs. Voluntary Training

The training mode might also influence the neuroplasticity underlying cognitive performance. Some studies have recently demonstrated that involuntary exercise (functional electrical stimulation), forced (treadmill) and voluntary (running wheel) training have similar beneficial effects on cognitive function after cerebral ischemia as indicated by improvement of both object recognition and location tests (Lin et al., 2015). Moreover, these three training regimens enhanced the levels of synapsin I, synaptophysin, PSD-95, MAP-2 and Tau protein in the hippocampus. It was confirmed by a previous study on healthy rats where 6 weeks of forced swimming or voluntary running resulted in similar increase of hippocampal BDNF level and in similar effect on learning capabilities and short/long term memories (Alomari et al., 2013). Nevertheless, other studies indicated divergent results. On one side, Hayes et al. (2008), demonstrated that, after 2-h of middle cerebral artery occlusion, forced treadmill training reduced infarct volume and increased the gene expression of heat shock proteins (Hsp), in particular the 27 kDa Hsp and the 70 kDa Hsp mRNA than voluntary exercise despite higher corticosterone level. The Hsp acts in the brain as molecular chaper ones with neuroprotective activities (Hayes et al., 2008). Other authors indicated that 12 weeks of forced treadmill training could protect against cognitive and biochemical impairments caused by CCAO in rat (Cechetti et al., 2012). Similar results were found after whole-brain irradiation where forced running training reduced the neurocognitive deficits but also the hippocampal neurogenesis impairments, i.e., the down-regulation of BDNF-mediated pathway (including TrkB receptors, Akt and CREB, for example; Ji et al., 2014). On other side, some authors indicated that voluntary exercise is the most effective training in up-regulating the hippocampal BDNF level (Luo et al., 2007; Ke et al., 2011). Indeed, Ke et al. (2011), compared the effect of voluntary, involuntary and forced training after cerebral ischemia in rat. Results indicated that 7-day intervention of voluntary training induced higher level of BDNF in the hippocampus than the other modes (Ke et al., 2011). Such divergent results might be attributable to variable experimental designs.

Motor Performance Improvement by Aerobic Training

Exercise Intensity

To date, post-stroke guidelines recommend moderate-intensity continuous aerobic training to improve aerobic capacity and motor recovery (40–80% of the maximum heart rate reserve; 3–5 sessions/week; 20–60 min/session). However, it was demonstrated that high-intensity exercise could improve aerobic fitness by increasing the peak oxygen uptake (VO_{2peak}) and 6-min walk performances, that remained higher 1 year after the end of training compared with baseline value (Globas et al., 2012). In addition, it has been found that the high-intensity interval training (HIT) could promote superior beneficial cardiovascular and muscular adaptations among persons with different cardiorespiratory disorders (Rognmo et al., 2004; Wisløff et al., 2007). HIT is defined as repeated series of brief and intense exercise separated by active or passive rest periods. This type of intense training is also well known to be a time-efficient strategy to promote metabolic adaptations because the total session duration is strongly reduced compared to traditional moderate-intensity continuous aerobic training (Sun et al., 2014b). Such finding is important given that "lack of time" remains the most cited barrier to regular aerobic exercise participation.

It was observed that HIT is well accepted for ambulatory chronic stroke and could induce encouraging improvements of quality of life as observed by improvements of VO_{2peak} and work economy (Gjellesvik et al., 2012; Boyne et al., 2013; Mattlage et al., 2013). Recently, only one study has compared HIT (series of 30 s at maximum tolerated treadmill speed separated by 30–60 s rest periods) and traditional moderate-intensity continuous aerobic training (Boyne et al., 2016). Authors indicated that no clear difference between HIT and moderate-intensity continuous aerobic training was observed because of a small sample size. Nevertheless, this type of training seems to be feasible and safe because no adverse events occurred.

Timing of Training Initiation

It was postulated in human studies that starting rehabilitation program in the acute-subacute phase after stroke could prevent complications relating to prolonged inactivity (i.e., deconditioning period) and presented a low relative risk for adverse effects (Musicco et al., 2003). Numerous studies in rodents with cerebral ischemia have also observed that an early starting aerobic exercise (from days 1 to 5) was more effective to improve the running performance and to reduce the infarct volume compared to late training (Bland et al., 2000; Luo et al., 2007; Schmidt et al., 2014). For example, Park et al. (2010), indicated that early treadmill training could better improve the motor performance, using the Rotarod test, than late treadmill training after hemorrhagic stroke (Park et al., 2010). Such early training did not increase the infarct volume or brain edema in accordance to other studies (Matsuda et al., 2011; Zhang et al., 2013b). Likewise, an early treadmill exercise increased the cellular expression levels of some neurotrophic factors, promoted cell growth and reduced the expression of apoptosis markers (Mizutani et al., 2010; Matsuda et al., 2011). Moreover, an early endurance exercise improved blood flow in the ischemic region and promoted angiogenesis (Zhang et al., 2013b). We may also add that sensorimotor deficits and cortical infarct volume were aggravated on a longer-term when training started too soon i.e., before 24 h post-ischemia (Kozlowski et al., 1996; Risedal et al., 1999; Bland et al., 2000; DeBow et al., 2004; Schmidt et al., 2014).

Forced vs. Voluntary Training

Numerous studies highlighted that forced treadmill training is more effective than all the other types of exercise, included voluntary exercise, to improve running function, aerobic fitness and to reduce infarct volume (Takamatsu et al., 2010, 2016; Schmidt et al., 2014). However, some authors indicated that voluntary exercise is more effective to improve motor recovery using the De Ryck's behavioral test (Ke et al., 2011). These controversial results might be explained by the use of different motor behavioral tests between studies as well as by a different training protocol (variable speed and timing of training initiation).

Concomitant Improvement of Cognitive and Motor Functions Induced by Aerobic Exercise

Interestingly, Sun et al. (2014), might find a compromise in rats by proving that training with gradually increased intensity on treadmill (from 5 to 26 m/min) could better improve motor function and produce higher hippocampal BDNF with lower stress compared to both stably low and high intensity training (Sun et al., 2014a). These results were in accordance with Zhang et al. (2012), study in which both motor performance (forelimb placing, stepping coordination) and spatial memory in rats with middle cerebral artery occlusion-reperfusion were improved after progressive intensity aerobic training (Zhang et al., 2012).

On the basis of these findings, it appears that training might alternate between high- and low-intensity sessions or might progressively reach high-intensity to accentuate improvement of either cognitive or motor performance. It also suggested that treadmill training might be appropriate for improving these two functions. However, it is more difficult to find a compromise for the timing of training initiation. Indeed, an early training seems to be more appropriate to promote motor recovery while cognitive performances were improved when aerobic training started later. Therefore, the influence of aerobic training on cognitive deficits might be considered to complete the actual exercise recommendations.

METHODOLOGICAL CONSIDERATIONS

Although it is currently admitted that aerobic training positively affects neuro-cognitive impairments, available studies reveal a great heterogeneity in the methods used and for some, weaknesses, which make results difficult to compare (Cumming et al., 2012). These methodological limitations, which are either specific or common to human and animal models, need to be considered before interpreting results.

Methodological Considerations Concerning Exercise Parameters in both Animal and Human Studies

Available studies strongly differ in the parameters related to exercise during aerobic training: duration, intensity, frequency, mode and timing of rehabilitation initiation. In particular, exercise intensity, which is a critical parameter of aerobic training effectiveness, deserves to be questioned (Pin-Barre and Laurin, 2015). For both human and animal models, intensity is frequently based on empirical speed/power (Ploughman et al., 2008; Kluding et al., 2011; Påhlman et al., 2012; Shih et al., 2013; Shimada et al., 2013). In some human studies, the intensity was determined from subjective parameters such as level of exertion perceived by the patient (Ploughman et al., 2008; Kluding et al., 2011; Påhlman et al., 2012). In these conditions, exercise intensity (moderate, intense and severe) could not be precisely determined because no physiological markers were recorded (Xu and Rhodes, 1999). Therefore, a given absolute intensity was considered as moderate for some authors but as severe for others. When training intensity was based on physiological markers, percentages of maximal heart rate or the maximal oxygen uptake (VO_{2peak}) were the most frequently used parameters (Ploughman et al., 2008; Quaney et al., 2009; Kluding et al., 2011; El-Tamawy et al., 2014). However, these methods are insufficiently reliable to distinguish between high and moderate training intensities. Indeed, patients barely reach their maximal aerobic capabilities during an incremental test. Recently, submaximal parameters such as ventilatory or lactic threshold have been recognized to be more suitable than VO_{2peak} to induce a higher inter-individual reproducibility in physiological response to exercise (Faude et al., 2009; Marzolini et al., 2013; Bosch et al., 2015). It is noticeable however that there is no consensus on the methods used to measure these physiological parameters from an incremental exercise test (Bentley et al., 2007). Indeed, depending on the type of incremental test, the performance and the related physiological parameters could be altered. The chosen ergometer (ergocycle or treadmill), stage duration as well as the magnitude of intensity increment between each stage are known to affect the performance (for review see, Bentley et al., 2007). Moreover, the progressive increase of exercise intensity on treadmill could be induced either by an elevation of speed (m/s) and/or inclination (percentage). The speed increment is not systematically reported in literature but some authors indicated that the grade increment was increased of 2% every 2 min with a constant (high) walking speed (Voss et al., 2013). Increase in the slope of the treadmill needs to be considered to improve the validity and the relevance of the chosen incremental test on treadmill for aging subjects. Indeed, the increment of treadmill inclination seems to be more appropriate for aging people and/or for the individuals for whom running is impossible or difficult. For instance, a lower running/walking speed on treadmill could reduce the perceived exertion of the exercise for some individuals and thus might reach highest intensities (Ehlen et al., 2011). Moreover, it was reported on obese persons that faster walking speeds might increase the risk of musculoskeletal injuries because of higher reaction forces and loading rates (Ehlen et al., 2011) in lower extremities tendons, joints and ligaments (Puga et al., 2012). Finally, most authors frequently used a stationary cycle ergometer for aging people (Maass et al., 2015) because measurements of physiological parameters during the test are more stable using this device compared to treadmill. The risk of falls is also lower on cycle ergometer. For the rodent model, some studies have proposed different treadmill protocol in order to reach the highest VO_{2peak} by modifying the treadmill inclination. It has been found in both rats and mice that the highest VO_{2peak} was reached at 25° because a distinct leveling-off of VO_2 was mainly observed at this inclination (Wisløff et al., 2001; Kemi et al., 2002).

In addition, among different studies, intensities are rarely individualized, especially in rodents, while training individualization is one of the most important recommendations of stroke rehabilitation (Pang et al., 2013; Schmidt et al., 2014). This limitation might attenuate the "real" effectiveness of aerobic training. Finally, it is commonly considered in exercise physiology studies that energy expenditure needs to be equivalent between exercise types in order to compare the different effects of a specific training parameter (such as intensity or duration). In this way, all the experimental groups have the same energy expenditure and thus only the influence of a tested exercise parameter is assessed (Rognmo et al., 2004; Wisløff et al., 2007). However, it has never been applied in animal as well as in human stroke studies.

Specific Methodological Considerations in Human

Inter-individual differences in cerebral ischemia location and/or aerobic fitness level may affect, positively or negatively, cognitive impairments. However, they remain difficult to counteract (Tang et al., 2013; Sun et al., 2014b). For example, it was found that patients with infarction located within cortical regions, middle cerebral artery territory and/or on left hemisphere were more prone to cognitive impairments (Sun et al., 2014b).

Otherwise, using a cognitive test that did not detect the specific cognitive impairments of a patient might hide some potential effect of a training intervention (McDonnell et al., 2011; Cumming et al., 2012). For instance, cognitive measurements are frequently limited to clinical tests, as functional independence measures (FIM), that are not enough sensitive. Likewise, mini-mental state examination (MMSE) may underestimate stroke-related cognitive deficits because it presents a lack of sensitivity for identifying disorders of visual perception and of high-order executive functions (Nys et al., 2006; Pendlebury et al., 2010; Cumming et al., 2012). This might be problematic given that these latter cognitive functions are frequently affected by stroke (Sun et al., 2014b; Tiozzo et al., 2015). In this respect, the MoCA can assess numerous cognitive impairments such as executive function, attention and delayed recall disorders that appear to be more suitable for stroke patient (Pendlebury et al., 2010). Some studies have also used specific neuropsychological tests such as Trail-making part A and B, Symbol digit test, Stroop test, Digit backward test, which allow to better detect cognitive deficits induced by stroke (Ploughman et al., 2008; Quaney et al., 2009; Rand et al., 2010; Kluding et al., 2011).

To ensure that cognitive performance improvements are related to aerobic training effectiveness, an increase of aerobic fitness needs to be observed at the end of the intervention. However, change in cardiorespiratory fitness after aerobic training is not systematically reported in the different studies. Thus, caution is often required when it is claimed that cognitive improvements are associated with aerobic training rather than other interventions or environmental factors.

The issue of cognitive-motor interactions in stroke patients also deserves to be considered. Indeed, cognitive and motor processes are classically considered as functionally independent and then, explored separately in the literature. However, the control and learning of complex goal-directed movements require a close cooperation between sensorimotor control processes and higher cognitive functions. This is even more marked in older adults, for which cognitive and motor processes become less differentiated by virtue of functional reorganization of brain activation patterns. Thus, change in cognitive-motor interplay expresses an important facet of age-related intrinsic plasticity of brain and cognition. Strategic variations might be thus analyzed to assess behavioral adaptability in cognitive (Lemaire and Hinault, 2014) and sensorimotor tasks (Poletti et al., 2015, 2016).

Specific Methodological Considerations in Animal Models

Animal experiments can provide information about underlying mechanisms of neuroplasticity that could not be investigated in human. However, several drawbacks are often observed in some studies. For instance, it is impossible to investigate the large range of cognitive functions identified in human, such as verbal learning and memory for example (Voss et al., 2013). Cognitive dysfunctions after cerebral ischemia are limited to spatial and working memory, recognition and motor learning skills (Morris water maze, passive avoidance test, object recognition or location test; Luo et al., 2007; Griesbach et al., 2009; Cechetti et al., 2012; Shih et al., 2013; Shimada et al., 2013).

In addition, exercise-induced neuroplasticity are mainly explored within hippocampus (CA1 and CA3 areas and dentate gyrus), which is related to memory and learning (Vaynman et al., 2003). However, other areas such as basal ganglia, prefrontal cortex, thalamus and cerebellum are also involved in learning and memory processes, executive functions and motor control (Graybiel, 1995; Doya, 2000; Johnson and Ojemann, 2000). Except the hippocampus, other regions, remote away from the lesion zone, are connected to the affected structures and thus might also be disturbed after stroke (i.e., diaschisis effect and synaptic inhibition). For example, inflammatory responses could be observed within thalamus or substantia nigra after cortical brain injury that might partially contribute to explain the cognitive deficits (Block et al., 2005). It could be relevant to investigate the effect of aerobic training on the cognitive functions of these cerebral areas (Carmichael et al., 2004).

CONCLUSION

This present article provides an overview of the positive effect of aerobic training on cognitive functions. It seems that training could increase the release of the same neurotrophic factors (BDNF and VEGF) in both elderly and stroke people that mediate beneficial neuroplasticity in brain areas involved in cognitive functions. We also identify some methodological limitations in both human and animal studies such as the standardization procedure of aerobic exercise intensity and the chosen cognitive tests, depending on the target population, that remain one of the most important concerns. Moreover, our review article suggests that the combination of aerobic training with other exercises/therapies or treatments represent a promising strategy with strong clinical perspectives. Importantly, this review highlights the lack of a firm guideline for exercise recommendations targeting recovery of cognition in stroke patient. Therefore, no standard aerobic protocol has yet been established as a commonly accepted reference regarding intensity, timing of training initiation and exercise type. It also appears that investigating changes in cognitive-motor interplay are critical to develop appropriate rehabilitation to improve both cognition and motor control after stroke.

AUTHOR CONTRIBUTIONS

All authors listed, have made substantial, direct, and intellectual contribution to the work, and approved its final version for publication. JL and J-JT: conceived the review focus, conducted literature review, summarized, and finalized the manuscript. PD: summarized, and finalized the manuscript. AC, CP-B and JL: reviewed literature, wrote first draft, and finalized the manuscript. All authors approved final version of manuscript.

FUNDING

This work was supported by Aix-Marseille Université (AMU) and Centre National de la Recherche Scientifique (CNRS).

REFERENCES

Alomari, M. A., Khabour, O. F., Alzoubi, K. H., and Alzubi, M. A. (2013). Forced and voluntary exercises equally improve spatial learning and memory and hippocampal BDNF levels. *Behav. Brain Res.* 247, 34–39. doi: 10.1016/j.bbr.2013.03.007

Alvarez-Sabín, J., and Román, G. C. (2011). Citicoline in vascular cognitive impairment and vascular dementia after stroke. *Stroke* 42, S40–S43. doi: 10.1161/STROKEAHA.110.606509

Ang, E. T., Wong, P. T. H., Moochhala, S., and Ng, Y. K. (2003). Neuroprotection associated with running: is it a result of increased endogenous neurotrophic factors? *Neuroscience* 118, 335–345. doi: 10.1016/s0306-4522(02)00989-2

Bartolo, M., Zucchella, C., Capone, A., Sandrini, G., and Pierelli, F. (2015). An explorative study regarding the effect of l-deprenyl on cognitive and functional recovery in patients after stroke. *J. Neurol. Sci.* 349, 117–123. doi: 10.1016/j.jns.2014.12.039

Béjot, Y., Mossiat, C., Giroud, M., Prigent-Tessier, A., and Marie, C. (2011). Circulating and brain BDNF levels in stroke rats. Relevance to clinical studies. *PLoS One* 6:e29405. doi: 10.1371/journal.pone.0029405

Bentley, D. J., Newell, J., and Bishop, D. (2007). Incremental exercise test design and analysis: implications for performance diagnostics in endurance athletes. *Sports Med.* 37, 575–586. doi: 10.2165/00007256-200737070-00002

Berthier, M. L., Pulvermüller, F., Dávila, G., Casares, N. G., and Gutiérrez, A. (2011). Drug therapy of post-stroke aphasia: a review of current evidence. *Neuropsychol. Rev.* 21, 302–317. doi: 10.1007/s11065-011-9177-7

Bherer, L., Erickson, K. I., and Liu-Ambrose, T. (2013). A review of the effects of physical activity and exercise on cognitive and brain functions in older adults. *J. Aging Res.* 2013:657508. doi: 10.1155/2013/657508

Billinger, S. A., Arena, R., Bernhardt, J., Eng, J. J., Franklin, B. A., Johnson, C. M., et al. (2014). Physical activity and exercise recommendations for stroke survivors: a statement for healthcare professionals from the American Heart Association/American Stroke Association. *Stroke* 45, 2532–2553. doi: 10.1161/STR.0000000000000022

Billinger, S. A., Coughenour, E., Mackay-Lyons, M. J., and Ivey, F. M. (2012). Reduced cardiorespiratory fitness after stroke: biological consequences and exercise-induced adaptations. *Stroke Res. Treat.* 2012:959120. doi: 10.1155/2012/959120

Bland, S. T., Schallert, T., Strong, R., Aronowski, J., Grotta, J. C., and Feeney, D. M. (2000). Early exclusive use of the affected forelimb after moderate transient focal ischemia in rats: functional and anatomic outcome. *Stroke* 31, 1144–1152. doi: 10.1161/01.str.31.5.1144

Block, F., Dihné, M., and Loos, M. (2005). Inflammation in areas of remote changes following focal brain lesion. *Prog. Neurobiol.* 75, 342–365. doi: 10.1016/j.pneurobio.2005.03.004

Bosch, P. R., Holzapfel, S., and Traustadottir, T. (2015). Feasibility of measuring ventilatory threshold in adults with stroke-induced hemiparesis: implications for exercise prescription. *Arch. Phys. Med. Rehabil.* 96, 1779–1784. doi: 10.1016/j.apmr.2015.04.023

Boyne, P., Dunning, K., Carl, D., Gerson, M., Khoury, J., and Kissela, B. (2013). High-intensity interval training in stroke rehabilitation. *Top. Stroke Rehabil.* 20, 317–330. doi: 10.1310/tsr2004-317

Boyne, P., Dunning, K., Carl, D., Gerson, M., Khoury, J., Rockwell, B., et al. (2016). High-intensity interval training and moderate-intensity continuous training in ambulatory chronic stroke: a feasibility study. *Phys. Ther.* doi: 10.2522/ptj.20150277 [Epub ahead of print].

Carmichael, S. T., Tatsukawa, K., Katsman, D., Tsuyuguchi, N., and Kornblum, H. I. (2004). Evolution of diaschisis in a focal stroke model. *Stroke* 35, 758–763. doi: 10.1161/01.str.0000117235.11156.55

Cassilhas, R. C., Lee, K. S., Fernandes, J., Oliveira, M. G. M., Tufik, S., Meeusen, R., et al. (2012). Spatial memory is improved by aerobic and resistance exercise through divergent molecular mechanisms. *Neuroscience* 202, 309–317. doi: 10.1016/j.neuroscience.2011.11.029

Cechetti, F., Worm, P. V., Elsner, V. R., Bertoldi, K., Sanches, E., Ben, J., et al. (2012). Forced treadmill exercise prevents oxidative stress and memory deficits following chronic cerebral hypoperfusion in the rat. *Neurobiol. Learn. Mem.* 97, 90–96. doi: 10.1016/j.nlm.2011.09.008

Chae, C.-H., and Kim, H.-T. (2009). Forced, moderate-intensity treadmill exercise suppresses apoptosis by increasing the level of NGF and stimulating phosphatidylinositol 3-kinase signaling in the hippocampus of induced aging rats. *Neurochem. Int.* 55, 208–213. doi: 10.1016/j.neuint.2009.02.024

Chang, Y.-K., Pan, C.-Y., Chen, F.-T., Tsai, C.-L., and Huang, C.-C. (2012). Effect of resistance-exercise training on cognitive function in healthy older adults: a review. *J. Aging Phys. Act.* 20, 497–517.

Chapman, S. B., Aslan, S., Spence, J. S., DeFina, L. F., Keebler, M. W., Didehbani, N., et al. (2013). Shorter term aerobic exercise improves brain, cognition and cardiovascular fitness in aging. *Front. Aging Neurosci.* 5:75. doi: 10.3389/fnagi.2013.00075

Cherry, K. M., Lenze, E. J., and Lang, C. E. (2014). Combining D-cycloserine with motor training does not result in improved general motor learning in neurologically intact people or in people with stroke. *J. Neurophysiol.* 111, 2516–2524. doi: 10.1152/jn.00882.2013

Churchill, J. D., Galvez, R., Colcombe, S., Swain, R. A., Kramer, A. F., and Greenough, W. T. (2002). Exercise, experience and the aging brain. *Neurobiol. Aging* 23, 941–955. doi: 10.1016/s0197-4580(02)00028-3

Clark, P. J., Brzezinska, W. J., Thomas, M. W., Ryzhenko, N. A., Toshkov, S. A., and Rhodes, J. S. (2008). Intact neurogenesis is required for benefits of exercise on spatial memory but not motor performance or contextual fear conditioning in C57BL/6J mice. *Neuroscience* 155, 1048–1058. doi: 10.1016/j.neuroscience.2008.06.051

Coelho, F. G., Gobbi, S., Andreatto, C. A. A., Corazza, D. I., Pedroso, R. V., and Santos-Galduróz, R. F. (2013). Physical exercise modulates peripheral levels of brain-derived neurotrophic factor (BDNF): a systematic review of experimental studies in the elderly. *Arch. Gerontol. Geriatr.* 56, 10–15. doi: 10.1016/j.archger.2012.06.003

Cohen, J. A., Verghese, J., and Zwerling, J. L. (2016). Cognition and gait in older people. *Maturitas* doi: 10.1016/j.maturitas.2016.05.005 [Epub ahead of print].

Colcombe, S. J., Erickson, K. I., Scalf, P. E., Kim, J. S., Prakash, R., McAuley, E., et al. (2006). Aerobic exercise training increases brain volume in aging humans. *J. Gerontol. A Biol. Sci. Med. Sci.* 61, 1166–1170. doi: 10.1093/gerona/61.11.1166

Colcombe, S., and Kramer, A. F. (2003). Fitness effects on the cognitive function of older adults a meta-analytic study. *Psychol. Sci.* 14, 125–130. doi: 10.1111/1467-9280.t01-1-01430

Colcombe, S. J., Kramer, A. F., Erickson, K. I., Scalf, P., McAuley, E., Cohen, N. J., et al. (2004a). Cardiovascular fitness, cortical plasticity and aging. *Proc. Natl. Acad. Sci. U S A* 101, 3316–3321. doi: 10.1073/pnas.0400266101

Colcombe, S. J., Kramer, A. F., McAuley, E., Erickson, K. I., and Scalf, P. (2004b). Neurocognitive aging and cardiovascular fitness: recent findings and future directions. *J. Mol. Neurosci.* 24, 9–14. doi: 10.1385/jmn:24:1:009

Corriveau, R. A., Bosetti, F., Emr, M., Gladman, J. T., Koenig, J. I., Moy, C. S., et al. (2016). The science of vascular contributions to cognitive impairment and dementia (VCID): a framework for advancing research priorities in the cerebrovascular biology of cognitive decline. *Cell. Mol. Neurobiol.* 36, 281–288. doi: 10.1007/s10571-016-0334-7

Cotman, C. W., and Berchtold, N. C. (2002). Exercise: a behavioral intervention to enhance brain health and plasticity. *Trends Neurosci.* 25, 295–301. doi: 10.1016/s0166-2236(02)02143-4

Cotman, C. W., Berchtold, N. C., and Christie, L.-A. (2007). Exercise builds brain health: key roles of growth factor cascades and inflammation. *Trends Neurosci.* 30, 464–472. doi: 10.1016/j.tins.2007.06.011

Cumming, T. B., Marshall, R. S., and Lazar, R. M. (2013). Stroke, cognitive deficits and rehabilitation: still an incomplete picture. *Int. J. Stroke* 8, 38–45. doi: 10.1111/j.1747-4949.2012.00972.x

Cumming, T. B., Tyedin, K., Churilov, L., Morris, M. E., and Bernhardt, J. (2012). The effect of physical activity on cognitive function after stroke: a systematic review. *Int. Psychogeriatr.* 24, 557–567. doi: 10.1017/s1041610211001980

Cupini, L. M., Diomedi, M., Placidi, F., Silvestrini, M., and Giacomini, P. (2001). Cerebrovascular reactivity and subcortical infarctions. *Arch. Neurol.* 58, 577–581. doi: 10.1001/archneur.58.4.577

Deary, I. J., Corley, J., Gow, A. J., Harris, S. E., Houlihan, L. M., Marioni, R. E., et al. (2009). Age-associated cognitive decline. *Br. Med. Bull.* 92, 135–152. doi: 10.1093/bmb/ldp033

DeBow, S. B., McKenna, J. E., Kolb, B., and Colbourne, F. (2004). Immediate constraint-induced movement therapy causes local hyperthermia that exacerbates cerebral cortical injury in rats. *Can. J. Physiol. Pharmacol.* 82, 231–237. doi: 10.1139/y04-013

Decourcelle, A., Moulin, S., Sibon, I., Murao, K., Ronzière, T., Godefroy, O., et al. (2015). Influence of previous physical activity on the outcome of patients treated by thrombolytic therapy for stroke. *J. Neurol.* 262, 2513–2519. doi: 10.1007/s00415-015-7875-4

Ding, Y.-H., Li, J., Zhou, Y., Rafols, J. A., Clark, J. C., and Ding, Y. (2006). Cerebral angiogenesis and expression of angiogenic factors in aging rats after exercise. *Curr. Neurovasc. Res.* 3, 15–23. doi: 10.2174/156720206775541787

Doya, K. (2000). Complementary roles of basal ganglia and cerebellum in learning and motor control. *Curr. Opin. Neurobiol.* 10, 732–739. doi: 10.1016/s0959-4388(00)00153-7

Driscoll, I., Martin, B., An, Y., Maudsley, S., Ferrucci, L., Mattson, M. P., et al. (2012). Plasma BDNF is associated with age-related white matter atrophy but not with cognitive function in older, non-demented adults. *PLoS One* 7:e35217. doi: 10.1371/journal.pone.0035217

Duzel, E., van Praag, H., and Sendtner, M. (2016). Can physical exercise in old age improve memory and hippocampal function? *Brain* 139, 662–673. doi: 10.1093/brain/awv407

Ehlen, K. A., Reiser, R. F. II, and Browning, R. C. (2011). Energetics and biomechanics of inclined treadmill walking in obese adults. *Med. Sci. Sports Exerc.* 43, 1251–1259. doi: 10.1249/MSS.0b013e3182098a6c

Elfving, B., Plougmann, P. H., Müller, H. K., Mathé, A. A., Rosenberg, R., and Wegener, G. (2010). Inverse correlation of brain and blood BDNF levels in a genetic rat model of depression. *Int. J. Neuropsychopharmacol.* 13, 563–572. doi: 10.1017/S1461145709990721

El-Tamawy, M. S. S., Abd-Allah, F., Ahmed, S. M., Darwish, M. H., and Khalifa, H. A. (2014). Aerobic exercises enhance cognitive functions and brain derived neurotrophic factor in ischemic stroke patients. *NeuroRehabilitation* 34, 209–213. doi: 10.3233/NRE-131020

Erickson, K. I., and Kramer, A. F. (2009). Aerobic exercise effects on cognitive and neural plasticity in older adults. *Br. J. Sports Med.* 43, 22–24. doi: 10.1136/bjsm.2008.052498

Erickson, K. I., Miller, D. L., and Roecklein, K. A. (2012). The aging hippocampus: interactions between exercise, depression and BDNF. *Neuroscientist* 18, 82–97. doi: 10.1177/1073858410397054

Faude, O., Kindermann, W., and Meyer, T. (2009). Lactate threshold concepts: how valid are they? *Sports Med.* 39, 469–490. doi: 10.2165/00007256-200939060-00003

Feeney, D. M., Gonzalez, A., and Law, W. A. (1982). Amphetamine, haloperidol and experience interact to affect rate of recovery after motor cortex injury. *Science* 217, 855–857. doi: 10.1126/science.7100929

Gao, Y., Zhao, Y., Pan, J., Yang, L., Huang, T., Feng, X., et al. (2014). Treadmill exercise promotes angiogenesis in the ischemic penumbra of rat brains through caveolin-1/VEGF signaling pathways. *Brain Res.* 1585, 83–90. doi: 10.1016/j.brainres.2014.08.032

Gjellesvik, T. I., Brurok, B., Hoff, J., Tørhaug, T., and Helgerud, J. (2012). Effect of high aerobic intensity interval treadmill walking in people with chronic stroke:

a pilot study with one year follow-up. *Top. Stroke Rehabil.* 19, 353–360. doi: 10.1310/tsr1904-353

Globas, C., Becker, C., Cerny, J., Lam, J. M., Lindemann, U., Forrester, L. W., et al. (2012). Chronic stroke survivors benefit from high-intensity aerobic treadmill exercise: a randomized control trial. *Neurorehabil. Neural Repair* 26, 85–95. doi: 10.1177/1545968311418675

Gordon, B. A., Rykhlevskaia, E. I., Brumback, C. R., Lee, Y., Elavsky, S., Konopack, J. F., et al. (2008). Neuroanatomical correlates of aging, cardiopulmonary fitness level and education. *Psychophysiology* 45, 825–838. doi: 10.1111/j.1469-8986.2008.00676.x

Graybiel, A. M. (1995). Building action repertoires: memory and learning functions of the basal ganglia. *Curr. Opin. Neurobiol.* 5, 733–741. doi: 10.1016/0959-4388(95)80100-6

Greenwood, P. M., and Parasuraman, R. (2010). Neuronal and cognitive plasticity: a neurocognitive framework for ameliorating cognitive aging. *Front. Aging Neurosci.* 2:150. doi: 10.3389/fnagi.2010.00150

Griesbach, G. S., Hovda, D. A., and Gomez-Pinilla, F. (2009). Exercise-induced improvement in cognitive performance after traumatic brain injury in rats is dependent on BDNF activation. *Brain Res.* 1288, 105–115. doi: 10.1016/j.brainres.2009.06.045

Griesbach, G. S., Hovda, D. A., Molteni, R., Wu, A., and Gomez-Pinilla, F. (2004). Voluntary exercise following traumatic brain injury: brain-derived neurotrophic factor upregulation and recovery of function. *Neuroscience* 125, 129–139. doi: 10.1016/j.neuroscience.2004.01.030

Hajjar, K., Fulton, R. L., Diener, H.-C., Lees, K. R., and the VISTA Collaborators. (2013). Does the cognitive measure Cog-4 show improvement among patients treated with thrombolysis after acute stroke? *Int. J. Stroke* 8, 652–656. doi: 10.1111/j.1747-4949.2012.00848.x

Harada, C. N., Natelson Love, M. C., and Triebel, K. L. (2013). Normal cognitive aging. *Clin. Geriatr. Med.* 29, 737–752. doi: 10.1016/j.cger.2013.07.002

Harris, I. M., Wong, C., and Andrews, S. (2015). Visual field asymmetries in object individuation. *Conscious. Cogn.* 37, 194–206. doi: 10.1016/j.concog.2015.09.004

Hayes, K., Sprague, S., Guo, M., Davis, W., Friedman, A., Kumar, A., et al. (2008). Forced, not voluntary, exercise effectively induces neuroprotection in stroke. *Acta Neuropathol.* 115, 289–296. doi: 10.1007/s00401-008-0340-z

Ivey, F. M., Macko, R. F., Ryan, A. S., and Hafer-Macko, C. E. (2005). Cardiovascular health and fitness after stroke. *Top. Stroke Rehabil.* 12, 1–16. doi: 10.1310/geeu-yruy-vj72-lear

Ji, J., Ji, S., Sun, R., Li, K., Zhang, Y., Zhang, L., et al. (2014). Forced running exercise attenuates hippocampal neurogenesis impairment and the neurocognitive deficits induced by whole-brain irradiation via the BDNF-mediated pathway. *Biochem. Biophys. Res. Commun.* 443, 646–651. doi: 10.1016/j.bbrc.2013.12.031

Johnson, M. D., and Ojemann, G. A. (2000). The role of the human thalamus in language and memory: evidence from electrophysiological studies. *Brain Cogn.* 42, 218–230. doi: 10.1006/brcg.1999.1101

Joseph, J. A., Shukitt-Hale, B., Casadesus, G., and Fisher, D. (2005). Oxidative stress and inflammation in brain aging: nutritional considerations. *Neurochem. Res.* 30, 927–935. doi: 10.1007/s11064-005-6967-4

Karbe, H., Szelies, B., Herholz, K., and Heiss, W.-D. (1990). Impairment of language is related to left parieto-temporal glucose metabolism in aphasic stroke patients. *J. Neurol.* 237, 19–23. doi: 10.1007/bf00319662

Karege, F., Schwald, M., and Cisse, M. (2002). Postnatal developmental profile of brain-derived neurotrophic factor in rat brain and platelets. *Neurosci. Lett.* 328, 261–264. doi: 10.1016/s0304-3940(02)00529-3

Kauranen, T., Turunen, K., Laari, S., Mustanoja, S., Baumann, P., and Poutiainen, E. (2013). The severity of cognitive deficits predicts return to work after a first-ever ischaemic stroke. *J. Neurol. Neurosurg. Psychiatry* 84, 316–321. doi: 10.1136/jnnp-2012-302629

Ke, Z., Yip, S.-P., Li, L., Zheng, X.-X., Tam, W.-K., and Tong, K.-Y. (2011). The effects of voluntary, involuntary and forced exercises on motor recovery in a stroke rat model. *Conf. Proc. IEEE Eng. Med. Biol. Soc.* 2011, 8223–8226. doi: 10.1109/IEMBS.2011.6092028

Kemi, O. J., Loennechen, J. P., Wisløff, U., and Ellingsen, Ø. (2002). Intensity-controlled treadmill running in mice: cardiac and skeletal muscle hypertrophy. *J. Appl. Physiol. (1985)* 93, 1301–1309. doi: 10.1152/japplphysiol.00231.2002

Kirchner, L., Chen, W.-Q., Afjehi-Sadat, L., Viidik, A., Skalicky, M., Höger, H., et al. (2008). Hippocampal metabolic proteins are modulated in voluntary and treadmill exercise rats. *Exp. Neurol.* 212, 145–151. doi: 10.1016/j.expneurol.2008.03.014

Kluding, P. M., Tseng, B. Y., and Billinger, S. A. (2011). Exercise and executive function in individuals with chronic stroke: a pilot study. *J. Neurol. Phys. Ther.* 35, 11–17. doi: 10.1097/NPT.0b013e318208ee6c

Komulainen, P., Pedersen, M., Hänninen, T., Bruunsgaard, H., Lakka, T. A., Kivipelto, M., et al. (2008). BDNF is a novel marker of cognitive function in ageing women: the DR's EXTRA study. *Neurobiol. Learn. Mem.* 90, 596–603. doi: 10.1016/j.nlm.2008.07.014

Kozlowski, D. A., James, D. C., and Schallert, T. (1996). Use-dependent exaggeration of neuronal injury after unilateral sensorimotor cortex lesions. *J. Neurosci.* 16, 4776–4786.

Kramer, A. F., and Erickson, K. I. (2007). Capitalizing on cortical plasticity: influence of physical activity on cognition and brain function. *Trends Cogn. Sci.* 11, 342–348. doi: 10.1016/j.tics.2007.06.009

Kremer, C., Perren, F., Kappelin, J., Selariu, E., and Abul-Kasim, K. (2013). Prognosis of aphasia in stroke patients early after iv thrombolysis. *Clin. Neurol. Neurosurg.* 115, 289–292. doi: 10.1016/j.clineuro.2012.05.019

Kwiatkowski, T. G., Libman, R. B., Frankel, M., Tilley, B. C., Morgenstern, L. B., Lu, M., et al. (1999). Effects of tissue plasminogen activator for acute ischemic stroke at one year. National institute of neurological disorders and stroke recombinant tissue plasminogen activator stroke study group. *N. Engl. J. Med.* 340, 1781–1787. doi: 10.1056/NEJM199906103402302

Leckie, R. L., Oberlin, L. E., Voss, M. W., Prakash, R. S., Szabo-Reed, A., Chaddock-Heyman, L., et al. (2014). BDNF mediates improvements in executive function following a 1-year exercise intervention. *Front. Hum. Neurosci.* 8:985. doi: 10.3389/fnhum.2014.00985

Lemaire, P., and Hinault, T. (2014). Age-related differences in sequential modulations of poorer-strategy effects. *Exp. Psychol.* 61, 253–262. doi: 10.1027/1618-3169/a000244

Leśniak, M., Bak, T., Czepiel, W., Seniów, J., and Czonkowska, A. (2008). Frequency and prognostic value of cognitive disorders in stroke patients. *Dement. Geriatr. Cogn. Disord.* 26, 356–363. doi: 10.1159/000162262

Lin, Y., Lu, X., Dong, J., He, X., Yan, T., Liang, H., et al. (2015). Involuntary, forced and voluntary exercises equally attenuate neurocognitive deficits in vascular dementia by the BDNF-pCREB mediated pathway. *Neurochem. Res.* 40, 1839–1848. doi: 10.1007/s11064-015-1673-3

Lövdén, M., Bäckman, L., Lindenberger, U., Schaefer, S., and Schmiedek, F. (2010). A theoretical framework for the study of adult cognitive plasticity. *Psychol. Bull.* 136, 659–676. doi: 10.1037/a0020080

Luo, C. X., Jiang, J., Zhou, Q. G., Zhu, X. J., Wang, W., Zhang, Z. J., et al. (2007). Voluntary exercise-induced neurogenesis in the postischemic dentate gyrus is associated with spatial memory recovery from stroke. *J. Neurosci. Res.* 85, 1637–1646. doi: 10.1002/jnr.21317

Maass, A., Düzel, S., Goerke, M., Becke, A., Sobieray, U., Neumann, K., et al. (2015). Vascular hippocampal plasticity after aerobic exercise in older adults. *Mol. Psychiatry* 20, 585–593. doi: 10.1038/mp.2014.114

Macko, R. F., Ivey, F. M., Forrester, L. W., Hanley, D., Sorkin, J. D., Katzel, L. I., et al. (2005). Treadmill exercise rehabilitation improves ambulatory function and cardiovascular fitness in patients with chronic stroke: a randomized, controlled trial. *Stroke* 36, 2206–2211. doi: 10.1161/01.str.0000181076.91805.89

Marosi, K., Bori, Z., Hart, N., Sárga, L., Koltai, E., Radák, Z., et al. (2012). Long-term exercise treatment reduces oxidative stress in the hippocampus of aging rats. *Neuroscience* 226, 21–28. doi: 10.1016/j.neuroscience.2012.09.001

Marsden, D. L., Dunn, A., Callister, R., Levi, C. R., and Spratt, N. J. (2013). Characteristics of exercise training interventions to improve cardiorespiratory fitness after stroke: a systematic review with meta-analysis. *Neurorehabil. Neural Repair* 27, 775–788. doi: 10.1177/1545968313496329

Marshall, R. S. (2015). Progress in intravenous thrombolytic therapy for acute stroke. *JAMA Neurol.* 72, 928–934. doi: 10.1001/jamaneurol.2015.0835

Martin, H. G. S., and Wang, Y. T. (2010). Blocking the deadly effects of the NMDA receptor in stroke. *Cell* 140, 174–176. doi: 10.1016/j.cell.2010.01.014

Marzolini, S., Oh, P., McIlroy, W., and Brooks, D. (2013). The effects of an aerobic and resistance exercise training program on cognition following stroke. *Neurorehabil. Neural Repair* 27, 392–402. doi: 10.1177/1545968312465192

Matsuda, F., Sakakima, H., and Yoshida, Y. (2011). The effects of early exercise on brain damage and recovery after focal cerebral infarction in rats. *Acta Physiol. (Oxf.)* 201, 275–287. doi: 10.1111/j.1748-1708.2010.02174.x

Mattlage, A. E., Ashenden, A. L., Lentz, A. A., Rippee, M. A., and Billinger, S. A. (2013). Submaximal and peak cardiorespiratory response after moderate-high intensity exercise training in subacute stroke. *Cardiopulm. Phys. Ther. J.* 24, 14–20.

McAuley, E., Kramer, A. F., and Colcombe, S. J. (2004). Cardiovascular fitness and neurocognitive function in older adults: a brief review. *Brain Behav. Immun.* 18, 214–220. doi: 10.1016/j.bbi.2003.12.007

McDonnell, M. N., Bryan, J., Smith, A. E., and Esterman, A. J. (2011). Assessing cognitive impairment following stroke. *J. Clin. Exp. Neuropsychol.* 33, 945–953. doi: 10.1080/13803395.2011.575769

Mizutani, K., Sonoda, S., Hayashi, N., Takasaki, A., Beppu, H., Saitoh, E., et al. (2010). Analysis of protein expression profile in the cerebellum of cerebral infarction rats after treadmill training. *Am. J. Phys. Med. Rehabil.* 89, 107–114. doi: 10.1097/PHM.0b013e3181b3323b

Monteleone, P., Tortorella, A., Martiadis, V., Serritella, C., Fuschino, A., and Maj, M. (2004). Opposite changes in the serum brain-derived neurotrophic factor in anorexia nervosa and obesity. *Psychosom. Med.* 66, 744–748. doi: 10.1097/01.psy.0000138119.12956.99

Murao, K., Leys, D., Jacquin, A., Kitazono, T., Bordet, R., Béjot, Y., et al. (2014). Thrombolytic therapy for stroke in patients with preexisting cognitive impairment. *Neurology* 82, 2048–2054. doi: 10.1212/WNL.0000000000000493

Musicco, M., Emberti, L., Nappi, G., Caltagirone, C., and Italian Multicenter Study on Outcomes of Rehabilitation of Neurological Patients. (2003). Early and long-term outcome of rehabilitation in stroke patients: the role of patient characteristics, time of initiation and duration of interventions. *Arch. Phys. Med. Rehabil.* 84, 551–558. doi: 10.1053/apmr.2003.50084

Ni, G.-X., Lei, L., and Zhou, Y.-Z. (2012). Intensity-dependent effect of treadmill running on lubricin metabolism of rat articular cartilage. *Arthritis Res. Ther.* 14:R256. doi: 10.1186/ar4101

Nys, G. M. S., van Zandvoort, M. J., Algra, A., Kappelle, L. J., and de Haan, E. H. (2006). Cognitive and functional outcome after intravenous recombinant tissue plasminogen activator treatment in patients with a first symptomatic brain infarct. *J. Neurol.* 253, 237–241. doi: 10.1007/s00415-005-0966-x

Påhlman, U., Sävborg, M., and Tarkowski, E. (2012). Cognitive dysfunction and physical activity after stroke: the Gothenburg cognitive stroke study in the elderly. *J. Stroke Cerebrovasc. Dis.* 21, 652–658. doi: 10.1016/j.jstrokecerebrovasdis.2011.02.012

Pan, W., Banks, W. A., Fasold, M. B., Bluth, J., and Kastin, A. J. (1998). Transport of brain-derived neurotrophic factor across the blood-brain barrier. *Neuropharmacology* 37, 1553–1561. doi: 10.1016/s0028-3908(98)00141-5

Pang, M. Y. C., Charlesworth, S. A., Lau, R. W. K., and Chung, R. C. K. (2013). Using aerobic exercise to improve health outcomes and quality of life in stroke: evidence-based exercise prescription recommendations. *Cerebrovasc. Dis.* 35, 7–22. doi: 10.1159/000346075

Park, J.-W., Bang, M.-S., Kwon, B.-S., Park, Y.-K., Kim, D.-W., Shon, S.-M., et al. (2010). Early treadmill training promotes motor function after hemorrhagic stroke in rats. *Neurosci. Lett.* 471, 104–108. doi: 10.1016/j.neulet.2010.01.020

Patel, M. D., Coshall, C., Rudd, A. G., and Wolfe, C. D. A. (2002). Cognitive impairment after stroke: clinical determinants and its associations with long-term stroke outcomes. *J. Am. Geriatr. Soc.* 50, 700–706. doi: 10.1046/j.1532-5415.2002.50165.x

Pendlebury, S. T., Cuthbertson, F. C., Welch, S. J. V., Mehta, Z., and Rothwell, P. M. (2010). Underestimation of cognitive impairment by mini-mental state examination versus the montreal cognitive assessment in patients with transient ischemic attack and stroke: a population-based study. *Stroke* 41, 1290–1293. doi: 10.1161/STROKEAHA.110.579888

Pereira, A. C., Huddleston, D. E., Brickman, A. M., Sosunov, A. A., Hen, R., McKhann, G. M., et al. (2007). An *in vivo* correlate of exercise-induced neurogenesis in the adult dentate gyrus. *Proc. Natl. Acad. Sci. U S A* 104, 5638–5643. doi: 10.1073/pnas.0611721104

Petcu, E. B., Smith, R. A., Miroiu, R. I., and Opris, M. M. (2010). Angiogenesis in old-aged subjects after ischemic stroke: a cautionary note for investigators. *J. Angiogenesis Res.* 2:26. doi: 10.1186/2040-2384-2-26

Pin-Barre, C., and Laurin, J. (2015). Physical exercise as a diagnostic, rehabilitation and preventive tool: influence on neuroplasticity and motor recovery after stroke. *Neural Plast.* 2015:608581. doi: 10.1155/2015/608581

Pirmoradi, M., Jemel, B., Gallagher, A., Tremblay, J., D'Hondt, F., Nguyen, D. K., et al. (2016). Verbal memory and verbal fluency tasks used for language localization and lateralization during magnetoencephalography. *Epilepsy Res.* 119, 1–9. doi: 10.1016/j.eplepsyres.2015.11.015

Ploughman, M., McCarthy, J., Bossé, M., Sullivan, H. J., and Corbett, D. (2008). Does treadmill exercise improve performance of cognitive or upper-extremity tasks in people with chronic stroke? A randomized cross-over trial. *Arch. Phys. Med. Rehabil.* 89, 2041–2047. doi: 10.1016/j.apmr.2008.05.017

Poletti, C., Sleimen-Malkoun, R., Lemaire, P., and Temprado, J.-J. (2016). Sensori-motor strategic variations and sequential effects in young and older adults performing a Fitts' task. *Acta Psychol. (Amst.)* 163, 1–9. doi: 10.1016/j.actpsy.2015.10.003

Poletti, C., Sleimen-Malkoun, R., Temprado, J.-J., and Lemaire, P. (2015). Older and younger adults' strategies in sensorimotor tasks: insights from Fitts' pointing task. *J. Exp. Psychol. Hum. Percept. Perform.* 41, 542–555. doi: 10.1037/xhp0000033

Puga, G. M., Kokubun, E., Simões, H. G., Nakamura, F. Y., and Campbell, C. S. G. (2012). Aerobic fitness evaluation during walking tests identifies the maximal lactate steady state. *ScientificWorld Journal* 2012:769431. doi: 10.1100/2012/769431

Quaney, B. M., Boyd, L. A., McDowd, J. M., Zahner, L. H., He, J., Mayo, M. S., et al. (2009). Aerobic exercise improves cognition and motor function poststroke. *Neurorehabil. Neural Repair* 23, 879–885. doi: 10.1177/1545968309338193

Radák, Z., Kaneko, T., Tahara, S., Nakamoto, H., Pucsok, J., Sasvári, M., et al. (2001). Regular exercise improves cognitive function and decreases oxidative damage in rat brain. *Neurochem. Int.* 38, 17–23. doi: 10.1016/s0197-0186(00)00063-2

Radák, Z., Toldy, A., Szabo, Z., Siamilis, S., Nyakas, C., Silye, G., et al. (2006). The effects of training and detraining on memory, neurotrophins and oxidative stress markers in rat brain. *Neurochem. Int.* 49, 387–392. doi: 10.1016/j.neuint.2006.02.004

Rafnsson, S. B., Deary, I. J., and Fowkes, F. (2009). Peripheral arterial disease and cognitive function. *Vasc. Med.* 14, 51–61. doi: 10.1177/1358863X08095027

Rafnsson, S. B., Deary, I. J., Smith, F. B., Whiteman, M. C., Rumley, A., Lowe, G. D. O., et al. (2007). Cognitive decline and markers of inflammation and hemostasis: the Edinburgh artery study. *J. Am. Geriatr. Soc.* 55, 700–707. doi: 10.1111/j.1532-5415.2007.01158.x

Ramic, M., Emerick, A. J., Bollnow, M. R., O'Brien, T. E., Tsai, S.-Y., and Kartje, G. L. (2006). Axonal plasticity is associated with motor recovery following amphetamine treatment combined with rehabilitation after brain injury in the adult rat. *Brain Res.* 1111, 176–186. doi: 10.1016/j.brainres.2006.06.063

Rand, D., Eng, J. J., Liu-Ambrose, T., and Tawashy, A. E. (2010). Feasibility of a 6-month exercise and recreation program to improve executive functioning and memory in individuals with chronic stroke. *Neurorehabil. Neural Repair* 24, 722–729. doi: 10.1177/1545968310368684

Rasmussen, R. S., Overgaard, K., Hildebrandt-Eriksen, E. S., and Boysen, G. (2006). D-amphetamine improves cognitive deficits and physical therapy promotes fine motor rehabilitation in a rat embolic stroke model. *Acta Neurol. Scand.* 113, 189–198. doi: 10.1111/j.1600-0404.2005.00547.x

Risedal, A., Zeng, J., and Johansson, B. B. (1999). Early training may exacerbate brain damage after focal brain ischemia in the rat. *J. Cereb. Blood Flow Metab.* 19, 997–1003. doi: 10.1097/00004647-199909000-00007

Rognmo, Ø., Hetland, E., Helgerud, J., Hoff, J., and Slørdahl, S. A. (2004). High intensity aerobic interval exercise is superior to moderate intensity exercise for increasing aerobic capacity in patients with coronary artery disease. *Eur. J. Cardiovasc. Prev. Rehabil.* 11, 216–222. doi: 10.1097/01.hjr.0000131677.96762.0c

Sakakima, H., Khan, M., Dhammu, T. S., Shunmugavel, A., Yoshida, Y., Singh, I., et al. (2012). Stimulation of functional recovery via the mechanisms of neurorepair by S-nitrosoglutathione and motor exercise in a rat model of transient cerebral ischemia and reperfusion. *Restor. Neurol. Neurosci.* 30, 383–396. doi: 10.3233/RNN-2012-110209

Save-Pédebos, J., Pinabiaux, C., Dorfmuller, G., Sorbets, S. F., Delalande, O., Jambaqué, I., et al. (2016). The development of pragmatic skills in children after hemispherotomy: contribution from left and right hemispheres. *Epilepsy Behav.* 55, 139–145. doi: 10.1016/j.yebeh.2015.12.013

Schaaf, M. J., Sibug, R. M., Duurland, R., Fluttert, M. F., Oitzl, M. S., De Kloet, E. R., et al. (1999). Corticosterone effects on BDNF mRNA expression in the rat hippocampus during morris water maze training. *Stress* 3, 173–183. doi: 10.3109/10253899909001121

Schmidt, A., Wellmann, J., Schilling, M., Strecker, J.-K., Sommer, C., Schäbitz, W.-R., et al. (2014). Meta-analysis of the efficacy of different training strategies in animal models of ischemic stroke. *Stroke* 45, 239–247. doi: 10.1161/STROKEAHA.113.002048

Shen, X., Li, A., Zhang, Y., Dong, X., Shan, T., Wu, Y., et al. (2013). The effect of different intensities of treadmill exercise on cognitive function deficit following a severe controlled cortical impact in rats. *Int. J. Mol. Sci.* 14, 21598–21612. doi: 10.3390/ijms141121598

Shih, P.-C., Yang, Y.-R., and Wang, R.-Y. (2013). Effects of exercise intensity on spatial memory performance and hippocampal synaptic plasticity in transient brain ischemic rats. *PLoS One* 8:e78163. doi: 10.1371/journal.pone.0078163

Shimada, H., Hamakawa, M., Ishida, A., Tamakoshi, K., Nakashima, H., and Ishida, K. (2013). Low-speed treadmill running exercise improves memory function after transient middle cerebral artery occlusion in rats. *Behav. Brain Res.* 243, 21–27. doi: 10.1016/j.bbr.2012.12.018

Silhol, M., Bonnichon, V., Rage, F., and Tapia-Arancibia, L. (2005). Age-related changes in brain-derived neurotrophic factor and tyrosine kinase receptor isoforms in the hippocampus and hypothalamus in male rats. *Neuroscience* 132, 613–624. doi: 10.1016/j.neuroscience.2005.01.008

Sleimen-Malkoun, R., Temprado, J.-J., and Berton, E. (2013). Age-related dedifferentiation of cognitive and motor slowing: insight from the comparison of Hick-Hyman and Fitts' laws. *Front. Aging Neurosci.* 5:62. doi: 10.3389/fnagi.2013.00062

Sleimen-Malkoun, R., Temprado, J.-J., Huys, R., Jirsa, V., and Berton, E. (2012). Is Fitts' law continuous in discrete aiming? *PLoS One* 7:e41190. doi: 10.1371/journal.pone.0041190

Sopova, K., Gatsiou, K., Stellos, K., and Laske, C. (2014). Dysregulation of neurotrophic and haematopoietic growth factors in Alzheimer's disease: from pathophysiology to novel treatment strategies. *Curr. Alzheimer Res.* 11, 27–39. doi: 10.2174/1567205010666131120100743

Soya, H., Nakamura, T., Deocaris, C. C., Kimpara, A., Iimura, M., Fujikawa, T., et al. (2007). BDNF induction with mild exercise in the rat hippocampus. *Biochem. Biophys. Res. Commun.* 358, 961–967. doi: 10.1016/j.bbrc.2007.04.173

Sun, J.-H., Ke, Z., Yip, S. P., Hu, X., Zheng, X., and Tong, K. (2014a). Gradually increased training intensity benefits rehabilitation outcome after stroke by BDNF upregulation and stress suppression. *Biomed Res. Int.* 2014:925762. doi: 10.1155/2014/925762

Sun, J.-H., Tan, L., and Yu, J.-T. (2014b). Post-stroke cognitive impairment: epidemiology, mechanisms and management. *Ann. Transl. Med.* 2:80. doi: 10.3978/j.issn.2305-5839.2014.08.05

Sun, M.-W., Qian, F.-L., Wang, J., Tao, T., Guo, J., Wang, L., et al. (2008). Low-intensity voluntary running lowers blood pressure with simultaneous improvement in endothelium-dependent vasodilatation and insulin sensitivity in aged spontaneously hypertensive rats. *Hypertens. Res.* 31, 543–552. doi: 10.1291/hypres.31.543

Swain, R. A., Harris, A. B., Wiener, E. C., Dutka, M. V., Morris, H. D., Theien, B. E., et al. (2003). Prolonged exercise induces angiogenesis and increases cerebral blood volume in primary motor cortex of the rat. *Neuroscience* 117, 1037–1046. doi: 10.1016/s0306-4522(02)00664-4

Takamatsu, Y., Ishida, A., Hamakawa, M., Tamakoshi, K., Jung, C.-G., and Ishida, K. (2010). Treadmill running improves motor function and alters dendritic morphology in the striatum after collagenase-induced intracerebral hemorrhage in rats. *Brain Res.* 1355, 165–173. doi: 10.1016/j.brainres.2010.07.070

Takamatsu, Y., Tamakoshi, K., Waseda, Y., and Ishida, K. (2016). Running exercise enhances motor functional recovery with inhibition of dendritic regression in the motor cortex after collagenase-induced intracerebral hemorrhage in rats. *Behav. Brain Res.* 300, 56–64. doi: 10.1016/j.bbr.2015.12.003

Tang, A., Marzolini, S., Oh, P., McIlroy, W. E., and Brooks, D. (2013). Factors associated with change in aerobic capacity following an exercise program for individuals with stroke. *J. Rehabil. Med.* 45, 32–37. doi: 10.2340/16501977-1053

Tatemichi, T. K., Desmond, D. W., Mayeux, R., Paik, M., Stern, Y., Sano, M., et al. (1992). Dementia after stroke Baseline frequency, risks and clinical features in a hospitalized cohort. *Neurology* 42, 1185–1193. doi: 10.1212/wnl.42.6.1185

Tatemichi, T. K., Desmond, D. W., Stern, Y., Paik, M., Sano, M., and Bagiella, E. (1994). Cognitive impairment after stroke: frequency, patterns and relationship to functional abilities. *J. Neurol. Neurosurg. Psychiatry* 57, 202–207. doi: 10.1136/jnnp.57.2.202

Temprado, J.-J., Sleimen-Malkoun, R., Lemaire, P., Rey-Robert, B., Retornaz, F., and Berton, E. (2013). Aging of sensorimotor processes: a systematic study in Fitts' task. *Exp. Brain Res.* 228, 105–116. doi: 10.1007/s00221-013-3542-0

Temprado, J.-J., Zanone, P.-G., Monno, A., and Laurent, M. (1999). Attentional load associated with performing and stabilizing preferred bimanual patterns. *J. Exp. Psychol. Hum. Percept. Perform.* 25, 1579–1594. doi: 10.1037/0096-1523.25.6.1579

Thompson, B. J., and Ronaldson, P. T. (2014). Drug delivery to the ischemic brain. *Adv. Pharmacol.* 71, 165–202. doi: 10.1016/bs.apha.2014.06.013

Tiozzo, E., Youbi, M., Dave, K., Perez-Pinzon, M., Rundek, T., Sacco, R. L., et al. (2015). Aerobic, resistance and cognitive exercise training poststroke. *Stroke* 46, 2012–2016. doi: 10.1161/STROKEAHA.114.006649

Unal, I., Gürsoy-Ozdemir, Y., Bolay, H., Söylemezoglu, F., Saribaş, O., and Dalkara, T. (2001). Chronic daily administration of selegiline and EGb 761 increases brain's resistance to ischemia in mice. *Brain Res.* 917, 174–181. doi: 10.1016/s0006-8993(01)02914-6

Vaynman, S., Ying, Z., and Gomez-Pinilla, F. (2003). Interplay between brain-derived neurotrophic factor and signal transduction modulators in the regulation of the effects of exercise on synaptic-plasticity. *Neuroscience* 122, 647–657. doi: 10.1016/j.neuroscience.2003.08.001

Vaynman, S., Ying, Z., and Gomez-Pinilla, F. (2004). Hippocampal BDNF mediates the efficacy of exercise on synaptic plasticity and cognition. *Eur. J. Neurosci.* 20, 2580–2590. doi: 10.1111/j.1460-9568.2004.03720.x

Ventriglia, M., Zanardini, R., Bonomini, C., Zanetti, O., Volpe, D., Pasqualetti, P., et al. (2013). Serum brain-derived neurotrophic factor levels in different neurological diseases. *Biomed Res. Int.* 2013:901082. doi: 10.1155/2013/901082

Voss, M. W., Erickson, K. I., Prakash, R. S., Chaddock, L., Kim, J. S., Alves, H., et al. (2013). Neurobiological markers of exercise-related brain plasticity in older adults. *Brain Behav. Immun.* 28, 90–99. doi: 10.1016/j.bbi.2012.10.021

Voss, M. W., Erickson, K. I., Prakash, R. S., Chaddock, L., Malkowski, E., Alves, H., et al. (2010a). Functional connectivity: a source of variance in the association between cardiorespiratory fitness and cognition? *Neuropsychologia* 48, 1394–1406. doi: 10.1016/j.neuropsychologia.2010.01.005

Voss, M. W., Prakash, R. S., Erickson, K. I., Basak, C., Chaddock, L., Kim, J. S., et al. (2010b). Plasticity of brain networks in a randomized intervention trial of exercise training in older adults. *Front. Aging Neurosci.* 2:32. doi: 10.3389/fnagi.2010.00032

Waldstein, S. R., and Wendell, C. R. (2010). Neurocognitive function and cardiovascular disease. *J. Alzheimers Dis.* 20, 833–842. doi: 10.3233/JAD-2010-091591

Wang, Q., Tang, X. N., and Yenari, M. A. (2007). The inflammatory response in stroke. *J. Neuroimmunol.* 184, 53–68. doi: 10.1016/j.jneuroim.2006.11.014

Wiesmann, C., and de Vos, A. M. (2001). Nerve growth factor: structure and function. *Cell. Mol. Life Sci.* 58, 748–759. doi: 10.1007/PL00000898

Wilcock, G. K., Birks, J., Whitehead, A., and Evans, S. J. G. (2002). The effect of selegiline in the treatment of people with Alzheimer's disease: a meta-analysis of published trials. *Int. J. Geriatr. Psychiatry* 17, 175–183. doi: 10.1002/gps.545

Wisløff, U., Helgerud, J., Kemi, O. J., and Ellingsen, O. (2001). Intensity-controlled treadmill running in rats: VO(2 max) and cardiac hypertrophy. *Am. J. Physiol. Heart Circ. Physiol.* 280, H1301–H1310.

Wisløff, U., Støylen, A., Loennechen, J. P., Bruvold, M., Rognmo, Ø., Haram, P. M., et al. (2007). Superior cardiovascular effect of aerobic interval training versus moderate continuous training in heart failure patients: a randomized study. *Circulation* 115, 3086–3094. doi: 10.1161/circulationaha.106.675041

Wogensen, E., Malá, H., and Mogensen, J. (2015). The effects of exercise on cognitive recovery after acquired brain injury in animal models: a systematic review. *Neural Plast.* 2015:830871. doi: 10.1155/2015/830871

Wurm, F., Keiner, S., Kunze, A., Witte, O. W., and Redecker, C. (2007). Effects of skilled forelimb training on hippocampal neurogenesis and spatial learning after focal cortical infarcts in the adult rat brain. *Stroke* 38, 2833–2840. doi: 10.1161/strokeaha.107.485524

Xu, F., and Rhodes, E. C. (1999). Oxygen uptake kinetics during exercise. *Sports Med.* 27, 313–327. doi: 10.2165/00007256-199927050-00003

Yaka, R., Biegon, A., Grigoriadis, N., Simeonidou, C., Grigoriadis, S., Alexandrovich, A. G., et al. (2007). D-cycloserine improves functional recovery and reinstates long-term potentiation (LTP) in a mouse model of closed head injury. *FASEB J.* 21, 2033–2041. doi: 10.1096/fj.06-7856com

Zhang, P., Yu, H., Zhou, N., Zhang, J., Wu, Y., Zhang, Y., et al. (2013a). Early exercise improves cerebral blood flow through increased angiogenesis in experimental stroke rat model. *J. Neuroeng. Rehabil.* 10:43. doi: 10.1186/1743-0003-10-43

Zhang, P., Zhang, Y., Zhang, J., Wu, Y., Jia, J., Wu, J., et al. (2013b). Early exercise protects against cerebral ischemic injury through inhibiting neuron apoptosis in cortex in rats. *Int. J. Mol. Sci.* 14, 6074–6089. doi: 10.3390/ijms14036074

Zhang, P., Zhang, Q., Pu, H., Wu, Y., Bai, Y., Vosler, P. S., et al. (2012). Very early-initiated physical rehabilitation protects against ischemic brain injury. *Front. Biosci. (Elite Ed).* 4, 2476–2489. doi: 10.2741/e559

17

ROCK1 is Associated with Alzheimer's Disease-Specific Plaques, as well as Enhances Autophagosome Formation But not Autophagic Aβ Clearance

Yong-Bo Hu[1†], Yang Zou[1†], Yue Huang[2†], Yong-Fang Zhang[3], Guinevere F. Lourenco[2], Sheng-Di Chen[1], Glenda M. Halliday[2], Gang Wang[1*] and Ru-Jing Ren[1*]*

[1] Department of Neurology and Neuroscience Institute, Ruijin Hospital Affiliated to Shanghai Jiao Tong University School of Medicine, Shanghai, China, [2] Neuroscience Research Australia and Faculty of Medicine, University of New South Wales (UNSW), Sydney, NSW, Australia, [3] Research Laboratory of Cell Regulation, School of Medicine, Shanghai Jiao Tong University, Shanghai, China

Edited by:
Andrew Harkin,
Trinity College Dublin, Ireland

Reviewed by:
Kah-Leong Lim,
National Neuroscience Institute,
Singapore
Lei Liu,
University of Florida, USA

****Correspondence:***
Glenda M. Halliday
g.halliday@neura.edu.au
Gang Wang
wgneuron@hotmail.com
Ru-Jing Ren
docotorren2001@126.com

[†]These authors have contributed equally to this work.

Alzheimer's disease (AD) is the most prevalent form of late-life dementia in the population, characterized by amyloid plaque formation and increased tau deposition, which is modulated by Rho-associated coiled-coil kinase 1 (ROCK1). In this study, we further analyze whether ROCK1 regulates the metabolism of amyloid precursor protein (APP). We show that ROCK1 is colocalized with mature amyloid-β (Aβ) plaques in patients with AD, in that ROCK1 enhances the amyloidogenic pathway, and that ROCK1 mediated autophagy enhances the intracellular buildup of Aβ in a cell model of AD (confirmed by increased ROCK1 and decreased Beclin 1 protein levels, with neuronal autophagosome accumulation in prefrontal cortex of AD APP/PS1 mouse model). *In vitro* over-expression of ROCK1 leads to a decrease in Aβ secretion and an increase in the expression of autophagy-related molecules. ROCK1 interacts with Beclin1, an autophagy initiator, and enhances the intracellular accumulation of Aβ. Reciprocally, overexpression of APP/Aβ promotes ROCK1 expression. Our data suggest ROCK1 participates in regulating Aβ secretion, APP shedding and autophagosome accumulation, and that ROCK1, rather than other kinases, is more likely to be a targetable enzyme for AD therapy.

Keywords: Alzheimer's disease, ROCK1, autophagy, Aβ, Beclin1

INTRODUCTION

Alzheimer's disease (AD) is the leading cause of dementia, characterized by the accumulation of extracellular and vascular amyloid in the brain. Amyloid plaques are composed of amyloid-β (Aβ) peptides, and they are derived from the sequential cleavage of the amyloid precursor protein (APP) by a set of proteases. The cleavage of APP occurs through two different pathways:

Abbreviations: AD, Alzheimer's disease; APP, amyloid precursor protein; Aβ, amyloid-β; CoIP, co-immunoprecipitation; PtdIns3KC3, phosphatidylinositol 3-kinase class III; ROCK1, Rho-associated coiled-coil kinase 1; 3-MA, 3-methyladenine.

a non-amyloidogenic pathway mediated by α-secretase and an amyloidogenic pathway mediated by β-secretase (Tang, 2005). α-Secretase is a metalloprotease and disintegrin enzyme that cleaves within the Aβ sequence to generate a secreted APP fragment (sAPPα). sAPPα has neurotrophic properties and promotes neurite outgrowth modulating the efficacy of synaptic neurotransmission (Ma et al., 2009). Conversely, APP cleavage by β-secretase occurs at the N-terminus with the C-terminal APP fragment subsequently cleaved by γ-secretase leading to the production of Aβ peptides.

Rho-associated coiled-coil kinases (ROCKs) are Ser/Thr kinases and the first identified effectors of Rho GTPase. They are involved in several aspects of cell behavior, such as cell motility, cell proliferation and apoptosis (Chang et al., 2006; Yang et al., 2013; Loirand, 2015; Swanger et al., 2015). Research indicates that ROCKs are potential therapeutic targets for Aβ metabolism modulation (Weggen et al., 2001; Jacobs et al., 2006; Salminen et al., 2008). Two constitutively-expressed ROCK enzymes have been identified—ROCK1 and ROCK2 that share 92% homology in their kinase domain and differ most in their regulatory domains and subcellular localization (Ishizaki et al., 1997; Shi et al., 2013; Chong et al., 2016). Recent studies show that ROCK1 modulates the shedding of the α-secretase-cleaved soluble APP ectodomain (sAPPα) from cultured cells, and that ROCK1 depletion reduces the levels of Aβ (Herskowitz et al., 2013; Henderson et al., 2016). The buildup of internal Aβ rather than its external deposition is associated with neuronal loss in APP/PS1 knock-in mice suggesting externalization of cellular Aβ is protective (Christensen et al., 2008). However, the mechanism by which ROCK1 externalizes Aβ or regulates Aβ production remains to be determined.

In AD, autophagy directly affects the secretion of Aβ and amyloid plaque formation (Nilsson et al., 2013), and long-term rapamycin treatment reduces Aβ plaque load by the induction of autophagy in an AD mouse model (Nilsson et al., 2013). The pivotal role for autophagy in the clearance of aggregate-prone proteins also manifests with an accumulation of autophagic vacuoles (autophagosomes and autolysosomes) in several neurodegenerative diseases (Zhang et al., 2016). Beclin1-mediated autophagy is the major cellular pathway for degradation of aggregated proteins and is required for the formation of double-membrane vesicles, cytoplasmic organelles called an autophagosome (McLeland et al., 2011). This dynamic process involves autophagosome formation, autophagosome-lysosome fusion and the degradation of autophagosomal contents by all kinds of hydrolases (Hong et al., 2016). During the process of autophagosome biogensis, Beclin1 plays a central role and governs the autophagic process by binding to phosphatidylinositol 3-kinase class III (PtdIns3KC3), which recruits additional autophagic proteins for autophagosome formation (Miki et al., 2016). ROCK1 phosphorylation of Beclin1 is the critical regulator for stress-induced autophagy (Gurkar et al., 2013). A reduction in ROCK1 is thought to diminish Aβ levels by enhancing lysosomal degradation of APP (Henderson et al., 2016).

To investigate the involvement of ROCK1 in the Aβ pathology diagnostic features for AD, the levels of and location of ROCK1 in brain tissue from preclinical and clinical AD patients were examined. Aβ production and autophagosome formation following increases or decreases in ROCK1 levels were tested using cell culture methods. We showed that ROCK1 is deposited with highly aggregated Aβ in human brain tissue, and that activated ROCK1 inhibits autophagic Aβ clearance via interaction with Beclin1, increasing Aβ burden during AD progression.

MATERIALS AND METHODS

Pathological Cohort

The human ethics committee of the University of New South Wales approved this tissue study. Following institutional approvals, 10 μm formalin-fixed paraffin-embedded temporal cortex sections from 17 cases with different severities of AD pathology (female: male = 13:4, age = 87 ± 9.5 (years old), post mortem delay = 15 ± 11 (h), low severity, Braak stages 0–2 and not demented: intermediate severity and Braak stages 3–4: high severity, Braak stages 5–6 and dementia = 5:3:9) were obtained from the Sydney Brain Bank which collects brain tissue with informed consent from longitudinally followed research participants. Subjects were characterized according to recent criteria for the pathological diagnosis of AD. One of the cases with an intermediate severity had a diagnosis of AD for 3 years, while all those with a high probability of AD had dementia for between 5 and 17 years. Exclusion criteria were alternate neurodegenerative disorders or a dominant family history of neurodegenerative disorder.

Immunofluorescence

For immunofluorescence, the 10 μm formalin-fixed, paraffin-embedded sections underwent heat-induced antigen retrieval with Citrate Buffer pH 6 for 3 min, followed by formic acid pre-treatment for 3 min. Tissue sections were double-labeled with rabbit anti-ROCK1 (1:50, Abcam) and mouse monoclonal anti-human Aβ1–42 (1:200, M0872, Dako, Glostrup, Denmark), and visualized with goat anti-rabbit Alexa Fluor 488 (1:500, A-11008, Life Technologies) and goat anti-mouse Alexa Fluor® 594 (1:500, A-11005, Life Technologies), respectively. Sections were coverslipped with Vectashield HardSet Antifade Mounting Medium with DAPI (H-1500, Vector Laboratories, Burlingame, CA, USA) and examined on confocal microscope (Nikon Eclipse E400).

Quantitative Analysis of Aβ and ROCK1 Colocalization

For quantification, 10 images were made for each case where plaques were present. All diffuse and cored plaques on each image was identified using the Aβ1-42 immunofluorescence, and the proportion that had ROCK1 co-localization recorded separately for both diffuse and core plaques. In total, an average of 40 ± 17 plaques were examined per case, with 66% on average being diffuse and 36% being cored. Multivariate statistics were performed in SPSS (IBM, v23) to assess differences between the percentages of plaques colocalizing ROCK1 immunoreactivity and the severity of cortical plaques observed, as assessed by the CERAD score (0 = none, 1 = mild or 1–5/image, 2 = moderate or 6–15/image and 3 = severe or more than 15/image), as well as to case diagnosis based on pathological load of different plaque types and neurofibrillary tangles (control, preclinical AD and AD).

Cell Lines and Cell Culture

HEK293 cells stably transfected with human APP695 harboring the "Swedish" mutation (HEK293 APP695sw) and SH-SY5Y human neuroblastoma were maintained in Eagle's minimal essential media or DMEM (Gibco), respectively, with 10% fetal bovine serum, and 1% penicillin/streptomycin. Cells were plated at 100,000 cells/cm^2 density in 6-well dishes that were coated with 100 μg/ml poly-lysine. On day 2 post plating, cells were transduced with indicated lentivirus with a multiplicity of infection of 1. For all studies, cells were treated with drugs at 72 h post-transduction in conditioned media for 16 h. For RNAi knockdown of ROCK1, cells were harvested 96 h post-transduction. For transductions or transfections, equivalent amounts of cells were plated, and transfections were performed using Lipofectamine 2000 (Invitrogen) according to the manufacturer's instructions. At 72 h post-transfection, cells were treated as indicated and then processed for western blot analysis or fluorescence imaging.

Cell Proliferation Assay

Cell proliferation was measured by the CCK-8 Kit (Beyotime) according to the manufacturer's instructions. Cells in 100 μl media were treated with 10 μl CCK-8 reagent at 37°C for 2 h, followed by measuring the absorbance at 450 nm on a microplate reader.

Plasmid Construct, RNA Interface and Transfection

ROCK1 plasmid (pCAG-myc-ROCK1$^{myc\text{-}727}$ Δ3, ROCK1 CA) was constructed as previously reported (Ishizaki et al., 1997). The siRNA sequence against ROCK1 (sense 5′-GGCAGAGGAAGAAUAUAAATT-3′; antisense 5′-UUUAUAUUCUUCCUCUGCCTT-3′) and scrambled siRNA was synthesized by GenePharma (Shanghai, China). Cells were transfected with ROCK1 plasmid, ROCK1 siRNA or scrambled siRNA using Lipofectamine 2000 reagent according to the manufacturer's instructions. At 72 h post-transfection, cells and supernatant were harvested and then processed for western blot analysis.

Aβ Measurements

For all cells, conditioned media were used for 48 h, and then the cells and media collected separately for biochemical analyses. Aβ40 was detected using a sandwich ELISA for human Aβ40 following the manufacturer's instructions. Plates were read at 450 nm on a Synergy MX plate reader (BioTeck, Winooski, VT, USA).

Immunoblotting

Cells were lysed with 1% RIPA Lysis Buffer (Beyotime, China). Cell lysate was subjected to a 13,000 rpm spin to remove nuclei and debris. Cleared lysate was used for the indicated biochemical assay. Protein concentrations were determined using the Enhanced BCA Protein Assay Reagent (Beyotime). Equal amounts of cell lysate were loaded onto SDS-PAGE gels and then transferred to PVDF membranes. Membranes were blocked with 5% fat-free dry milk in Tris buffered saline (TBS), containing 0.05% Tween-20, and incubated with primary antibodies. Protein bands were detected by horseradish peroxidase-conjugated species-specific secondary antibodies. Actin was used as loading control. Images were captured using an Odyssey Image Station (LI-COR), and band intensities were quantified using Scion Image.

mCherry-GFP-LC3B Assay

In order to evaluate the effects of ROCK1 plasmid on GFP–LC3B puncta formation, SH-SY5Y cells were plated on poly-lysine-coated 96-well plates and transduced with adenovirus expressing mCherry-GFP-LC3B fusion protein. After 24 h and 48 h, cell images were obtained by EVOS fl Auto (Life, USA).

Co-Immunoprecipitation

Co-immunoprecipitation (CoIP) was performed as previously described (Rijal Upadhaya et al., 2014). HEK293 cells in 60-mm dishes were co-transfected with pCAG-myc-ROCK1$^{myc\text{-}727}$ Δ3 plasmid. Forty eight hours later, the cells were lysed with 1% RIPA Lysis Buffer (Beyotime). After clarification by centrifugation at 4°C for 30 min at 12,000 rpm, 500 μl cell lysates were incubated with 20 μl of protein A + G agarose beads (Beyotime, China) for 4 h with gentle rotation at 4°C. The beads were washed four times with the cell lysis buffer and precipitates were eluted with 2× SDS-PAGE sample buffer, and then analyzed by western blot for anti-Myc and anti-Beclin1 immunoreactivity, respectively.

Primary Neuron Culture, Transfection and Immunofluorescence

Primary cortical neurons were prepared from E16 to E18 days of Sprague-Dawley rat brain tissues. Briefly, cerebral cortex was removed aseptically, and then digested and dispersed into single cells; then neurons were re-suspended in neuro-basal medium with 2% B27 supplement (Invitrogen), 2 mM glutamine and 1% penicillin and streptomycin (Invitrogen, Carlsbad, CA, USA) and then seeded at 1.25 × 10^5 cells per cm^2 on 12-well plates (Corning Inc., Midland, NC, USA) coated with 100 μg/ml poly-l-lysine and incubated in humidified atmosphere with 5% CO_2 at 37 °C. Transfection using Lipofectamine 2000 (Invitrogen) was carried out on acutely dissociated neurons before plating, and 4 h later, the whole medium was replaced with NB/B27 and immunofluorescence experiment was performed after 48 h transfection.

For immunofluorescence, primary neurons were cultured on a cover glass and fixed with 4% paraformaldehyde in PBS for 10 min at room temperature. Permeabilization was performed in PBS with 0.3% Triton X-100 for 10 min at room temperature. After blocking for 30 min with 5% normal donkey serum, neurons were incubated with rabbit anti-LC3 (1:100, CST) antibody or mouse anti-ROCK1 (1:500, Abcam) antibody overnight at 4°C. After washing three times with 0.1 M PBS, the sections were incubated with AlexaFluor 488-conjugated donkey anti-rabbit or anti-mouse IgG secondary antibodies (Invitrogen), respectively, and the sections were visualized with a confocal microscope (FV-1000).

Immunohistochemistry and Histology

APP/PS1 mice were provided by Model Animal Research Center of Nanjing University. APP/PS1 mice have been intensively characterized for Aβ plaques load and AD behavioral phenotypes. In this experiment, 10-month-old APP/PS1 transgenic mice and age-matched C57BL/6J were used. Mice were deeply anesthetized and perfused with 10% formalin, and their brains were removed and fixed in 4% paraformaldehyde in PBS overnight at 4°C. Whole brains were cryoprotected in 25% sucrose in 0.1M PBS at 4°C until sectioning. The brain tissues were cut in to coronal 30 μm sections. Immunohistochemistry (IHC) for APP and Beclin1 were performed using primary antibodies of 6E10 (1:100, Novus) and rabbit anti-Beclin1 (1:100, Novus) respectively (Sugrue et al., 2010). APP and Beclin1 immunopositive neurons were quantified according to the previously established method (Dlugos and Pentney, 2002).

Antibodies and Reagents

Mouse anti-ROCK1 antibody (Abcam, 1:500 dilution), rabbit anti-Beclin1 (Novus, 1:10,000), rabbit anti-APP-CTF (Sigma-Aldrich, 1:5000), anti-mouse sAPPα (IBL, 1:50), anti-mouse myc (Abcam, 1:1000), anti-rabbit LC3 (Cell Signaling, 1:100) and mouse anti-β-actin (Sigma-Aldrich, 1:1000) were used. Loading controls (β-actin) were used for Western blot standardization. Lipofectamine 2000 was sourced from Invitrogen. 3-methyladenine (3-MA) was purchased from Sigma Aldrich (St. Louis, MO, USA) and 3-MA was dissolved in double distilled water and titrated to 1 mM.

Statistical Analysis of the Cell Culture Experiments

Data are reported as mean ± SEM. Comparisons between experimental groups were analyzed by Student's *t*-test or ANOVA as appropriate, with $p < 0.05$ considered as significant.

RESULTS

ROCK1 is Associated with Aβ Plaques in the Brains of AD Patients

To determine whether Aβ associates with ROCK1 in the brains of patients with AD, co-localization studies were performed using specific antibodies in healthy aged controls ($n = 5$ aged 89 ± 4 years, Braak neuritic stages 0–2), preclinical AD ($n = 4$ aged 85 ± 3 years, Braak neuritic stages 3–4) and clinical end-stage AD ($n = 8$ aged 86 ± 4 years, Braak neuritic stages 5–6). Consistent with this finding, ROCK1 immunoreactivity was identified in more cored than diffuse plaques (**Figure 1**). Quantitation showed that the majority of cored plaques contained ROCK1 immunoreactivity, and that colocalization increased with increasing severity of cortical Aβ deposition as assessed by CERAD plaque score (**Figure 1J**, Wilks' Lambda $p < 0.0001$ covarying for age and brain size, *post hoc* Bonferroni $p = < 0.002$). Nearly half of all Aβ plaques in preclinical AD contained ROCK1 immunoreactivity, with significantly higher numbers of ROCK1-immunopositive Aβ plaques found in AD patients (**Figure 1K**, Wilks' Lambda $p = 0.03$ covarying for age and brain size, *post hoc* Bonferroni $p = 0.003$ for AD diagnosis). These results demonstrate a close relationship between ROCK1 localization and pathological Aβ plaque in both preclinical and clinical AD.

ROCK1 Regulates Aβ Secretion

To further explore the effects of ROCK1 cleavage on the production of Aβ, we constructed a plasmid expressing this constitutively active ROCK1 fragment (ROCK1 CA), as previously reported (Ishizaki et al., 1997). In HEK 293T cells stably transfected with the APP695 Swedish mutation (APPsw), ROCK1 levels were manipulated by transfection with ROCK1 CA plasmid, ROCK1 siRNA or scrambled siRNA. Forty eight hours after transfections, the levels of secreted Aβ40 in the cell culture medium were measured by ELISA. As shown in **Figure 2**, secreted Aβ40 levels were increased by 80% compared to the control after depletion of ROCK1 (**Figures 2A,B**), which is consistent with a recent study. In contrast, secreted Aβ40 levels were decreased following ROCK1 CA over-expression in HEK293T APPsw cells (**Figures 2C,D**). The Aβ42 level was too low to be detected by ELISA. ROCK1 CA plasmid transfection did not change cell proliferation (**Figure 2E**). These results confirm that ROCK1 influences Aβ secretion.

ROCK1 Modulates APP Shedding

Given that there is an established relationship between ROCK1 and Aβ secretion, we next investigated the effects of ROCK1 on APP cleavage. After transfection of ROCK1-targeted siRNA or ROCK1 CA plasmid to HEK293T APPsw cells, cells were harvested 48 h later and lysates were analyzed. The holo-APP and sAPPα were examined by Western Blot with the mAb 6E10, specific for residues 1–17 of the Aβ sequence (**Figure 3A**). Electrophoresis revealed no significant difference of full-length APP (**Figure 3C**), however the amount of sAPPα was higher after ROCK1 depletion (**Figure 3D**). In cells with increased ROCK1 CA levels, sAPPα was significantly decreased (**Figure 3D**). These results confirm that ROCK1 modulates the metabolism of APP. To further explore the interaction between ROCK1 and APP/Aβ, we performed normal HEK293T cell culture with Aβ40 treatment or APP695 plasmid transfection. Addition of Aβ40 or APP695 over-expression promoted endogenous ROCK1 expression in normal HEK293T cells (**Figures 3B,E**).

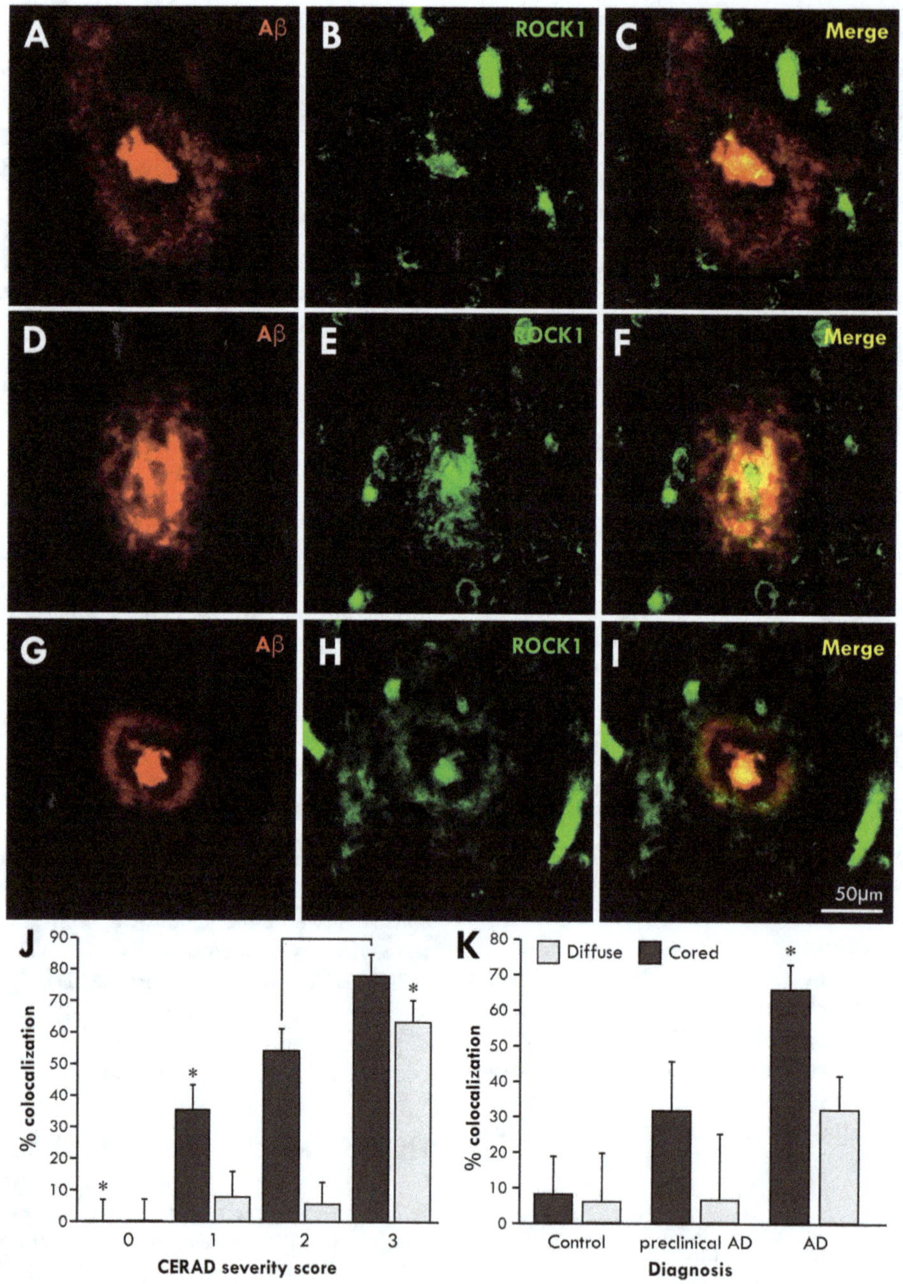

FIGURE 1 | Co-localization of Rho-associated coiled-coil kinase 1 (ROCK1) and amyloid-β (Aβ) in cortical plaques. Confocal microscopy using specific antibodies to Aβ (red) and ROCK1 (green) revealed a high degree of co-localization in the dense cores of cortical Aβ plaques and less overlap with diffuse Aβ depositions in the cortex **(A–I)**. Quantitation of the degree of colocalization in Aβ plaques was assessed in 40 ± 17 temporal lobe plaques in each case with Aβ plaque deposition ($n = 14/17$). Multivariate analysis identified a significant increase ($^*p < 0.02$) in ROCK1 and Aβ colocalization in plaques with increasing cortical deposition of Aβ plaques, as assessed by the CERAD plaque score **(J)**. With increasing CERAD plaque severity, more cored plaques contained ROCK1 immunoreactivity, whereas colocalization of ROCK1 and Aβ in diffuse plaques was mainly observed when there was a high cortical load of Aβ **(J)**. Multivariate analysis revealed that the degree of colocalization of ROCK1 and Aβ in cored plaques was highest in patients with clinical Alzheimer's disease (AD; $^*p = 0.003$), although significant numbers of Aβ plaques contained ROCK1 immunoreactivity in preclinical AD **(K)**.

Identification of ROCK1 as an Enhancer of Beclin1 Dependent Autophagy

In further experiments, we explored the mechanism of ROCK1 as an enhancer of Beclin 1 dependent autophagy. When ROCK1 was depleted, the expression of Beclin1 was decreased, and when ROCK1 CA was over-expressed by plasmid transfection, the level of Beclin1 was also increased. To determine whether autophagy is involved in the mechanism

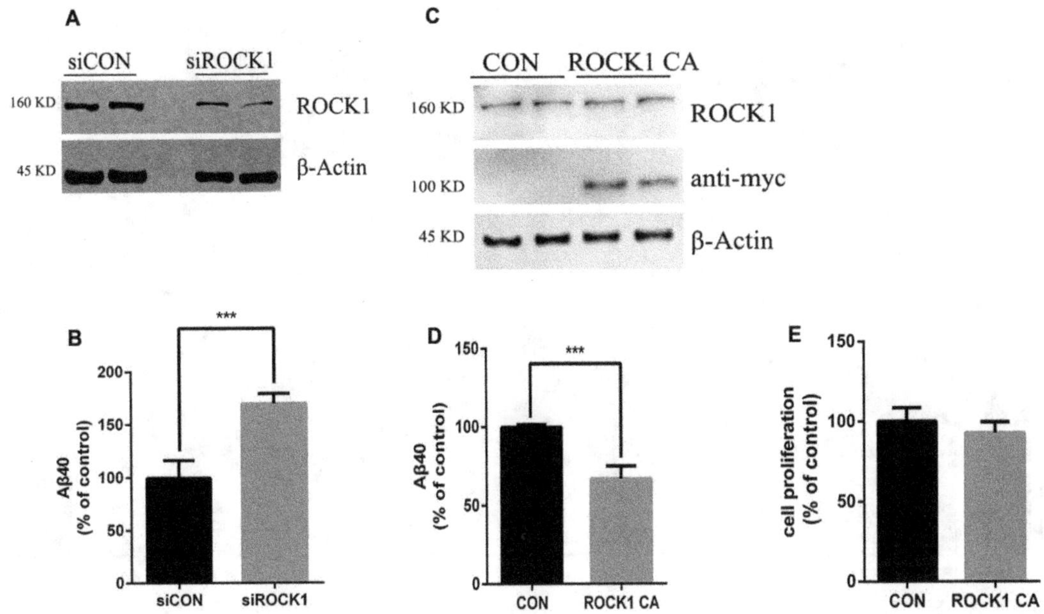

FIGURE 2 | ROCK1 levels modulate Aβ secretion. (A,C) Effects of knocking down ROCK1 levels **(A)** and increasing constitutively activated ROCK1 (ROCK1 CA) levels **(C)** on secreted Aβ. HEK293 cells were transfected with ROCK1 siRNA (siROCK1), scramble siRNA (siCON), ROCK1 CA plasmid and pcDNA (Con) and 48 h post-transfection secreted Aβ40 was measured by ELISA. **(B,D)** Representative immunoblot confirms ROCK1 knockdown **(B)** and increase **(D)**. **(E)** Cell proliferation assay following ROCK1 CA plasmid transfection. Data are presented as Mean ± SEM. Graphs represent % of control groups, $n = 10$; students' t test, $^{***}p < 0.01$.

by which ROCK1 depletion increases Aβ secretion, SH-SY5Y cells were co-transfected with mCherry-LC3B adenovirus and ROCK1 CA plasmid and the patterns of LC3 puncta were analyzed by immunoflouresence. **Figure 4A** shows an increase in LC3 puncta after ROCK1 CA plasmid transfection. LC3 was also assessed in HEK293T cells and, as the results show, the LC3II/I ratio was increased in cells when ROCK1 CA was over-expressed and decreased following ROCK1 depletion (**Figures 4E,G**). We also explored whether ROCK1 interacted with Beclin1 during autophagy (**Figures 4B,C**). HEK293T cells transfected with myc-tagged human ROCK1 were lysed and the proteins subjected to co-immunoprecipitation with anti-ROCK1 and anti-myc antibody. Our results showed that endogenous ROCK1 and Beclin1 interacted with each other. Moreover, when ROCK1 CA was over-expressed, this interaction was enhanced (**Figures 4D,F**). These results showed that an interaction between ROCK1 and Beclin1 triggered the autophagic build-up of intracellular Aβ and a decrease in Aβ secretion.

To further elucidate ROCK1 influence on autophagy, 3-MA was used as an inhibitor of autophagy. After HEK293T APPsw cells were treated with 3-MA for 6 h, they were transfected with ROCK1 CA plasmid for 48 h. To test whether ROCK1 CA over-expression rescued 3-MA-induced autophagy inhibition, the cells were lysed and proteins analyzed by ELISA and Western blot. Inhibiting autophagy increased intracellular Aβ40 levels (**Figure 4J**), and over-expression of ROCK1 by transfection with ROCK1 CA plasmid reversed this effect even though 3-MA treatment decreased Beclin1 levels (**Figures 4H,I**).

APP/PS1 Mice have Increased ROCK1 and Neuronal Autophagosome Accumulation

After confirming the relationship between ROCK1 and autophagosome formation *in vitro*, we next assessed whether ROCK1 and autophagosome proteins are upregulated with Aβ *in vivo* by conducting immunofluorescence and IHC staining of brain sections from 10 months old APP/PS1 transgenic C57BL/6 mice. Our data showed that ROCK1 was increased significantly with neuronal autophagosomes accumulation (**Figures 5A,C**) and that Beclin1 was decreased in the AD mouse model (**Figures 5B,D**). These observations suggested that autophagy was impaired in neurons and increased ROCK1 inhibited Aβ secretion, resulting in intracellular Aβ accumulation and neurotoxicity. Taken together, these data demonstrated the same associations between ROCK1, intracellular Aβ and autophagosomes accumulation as we identified in our *in vitro* experiments.

DISCUSSION

The critical events that trigger or cause increased Aβ levels and post-translational modifications that increase Aβ insolubility are still under debate. However, modulation of the production, metabolism and fibrilization of the protein are key pathogenic aspects. Our results show that ROCK1 levels regulate Aβ clearance by modulating the autophagy pathway via an interaction with its substrate, Beclin1, that initiates autophagosome formation that then accumulate

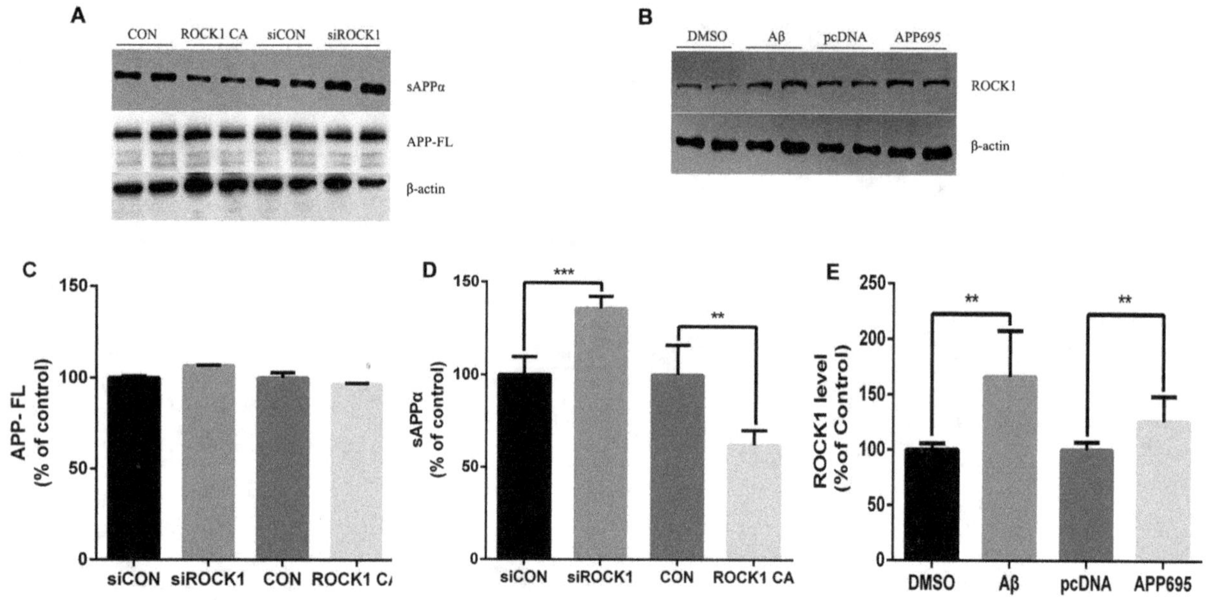

FIGURE 3 | ROCK1 modulates amyloid precursor protein (APP) shedding. (A) Immunoblot analysis of sAPPα and APP full-length (APP FL) following ROCK1 knockdown and ROCK1 increase. **(B)** Immunoblot of ROCK1 after Aβ40 treatment and APP695 plasmid transfection in HEK 293T cells. **(C–E)** Quantification of APP FL **(C)**, sAPPα **(D)** and ROCK1. Data are presented as Mean ± SEM, $n = 12$, students' t test, $^{***}p < 0.001$, $^{**}p < 0.01$.

intracellularly. This is consistent with previous studies showing that ROCK1 regulates autophagosome formation (Gurkar et al., 2013), that autophagosomes accumulate in AD and that ROCK1 inhibition reduces Aβ levels in brain (Nixon and Yang, 2011). Our data also show that ROCK1 collocates with fibrilized Aβ. It has recently been shown that different post-translational modifications of Aβ occur in different types of plaques (Rijal Upadhaya et al., 2014). The cases in this study have been previously analyzed using Western blotting for ROCK1 with no reduction in membrane associated SDS-soluble ROCK1 protein levels by end-stage AD (Wang et al., 2016). Taken together, our data indicate that ROCK1 may be involved in Aβ modification.

Phosphorylation of Aβ at serine 8 at the cell surface has recently been identified to dramatically increase the rate and amount of Aβ oligomerization and amyloid fibril formation (Rezaei-Ghaleh et al., 2016). In fact, AD patients are distinguished from those without clinical AD by selectively accumulating this phosphorylated form of Aβ (Rijal Upadhaya et al., 2014). The kinases that are involved in phosphorylating Aβ are poorly understood, but are thought to be of the AGC kinase family of serine-threonine kinases (Rezaei-Ghaleh et al., 2016), which includes ROCK1. Unlike ROCK2, ROCK1 interacts with a number of proteins in the plasma membrane (Stroeken et al., 2006) and we show that ROCK1 co-localizes with highly fibrilized Aβ in human brain. The localization and association of ROCK1-associated Aβ with clinical AD mirrors the data observed for serine 8 phosporylated Aβ (Rijal Upadhaya et al., 2014) and suggests that ROCK1 may be the kinase involved in this disease-specific Aβ phosphorylation.

We provide further evidence that ROCK1 has a role in the plasma membrane in its influence on APP shedding. APP shedding is directly mediated by α- and β-secretase generating either non-amyloidogenic (sAPPα) or amyloidogenic fragments (Tang, 2005). Our data show that ROCK1 activation enhances the amyloidogenic pathway, consistent with recent data (Henderson et al., 2016). However, we demonstrate that ROCK1 decreased sAPPα shedding in cultured cells, but also reduced rather than increased Aβ secretion from the cells, suggesting that ROCK1 may also play a role in Aβ secretion at the plasma membrane (potentially associated with the aberrant phosphorylation of Aβ, see above). Together these results are also consistent with ROCK1 activation increasing intracellular Aβ.

We show that activated ROCK1 inhibits the autophagic clearance of Aβ via its interaction with Beclin1, increasing Aβ burden during AD progression. Autophagy is a critical clearance system for cellular toxic protein aggregates and it is crucial for the physiological regulation of normal cell function, which can be induced by extracellular and intracellular signals, including oxidative stress, starvation and endoplasmic reticulum stress (Wang and Mao, 2014). In the brain, the complex axonal and dendritic structures are highly dependent on efficient autophagic turnover (Wong and Holzbaur, 2015; Hong et al., 2016). In AD, autophagy is upregulated at early disease stages, as evidenced by swollen endosomes and the accumulation of autophagosomes (Wong and Holzbaur, 2015). At the transcriptional level, autophagy-activating factors are also upregulated in AD (Jiang et al., 2013). ROCK1 phosphorylation of Beclin1 is known to be the critical regulator for stress-induced autophagy (Gurkar et al., 2013). We confirm that Beclin1 is a

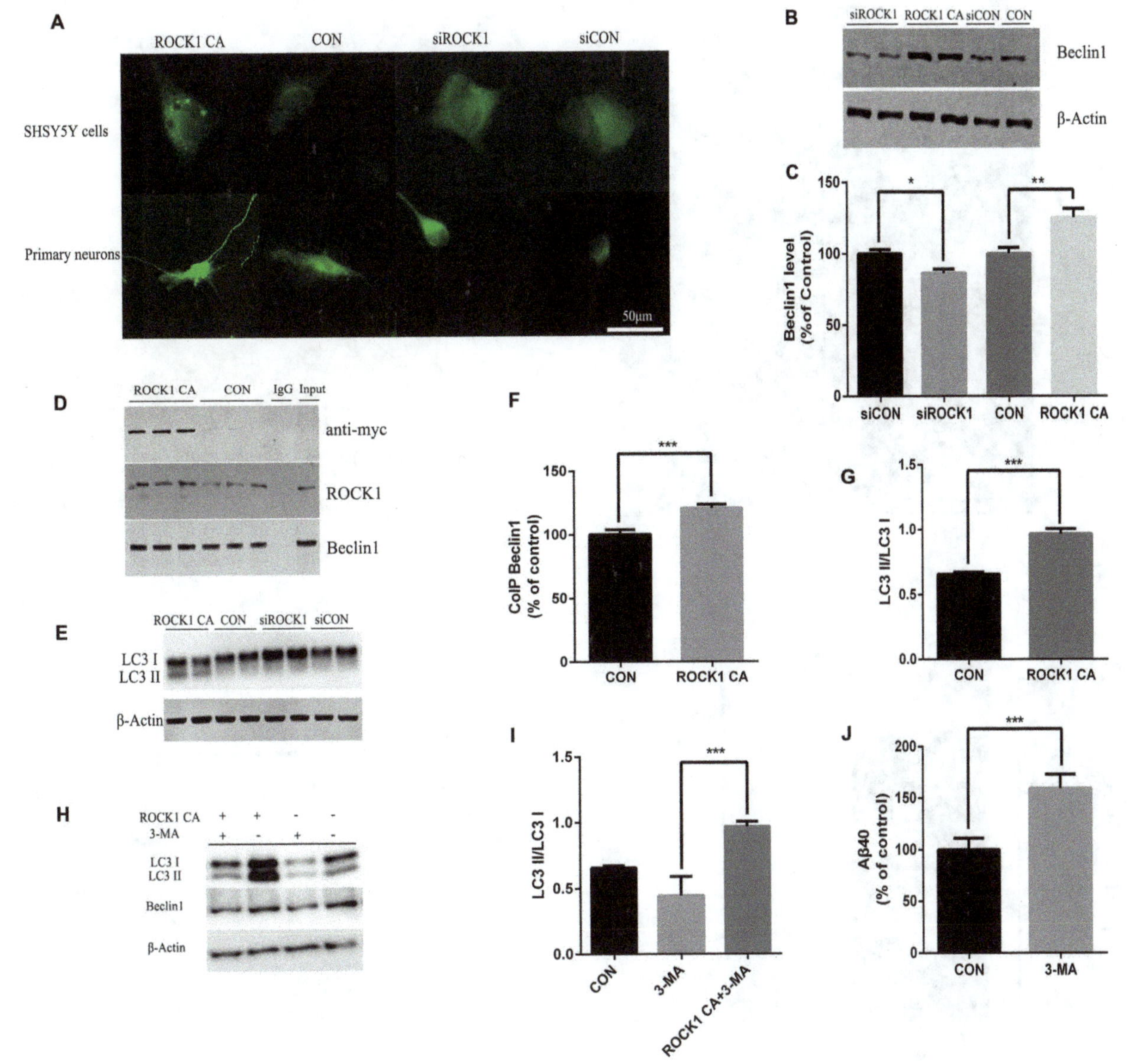

FIGURE 4 | ROCK1 increases autophagy via an interaction with Beclin1. (A) Increased ROCK1 CA levels induced an increase in the intracellular autophagosome formation and accumulation. SH-SY5Y cells (upper panels) and primary neurons (lower panels) were co-transfected with ROCK1 CA plasmid and mCherry-GFP-LC3B adenovirus (pcDNA was used as a control). Fluorescence microscopy was used to detect the formation of GFP-LC3 puncta after 24 h post-transfection. **(B)** Expression of Beclin1 following ROCK1 knockdown and ROCK1 CA over-expression. **(C)** Quantification of Beclin1 following ROCK1 knockdown and ROCK1 CA over-expression. **(D)** HEK293 cells transfected with ROCK1 CA plasmid and pcDNA. Forty eight hours post-transfection co-immunoprecipitation (CoIP) was performed with cell lysates by using ROCK1 crosslinked agarose and then blotted with antibodies. **(E)** Representative immunoblot of LC3 II/LC3 I after ROCK1 CA over-expression and ROCK1 knockdown. **(F)** Quantification of CoIP Beclin1 levels. **(G)** Representative immunoblot of LC3 II/LC3 I after ROCK1 CA over-expression and ROCK1 knockdown. **(H)** Representative immunoblot of LC3 II/LC3 I after ROCK1 CA over-expression and ROCK1 knockdown. **(I)** ROCK1 CA plasmid transfection reverses 3-methyladenine (3-MA) induced autophagy inhibition. Representative immunoblot of LC3 II/LC3 I. **(J)** Increased Aβ40 secretion after 3-MA treatment (48 h) by ELISA. Data are presented as Mean ± SEM, students' *t* test, $^{*}p < 0.05$, $^{**}p < 0.01$, $^{***}p < 0.001$.

substrate of ROCK1 and that the interaction of ROCK1 and Beclin1 results in the inhibition of autophagic Aβ clearance. It is well known that Beclin1 is a critical regulator of autophagy and several lines of investigation have demonstrated that autophagy plays an important role in Aβ clearance (also known as "autophagic Aβ clearance"; Wirawan et al., 2012). Although ROCK1 phosphorylation of Beclin1 activates autophagosome production, our data show that these organelles accumulate intracellularly with enhanced intracellular Aβ and a reduction in secreted Aβ. This is consistent with previous reports showing that autophagosome maturation to autolysosomes is the main problem with autophagy in AD and results in accumulating intracellular Aβ (Nixon and Yang, 2011).

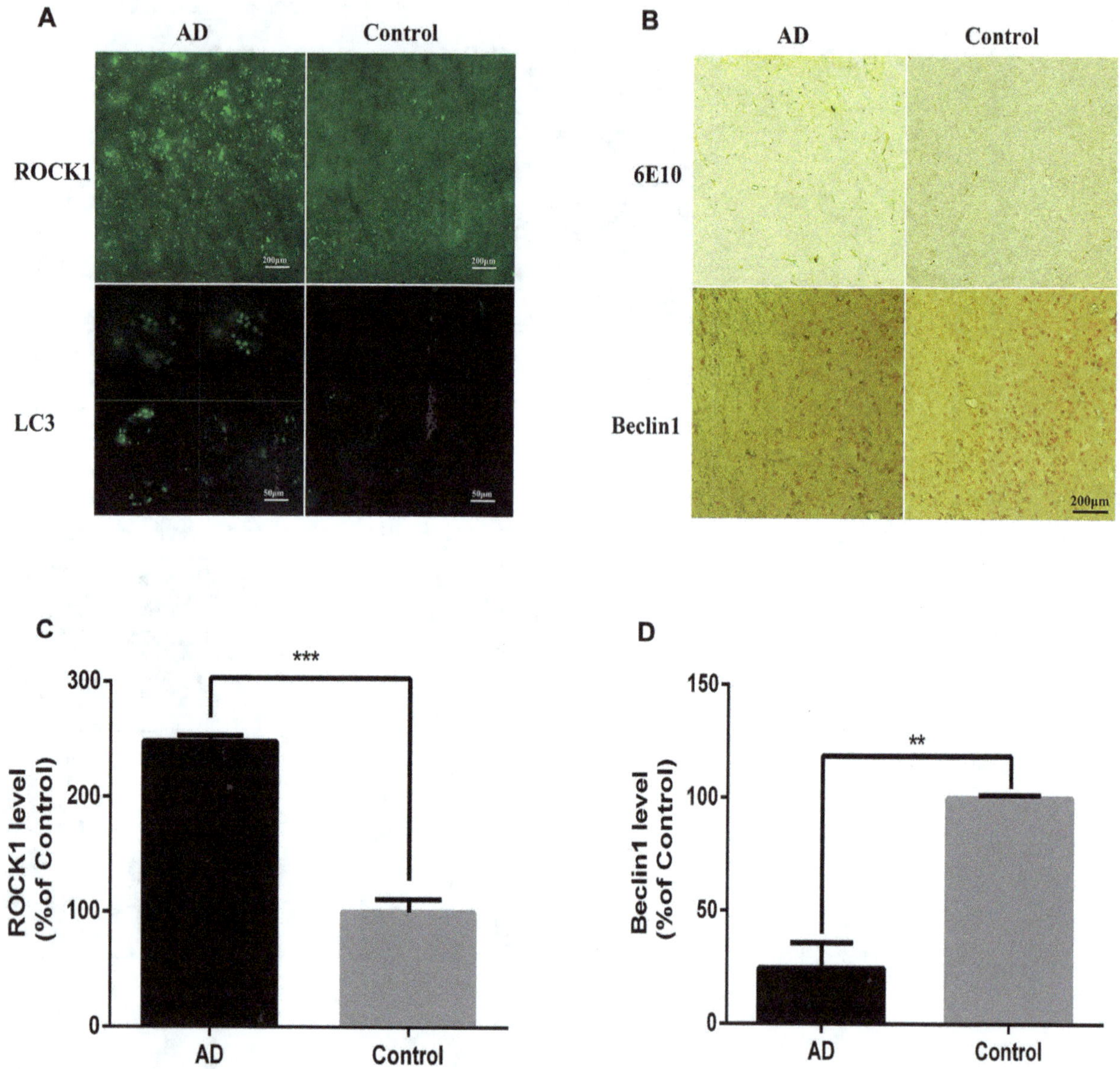

FIGURE 5 | ROCK1 is up-regulated with neuronal autophagosome accumulation in AD mice. (A) Representative ROCK1 (upper panels) and LC3 (lower panels) immunofluorescence in AD and normal mouse brain sections. **(B)** Representative immunohistochemical (IHC) micrographs of Aβ (6E10, upper panels) and Beclin1 (lower panels) immunofluorescence in AD and normal mouse brain sections. **(C)** Quantification of ROCK1 immunopositive neurons in AD mouse brain sections compared to control sections ($n = 4$). **(D)** Quantification of Beclin1 immunopositive neurons in AD mouse brain sections compared to control sections ($n = 4$). Data are expressed as mean ± SEM; $^{**}p < 0.01$, $^{***}p < 0.001$.

Overall our data suggest a role for ROCK1 in regulating Aβ production, secretion and post-translational modification at the plasma membrane, as well as its important role in intracellular autophagosome induction. The location of ROCK1 to the plasma membrane (Stroeken et al., 2006), and also in extracellular plaques (as shown in this study), makes this kinase potentially more easily targetable and relevant for therapeutic manipulations than others. If as suggested, Aβ phosphorylation at serine 8 enhances plaque maturation to progress presymptomatic pathology to symptomatic AD (Rijal Upadhaya et al., 2014), then inhibition of ROCK1 and/or Aβ dephosphorylating enzymes, may provide the most relevant treatments. Taken together, our findings outline a critical role of ROCK1 in the progression of Aβ pathology, highlighting its potential as a therapeutic target.

AUTHOR CONTRIBUTIONS

Y-BH and YZ performed most experiments, collected and analyzed data, and wrote the manuscript. YH and GFL performed pathological experiments. GW, R-JR, S-DC and GMH participated in the design of the study. Manuscript was written by

Y-BH and YH, and critically reviewed by GW, R-JR, Y-FZ, S-DC and GMH. All authors read and approved the final manuscript.

ACKNOWLEDGMENTS

This study was supported by the National Basic Research Development Program of China (Nos. 2010CB945200, 2011CB504104), the National Natural Science Foundation of China (Nos. 81001426, 81171027, 81200842, 91332107), Shanghai Pujiang Program (No. 15PJ1405400) and the National Health and Medical Research Council of Australia (program grant #1037746 and senior principal research fellowship grant #1079679). Human brain tissue was received from the Sydney Brain Bank at Neuroscience Research Australia that is supported by the University of New South Wales and Neuroscience Research Australia.

REFERENCES

Chang, J., Xie, M., Shah, V. R., Schneider, M. D., Entman, M. L., Wei, L., et al. (2006). Activation of Rho-associated coiled-coil protein kinase 1 (ROCK-1) by caspase-3 cleavage plays an essential role in cardiac myocyte apoptosis. *Proc. Natl. Acad. Sci. U S A* 103, 14495–14500. doi: 10.1073/pnas.0601911103

Chong, C. M., Ai, N., and Lee, S. M. (2016). ROCK in CNS: different roles of isoforms and therapeutic target for neurodegenerative disorders. *Curr. Drug Targets* 17. doi: 10.2174/1389450117666160401123825 [Epub ahead of print]

Christensen, D. Z., Kraus, S. L., Flohr, A., Cotel, M. C., Wirths, O., and Bayer, T. A. (2008). Transient intraneuronal A beta rather than extracellular plaque pathology correlates with neuron loss in the frontal cortex of APP/PS1KI mice. *Acta Neuropathol.* 116, 647–655. doi: 10.1007/s00401-008-0451-6

Dlugos, C. A., and Pentney, R. J. (2002). Quantitative immunocytochemistry of GABA and synaptophysin in the cerebellar cortex of old ethanol-fed rats. *Alcohol. Clin. Exp. Res.* 26, 1728–1733. doi: 10.1111/j.1530-0277.2002.tb02477.x

Gurkar, A. U., Chu, K., Raj, L., Bouley, R., Lee, S. H., Kim, Y. B., et al. (2013). Identification of ROCK1 kinase as a critical regulator of Beclin1-mediated autophagy during metabolic stress. *Nat. Commun.* 4:2189. doi: 10.1038/ncomms3189

Henderson, B. W., Gentry, E. G., Rush, T., Troncoso, J. C., Thambisetty, M., Montine, T. J., et al. (2016). Rho-associated protein kinase 1 (ROCK1) is increased in Alzheimer's disease and ROCK1 depletion reduces amyloid-β levels in brain. *J. Neurochem.* 138, 525–531. doi: 10.1111/jnc.13688

Herskowitz, J. H., Feng, Y., Mattheyses, A. L., Hales, C. M., Higginbotham, L. A., Duong, D. M., et al. (2013). Pharmacologic inhibition of ROCK2 suppresses amyloid-beta production in an Alzheimer's disease mouse model. *J. Neurosci.* 33, 19086–19098. doi: 10.1523/JNEUROSCI.2508-13.2013

Hong, C. J., Park, H., and Yu, S. W. (2016). Autophagy for the quality control of adult hippocampal neural stem cells. *Brain Res.* 1649, 166–172. doi: 10.1016/j.brainres.2016.02.048

Ishizaki, T., Naito, M., Fujisawa, K., Maekawa, M., Watanabe, N., Saito, Y., et al. (1997). p160ROCK, a Rho-associated coiled-coil forming protein kinase, works downstream of Rho and induces focal adhesions. *FEBS Lett.* 404, 118–124. doi: 10.1016/s0014-5793(97)00107-5

Jacobs, M., Hayakawa, K., Swenson, L., Bellon, S., Fleming, M., Taslimi, P., et al. (2006). The structure of dimeric ROCK I reveals the mechanism for ligand selectivity. *J. Biol. Chem.* 281, 260–268. doi: 10.1074/jbc.M508847200

Jiang, W., Zhang, Y., Meng, F., Lian, B., Chen, X., Yu, X., et al. (2013). Identification of active transcription factor and miRNA regulatory pathways in Alzheimer's disease. *Bioinformatics* 29, 2596–2602. doi: 10.1093/bioinformatics/btt423

Loirand, G. (2015). Rho kinases in health and disease: from basic science to translational research. *Pharmacol. Rev.* 67, 1074–1095. doi: 10.1124/pr.115.010595

Ma, T., Zhao, Y., Kwak, Y. D., Yang, Z., Thompson, R., Luo, Z., et al. (2009). Statin's excitoprotection is mediated by sAPP and the subsequent attenuation of calpain-induced truncation events, likely via rho-ROCK signaling. *J. Neurosci.* 29, 11226–11236. doi: 10.1523/JNEUROSCI.6150-08.2009

McLeland, C. B., Rodriguez, J., and Stern, S. T. (2011). Autophagy monitoring assay: qualitative analysis of MAP LC3-I to II conversion by immunoblot. *Methods Mol. Biol.* 697, 199–206. doi: 10.1007/978-1-60327-198-1_21

Miki, Y., Tanji, K., Mori, F., Utsumi, J., Sasaki, H., Kakita, A., et al. (2016). Alteration of upstream autophagy-related proteins (ULK1, ULK2, Beclin1, VPS34 and AMBRA1) in lewy body disease. *Brain Pathol.* 26, 359–370. doi: 10.1111/bpa.12297

Nilsson, P., Loganathan, K., Sekiguchi, M., Matsuba, Y., Hui, K., Tsubuki, S., et al. (2013). Aβ secretion and plaque formation depend on autophagy. *Cell Rep.* 5, 61–69. doi: 10.1016/j.celrep.2013.08.042

Nixon, R. A., and Yang, D. S. (2011). Autophagy failure in Alzheimer's disease–locating the primary defect. *Neurobiol. Dis.* 43, 38–45. doi: 10.1016/j.nbd.2011.01.021

Rezaei-Ghaleh, N., Amininasab, M., Kumar, S., Walter, J., and Zweckstetter, M. (2016). Phosphorylation modifies the molecular stability of beta-amyloid deposits. *Nat. Commun.* 7:11359. doi: 10.1038/ncomms11359

Rijal Upadhaya, A., Kosterin, I., Kumar, S., von Arnim, C. A., Yamaguchi, H., Fändrich, M., et al. (2014). Biochemical stages of amyloid-beta peptide aggregation and accumulation in the human brain and their association with symptomatic and pathologically preclinical Alzheimer's disease. *Brain* 137, 887–903. doi: 10.1093/brain/awt362

Salminen, A., Suuronen, T., and Kaarniranta, K. (2008). ROCK, PAK and Toll of synapses in Alzheimer's disease. *Biochem. Biophys. Res. Commun.* 371, 587–590. doi: 10.1016/j.bbrc.2008.04.148

Shi, J., Wu, X., Surma, M., Vemula, S., Zhang, L., Yang, Y., et al. (2013). Distinct roles for ROCK1 and ROCK2 in the regulation of cell detachment. *Cell Death Dis.* 4:e483. doi: 10.1038/cddis.2013.10

Stroeken, P. J., Alvarez, B., Van Rheenen, J., Wijnands, Y. M., Geerts, D., Jalink, K., et al. (2006). Integrin cytoplasmic domain-associated protein-1 (ICAP-1) interacts with the ROCK-I kinase at the plasma membrane. *J. Cell. Physiol.* 208, 620–628. doi: 10.1002/jcp.20699

Sugrue, M. L., Vella, K. R., Morales, C., Lopez, M. E., and Hollenberg, A. N. (2010). The thyrotropin-releasing hormone gene is regulated by thyroid hormone at the level of transcription *in vivo*. *Endocrinology* 151, 793–801. doi: 10.1210/en.2009-0976

Swanger, S. A., Mattheyses, A. L., Gentry, E. G., and Herskowitz, J. H. (2015). ROCK1 and ROCK2 inhibition alters dendritic spine morphology in hippocampal neurons. *Cell. Logist.* 5:e1133266. doi: 10.1080/21592799.2015.1133266

Tang, B. L. (2005). Alzheimer's disease: channeling APP to non-amyloidogenic processing. *Biochem. Biophys. Res. Commun.* 331, 375–378. doi: 10.1016/j.bbrc.2005.03.074

Wang, G., Huang, Y., Wang, L. L., Zhang, Y. F., Xu, J., Zhou, Y., et al. (2016). MicroRNA-146a suppresses ROCK1 allowing hyperphosphorylation of tau in Alzheimer's disease. *Sci. Rep.* 6:26697. doi: 10.1038/srep26697

Wang, G., and Mao, Z. (2014). Chaperone-mediated autophagy: roles in neurodegeneration. *Transl. Neurodegener.* 3:20. doi: 10.1186/2047-9158-3-20

Weggen, S., Eriksen, J. L., Das, P., Sagi, S. A., Wang, R., Pietrzik, C. U., et al. (2001). A subset of NSAIDs lower amyloidogenic Aβ42 independently of cyclooxygenase activity. *Nature* 414, 212–216. doi: 10.1038/35102591

Wirawan, E., Lippens, S., Vanden Berghe, T., Romagnoli, A., Fimia, G. M., Piacentini, M., et al. (2012). Beclin1: a role in membrane dynamics and beyond. *Autophagy* 8, 6–17. doi: 10.4161/auto.8.1.16645

Wong, Y. C., and Holzbaur, E. L. (2015). Autophagosome dynamics in neurodegeneration at a glance. *J. Cell Sci.* 128, 1259–1267. doi: 10.1242/jcs.161216

Yang, H., Wittnam, J. L., Zubarev, R. A., and Bayer, T. A. (2013). Shotgun brain proteomics reveals early molecular signature in presymptomatic mouse model of Alzheimer's disease. *J. Alzheimers Dis.* 37, 297–308. doi: 10.3233/JAD-130476

Zhang, Z., Miah, M., Culbreth, M., and Aschner, M. (2016). Autophagy in neurodegenerative diseases and metal neurotoxicity. *Neurochem. Res.* 41, 409–422. doi: 10.1007/s11064-016-1844-x

Permissions

All chapters in this book were first published in BBD, by Frontiers; hereby published with permission under the Creative Commons Attribution License or equivalent. Every chapter published in this book has been scrutinized by our experts. Their significance has been extensively debated. The topics covered herein carry significant findings which will fuel the growth of the discipline. They may even be implemented as practical applications or may be referred to as a beginning point for another development.

The contributors of this book come from diverse backgrounds, making this book a truly international effort. This book will bring forth new frontiers with its revolutionizing research information and detailed analysis of the nascent developments around the world.

We would like to thank all the contributing authors for lending their expertise to make the book truly unique. They have played a crucial role in the development of this book. Without their invaluable contributions this book wouldn't have been possible. They have made vital efforts to compile up to date information on the varied aspects of this subject to make this book a valuable addition to the collection of many professionals and students.

This book was conceptualized with the vision of imparting up-to-date information and advanced data in this field. To ensure the same, a matchless editorial board was set up. Every individual on the board went through rigorous rounds of assessment to prove their worth. After which they invested a large part of their time researching and compiling the most relevant data for our readers.

The editorial board has been involved in producing this book since its inception. They have spent rigorous hours researching and exploring the diverse topics which have resulted in the successful publishing of this book. They have passed on their knowledge of decades through this book. To expedite this challenging task, the publisher supported the team at every step. A small team of assistant editors was also appointed to further simplify the editing procedure and attain best results for the readers.

Apart from the editorial board, the designing team has also invested a significant amount of their time in understanding the subject and creating the most relevant covers. They scrutinized every image to scout for the most suitable representation of the subject and create an appropriate cover for the book.

The publishing team has been an ardent support to the editorial, designing and production team. Their endless efforts to recruit the best for this project, has resulted in the accomplishment of this book. They are a veteran in the field of academics and their pool of knowledge is as vast as their experience in printing. Their expertise and guidance has proved useful at every step. Their uncompromising quality standards have made this book an exceptional effort. Their encouragement from time to time has been an inspiration for everyone.

The publisher and the editorial board hope that this book will prove to be a valuable piece of knowledge for researchers, students, practitioners and scholars across the globe.

List of Contributors

Dean Carcone and Anthony C. Ruocco
Departments of Psychology and Psychological Clinical Science, University of Toronto, Toronto, ON, Canada

Lancelot J. Millar, Anna Hoerder-Suabedissen and Zoltán Molnár
Molnár Group, Department of Physiology, Anatomy and Genetics, University of Oxford, Oxford, UK

Lei Shi
Molnár Group, Department of Physiology, Anatomy and Genetics, University of Oxford, Oxford, UK
JNU-HKUST Joint Laboratory for Neuroscience and Innovative Drug Research, College of Pharmacy, Jinan University, Guangzhou, China

Elizabeth P. Crowe, Ferit Tuzer, Justin Cohen, Emre Yetkin, Christian Sell and Claudio Torres
Department of Pathology and Laboratory Medicine, Drexel University College of Medicine, Philadelphia, PA, USA

Brian D. Gregory, Sager J. Gosai and Nancy M. Bonini
Department of Biology, Penn Genome Frontiers Institute, University of Pennsylvania, Philadelphia, PA, USA

Greg Donahue, Raffaella Nativio and Shelley L. Berger
Epigenetics Program, Department of Cell and Developmental Biology, Perelman School of Medicine, University of Pennsylvania, Philadelphia, PA, USA

Yuk Y. Leung, Li-San Wang and F. Brad Johnson
Department of Pathology and Laboratory Medicine, Perelman School of Medicine, University of Pennsylvania, Philadelphia, PA, USA

Vanessa M. Machado and Ana Sofia Lourenço
Center for Neuroscience and Cell Biology, University of Coimbra, Coimbra, Portugal
Center for Biomedical Research, CBMR, University of Algarve, Faro, Portugal
Regenerative Medicine Program, Department of Biomedical Sciences and Medicine, University of Algarve, Faro, Portugal

Cláudia Florindo
Center for Biomedical Research, CBMR, University of Algarve, Faro, Portugal
Regenerative Medicine Program, Department of Biomedical Sciences and Medicine, University of Algarve, Faro, Portugal

Raquel Fernandes
Regenerative Medicine Program, Department of Biomedical Sciences and Medicine, University of Algarve, Faro, Portugal

Caetana M. Carvalho
Center for Neuroscience and Cell Biology, University of Coimbra, Coimbra, Portugal

Inês M. Araújo
Center for Biomedical Research, CBMR, University of Algarve, Faro, Portugal
Regenerative Medicine Program, Department of Biomedical Sciences and Medicine, University of Algarve, Faro, Portugal
Algarve Biomedical Center, University of Algarve, Faro, Portugal

Marija Kojic and Brandon Wainwright
Genomics of Development and Disease Division, Institute for Molecular Bioscience, The University of Queensland, Brisbane, QLD, Australia

Jessica Di Re
Neuroscience Graduate Program, University of Texas Medical Branch, Galveston, TX, USA
Department of Pharmacology and Toxicology, University of Texas Medical Branch, Galveston, TX, USA

Paul A. Wadsworth
Biochemistry and Molecular Biology Graduate Program, The University of Texas Medical Branch, Galveston, TX, USA

Fernanda Laezza
Department of Pharmacology and Toxicology, University of Texas Medical Branch, Galveston, TX, USA
Mitchell Center for Neurodegenerative Diseases, The University of Texas Medical Branch, Galveston, TX, USA
Center for Addiction Research, The University of Texas Medical Branch, Galveston, TX, USA

Shayne Mason
Centre for Human Metabolomics, North-West University, Potchefstroom, South Africa

Huamin Xu, Hong Jiang and Junxia Xie
Collaborative Innovation Center for Brain Science, Department of Physiology, Shandong Provincial Key Laboratory of Pathogenesis and Prevention of Neurological Disorders and State Key Disciplines: Physiology, Medical College of Qingdao University, Qingdao, China
Shandong Provincial Collaborative Innovation Center for Neurodegenerative Disorders, Qingdao University, Qingdao, China

Sarah Wrigley and Donia Arafa
School of Medicine, Trinity College Dublin, Dublin, Ireland

Daniela Tropea
Neuropsychiatric Genetics, Trinity Translational Medicine Institute St. James Hospital, Dublin, Ireland
Institute of Neuroscience, Trinity College Dublin, Dublin, Ireland

Xiaoyu Yang, Qimei Wu, Lei Zhang and Linyin Feng
CAS Key Laboratory of Receptor Research, Shanghai Institute of Materia Medica, Chinese Academy of Sciences, Shanghai, China

Anton R. Lord
Department of Behavioral Neurology, Leibniz Institute for Neurobiology, Magdeburg, Germany
Clinical Affective Neuroimaging Laboratory, Otto-von-Guericke University, Magdeburg, Germany
QIMR Berghofer Medical Research Institute, Brisbane, QLD, Australia

Meng Li
Clinical Affective Neuroimaging Laboratory, Otto-von-Guericke University, Magdeburg, Germany
Department of Neurology, Otto-von-Guericke University, Magdeburg, Germany

Liliana R. Demenescu
Department of Behavioral Neurology, Leibniz Institute for Neurobiology, Magdeburg, Germany
Clinical Affective Neuroimaging Laboratory, Otto-von-Guericke University, Magdeburg, Germany

Johan van den Meer
Clinical Affective Neuroimaging Laboratory, Otto-von-Guericke University, Magdeburg, Germany
Department of Neurology, Otto-von-Guericke University, Magdeburg, Germany
Department of Cognition and Emotion, Netherlands Institute for Neuroscience, An Institute of the Royal Academy of Arts and Sciences, Amsterdam, Netherlands

Viola Borchardt
Clinical Affective Neuroimaging Laboratory, Otto-von-Guericke University, Magdeburg, Germany

Anna Linda Krause
Clinical Affective Neuroimaging Laboratory, Otto-von-Guericke University, Magdeburg, Germany
Department of Psychiatry and Psychotherapy, Otto-von-Guericke University, Magdeburg, Germany

Hans-Jochen Heinze
Department of Behavioral Neurology, Leibniz Institute for Neurobiology, Magdeburg, Germany
Department of Neurology, Otto-von-Guericke University, Magdeburg, Germany
Center of Behavioral Brain Sciences, Otto-von-Guericke University, Magdeburg, Germany

Michael Breakspear
QIMR Berghofer Medical Research Institute, Brisbane, QLD, Australia
Metro North Mental Health Service, Royal Brisbane and Women's Hospital, Brisbane, QLD, Australia

Martin Walter
Department of Behavioral Neurology, Leibniz Institute for Neurobiology, Magdeburg, Germany
Clinical Affective Neuroimaging Laboratory, Otto-von-Guericke University, Magdeburg, Germany
Department of Psychiatry and Psychotherapy, Otto-von-Guericke University, Magdeburg, Germany
Center of Behavioral Brain Sciences, Otto-von-Guericke University, Magdeburg, Germany
Department of Psychiatry, Eberhad Karls University Tuebingen, Tuebingen, Germany

Chuanjun Zhuo
Department of Psychiatry, Wenzhou Seventh People's Hospital, Wenzhou, China
Department of Psychiatry, Tianjin Mental Health Center, Tianjin Anding Hospital, Tianjin, China
Department of Psychiatry, Tianjin Anning Hospital, Tianjin, China

Weihong Hou
Department of Biology, University of North Carolina at Charlotte, Charlotte, NC, USA

Lirong Hu, Chongguang Lin, Ce Chen and Xiaodong Lin
Department of Psychiatry, Wenzhou Seventh People's Hospital, Wenzhou, China

Hyeyeon Kang, Kyung Ah Han, Young-Ho Lee and Ji Won Um
Department of Physiology and BK21 PLUS Project for Medical Science, Yonsei University College of Medicine, Seoul, Korea

Seoung Youn Won
Department of Chemistry, Korea Advanced Institute of Science and Technology, Daejeon, Korea

Ho Min Kim
Graduate School of Medical Science and Engineering, Korea Advanced Institute of Science and Technology, Daejeon, Korea

Jaewon Ko
Department of Biochemistry, College of Life Science and Biotechnology, Yonsei University, Seoul, Korea

Tingting Zhang, Juan Hong and Ling Chen
State Key Lab of Reproductive Medicine, Nanjing Medical University, Nanjing, China
Department of Physiology, Nanjing Medical University, Nanjing, China

Tingting Di
Department of Physiology, Nanjing Medical University, Nanjing, China

Sara Redenšek and Vita Dolžan
Pharmacogenetics Laboratory, Institute of Biochemistry, Faculty of Medicine, University of Ljubljana, Ljubljana, Slovenia

Maja Trošt
Department of Neurology, University Medical Centre Ljubljana, Ljubljana, Slovenia

Annabelle Constans, Jean-Jacques Temprado, Patrick Decherchi and Jérôme Laurin
Aix-Marseille Université, CNRS, ISM, UMR 7287, Marseille, France

Caroline Pin-barre
Aix-Marseille Université, CNRS, ISM, UMR 7287, Marseille, France
Université Nice Sophia Antipolis, LAMHESS, UPRES EA 6309, Nice, France

Yong-Bo Hu, Yang Zou, Sheng-Di Chen, Gang Wang and Ru-Jing Ren
Department of Neurology and Neuroscience Institute, Ruijin Hospital Affiliated to Shanghai Jiao Tong University School of Medicine, Shanghai, China

Yue Huang, Guinevere F. Lourenco and Glenda M. Halliday
Neuroscience Research Australia and Faculty of Medicine, University of New South Wales (UNSW), Sydney, NSW, Australia

Yong-Fang Zhang
Research Laboratory of Cell Regulation, School of Medicine, Shanghai Jiao Tong University, Shanghai, China

Index

P

R

S

T

www.ingramcontent.com/pod-product-compliance
Lightning Source LLC
LaVergne TN
LVHW080953210926
848485LV00004B/830